Mental Health Nursing

Applying Theory to Practice

Gylo (Julie) Hercelinskyj
& Louise Alexander

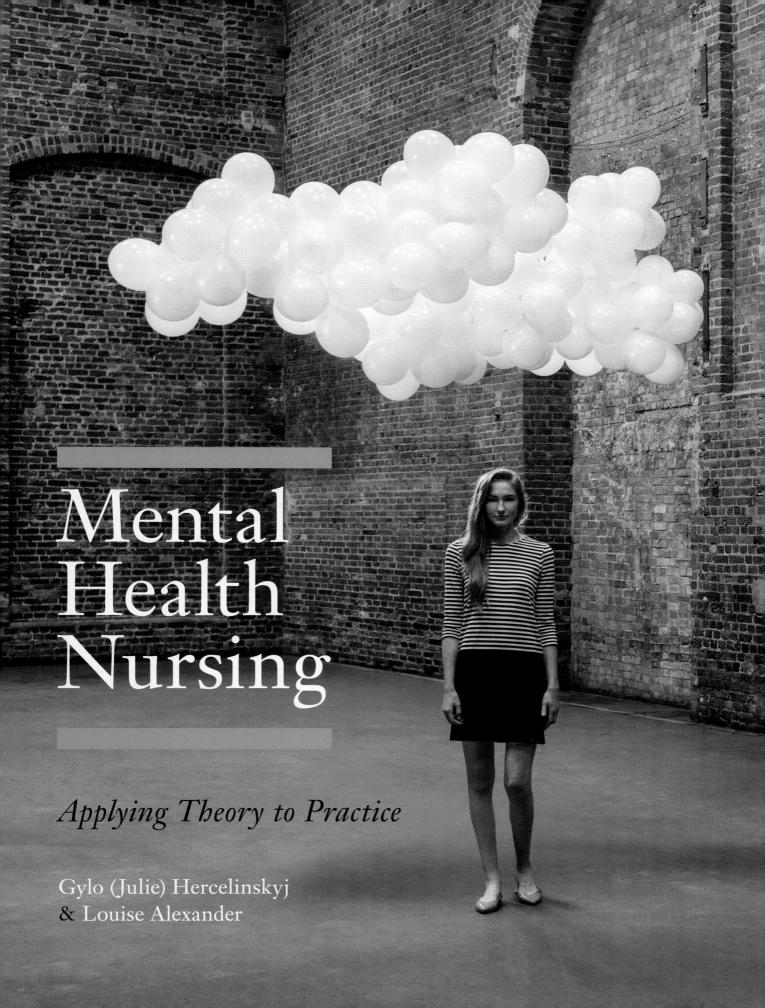

Mental Health Nursing

Applying Theory to Practice

Gylo (Julie) Hercelinskyj
& Louise Alexander

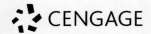

Mental health nursing: Applying theory to practice
1st Enhanced Edition
Gylo (Julie) Hercelinskyj
Louise Alexander

Senior content manager: Michelle Aarons
Content developer: Eleanor Yeoell
Senior project editor: Nathan Katz
Cover designer: Danielle Maccarone
Text designer: Norma Van Rees
Permissions/Photo researcher: Mira Fatin; Corrina Gilbert
Editor: Anne Mulvaney
Indexer: Julie King
Art direction: Nikita Bansal
Cover: Cover image courtesy of Stocksy.com/Lumina Images
Typeset by KnowledgeWorks Global Ltd.

Any URLs contained in this publication were checked for currency during the production process. Note, however, that the publisher cannot vouch for the ongoing currency of URLs.

Notice to the Reader

Publisher does not warrant or guarantee any of the products described herein or perform any independent analysis in connection with any of the product information contained herein. Publisher does not assume, and expressly disclaims, any obligation to obtain and include information other than that provided to it by the manufacturer. The reader is expressly warned to consider and adopt all safety precautions that might be indicated by the activities described herein and to avoid all potential hazards. By following the instructions contained herein, the reader willingly assumes all risks in connection with such instructions. The publisher makes no representations or warranties of any kind, including but not limited to, the warranties of fitness for particular purpose or merchantability, nor are any such representations implied with respect to the material set forth herein, and the publisher takes no responsibility with respect to such material. The publisher shall not be liable for any special, consequential, or exemplary damages resulting, in whole or part, from the readers' use of, or reliance upon, this material.

This 1st Enhanced edition published in 2022.

For product information and technology assistance,
in Australia call **1300 790 853**;
in New Zealand call **0800 449 725**

For permission to use material from this text or product, please email **aust.permissions@cengage.com**

National Library of Australia Cataloguing-in-Publication Data
ISBN: 9780170458610
A catalogue record for this book is available from the National Library of Australia.

Cengage Learning Australia
Level 7, 80 Dorcas Street
South Melbourne, Victoria Australia 3205

Cengage Learning New Zealand
Unit 4B Rosedale Office Park
331 Rosedale Road, Albany, North Shore 0632, NZ

For learning solutions, visit **cengage.com.au**

Printed in Singapore by C.O.S. Printers Pte Ltd.
1 2 3 4 5 6 7 25 24 23 22 21

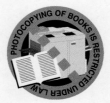

BRIEF CONTENTS

CONTENTS

Guide to the text

As you read this text you will find a number of features in every chapter to enhance your study of mental health nursing and help you understand how the theory is applied in the real world.

CHAPTER-OPENING FEATURES

Identify the key concepts that the chapter will cover with the **Learning outcomes** at the start of each chapter.

Challenge your perspective on mental health nursing in the real world with the **Learning from Practice vignette** and reflective questions. Then, consider how the chapter has impacted your understanding, with the **Reflection on Learning from Practice** at the end of chapter.

LEARNING OUTCOMES

Upon completion of this chapter, you should be able to:

2.1 Define the terms health, mental health, human behaviour and personality
2.2 Describe biomedical theories of personality, their application and relevance to mental health nursing practice and some of the major critiques of these theories
2.3 Describe psychodynamic theories of personality, their application and relevance to mental health nursing practice and some of the major critiques of these theories
2.4 Describe behavioural/social cognitive theories of personality, their application and relevance to mental health nursing practice and some of the major critiques of these theories
2.5 Describe humanistic theories of personality, their application and relevance to mental health nursing practice and some of the major critiques of these theories
2.6 Describe how nursing theorists have drawn from psychological and sociological theorists to understand human behaviour and how this influences the role of the mental health nurse
2.7 Reflect on which psychological and/or nursing theories would be relevant to your nursing practice

LEARNING FROM PRACTICE

Shelley is a 21-year old woman who lives at home with her mother. Shelley has been admitted for the first time to the inpatient unit at the local acute inpatient mental health facility. Shelley's first 36 hours in the unit were unsettled as she was extremely suspicious of the nursing staff and resisted efforts by the nurses to engage with her. Shelley did not believe she needed to be in hospital and became extremely agitated when staff attempted to administer prescribed medication, saying that everyone was trying to

At the end of the second visit, a registered nurse approached Rose as she was leaving the unit. Indicating that she was concerned that Rose appears uncomfortable while in the unit and that she was very happy to answer any questions Rose may have, Rose's whole body appeared to stiffen and with a trembling voice she replied, 'Why would you care, my daughter is lost to me and places like this don't help. I know what these places are like and the sooner she is out of here the better for her!'

FEATURES WITHIN CHAPTERS

Recognise the core DSM V Diagnostic Criteria for specific mental health conditions with the **Diagnostic criteria** boxes.

DIAGNOSTIC CRITERIA

General personality disorder

TABLE 12.2
Diagnostic criteria general personality disorder

A. An enduring pattern of inner experience and behavior that deviates markedly from the expectations of the individual's culture. This pattern is manifested in two (or more) of the following areas:
1. Cognition (i.e., ways of perceiving and interpreting self, other people, and events).
2. Affectivity (i.e., the range, intensity, lability, and appropriateness of emotional response).

Consider approaches to respectful care for clients from diverse backgrounds with the **Cultural considerations** boxes.

CULTURAL CONSIDERATIONS

Mental illness and European settlement of Australia
Prior to the settlement of Europeans in Australia, mental illness was almost unheard of in Aboriginal and Torres Strait Islander cultures. With the colonisation of Australia came disease and the introduction of many substances previously unknown to Indigenous cultures (such as alcohol). Since European settlement, rates of mental health challenges in Aboriginal and Torres Strait Islander people have increased to an extent that significantly passes the rates of mental health conditions among non-

Identify important client health and safety issues, and the appropriate response to critical situations with the **Safety first** boxes.

SAFETY FIRST

DON'T JUST FOCUS ON THE PROBLEM!
In the context of the therapeutic relationship, it can be easy to think that mental health nurses only listen to problems. But this is not the case. Practising within a recovery-oriented framework means listening for the consumer's strengths, what worked previously, what their hopes are, and not just what they feel went wrong.

Highlight specific key aspects of clinical presentation relevant to a specific mental health condition with the **Clinical observations** boxes.

CLINICAL OBSERVATIONS

Possible early symptoms of the prodrome
Possible early symptoms are:
- strange beliefs, perceptions or bodily sensations
- issues with maintaining concentration
- suspicious thoughts
- superstitious beliefs
- changes to affect

FEATURES WITHIN CHAPTERS

Analyse **Case studies** that present mental health nursing issues in context, encouraging you to integrate and apply the concepts discussed in the chapter.

CASE **STUDY**

A NEW CLIENT

Tomas is a 19-year-old client recently diagnosed with schizophrenia and living with his mother. He has been unable to return to his study course or find work since dropping out of his VET course the previous semester. He is reluctant to accept the diagnosis and struggles to agree with a need to take his olanzapine. His mother has expressed worries that she 'cannot talk to him any more' and get him to take his medication. She says he is becoming worse and

with Tomas and support his mother. You decide to locate and review the most current and best evidence to develop your response.

Questions

1   What background questions need to be answered in order to then develop the specific foreground question?
2   Develop a searchable and answerable foreground question using the PICO format to locate the highest

Identify commonalities that you may see with consumers experiencing a specific mental health condition with the **Commonalities of the MSE** section in each chapter of Unit 2.

COMMONALITIES OF THE MSE: SCHIZOPHRENIA

General appearance and behaviour

An individual with schizophrenia *may* present with the following anomalies in their appearance and behaviour:

- dishevelled (due to disorganisation, issues with EF, motivation due to negative symptoms, etc.)
- uncooperative with interview (due to poor **insight** into illness and belief in the need to require intervention) or suspiciousness and **paranoia**

voices for some individuals may be negative ('You are worthless, you should kill yourself') or positive in nature ('You are important and special; this is why you have been chosen'). Voices can be male or female (and less frequently, childlike), although McCarthy-Jones et al. (2014) note in their study exploring hallucinations that male voices were more common. While the individual may recognise the voice as someone who is known to them, unknown voices are just as common.

Learn about the importance of evidence and clinical research in nursing with the **Evidence-based practice** boxes, which link research to nursing practice.

EVIDENCE-BASED PRACTICE

Seasons and bipolar disorders?

Title of study

Seasonal variations in rates of hospitalization for mania and hypomania in psychiatric hospitals in NSW

Authors

Gordon Parker and Rebecca Graham

Background

A number of studies have suggested that individuals with bipolar disorder experience higher rates of hospitalisation in

spring; however, the same information about hypomania is not readily available.

Design

Quantitative data collected in New South Wales from December 1999 to January 2014 was extrapolated using ICD classification labels.

Participation

Admission information on 27 255 mental health patients with mania and hypomania in all NSW mental health facilities was explored.

Follow an individual person's case and the process of planning care, identifying problems, performing interventions and evaluating outcomes for that person with the detailed **Nursing care plans**.

NURSING **CARE PLAN**

MANAGING PANIC ATTACKS

Consumer Diagnosis: Panic Attacks

Nursing Diagnosis: Extreme fear/panic whereby Maeve experiences feelings of intense dread and anxiety, tightness in the chest, palpitations, sweating and difficulty breathing.

Outcomes: Develop strategies to manage any future episodes of panic.

Maeve is a 42-year-old woman who recently presented to the emergency department. Maeve was driving to work along a busy arterial road when she suddenly felt faint and experienced

tightness in her chest and difficulty breathing. She managed to turn into a side street, where she continued to experience these symptoms for several minutes before they subsided. Eventually, the symptoms settled down, which enabled Maeve to contact her partner. She attended the emergency department, where a range of tests was performed with all results being within normal parameters. Since this first visit, Maeve has experienced several more of these episodes. As nothing physiological was identified, Maeve has been asked to visit her local GP, who has referred her for assessment to the practice nurse.

END-OF-CHAPTER FEATURES

At the end of each chapter you will find several tools to help you to review, practise and extend your knowledge of the key learning outcomes.

Review your understanding of the key chapter topics with the **Summary**.

SUMMARY

- This chapter has explored the legal and ethical contexts for nurses working in the field of mental health in the context of mental health legislation in Australia.
- Mental health legislation in various jurisdictions of Australia is varied. However, commonalities lie in the preservation of dignity, upholding duty of care, and providing mental health

- Law and ethics apply in the context of nursing in Australia and all nurses working in health care need to be familiar with local Mental Health Acts and other relevant legislation.
- Of supreme importance are the issues of informed consent and involuntary or compulsory treatment, and the mental

Test your knowledge and consolidate your learning through the **Review questions**.

REVIEW QUESTIONS

1 Choose the statement that best defines the difference between law and ethics:
   a Ethics dictates behaviour, but law does not
   b Law is 'prescriptive' and ethics is 'guiding'
   c Ethics is based on law
   d A person can be punished for breaching ethics
2 Where there is an actual or perceived conflict between the code of conduct for nurses and the law:

3 The following requirements are necessary for all patient consent:
   a The consent must be voluntary, specific to the intervention/treatment, informed and the person must have capacity
   b The consent does not need to be voluntary as long as the person has the legal capacity
   c The consent can be considered valid if obtained

Challenge yourself to reflect on and discuss complex issues in relation to nursing with the **Critical thinking** questions.

CRITICAL THINKING

1 What factors would a mental health nurse take into account when considering which theoretical perspective might help them to understand a consumer's behaviour?
2 Jennifer has been receiving chemotherapy as part of her breast cancer treatment. The nurse notes that when her husband attends the appointment with her there is very

They are sleeping in separate rooms and she will not let him see her undressed. 'I just want to be there for her… but she's locking me out', Ivan states. 'I have no-one I can speak to.' Using a psychodynamic perspective, how could the nurse understand Jennifer's current behaviour?
3 Using Erikson's theory, identify what factors impact on a

Start your online reading and research using the short list of **Useful websites**.

USEFUL WEBSITES

- Approaches to Psychology – the humanistic approach: https://www.ryerson.ca/~glassman/humanist.html
- Australian Psychological Society: https://www.psychology.org.au

- Hildegard Peplau's interpersonal relations theory: https://nurseslabs.com/hildegard-peplaus-interpersonal-relations-theory

Reflect on this boxes encourage you to reflect on your learning and experience by drawing on real-world examples and concepts.

REFLECT ON THIS

Using the Cochrane Library to research COVID-19
There is a great deal of attention being paid to the evidence underpinning our developing understanding of coronavirus and the COVID-19 pandemic. While our understanding continues to develop, the Cochrane Library has begun to

2 Did the reviewers provide assistance in translating the results into your own practice?
3 Read the synopsis of evidence article 'Educational interventions for patients receiving psychotropic medication' (Joanna Briggs Institute, 2007).

Guide to the online resources

FOR THE INSTRUCTOR

Cengage is pleased to provide you with a selection of resources that will help you prepare your lectures and assessments. These teaching tools are accessible via cengage.com.au/instructors for Australia or cengage.co.nz/instructors for New Zealand.

INSTRUCTOR'S MANUAL

The Instructor's manual includes:

- Learning outcomes
- Key words and definitions
- Cases and case question solutions (including additional questions for instructors).
- Solutions to end-of-chapter review and critical thinking questions.

- Video activities for classroom teaching
- Websites and readings
- Search me! key terms and activities.

WORD-BASED TEST BANK AND STUDENT REVISION QUIZ

This bank of questions has been developed in conjunction with the text for creating quizzes, tests and exams for your students. Deliver these through your LMS and in your classroom. An additional bank of questions has been created to provide direct to students for their own revision and self-assessment.

POWERPOINT™ PRESENTATIONS

Use the chapter-by-chapter PowerPoint slides to enhance your lecture presentations and handouts by reinforcing the key principles of your subject.

ARTWORK FROM THE TEXT

Add the digital files of graphs, pictures and flow charts into your course management system, use them in student handouts, or copy them into your lecture presentations.

PREFACE

ABOUT THIS BOOK

Florence Nightingale once said, 'nursing is an art *and* a science'. This point perhaps best describes the dichotomy for students when entering mental health. For many students their previous learning has focused on technical psychomotor skill acquisition. For example, undertaking a physical assessment, blood pressure, or administration of sub-cutaneous medication. Mental health nursing requires a uniquely different, and *human* set of skills that can be very challenging for some. Mental health nursing centres on the individual, their needs, their challenges, their hopes and their goals, and nurses require competent therapeutic communication skills to help.

Mental health nursing proficiency is a standard requirement of every nursing graduate. Individuals with a lived experience of a mental health condition are understood to experience discrimination, stigmatisation and disadvantage that results in worsening of mental and physical health. While mental health nursing is a highly specialised sector of healthcare, the increasing prevalence of mental health conditions means that *all* nurses must be suitably equipped to engage therapeutically with someone experiencing a mental health challenge. This requires a combination of theoretical understanding of mental health and mental ill health, and how the person's lived experience of a mental health condition is central to working collaboratively with them. This understanding is then applied in practice through the multidisciplinary team by safely applying therapeutic skills in interactions with consumers experiencing a mental health condition. This text provides a comprehensive exploration of mental healthcare that enables practical application of skills.

Areas comprehensively covered in this text include:
- historical perspectives of mental healthcare
- recovery and trauma informed practice
- theory of communication
- legal and ethical considerations
- extensive exploration of conditions (e.g., schizophrenia, depression, personality disorders etc.)
- complements the acclaimed DSM5 (2013)
- therapeutic use of medicines
- suicide and non-suicidal self-injury
- non-pharmacological approaches to intervention
- community mental health
- carer and family input
- Indigenous perspectives
- mental health first aid.

One of the most difficult aspects of mental health nursing for students is applying what they have leaned into a clinical context. For example, how to undertake a mental state examination. This text has been developed with these issues specifically in mind by:
- providing examples of common mental state examination presentations specifically according to the mental health condition
- comprehensive exploration of mental state examination including provision of questions and definitions
- the use of clinical observation and Safety First boxes to highlight specific areas of practice that students must be familiar with.

This text provides a comprehensive introduction to mental health nursing where the consumer is central to the caring process, and how care is delivered by the multidisciplinary team. Core features of this text will provide students with the foundation knowledge and skills they can apply during their clinical placement and future nursing career.

Gylo (Julie) Hercelinskyj and
Louise Alexander

ABOUT THE AUTHORS

Gylo (Julie) Hercelinskyj is an Honorary fellow at Australian Catholic University (ACU), Melbourne. Julie's clinical, teaching and research background is in older person's mental health, perinatal mental health, interpersonal skills and psychosocial nursing practice. Julie completed her original nursing education in general nursing and then specialised in mental health nursing. Julie has a Masters in Nursing Studies and completed her PhD in philosophy in 2011, which explored professional identity in mental health nursing. She has presented at national and international conferences and has published in a number of areas, including the use of educational technologies, professional identity, and emotional labour in mental health nursing.

Julie believes that all nurses need to incorporate promoting mental health into their practice. This requires a clear understanding of mental health and mental distress, and how nurses work collaboratively with people who have a lived experience of mental distress, and their families and significant others.

Louise Alexander is a senior lecturer in mental health nursing at Australian Catholic University (ACU), Melbourne. Louise has a background in forensic mental health nursing in acute, subacute and rehabilitation areas. Louise is a registered nurse with post-graduate qualifications in psychiatric nursing, and professional education and training. She also has a Masters in Education, and a PhD in Psychology. Louise also remains active in mental health nursing research, and continues to publish her research in this field. Louise has presented at conferences both nationally and internationally about teaching mental health nursing and has a special interest in the use of simulation in mental health teaching.

Louise is passionate about students' developing a comprehensive understanding of the theoretical underpinnings of mental health nursing. In particular, students' understanding and ability to undertake a mental state examination, and activities that alleviate pre-clinical placement anxiety. Louise currently oversees the mental health nursing unit within the Bachelor of Nursing program and is the national course coordinator for postgraduate mental health nursing at ACU.

Contributing authors
Cengage would like to thank the numerous contributors who assisted in this publication.

Melody Carter
PhD, MSc (ECON), PGCE(HE), BSc (HONS), RGN, DN, Senior Fellow of the Higher Education Academy, Principal Lecturer Nursing, Three Counties School of Nursing and Midwifery, University of Worcester/ Associate Professor (adjunct) School of Nursing and Midwifery, La Trobe University
- **Chapter 18:** Trauma and stressor-related disorders, with Louise Ward.

Glen Collett
Ad. Dip Nursing Studies, Facilitating Learning in Clinical Practice, P.Grad Certificate of Nursing, Papers in Alcohol and Drug Rehabilitation and Clinical Speciality in Mental Health. Prior Nurse Unit Manager for Addictions, Healthscope, Clinical Facilitator
- **Chapter 14:** Substance-related and addictive disorders, with Desiree Smith

Doseena Fergie
PhD. FCATSINaM. 2016 Churchill Fellow. Project Lead, Indigenous Recruitment and Retention, (Postgraduate & Academic), Australian Catholic University
- **Chapter 25:** Cultural context in practice in Australia

Terry Froggatt
PhD. MSc. BHA (UNSW). RN.CMHN, Head – Faculty of Health and Social Wellbeing, Honorary Fellow University of Wollongong, Nan Tien Institute
- **Chapter 3:** Ethics, law and mental health nursing practice, with Alison Hansen
- **Chapter 7:** Assessment and diagnosis, with Louise Alexander
- **Chapter 26:** Mental health first aid, with Nygell Topp.

Karen Hall
RN, Dip VET, MMentHlth, PhD (cand.), Swinburne University.
- **Chapter 24:** Community mental health context

Alison Hansen
RN, MAdvNursPrac (Mental Health), GCHE, PhD (Cand.), Lecturer, Monash University
- **Chapter 3:** Ethics, law and mental health nursing practice, with Terry Froggatt

Peri O'Shea
PhD, M. Soc. Pol., Psyc. Hon., B. Soc. Sc. Lived Experience Researcher and Consultant – xperienhance
- **Chapter 21:** Recovery and resilience in mental health

Brian Phillips

DipSc, MSc, PhD, RN, Senior Lecturer in Nursing, Charles Darwin University

- **Chapter 6:** Using evidence to guide mental health nursing practice

Desiree Smith

RN, BHSc (Nursing), GCPNP, MPH, Sessional Tertiary Educator, Intake Clinician: The Melbourne Clinic

- **Chapter 14:** Substance-related and addictive disorders, with Glen Collett

Nygell Topp

RN, B.N, PGD Adult Ed, Accredited mental health first aid instructor

- **Chapter 26:** Mental health first aid, with Terry Froggatt

Louise Ward

PhD, MN (Mental health), PGDip Arts therapy, PGCert ed. BN (Hons), RN, Associate Professor Clinical practice, School of Nursing and Midwifery, La Trobe University Australia.

- **Chapter 18:** Trauma and stressor-related disorders, with Melody Carter

Cengage would also like to extend thanks for partial chapter contributions to:

Russell Fremantle

- **Chapter 15:** Neurodevelopmental disorders

Scott Truman

- **Chapter 17:** Obsessive compulsive and related disorders.

ACKNOWLEDGEMENTS

Gylo (Julie): This has been a journey shared with a number of people. Thanks to Louise for agreeing to go on this rollercoaster ride with me. To my amazing husband Peter – your support, love and friendship have always been the mainstay in my life. You are my 'rock'. Here's to the future. To my children Ayisha and Shae and my amazing grandson Ralph, I am immensely proud of the people you are, and that I get to be your mum and grandma. Mum, your indomitable spirit inspires me to be best I can be personally and professionally. To my father, sister and brother, I miss you all. This book is dedicated to you.

Louise: I would like to thank my family for their support during this journey. You have all had to put up with an awful lot of literary suffering, far in excess of the usual undertakings of an academic: manuscripts, PhD thesis and this book. In particular, I want to thank my husband Christian, and children Madeleine and Charlotte. Christian, thank you for your support during this process, and for believing in me. I love you. To my daughters, I know it always seems like mum is always busy 'doing something' but I do hope you understand that I do it for you both.

You are both my biggest motivation, and my proudest achievement. I love you both very much. Finally, I would like to dedicate this book to my nephew James. Never forgotten.

Cengage and the authors would like to thank the following reviewers for their incisive and helpful feedback:
- Trudy Atkinson – Central Queensland University
- Rhonda Dawson – University of Southern Queensland
- Cheryl Green – University of Adelaide
- Phillip Maude – RMIT University
- Eddie Robinson – Monash University
- Tracy Robinson – University of Canberra
- Susan Sumskis – University of Wollongong
- Sione Vaka – Massey University
- Philip Warelow – Federation University.

UNDERPINNINGS OF MENTAL HEALTH NURSING

From the days of the asylum and work of attendants through to contemporary mental health service delivery, mental health nursing has evolved into a discipline that is guided by humanistic principles and evidence for practice. Practice is founded on a range of theoretical perspectives, legislative requirements, a variety of treatment and management options and therapeutic processes. Section 1 explores these foundational ideas in order to set the scene for the remainder of the book.

To understand the role of the mental health nurse as a member of the multidisciplinary team in delivering recovery-oriented and trauma-informed care, Chapter 1 provides a sense of the historical development of the discipline. Chapter 2 introduces some of the key theoretical frameworks that underpin mental health nursing practice. You will read about ideas from psychology and medicine as well as key contributions from mental health nursing theorists. These ideas will be applied to practice and critiqued. Chapter 3 presents essential knowledge regarding how mental health legislation underpins mental health service delivery, how recovery has influenced recent legislation and the consumer perspective of compulsory treatment and nursing practice, as well as key ethical considerations and issues related to practice and ethical frameworks to identity these issues. Chapter 4 explores the range of pharmacological and psychosocial treatment options currently used in contemporary practice. Core to effective practice in mental health is the capacity to listen to, respond and work collaboratively with consumers and their families. Chapter 5 explores the concept of mental health nursing as a therapeutic process. The fundamental components of the communication process, and the application of knowledge and skills to the therapeutic process are identified and explored. Section 1 concludes with Chapter 6, which looks at how mental health nurses understand, apply and critique evidence for practice. This includes consideration of clinical reasoning and decision-making.

CHAPTER 1

MENTAL HEALTH NURSING – THEN AND NOW

Louise Alexander and Gylo (Julie) Hercelinskyj

LEARNING OUTCOMES

Upon completion of this chapter, you should be able to:

1.1 Describe early human beliefs in illness and disease that affected how mental illness has been perceived

1.2 Describe factors behind the rise and growth of asylums throughout the world as well as the conditions that historically prevailed at asylums

1.3 Describe the history of asylums in Australia and the emergence of mental health nursing as a distinct profession within Australia

1.4 Describe treatments of mental health conditions throughout history, including the improvement of care, conditions and more humane perspectives on mental health and mental health nursing

1.5 Explore the role and identity of the mental health nurse in contemporary mental health service delivery

LEARNING FROM PRACTICE

To be honest, when I started nursing, I didn't even realise there was an area of practice dedicated to working in mental health. But even in the beginning of my education, I was always drawn to those ideas and concepts that explored the person's response to both health and illness. All the science was important, but it was learning about people that interested me the most. Having a clinical placement at a community mental health facility provided my first experience of a positive learning opportunity. I loved the learning, the teamwork, and seeing the way consumers experienced their recovery journey. I wasn't made to feel small or insignificant and no-one made me cry. But even then, I still did not see myself as a mental health nurse. I was going to be a midwife and thought completing mental health nursing after graduation would be useful in that work. I never became a midwife. The closest I came to holding an infant was the time spent working in paediatrics. My postgraduate year had clearly shown me that I wanted to be a mental health nurse. It was there that I felt I could contribute and make a difference as a registered nurse.

But when I told my parents of my decision my father's response was: 'Why can't you be a normal nurse and work with babies?'

Even now many years later, when I say I am a mental health nurse I wait for what seems to be the inevitable reaction from people. I watch their eyes widen, their jaw drop ever so slightly and then they say: 'But what do psych nurses actually do?', 'You're a mental health nurse? That must be so hard', 'You deserve a medal' or 'Why did you choose that?' So, I tell them my story and hope they take even a small level of understanding away.

JD, mental health nurse

JD has described her journey into mental health nursing, one she herself admits she was surprised to have enjoyed. You may find yourself in a similar position – contemplating your future as a nurse, and finding certain areas challenge your preconceived ideas. What is your understanding of mental health nursing? Reflect on how you feel about your upcoming mental health studies.

INTRODUCTION

To understand where we are going in the profession of mental health nursing, it is important to consider where we have come from. Often the history of mental health, or psychiatry as it has been referred to historically, is understood in terms of its historical development, treatment of people with a lived experienced of mental illness and the plethora of iconic or infamous events and images that surround it. Mental health nursing has been largely ignored, and seen only in relation to psychiatry and promulgated through literature, art, film and television in ways that perpetuate many of the myths that surround mental health. Mental health nursing has been overlooked by historians in terms of the contribution it has made to the care of people with a mental health condition in Australia, with only fleeting references to mental health nursing in their work (Maude, 2002). Nolan (1993) also believes much of the literature that does exist relates primarily to the history of psychiatric services, with nursing only considered in a marginal capacity. For example, the image of nursing is inevitably viewed through the lens of Florence Nightingale's exploits in the Crimea, her establishment of the first formalised nurse training school and the publication of her text 'Notes on nursing' in 1859.

It is most likely that mental health nursing evolved from what was historically a correctional or custodial position within an asylum. Asylums were notoriously inhumane places to reside and a significant portion of the history of mental illness encompasses this suffering. Workers within asylums monitored the whereabouts and cared for the inhabitants confined there. From around the mid-nineteenth century, the acceptable term for attendants was 'nurse' and this included both male and female attendants. This chapter explores some main historical perspectives of the causes of mental illness, historical mental health rituals, the establishment of asylums throughout the world and then in Australia, and the development of mental health treatments throughout human civilisation. In this chapter, we argue that to understand and value the role of mental health care and nursing practice today, it is essential to see how it evolved over the course of history. We approach this task by first looking at the history of mental health and then introducing the role of the mental health nurse in contemporary mental health service delivery, including introducing recent debates on the professional identity of the contemporary mental health nurse.

Historical terms

While today it is unacceptable to refer to individuals experiencing a mental health challenge as 'mad' or 'insane', historically such terms were widely acceptable and originated from actual medical diagnoses. Unlike their usage today, they were not intended to be derogatory.

The following terms were all socially appropriate and, in fact, diagnostic labels of early mental health conditions:

- lunatic
- idiot
- raving mad
- feebleminded
- insane
- incoherent
- intemperate
- hysterical.

The institution that housed the mentally ill of yesteryear was commonly called an 'insane asylum' or a 'lunatic asylum'.

BELIEF IN SUPERNATURAL ORIGINS OF ILLNESS AND DISEASE

In today's modern and civilised society, it seems abhorrent to consider that disease and ill health have a basis in any realm outside modern medicine. This was not the case in the fourteenth century, however. We consider a time where preoccupation with witchcraft, sorcery and demonology was a common justification for regular occurrences of that era: plagues, famine and general social unrest. By trusting in such supernatural concepts, believers of those times had something tangible on which to project their anger, fear and blame.

Witches

Witches and witchcraft were blamed for many events of the early and Middle Ages, ranging from simple misfortune (such as the death of a child, crop blighting or adverse weather events) to the bizarre that had no basis in fact (such as riding on a broomstick or changing form from human to animal). It is perhaps human nature to seek an understanding of why 'bad' things occur, and for many people ascribing blame to an evil, mythological being made sense. While there were varied and numerous reasons why women were ultimately tried as witches, many of which were purely matters of politics or the result of religious differences, it is understood that some of those who were persecuted were mentally unwell individuals who were probably suffering psychosis. In the majority of cases, there was no treatment offered to the suspected guilty party, and 'confessions' were obtained under torture or other duress; usually to make a deliberate example of the victim. Witches were burned at the stake (see **Figure 1.1**) or suffered what is known as the 'dunking test'. In this ultimate no-win situation (see **Figure 1.2**), the witch was tied to a chair and lowered into a body of water such as a river or lake. She was dunked in the water repeatedly, and if she died it was determined that she was *not* a witch. If she managed to survive the dunking, this meant that she *was* a witch, and she would be outed as a devil and killed regardless. Alternative recollections of this historical perspective also suggest that if she sank, she was deemed innocent (yet was now dead) and if she floated, she was guilty and was killed anyway. It is unknown how many women and clergymen died under the pretence of supernatural and/or spiritual causes of civil unrest, but it has been suggested that hundreds of thousands of people were killed due to such beliefs throughout the centuries (Elmer, 2016).

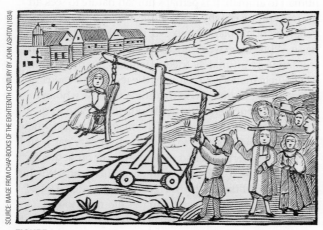

SOURCE: IMAGE FROM ALT- UND NEU-WIEN, GESCHICHTE DER KAISERSTADT UND IHRER UMGEBUNGEN, ETC BY MORIZ BERMANN (1880), BRITISH LIBRARY

FIGURE 1.1
Witch being burned at the stake

SOURCE: IMAGE FROM CHAP-BOOKS OF THE EIGHTEENTH CENTURY BY JOHN ASHTON (1834)

FIGURE 1.2
The dunking test

In Scotland in 1662, Isabel Gowdie was accused of being a witch and she readily confessed to this crime without requiring any torture. During her trial, Isabel was quoted as saying, 'He would have carnal dealing with us in the shape of a deer or any other shape that he would be in. We would never refuse him' (Zacks, 1994). Isabel described in great detail the intimate knowledge of her sexual encounters with the devil:

> And within a few days, he came to me, in the New Ward's of Inshoch, and there had carnal copulation with me. He was a very huge, black, rough man, very cold; and I found his nature [semen] within me all cold as spring well water. He will lie all heavy upon us, when he has carnal dealing with us, like a sack of barley malt. His member is exceedingly great and long; no man's member is so long and big as his. He would be among us like a stud horse among mares.
>
> The youngest and lustiest women will have very great pleasure in their carnal copulation with him, yea much more than with their own husbands; and they will have an exceedingly great desire for it with him, as much as he can give them and more, and never think shame of it. He is abler for us that way than any man can be (Alas! that I should compare him to any man!) only he is heavy like a sack of barley malt; a huge nature [outpouring of semen], very cold as ice.

Source: Zacks, 1994

Given the content of this extract, it is possible that Isabel was experiencing psychosis in the context of mania or schizophrenia. Her plight was met with the response that was common for the 'witches' of the Middle Ages: she was killed.

Exorcisms and spirit possession

Most religions have a history of exorcism and the history of such practices goes back thousands of years. Exorcism has a place in the management of the mentally ill in some countries even to this day, and demonic possession has been attributed to many strange beliefs or behaviours that now are commonly associated with psychosis or schizophrenia (Craig, 2014). In the Middle Ages countless people suffered painful treatments at the hands of clergymen seeking to exorcise spirits from their inhabitant and these frequently resulted in death (McNamara, 2011). **Figure 1.3** depicts St Francis Borgia providing the last rites to a dying man who appears haunted by demonic spirits.

While exorcism is predominantly associated with Catholic practices throughout history, there are many other historical examples in other cultures. Aboriginal Australians have an embryonic history of spiritual Dreamtime dating back 50 000 years, which includes entering spiritual dreamlands that have included possession (McNamara, 2011). Spirit possession is also recounted in the histories of Native America, pre-Columbian South America, West African Yoruba, Islam and Northern and Southern Asia (McNamara, 2011).

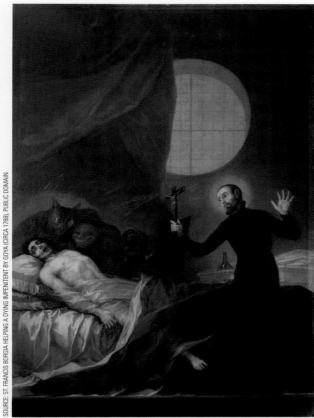

SOURCE: ST. FRANCIS BORGIA HELPING A DYING IMPENITENT BY GOYA (CIRCA 1788), PUBLIC DOMAIN

FIGURE 1.3
St Francis Borgia (1510–72) helping a dying impenitent Francisco José De Goya

ASYLUMS OF THE WORLD

An **asylum** was an institution where people with a mental health condition were housed. This process became colloquially known as **institutionalisation**. Asylums tended to be large buildings with dorms or rooms (which were locked) under the proviso that they were providing specialised care for people with mental illness. In reality, they were places of disease, distress and depravity (Arnold, 2009). The world's first hospital for the mentally insane was opened in Baghdad in 792 CE, and Europe soon followed suit, but prior to this, families were generally responsible for the keeping of mentally ill people, much to their immense shame and embarrassment.

The superstitions associated with mental illness rendered many families with disturbed family members deemed to be unlucky and cursed, thus resulting in them being isolated and ridiculed. Lunatic asylums began to emerge in the sixteenth century. These were not places of healing, but were locked penal colonies where the mentally ill could be abandoned by their long-suffering families, often never to be seen again. Conditions were appalling – vermin and disease were rife, the food insufficient, sanitation grossly inadequate and the caretakers sadistic – and overcrowding resulted in inmates being unable to lie down or move around (as they were almost always chained up anyway) (Arnold, 2009). Individuals with an intellectual disability were also housed in asylums in the same horrendous conditions, and this is hypothesised as being one of the more common reasons why many people wrongly think even today that those with a mental health condition are of lower intellect. These horrendous conditions continued worldwide until around the 1850s, although in some countries they continued well into the 1900s.

CASE **STUDY**

THE ROSENHAN EXPERIMENT

The Rosenhan experiment is a further example of subjectivity within psychiatry. David Rosenhan was a psychologist, and in 1972 he and seven colleagues presented to various hospitals across America fabricating mental illnesses of varying degrees. All were admitted to hospital for periods ranging from seven to 52 days, given invasive treatments against their will, and despite trying to convince doctors they were undertaking an experiment, they were only released when they appeared to comply with their diagnosis and subsequent treatment (Fontaine, 2013).

Questions

1   The participants of the Rosenhan experiment were trying to make a point about diagnostic subjectivity in psychiatry. What do you think this means?
2   Reflect on your understanding of general medical conditions. Is psychiatry unique to such ambiguity in diagnosis?

Bedlam

One of the most notorious and infamous asylums in the world was Saint Mary of Bethlehem, located in London in the mid-sixteenth century (see **Figure 1.4**). This asylum was quickly named 'Bedlam' and is in fact the origin of the moniker itself. Bedlam has a dark, well documented and researched history.

Locals were encouraged to come and view the 'lunatics' of Bedlam as entertainment, and on the first Tuesday of the month people could peer through holes in the stones for free. On other days, this outing would cost a penny. Around 100 000 people visited the site every year, and Bedlam remained a popular tourist attraction into the nineteenth century (Arnold, 2009).

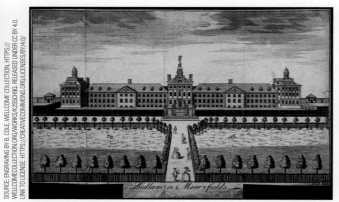

FIGURE 1.4
Saint Mary of Bethlehem, or 'Bedlam'

HISTORY OF AUSTRALIA'S ASYLUMS AND MENTAL HEALTH NURSING

The first lunatic asylum to operate in Australia was New South Wales' Castle Hill Asylum, which opened in 1811. Like many asylums of its time, Castle Hill has a dark history. Treatment of mental illness did not usually serve as part of the purpose of such asylums, and if it did, many 'treatments' were both inhumane and barbaric when they were instituted in similar asylums in Europe. A vast majority of the treatments of mental illness were experimental, and often formed the basis of a speculated theory. The purpose of these institutions was to contain the uncontainable – to control the uncontrollable. This included restricting (or preventing) access to the community (and thus eliminating perceived threats), as well as cohabitation of prisoners, those suffering dissolute or intemperate habits (such as alcoholism or sexual promiscuity) and intellectually disabled individuals.

The gold rush of the 1850s resulted in both an influx of migrants and serious increases in mental illness exacerbated by the use of alcohol and drugs such as opium. By the 1880s, more than 3% of Australia's population were identified as lunatics (this figure was more than three times higher than just 30 years prior) and services were ill-equipped to manage them. As a result, between 1811 and 1912 close to 30 asylums were opened across Australia. Despite this, it seemed nothing could keep up with the influx of those afflicted with 'diseases of the soul', and most asylums filled beyond capacity quickly, adding to the despair inhabitants were already experiencing.

While the personal tolls of drugs and alcohol provide a justifiable rationale for the increases in people committed to asylums across Australia, they are not the only cause. In fact, a more sinister reason exists. Being committed to an asylum was a seemingly easy task if you were a woman, married to a man who wanted to be rid of you. Getting out of such a facility was much harder (or seemingly impossible), and given the penchant for men

to hold the powerful and authoritarian roles in historical psychiatry; many women remained institutionalised for mere convenience (Toy, 2014).

Mental health nursing in Australia

Formerly custodial attendants, mental health nursing emerged as a distinct profession in Australia around 1890 with the increased medicalisation of mental health (Sands, 2009). Generally, men were responsible for the care of the mentally insane, until women were employed in the early twentieth century (Happell, 2007). Identification of nursing as a profession emerged in the mid- to late twentieth century and this resulted in the notion of specialisation in the field of psychiatry. With the development of psychotropic medication in the 1950s, psychiatry experienced changes in credibility and further interest in psychiatry as a nursing specialisation. The **deinstitutionalisation** of people with a mental health condition in the late 1980s saw a move from institutionalised care to community-based care, and thus the role and expertise of the psychiatric nurse also adapted (Happell, 2007).

Mental health nursing history and education

The history of psychiatry, or mental health as it is now referred to, has had a considerable impact on the development of nursing practice. The history of (psychiatric) mental health nursing differs significantly from that of other branches of nursing (Happell, 2007), where the influence of iconic figures such as Florence Nightingale and Lucy Osborne on the development of nursing services in the Colonies is clear and has been extensively documented (Bessant, 1999). Prior to the establishment of the first asylums in Australia, individuals with a mental health condition were confined to jails or cared for privately. There was no distinction between those individuals experiencing mental illness and those who were intellectually disabled (Happell, 2007). Jails were always custodial rather than treatment oriented, so incarceration of individuals with a mental health condition was obviously ineffective.

The introduction of the first Australian asylum at Castle Hill in 1811 failed to provide a feasible alternative to existing options in the lives of the mentally ill. Although the philosophy underpinning care was based on humane treatment, the day-to-day reality of caring for patients was primarily about containment. While this could partly be a consequence of the overcrowded conditions at Castle Hill (Curry, 1989), it also reflected the prevailing attitude that mental illness was incurable (Sands, 2009). The people who managed and cared for individuals with a mental health condition were referred to as 'attendants' and their work came under the control of the medical profession in Australia at the same time that the first legislation relating to mental health was enacted through the 1843 *Lunacy Act* (Curry, 1989). Prior to this, the first superintendent had been a layperson, whose approach to the care of individuals with a mental health condition was focused on using psychosocial care as a means for managing their behaviour.

The ideological conflict between proponents of such models of care and those who supported medical approaches to treatment 'based in neurophysiology and neuropathology' (Curry, 1989, p. 10) contributed to the establishment of the Select Committee on the Lunatic Asylum, Tarban Creek in 1846. The findings of this committee enabled medical practitioners to assume the responsibility for governance and treatment. This development meant that the lay superintendent was demoted to the position of senior warden. Curry (1989) argues that this arrangement established the medical and nursing systems for the asylums and was copied everywhere throughout the colonies.

The first facility for individuals with a mental health condition in Victoria was established in 1848 and was proclaimed a ward of the NSW asylum at Tarban Creek. It became locally known as the Merri Creek Lunatic Asylum. Following separation from New South Wales, it became known as the Yarra Bend Lunatic Asylum (Reischel, 2001). The first evidence of education for 'mental nurses' in Victoria was noted in the Annual Report for 1887 of the Kew asylum in Victoria (Reischel, 1974). This was the beginning of a formal training system for staff in asylums. Reischel (2001) observes that lectures were provided by medical staff who also oversaw and controlled the educative process. In 1902, a number of general trained nurses were employed at the Kew asylum and several trained and untrained female nurses were employed in the main male ward (Reischel, 1974). This was the first recorded occasion of female staff being involved in the care of individuals with a mental health condition. Women were specifically referred to as nurses now, defining them differently from their male colleagues who were known as **attendants** (Reischel, 1974). Education continued to be provided to attendants

and nurses by medical staff and a three-year training program approved by the relevant health authority in Victoria was introduced. However, this qualification was not recognised outside of Victoria, and nurses and attendants were not registered with the Nurses' Board of Victoria (Reischel, 1974).

Modern mental health nursing education commenced in the mid-twentieth century (Reischel, 2001); for example, recognised education and registration as psychiatric nurses commenced in Victoria with the passing of the Victorian *Nurses Act 1958* (Reischel, 1974). Parallel with these developments, statements regarding changes to health care delivery generally, and mental health care in particular, were also being reported. Holland (1978, p. 16) stated that 'A greater emphasis was emerging on health services outside institutions such as hospitals'. Since this time, nursing education in all disciplines has come under the control of nursing bodies such as the Nursing Board of Victoria and, in contemporary times, the Nursing and Midwifery Board of Australia. This organisation sets the requirements for accreditation of educational programs and defines the standards for nursing (and midwifery) practice. The development of the treatments for mental health disorders throughout history is dealt with in more detail in the following section.

CULTURAL CONSIDERATIONS

Mental illness and European settlement of Australia
Prior to the settlement of Europeans in Australia, mental illness was almost unheard of in Aboriginal and Torres Strait Islander cultures. With the colonisation of Australia came disease and the introduction of many substances previously unknown to Indigenous cultures (such as alcohol). Since European settlement, rates of mental health challenges in Aboriginal and Torres Strait Islander people have increased to an extent that significantly passes the rates of mental health conditions among non-Indigenous Australians. Currently, rates of psychological distress among Indigenous Australians are more than twice those of non-Indigenous Australians (AIHW, 2021).

CASE **STUDY**

PENNY'S 'CALLING'

I completed my nurse training in the 1970s, back when nurses trained in a hospital and also lived there too. I guess I sort of 'fell' into mental health. I did a rotation in the psychiatric ward and the nurse manager pulled me aside and told me I would be a good addition to their staff, and I haven't really looked back since. I certainly haven't regretted it. I've been nursing

so long that I have been fortunate enough to see the amazing progression of mental health care, to even play a part in this... things weren't always great in mental health when I first started, but we were doing the best we could with what we knew. I really believe I was able to help many of my patients even in the early days where medications were limited and care was almost custodial. It didn't feel like that at the time though. We thought we were cutting edge! Helping patients and their families has always been my motivation for staying in mental health nursing. Mental illness is so destructive, and the suffering and pain it causes is immense. To play a part in easing someone's distress is my calling.

I've seen deinstitutionalisation firsthand, and the benefits and challenges that this created. One of the big changes in my career was the move from hospital-based training to university-educated nursing. I remember there was a lot of resistance from some nurses when this happened. But I embraced it; change is inevitable, and I have had the firsthand experience of seeing a student realise their 'calling'. What advice would I give a student

nurse? Don't disregard mental health nursing… maybe it's your calling too.

Penny, registered nurse

Question

Penny has described the types of transitions that someone who has worked in health care for a long time will encounter. Her experience of change was welcomed and she was able to embrace it. Not everyone embraces change, however. Consumers in the mental health system also experience great adjustments during times of hospitalisation, diagnosis and treatment, and may be resistant to such change. How do you think you can support someone experiencing change?

TREATMENTS THROUGHOUT HISTORY

The term '**consumer**' is used to describe a person who identifies as having a lived experience of a mental health condition (Fuller Torrey, 2011). This experience may be past or current. The term consumer is preferred to 'patient', and throughout this book, you will see this term used frequently, and interchanged with other terms such as 'individual' or 'person'. Consumers of today are afforded a range of management options such as medication and talking therapies that have benefited from extensive testing prior to their use in human populations, and this is a strictly regimented requirement of pharmaceutical companies.

Recovery-oriented models of practice now place the person with a lived experience of a mental health condition at the centre of their care. It is understood that they are the experts on their lives. This, however was not always the case, and while consumers today have a central voice in how they are treated, patients of the past were exposed to brutal and barbaric 'treatments'. Some earlier treatments focused on Hippocrates' belief in the four 'humours' (blood, yellow bile, black bile and phlegm) and their imbalance as a precursor for all types of illness, including psychiatric illness. **Table 1.1** outlines many of the treatments for mental illness throughout history.

TABLE 1.1

Timeline of treatment of mental disorders through history

TREATMENT	TIME OR ERA	PERCEIVED BENEFITS
Trephination – the drilling of a small hole into the skull	8000 BCE to 600 BCE	It was believed that this process would allow evil spirits to exit the mind.
Fumigation of vagina – alleged to encourage the vagina to realign to its correct positioning	Ancient Egyptian and Greek	Fumigation of the vagina was thought to cure a 'wandering uterus', which was commonly associated with hysteria in women.
Imbalance of humours – use of leeches, laxatives and substances to induce vomiting	Middle Ages	This process purged the individual of melancholy and rebalanced their 'humours'.
Bloodletting or **scarification** – of brain, rectum, large leg veins	Middle Ages	It was believed that this resulted in the drawing away of poison from the brain.
Flogging – beating, sometimes in public	Middle Ages	People believed that poor behaviour could be 'beaten' out of the person.
Freezing or scalding – being immersed in hot or cold water, or throwing it at the individual	Middle Ages	This process was believed to shock the person back to sanity.
Gyrating chair – a chair that spun around wildly until the strapped patient lost consciousness (see **Figure 1.5**)	Mid-1700s	The spinning and gyrating was believed to result in mixing blood and tissues and re-establishing balance.
Straight jacket – a confining garment where the patient's arms were strapped securely across their body	1700s	Deemed to be a 'humane' treatment for a patient who needed to be restrained, as it permitted the individual to move about freely (from waist down) while preventing them from harming themself and others.

TREATMENT	TIME OR ERA	PERCEIVED BENEFITS
Tranquillising chair – a movement-restricting chair that included a box held over the person's head to keep them immobile	Late 1700s	Used the premise that agitation was a form of inflammation of the brain, exacerbated by movement. By preventing movement, the inflammation would diminish and the madness would be cured.
Rotary chair – a chair that turned on its axis and was propelled at high velocity, resulting in fright and painful cranial pressure	1850s	The chair resulted in feelings of terror, nausea, a sense of suffocation and distress and some believed that it would restore balance in the brain.
Utica crib – a fully enclosed 'cot' or crib where the opening was also sealed with bars	1860s	Resulted in containment and some perceived therapeutic calming benefits.
Shock treatments: **Insulin** – large doses of insulin injected over a period of weeks resulting in coma **Fever** – malaria was injected into the patient to induce fever **Medicine** – induced seizures	1920s to 1950s	Insulin shock was believed to effectively treat schizophrenia and the resulting coma and seizures were believed to reset the brain. It was believed that a severe episode of fever could restore a previously insane person, to calm and sanity. Seizures were induced with a variety of medicines (including metrazol) in persons with schizophrenia as it was falsely believed that schizophrenia and epilepsy could not coexist.
Lobotomy – prefrontal lobe lobotomy is a surgical intervention that severs the pathways between frontal lobes and lower regions of the brain. The physician would often gain access to the brain via the tear duct of the eye, or through the nose	1935	Usually reserved for those experiencing depression (and schizophrenia), the lobotomy was a highly invasive procedure that rendered the individual calm and compliant, and more frequently cognitively impaired. It was often used on patients who were violent, highly emotive and deemed too difficult to manage.

SOURCE: ADAPTED FROM VALENSTEIN, 2010

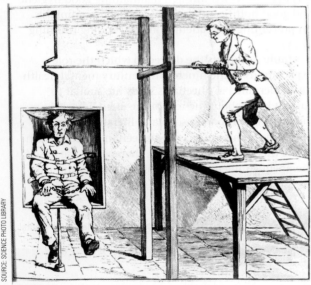

SOURCE: SCIENCE PHOTO LIBRARY

FIGURE 1.5
Dr Herman Boerhaave's gyrating chair

In the late eighteenth century, conditions began to improve in many asylums. Treatments became more focused on improving mental illness through humane treatment, fresh air and interaction. A number of **talk therapies** were developed in an effort to explore an individual's past experiences and consider the impact of these experiences on the person's current mental health. Pioneers of modern psychiatry included physicians such as Sigmund Freud and Carl Jung.

In the mid-twentieth century, the emergence of **psychotropic** medication resulted in a revolution in both the treatment and care of persons with a mental health condition, and in part helped facilitate the eventual deinstitutionalisation of people with a lived experience in the late 1980s. **Table 1.2** outlines the emergence of psychotropic medications in psychiatry.

TABLE 1.2
Timeline of psychotropic medications

YEAR	MEDICATION	USES
1952	Chlorpromazine (typical antipsychotic)	First antipsychotic used to treat schizophrenia
1952	Lithium	Bipolar disorder
Early 1950s	Monoamine oxidase inhibitors (MAOIs)	Depression
1958	Haloperidol (typical antipsychotic)	Schizophrenia
1958	Tricyclic antidepressants	Depression
1960s	Benzodiazepines	Anxiety and insomnia
1970s	Clozapine (atypical antipsychotic)	Treatment-resistive or refractory schizophrenia
1980s	Selective serotonin reuptake inhibitors (SSRIs)	Depression and anxiety
1990s	Atypical antipsychotics	Schizophrenia and mania

While the history of mental illness may make some believe that psychiatrists and nurses were motivated by experimenting on and hurting vulnerable people, the vast majority were working in a field that was highly criticised and even stigmatised by the medical profession as a whole. With the benefit of hindsight, we can now see how destructive many practices were; however, at the time it is likely that people were motivated to help ease suffering and improve people's lives. The next section explores the role of contemporary mental health nurses.

THE ROLE AND IDENTITY OF THE MENTAL HEALTH NURSE IN CONTEMPORARY SERVICE DELIVERY

Mental health nurses play a central role as clinicians, case managers, clinical nurse specialists and nurse practitioners in mental health care settings. They are increasingly involved in a range of psychosocial interventions and work within recovery-based models of care with consumers and carers.

Interventions include the development and implementation of psychosocial therapies for psychological distress, consumer participation in the development, implementation and evaluation of mental health services, and the development and coordination of aggression management programs in acute inpatient facilities (Sinclair et al., 2007). Recently, mental health nurses have also renewed their skills in the more traditional areas of medication administration and education (Hemingway, 2004, 2005; Hemingway et al., 2008). In 2001, the World Health Organization (WHO) stated that nurses, as part of the multidisciplinary team, are especially relevant in the management of mental illness (WHO, 2001).

Furthermore, population health approaches have identified that mental health nurses take up the bulk of the work with consumers in both community and inpatient settings (Raphael, 2000). This is verified by moves towards expanded practice roles for mental health nurses, particularly in the area of community mental health, which have occurred over the past decade (Elsom, Happell & Manias, 2005, 2007, 2009).

It is informative to consider how the role of the mental health nurse has evolved historically in line with the development of care and treatment options for consumers and carers, as well as changes in public expectations of the role of the mental health nurse. According to numerous authors, the public does hold perceptions about who nurses are and what they do (see Aber & Hawkins, 1992; Bridges, 1990; Brodie et al., 2004; Fiedler, 1998; Gordon, 2001; Gordon & Johnson, 2004; Kalisch, Kalisch & McHugh, 1980; Takase, Maude & Manias, 2006). This holds true also – although to a lesser degree – for mental health nurses (Kalisch & Kalisch, 1981; Rungapadiachy

et al., 2006). Some of the perceptions of nursing include:

- nurses are less powerful, and they are dependent on medical officers
- it is a 'good' career choice for women
- it is an occupation that requires patience, virtue and physical strength
- nurses are self-sacrificing
- it is a low-status career.

Some researchers have hypothesised that these social perceptions, media representations and professional attitudes converge and stigmatise the role of mental health nurses through a negative association with mental health (Halter, 2002).

Discussion about the role of the mental health nurse is not new. Sheehan's (1998) study reported on the role and rewards of asylum attendants at a West Yorkshire, England, asylum from 1852 to 1889. Defining their role as the list of functions an individual performs, Sheehan identifies those specific tasks that were prescribed for attendants. These functions included qualities such as kindness, gentleness and firmness. Attendants were expected to promote the safety, comfort and recovery of patients and every effort was to be made to secure the goodwill of the patient and friendship. Physical care was to be provided through maintaining good hygiene and good nutrition. There was also a large emphasis on preventing the patient from absconding (running away).

Table 1.3 charts the degree to which the role expectations of the nineteenth-century mental health nurse identified in Sheehan's study are similar to current ideas about the role of the mental health nurse in contemporary scholarly literature. Some immediate comparisons can be seen in concepts such as the therapeutic relationship, therapeutic use of self, therapeutic milieu, professional boundaries and risk assessment.

TABLE 1.3
Comparison between historical and contemporary roles of the mental health nurse

HISTORICAL PERIOD	ROLE DEFINITION
Role of the attendant 1852–89 (Sheehan, 1998)	• Kindness, gentleness and firmness • Securing the goodwill of the patient and friendship • Maintaining safety and comfort • Prevent patient from absconding • Physical care/nutrition/hygiene
Contemporary role functions (Crowe & Carlyle, 2003; Hewitt, 2009; Scanlon, 2006)	• Limit setting and boundaries • Therapeutic relationship/therapeutic use of self • Therapeutic milieu • Risk assessment/supervision • Support activities of daily living

SOURCE: ADAPTED FROM CROWE & CARLYLE, 2003; HEWITT, 2009; SCANLON, 2006; SHEEHAN, 1998.

Contemporary debates on the professional roles and identity of the mental health nurse

One debate that surrounds the knowledge and skills required for mental health nurses to carry out their role is centred on whether mental health nurses work within a biomedical or an interpersonal framework (Barker et al., 1997; Gournay, 1995; Peplau, 1962). Both of these approaches are explored in Chapter 2. The biomedical approach emphasises the diagnosis of an illness based on a set of signs and symptoms. Treatment is focused on removing or at least reducing these signs and symptoms. Mental health nursing practice is located in the administration of medications, education and symptom management.

The interpersonal approach views the relationship that develops between the nurse and consumer as the central feature of mental health nursing. It is through this relationship that the mental health nurse uses the therapeutic process to facilitate the consumer's change and growth and interventions are usually psychosocial rather than medicalised. The key questions are whether it is possible or even desirable to separate these two approaches to practice, or whether it is necessary to understand the role of the mental health nurses as encompassing both approaches.

Some researchers argue that describing the role of the mental health nurse is difficult. This difficulty lies in part with what is referred to as the 'invisibility' of the core skills of mental health nursing; that is, the nurse–consumer relationship rather than the execution of specific technical skills (Bray, 1999; Forchuk, 1994; Hamilton & Manias, 2007; O'Brien, 1999; Peplau, 1962; Welch, 2005). Hamilton and Manias (2007) believe that the invisibility of mental health nursing interventions, such as focused observation, has negative consequences for the capacity for mental health nurses to describe their role.

How do mental health nurses understand and explain their role? Work by Hercelinskyj et al. (2014) shows that mental health nurses do not define their role in one particular way. Mental health nurses work in increasingly diverse roles and clinical contexts that enable them to engage according to the needs of the consumers with whom they work. The role of the mental health nurse is seen through the therapeutic relationship they engage in with consumers. Mental health nursing practice is grounded in the structures of knowledge and skills through which nurses provide a supportive, empowering and recovery-oriented environment. The degree of support given is based on the identified needs of the individual consumer through partnership and collaboration.

Hildegard Peplau (1962), considered by many to be the founder of modern mental health nursing, viewed mental health nursing as an interpersonal and interactive process between the nurse and consumer. She described the nurse–consumer relationship as being the crux of mental health nursing. Through this relationship the nurse uses him/herself as the therapeutic facilitator of growth and development within collaborative engagement; that is, the nurse engages with consumers through a variety of psychosocial interventions to facilitate personal growth on the part of the consumer. Peplau (1962) also proposed the therapeutic relationship passed through several phases that evolved from the initial contact through to discharge. These phases are the orientation, working and resolution (Forchuk, 1994) and it is during each of these phases that the nurse will take on various roles in response to the emerging and identified needs of the consumer.

These roles involve various strategies such as risk assessment, therapeutic engagement or support with activities of daily living and promoting healthy lifestyles. Research also highlights the importance that consumers place on the therapeutic relationship, with communication, trust and respect being highly valued. Having time to develop positive relations, not holding stigmatising views and being non-judgemental, assisting consumers to find the balance between independence and the need for support are examples of ways in which the role of the mental health nurse is enacted (Gilburt, Rose & Slade, 2008; Johansson & Eklund, 2003). We consider the therapeutic relationship in depth in Chapter 5, and learn more about Peplau's ideas in Chapter 2.

The role of the mental health nurse and professional identity

When a person asks you, 'What do you do for a living?', you may say, 'I am a student nurse', 'I am a parent' or 'I work part time at a chemist'. Explaining what you do as a student nurse usually will be described in terms of where you study, what is expected of you, the specific tasks or functions you have to fulfil, who you study with and perhaps examples of what you are currently doing. What you are actually describing is your role. It is this process that is part of establishing your professional identity as an emerging nurse. The 'Reflect on this' box details some further ideas around the concept of professional identity in mental health nursing.

REFLECT ON THIS

We have undoubtedly come a long way in mental health nursing, but our journey is far from over. Our professional practice continues to evolve as we see the introduction of new treatments, therapies and findings about mental illness. In more recent times, we have seen a surge from consumer movement groups where there is a push to include more people with a lived experience of mental illness in peer support roles and in mental health policy and reform. This is an important step where the notion of 'expert by experience' is valued and respected as a fundamental contributor to the improvement of mental health services, the experiences of consumers within these services and future directions of mental health care.

Soon you will likely embark on your mental health clinical placement. You will encounter lots of people from diverse backgrounds, with an array of mental health challenges. Hopefully you will have the opportunity to meet a peer support worker. This is usually someone who has a lived experience of a mental health condition, and who uses this experience to provide guidance and help to people who are experiencing a mental health issue. Peer support workers have the unique perspective of personal experience of mental illness, but also working closely in the multidisciplinary team.

Think of three questions you could ask a peer support worker about what qualities they look for in a good nurse.

REFLECTION ON LEARNING FROM PRACTICE

As JD reflected at the beginning of this chapter, it can be challenging to accurately and clearly represent the role of the mental health nurse to people who have little to no understanding of mental health and mental illness generally, or who are only familiar with the images and stories of mental health practice from past years. JD's own journey illustrates the level of invisibility that mental health has and the narrow view that people have of the type of work that nurses undertake, and what even constitutes proper nursing work.

The history of mental health (psychiatry) is replete with stories of ignorance and inhumane treatment. But this chapter also highlights the way in which mental health nursing education and practice has evolved and represents new and diverse methods of practice. In the chapters that follow, we explore in greater detail how nurses contribute to and collaborate with consumers, carers and the multidisciplinary team in the delivery of contemporary mental health care.

CHAPTER RESOURCES

SUMMARY

- Historically humankind has attributed many adversities to supernatural origins. However, with the benefit of hindsight, we can safely assume that many of these experiences lay in mental illness.
- Asylums were erected in response to a need to contain and segregate people with mental illness, rather than treat them.
- The history of mental health nursing in Australian is closely linked to the development of psychiatry as a discipline. Education was historically controlled by medicine.

- Changes to nursing education and practice coincided with changes to the understanding of mental illness and its subsequent treatment.
- As future nurses, we need to ensure that we practise in an evidence-based environment and that this information is applied to our practice rigorously.

REVIEW QUESTIONS

1 How accurate do you believe the public perceptions of mental health nursing are? Discuss the factors that might contribute to these perceptions.

2 What do you consider to be the key attributes and qualities of a mental health nurse?

3 The deinstitutionalisation of mental health facilities in the 1990s in Australia has seen major changes to mental health services and improvements for consumers. Describe the many different benefits of moving from institutionalised care.

4 How does the role of the mental health nurse differ from other disciplines of nursing?

5 How would you explain the role of the mental health nurse to a fellow student?

CRITICAL THINKING

1 How has the education of nurses changed during the past 30 years? What impact do you believe this has had on mental health nursing?

2 You are currently attending a clinical learning placement at a mental health facility. How would you describe the role of the mental health nurse to a friend who is not studying nursing?

USEFUL WEBSITES

- Australian College of Mental Health Nurses: http://www.acmhn.org

- History of Psychiatry: http://journals.sagepub.com/home/hpy

REFLECT ON THIS

Time capsule

Hopefully you are reading this at the start of your mental health studies in your efforts to become a nurse. When you are caught up with study, sometimes it is hard to take stock of everything you have learned on your journey.

On a piece of paper, write down all the things you think a mental health nurse does. Now write down what you think are the causes of mental illness, and what it would be like to have a mental health condition. What do you know about schizophrenia, mania or depression, for example?

Place this piece of paper with your answers at the end of this book. When you have finished your mental health unit, go back to it and see just how much you've learned by reading your answers to the questions.

REFERENCES

Aber, C.S. & Hawkins, J.W. (1992). Portrayal of nurses in advertisements in medical and nursing journals. *IMAGE Journal of Nursing Scholarship*, 24(4 winter), 289–93.

Arnold, C. (2009). *Bedlam, London and Its Mad*. London: Simon & Schuster.

Australian Institute of Health & Welfare (2021). 1.18 Social and emotional wellbeing. *Aboriginal and Torres Strait Islander Health Performance Framework*. Retrieved from https://www.indigenoushpf.gov.au/measures/1-18-social-emotional-wellbeing#keyfacts

Barker, P.J., Reynolds, W. & Stevenson, C. (1997). The human science basis of psychiatric nursing: Theory and practice. *Journal of Advanced Nursing*, 25(4), 660–7.

Bessant, B. (1999). Milestones in Australian Nursing. *Collegian*, 6(4), suppl. 1–3.

Bray, J. (1999). An ethnographic study of psychiatric nursing. *Journal of Psychiatric and Mental Health Nursing*, 6(4), 297–305. doi:10.1046/j.1365-2850.1999.00215.x

Bridges, J.M. (1990). Literature review on the images of the nurse and nursing in the media. *Journal of Advanced Nursing*, 15(7), 850–4.

Brodie, D.A., Andrews, G.J., Andrews, J.P., Thomas, G.B., Wong, J. & Rixona, L. (2004). Perceptions of nursing: Confirmation, change and the student experience. *International Journal of Nursing Studies*, 41(7), 721–33.

Craig, L.A. (2014). The history of madness and mental illness in the Middle Ages: Directions and questions. *History Compass*, 12(9), 729–44.

Crowe, M. & Carlyle, D. (2003). Deconstructing risk assessment and management in mental health nursing. *Journal of Advanced Nursing*, 43(1), 19–27.

Curry, G. (1989). *The Select Committee on the Lunatic Asylum, Tarban Creek, 1846: The Medicalisation of Mental Nursing in NSW*. Lindfield: Kuring-gai College of Advanced Education.

Elmer, P. (2016). Witchcraft, witch-hunting, and politics in early modern England. *Oxford Scholarship Online*. doi:10.1093/acprof:oso/9780198717720.001.0001.

Elsom, S., Happell, B. & Manias, E. (2005). Mental health nurse practitioner: Expanded or advanced. *International Journal of Mental Health Nursing*, 14(3), 18–186.

Elsom, S., Happell, B. & Manias, E. (2007). Exploring the advanced practice roles of community mental health nurses. *Issues in Mental Health Nursing*, 28(4), 413–29.

Elsom, S., Happell, B. & Manias, E. (2009). Australian mental health nurses' attitudes to role expansion. *Perspectives in Psychiatric Care*, 45(2), 100–7.

Fiedler, L.A. (1998). Images of the nurse in fiction and popular culture. In A.H. Jones (ed.), *Images of Nurses, Perspectives from History, Art and Literature*. Philadelphia, PA: University of Pennsylvania Press.

Fontaine, M. (2013). On being sane in an insane place – the Rosenhan experiment in the laboratory of Plautus' Epidamnus. *Current Psychology*, 32(4), 348–65.

Forchuk, C. (1994). The orientation phase of the nurse–client relationship: Testing Peplau's theory. *Journal of Advanced Nursing*, 20(3), 532–7.

Fuller Torrey, E. (2011). Patients, clients, consumers, survivors et al: What's in a name? *Schizophrenia Bulletin*, 31(3), 466–8. doi:10.1093/schbul/sbq102

Gilburt, H., Rose, D. & Slade, M. (2008). The importance of relationships in mental health care. A qualitative study of service users' experiences of psychiatric hospital admission in the UK. *BMC Health Services Research*, 8(92). Retrieved from http://www.biomedcentral.com/1472-6963/8/92.

Gordon, S. (2001). Nurses speaking out about what they do. *Australian Nursing Journal*, 9(3), 46–7.

Gordon, S. & Johnson, R. (2004). How Hollywood portrays nurses. Report from the front row. *Revolution*, March–April, 15–21.

Gournay, K. (1995). Training and education in mental health nursing. *Mental Health Nursing*, 15(6), 12–15.

Hamilton, B.E. & Manias, E. (2007). Rethinking nurses' observations: Psychiatric nursing skills and invisibility in an acute inpatient setting. *Social Science and Medicine*, 65(2), 331–43. Retrieved from ScienceDirect Database.

Happell, B. (2007). Appreciating the importance of history: A brief historical overview of mental health, mental health nursing and education in Australia. *International Journal of Psychiatric Nursing Research*, 12(2), 1439–45.

Hemingway, S. (2004). The mental health nurse's perspective on implementing nurse prescribing. *Nurse Prescribing*, 2(1), 37–44.

Hemingway, S. (2005). An emerging picture of mental health nurses as non-medical prescribers. *Nurse Prescribing*, 3(6), 257–62.

Hemingway, S., White, J., Turner, J., Maginnis, R. & Gray, J. (2008). Medicines with respect. Collaboratively establishing the art and science of medicines administration. *International Journal of Mental Health Nursing*, 17, suppl. 1(A14).

Hewitt, J. (2009). Redressing the balance in mental health nursing education: Arguments for a values-based approach. *International Journal of Mental Health Nursing*, 18(5), 368–79.

Holland, J. (1978). New health body to take over. *The Age*, 6 December. Retrieved from Google News.

Johansson, H. & Eklund, M. (2003). Patients' opinion on what constitutes good psychiatric care. *Scandinavian Journal of Caring Science*, 17, 339–46. Retrieved from http://web.ebscohost.com.ezproxy-m.deakin.edu.au/ehost/pdf?vid=3&hid=7&sid=0d5a034d-d286-4358-885b-67dcfe6b61fc%40sessionmgr2.

Kalisch, B.J., Kalisch, P.A. & McHugh, M. (1980). Content analysis of film stereotypes of nurses. *International Journal of Women's Studies*, 3(6) 531–58.

Kalisch, P. & Kalisch, B.J. (1981). The image of psychiatric nurses in motion pictures. *Perspectives in Psychiatric Care*, XIX(3 & 4), 116–24.

Maude, P. (2002). Historians overlook the role of nurses. *Mental Health Practice*, 6(4), 5.

McNamara, P. (2011). *Spirit Possession and Exorcism: History, Psychology, and Neurobiology: Mental States and the Phenomenon of Possession*. Westport, CT: Greenwood Publishing Group.

New South Wales Health. (n.d.). *The Lunatic Asylums*. Retrieved from http://www.health.nsw.gov.au/about/history/Publications/h-asylums.pdf.

Nolan, P. (1993). *A History of Mental Health Nursing*. London: Chapman & Hall.

O'Brien, A.J. (1999). Negotiating the relationship: Mental health nurses' perceptions of their practice. *Australian and New Zealand Journal of Mental Health Nursing*, 8(4), 153–61.

Peplau, H.E. (1962). Interpersonal techniques: The crux of psychiatric nursing. *American Journal of Nursing*, 62(6), 50–4.

Reischel, H.J. (1974). Nurse education in mental health, Victoria past, present and future. *UNA Nursing Journal*, 72(2), 14–17.

Reischel, H.J. (2001). *The Care that Was*. Ebookland/Zeus Publications.

Rungapadiachy, D.M., Madill, A. & Gough, B. (2006). How newly qualified mental health nurses perceive their role. *Journal of Psychiatric and Mental Health Nursing*, 13(5), 533–42. doi:10.1111/ j.1365-2850.2006.00976.x

Sands, N. (2009). Round the bend: A brief history of mental health nursing in Victoria, Australia 1848 to 1950s. *Issues in Mental Health Nursing*, 30(6), 364–71.

Scanlon, A. (2006). Psychiatric nurses' perceptions of the constituents of the therapeutic relationship: A grounded theory study. *Journal of Psychiatric and Mental Health Nursing*, 13, 319–29.

Sheehan, J. (1998). The role and rewards of asylum attendants in Victorian England. *International History of Nursing Journal*, 3(4), 25–33.

Sinclair, E., Townsend, J., Keith, R., Hazelton, M. & Constable, J. (2007). Development, implementation and evaluation of a nursing delivered psychosocial intervention for psychological disease. Paper presented at the Nursing Innovations Showcase. NSW Department of Health: Nursing and Midwifery Office.

Takase, M., Maude, P. & Manias, E. (2006b). Role discrepancy: Is it a common problem among nurses? *Journal of Advanced Nursing*, 54(6), 751–9.

Toy, M. (2014). Victorian psychiatric patients' grim fate in hellish 1800s hospitals. *Herald Sun*, 9 December. Retrieved from https:// www.heraldsun.com.au/news/victoria/victorian-psychiatric-patients-grim-fate-in-hellish-1800s-hospitals/news-story/ c7928ebe8a9f527a941cce86e0990fef.

Valenstein, E.S. (2010). *Great and Desperate Cures: The Rise and Decline of Psychosurgery and Other Radical Treatments for Mental Illness*. New York: Basic Books.

Welch, M. (2005). Pivotal moments in the therapeutic relationship. *International Journal of Mental Health Nursing*, 14, 161–5.

Wikipedia. (2017). List of psychiatric hospitals in Australia. Retrieved from https://en.wikipedia.org/wiki/List_of_Australian_psychiatric_ institutions.

World Health Organization (WHO). (2001). *The World Health Report 2001: Mental Health – New Understanding, New Hope*. Geneva: WHO. Retrieved from http://www.who.int/whr/2001/en/whr01_ en.pdf.

Zacks, R. (1994). *History Laid Bare: Love, Sex and Perversity from the Ancient Etruscans to Warren G. Harding*. New York: HarperPerennial.

CHAPTER 2

THEORETICAL FRAMEWORKS UNDERPINNING PRACTICE

Gylo (Julie) Hercelinskyj

LEARNING OUTCOMES

Upon completion of this chapter, you should be able to:

2.1 Define the terms health, mental health, human behaviour and personality

2.2 Describe biomedical theories of personality, their application and relevance to mental health nursing practice and some of the major critiques of these theories

2.3 Describe psychodynamic theories of personality, their application and relevance to mental health nursing practice and some of the major critiques of these theories

2.4 Describe behavioural/social cognitive theories of personality, their application and relevance to mental health nursing practice and some of the major critiques of these theories

2.5 Describe humanistic theories of personality, their application and relevance to mental health nursing practice and some of the major critiques of these theories

2.6 Describe how nursing theorists have drawn from psychological and sociological theorists to understand human behaviour and how this influences the role of the mental health nurse

2.7 Reflect on which psychological and/or nursing theories would be relevant to your nursing practice

LEARNING FROM PRACTICE

Shelley is a 21-year old woman who lives at home with her mother. Shelley has been admitted for the first time to the inpatient unit at the local acute inpatient mental health facility. Shelley's first 36 hours in the unit were unsettled as she was extremely suspicious of the nursing staff and resisted efforts by nurses to engage with her. Shelley did not believe she needed to be in hospital and became extremely agitated when staff attempted to administer prescribed medication, saying that everyone was trying to poison her 'because she knew too much'. Shelley's mother Rose has been in twice to visit her. Nursing staff have asked several times to make a time to meet with Rose to discuss Shelley's progress and obtain additional information regarding the circumstances leading to Shelley's admission. On both occasions, staff have observed that Rose avoids eye contact with them, says very little to Shelley and seems ill at ease in the environment.

At the end of the second visit, a registered nurse approached Rose as she was leaving the unit. Indicating that she was concerned that Rose appeared uncomfortable while in the unit and that she was very happy to answer any questions Rose may have, Rose's whole body appeared to stiffen and with a trembling voice she replied, 'Why would you care, my daughter is lost to me and places like this don't help. I know what these places are like and the sooner she is out of here the better for her!'

Following Rose's abrupt departure, the registered nurse considered this interaction. What emotions, feelings and experiences could be behind Rose's response? How could an understanding of psychological theories assist the team to support and work collaboratively with Shelley and Rose during this time?

INTRODUCTION

This chapter explores theoretical frameworks common within mental health practice. Such theoretical frameworks permit the nurse to provide care that is evidence-based and provide a sound base that guides the nurse's practice and reflection. Working collaboratively with consumers and carers requires mental health nurses to understand:

- how people understand health
- how their understanding of health impacts on their health choices and health behaviours.

There are multiple ways to explain or predict personality or human behaviour. For example, perhaps we want to understand why some consumers agree to take regular medications and others will not. Where would we start? There are a variety of ways in which to understand this behaviour, and disciplines such as nursing and psychology have philosophical assumptions and focus on different aspects of human existence and experience (Bernstein, Penner, Clarke-Stewart & Roy, 2012). Theories comprise a range of concepts about a phenomenon studied within a discipline. They are based upon what has been observed and researched across larger populations. No theory is perfect, but a useful theory will give clinicians a structure that enables them to understand people's behaviour and health-related decisions and to plan strategies to implement in practice (Bernstein et al., 2018; Burger, 2011; Weiten, 2011). In this chapter, we consider foundational ideas regarding health, mental health, human behaviour and personality.

HEALTH, MENTAL HEALTH AND HUMAN BEHAVIOUR

The word 'health' in its broadest sense holds different meanings for different people at different times in history, in different cultures, in different social classes or even within the same family. Our understanding of **health** is therefore an evolving and dynamic process.

Traditional definitions of health have tended to have a biomedical focus where health was viewed as the absence of disease or pathology and health was achieved through the physical process of **homeostasis**. Illness was caused by the body being subjected to a range of factors (e.g. pathogens such as infections, trauma, biochemical changes or degenerative processes) that disrupted homeostasis. The World Health Organization (WHO) produced a seminal definition of health when it stated that health was a 'State of complete physical, mental and social well-being and not merely the absence of disease or infirmity' (WHO, 1946).

However, these understandings of health fail to acknowledge the broader cultural, psychological, sociological, political, economic and environmental factors that impact health in general and **mental health** specifically. This critique is important to framing our understanding of what constitutes mental health and mental illness.

What makes a person mentally healthy? Frisch and Frisch (2006) believe there is no clear single definition of mental health. While this might be so, we make judgements about a person's mental health from their behaviour. Using this framework, characteristics of mental health might include:

- self-determination and autonomy
- self-actualising and goal-directed behaviour
- flexibility and tolerance of uncertainty
- awareness of strengths and limitations to build self-esteem
- ability to maintain relationships and communicate directly with others
- respect for others
- actions grounded in reality
- managing stress appropriately
- capacity to meet basic needs (adapted from Frisch & Frisch, 2006).

As can be seen from this list, the process of defining what mental health is and ascribing this term to a person is far more complex than the WHO's original definition (Galderisi, Heinz, Kastrup, Beezhold & Sartorius, 2015). The remainder of this chapter looks at the different ways in which personality development is viewed and how this impacts on mental health.

Definitions of personality

Before we explore different theories of personality, it is important to have a working definition of the term. When we think of the term 'personality', different ideas come to mind, such as 'they have a great personality' or 'they have a really quirky way of behaving'. People differ in the ways they think, feel and behave – in short, everyone has a unique personality.

Personality can be defined as the set of cognitions, emotions and feelings that a person brings to their interactions with the total environment. It is this interaction that will influence the way in which an individual thinks, feels and subsequently behaves. These patterns of thinking, feeling and behaving in different circumstances are seen to be consistent or enduring over time and across situations. This means there will be distinct differences in the way people can respond to the same situation (Burger, 2011; Cervone & Pervin, 2013; Weiten, 2011).

BIOMEDICAL THEORIES OF PERSONALITY

Any discussion that focuses on understanding personality and its relationship to human behaviour would not be complete without a review of what must be considered the predominant approach to mental health; that is, the identification of mental illness.

The fundamental premise of the biomedical model of health and illness is that behaviour is the result of maintaining an internal (physiological) balance (or equilibrium). Normal behaviour represents this balance and abnormal behaviour represents a dysfunction (either pathological or neurological). A biomedical view of mental health and mental illness is fundamentally concerned with providing a physiological explanation of health, illness and resulting behaviour. Changes can be assessed by a clinician observing a series of signs and symptoms. The clinician then takes this constellation of signs and symptoms and classifies them as a diagnosis. Recovery from mental illness (discussed in greater detail in Chapter 21) traditionally has been conceptualised in terms of the elimination of symptomatology (Nye, 2003; Hogan, 2019).

Relevance of the biomedical orientation to mental health nursing practice

The **biomedical orientation** to mental health nursing practice allows clinicians to make sense of the range of symptoms a consumer can experience and their unique response to those signs and symptoms. Research into mental health and mental illness has paved the way for the development of specific treatment approaches, particularly in the area of psychotropic medication. The biomedical model also provides a clear framework for the mental health nurse to use when working with consumers and families, particularly in the area of psychoeducation.

Critique of the biomedical orientation to mental health nursing practice

From a Western cultural perspective, the biomedical orientation could be seen to be the dominant focus of clinical practice, research and education in mental health service delivery. The outcome has been the advent of drug therapies to treat mental illness. This focus on the use of drugs has led to the idea that it is possible to 'cure' mental illnesses. One critique of the biomedical orientation is that, as the dominant (Western) approach to understanding mental health and illness, it limits the capacity for other (non-biomedical) interventions or reduces their use to an adjunct status at best (Pickersgill, 2014).

There has been an increasing emphasis on the role of the nurse in the treatment of mental illnesses to focus increasingly on areas such as assessment and diagnosis, medication-prescribing privileges and educating consumers and carers about mental illnesses that are largely defined by and constructed on the biological model. However, according to Norman and Ryrie (2009), it is not possible to classify mental health nursing in such a distinct way, because the complexity of mental health nursing means there is a diversity of clinical contexts that mental health nurses work in and the role of expectations in these areas of practice.

CULTURAL CONSIDERATIONS

Are Western theoretical perspectives universally valid?

As mentioned above, the theoretical perspectives reviewed in this chapter were developed within a Western context. They also represent the social, economic and personal stories of each person who developed the theory. In today's culturally diverse world, there is ongoing debate regarding the utility of such models for people (a one-size-fits-all approach) as opposed to exploring and utilising a variety of models to best meet the needs of the individual person.

PSYCHODYNAMIC THEORIES OF PERSONALITY

There can be no discussion of Western models of personality without considering the **psychodynamic approach** and in particular the work of Sigmund Freud (1856–1939). Freud produced the first structured and formalised attempt to understand personality and human behaviour. While there is intense debate regarding the contemporary usefulness of his original ideas, all subsequent theory development, research and clinical application has developed from these core ideas. The core assumption of the psychodynamic orientation is that abnormal behaviour reflects unconscious conflicts within the person.

Key areas of Freud's theory relate to the psychosexual stages of development (human mind) psyche, the structure of personality and the use of defence mechanisms. We consider Freud's theory and then look at the key neo-Freudians who challenged and extended many aspects of Freud's theory.

Freud's theory

Freud (**Figure 2.1**) believed that all behaviour is purposeful. An individual's behaviour is determined by irrational forces, unconscious motivations, and biological and instinctual drives that develop through various psychosexual stages in the first six years of life. The childhood of a person was seen as crucial to

The notion of drives or instincts was central to Freud's ideas. These instinctual drives were Eros, which was described by Freud as the life drive, and Thanatos, which referred to the death/aggressive drive people held. These instincts served to assist the survival and growth of individuals and were oriented towards development and creativity. **Libido** was the term used to describe an individual's emotional energy derived from underlying instinct of Eros (Sigelman, Rider & De George-Walker, 2016).

Libido (emotional energy) is invested in different parts of a child's body as they pass through a rigid developmental stage. These stages were referred to by Freud as the psychosexual stages of development. **Table 2.1** provides an overview of the psychosexual stages of development.

Freud argued that an individual's psyche contained all their conscious and unconscious desires (e.g. wishes, fantasies, fears and intentions). It is the capacity of the psyche to maintain a balance between these conscious and unconscious forces that determines an individual's personality. Freud was specifically interested in how the mind (human psyche), especially the unconscious part of the human mind, is responsible for everyday behaviour.

Freud argued that behaviour was dictated by a person's personality, which was composed of three parts (in which the instinctual drives of Eros and Thanatos originate). According to Freud, these three components are distinct yet interrelated.

The **id** is the original system of personality. At birth, an individual is all id. The id operates at an unconscious level, is amoral and is governed by the **pleasure principle** in which the individual seeks to gratify their desires. These needs and their fulfilment might be in conflict with societal values and mores;

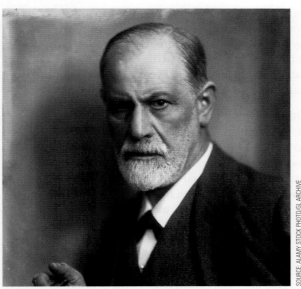

FIGURE 2.1
Sigmund Freud (1856–1939)

SOURCE: ALAMY STOCK PHOTO/GL ARCHIVE

the development of the adult personality. Abnormal behaviour in Freud's view resulted from anxiety due to unconscious conflicts. Behaviour was seen as a result of unconscious drives and needs and the mechanisms developed to satisfy or control them. An individual must repress or modify these basic drives when they come into conflict with socially developed cultural restraints. These mechanisms of control are developed in early childhood.

Freud believed these basic drives within the unconscious mind and past psychological events determined behaviour; that is, his theory of human personality and behaviour was a deterministic theory. This means that events from childhood can determine adult behaviour.

TABLE 2.1
Freud's stages of psychosexual development

STAGE	AGE	FEATURES
Oral	Birth to 18 months	Behaviour is governed by the id. The child seeks immediate gratification. This gratification is achieved through the mouth, lips and tongue.
Anal	18 months to three years	With the advent of toilet training, children begin to perceive the impact their behaviour has on others. For example, praise and rewards for successfully using the toilet and expressions of disappointment if they wet the bed. It is at this time that children begin to modify their behaviour to achieve a positive response from others.
Phallic	Three to six years	In this phase the penis or clitoris becomes the focus of attention of the libido. The Superego also begins to develop. It is at this stage that all children go through the **Oedipus complex** whereby the child represses their desire for the parent of the opposite gender and identifies with the same sex parent in order to avoid the same gender parent discovering their incestuous feelings towards the same sex parent. Freud argued that this process enabled children to develop those socially sanctioned behaviour attributes of male and female and it is also the time during which the Superego emerges.
Latent	Six years to puberty	There is little sexual motivation during this stage.
Genital	Puberty onwards	The focus of the libido is on the adult genital region.

SOURCE: ADAPTED FROM BURGER, 2011; RANA & UPTON, 2013; WEITEN, 2017

that is, its aim is to gain pleasure and avoid pain. The id operates to meet immediate needs for satisfaction. Think of a baby who is picked up by a person wearing brightly coloured glasses or perhaps a hair accessory. Their immediate response will be to reach for the object and grab it. This is the id in operation. It does not matter to the baby that the object belongs to someone else or that the infant may hurt the other person. Freud identified the concept of wish fulfilment to explain how the individual meets the needs of the id in a socially acceptable way. The instinctual drives of Eros and Thanatos are said to be housed in the id. Therefore, if a person is unable to meet the demands of the id, they must find a way to manage this that is socially acceptable, or they may find themselves in conflict with society (Sigelman, Rider & De George-Walker, 2016).

The next component of a person's personality is the **superego**. The superego develops as a child begins to internalise parental demands for socially acceptable behaviour. It is the 'moral guardian'. It strives for perfection. As Corey states, it is the 'judicial branch of the personality' (Corey, 2013, p. 65). Recall an instance where you have told someone (or even yourself) that something is right or wrong, or good or bad. These are two examples of what Freud saw as the superego. The easiest way to think of the superego is to think of it as the moral component of one's psyche; it operates using the **morality principle**. The superego represents society's views on what is right and wrong. Clearly, the superego develops through a child's interactions with people. The most significant people in a child's life in their developing years are, in Freud's view, the parents.

The **ego** emerges to deal with the real world; it operates on the **reality principle**. It acts as the mediator between the demands of the id and the moral expectations of the superego. It is viewed as the 'executive that governs, controls and regulates the personality' (Corey, 2013, p. 65). The ego controls perception, memory, thought and actions, and suffers

from anxiety. Much of our personality is unconscious, consisting of repressed memories not easily accessed by the ego. So when the ego uses the reality principle, it is attempting to adapt to the real world while still satisfying the psychic forces of both the id and the superego.

Defence mechanisms

If, as described earlier, behaviour results from the need to satisfy or modify needs, then it becomes easier to see how behaviour, in Freud's view, is goal directed. In essence, an individual experiences a need, which they seek to satisfy. This can be achieved in two ways:

- **conscious mental processes**: by direct methods
- **unconscious mental processes**: by the use of ego defence mechanisms.

Ego **defence mechanisms** are specific intra-psychic adjustments used to resolve emotional conflict, reduce anxiety and prevent the ego from being overwhelmed when it unsuccessfully attempts to meet an unresolved need. Essentially, defence mechanisms are coping mechanisms of the ego to protect the person from feelings of anxiety. They are unconscious and involve a degree of self-deception and reality distortion (Weiten, 2011).

While the use of defence mechanisms was traditionally seen as unhealthy, more contemporary work views the use of defence mechanisms as part of an individual's coping style when they attempt to address an emotional conflict or stressor. It is when defence mechanisms are overused and/or ineffective that they become maladaptive and can result in mental/emotional dysfunction. Defence mechanisms have two common features: they deny or distort reality, and they operate at an unconscious level (Corey, 2013; Rana & Upton, 2013; Weiten, 2011). Freud identified a number of ego defence mechanisms. Some of the key ones are listed and described in **Table 2.2**.

TABLE 2.2
Key ego defence mechanisms

DEFENCE MECHANISM	DESCRIPTION	EXAMPLE/COMMENTS
Repression	Seen as the primary defence mechanism used by the ego to push memories that are unacceptable/threatening to the ego into the unconscious. It is said that this process is unconscious	Memories of childhood abuse. Freud believed that repression was perhaps the most important defence mechanism. While these painful events are submerged in unconsciousness, they can continue to influence behaviour later in life.
Projection	Attributing personal impulses or desires that are socially unacceptable onto another person	Socially unacceptable impulses such as lust, aggression or greed are seen as being held by others, not the person themselves.

DEFENCE MECHANISM	DESCRIPTION	EXAMPLE/COMMENTS
Displacement	Transferring a strong emotion from the original object/person that would be unacceptable to express to another more socially acceptable (or 'safer') object or person	A person who is being bullied and feels unable to address this behaviour with the person concerned goes home and 'kicks the cat'.
Denial	Refusal to accept the reality of a situation that the ego would find threatening	Being charged with drink driving offences repeatedly but not accepting that there is an alcohol dependence issue.
Regression	Reverting back to an earlier developmental level of responding to a situation or event	Throwing a temper tantrum.
Rationalisation	Constructing plausible reasons/excuses to try and explain unreasonable behaviour	A person who binge drinks argues that they do not have an alcohol dependence as they do not drink every day.
Sublimation	A socially acceptable substitute replaces a socially unacceptable impulse	Sport or art are socially acceptable ways of replacing socially unacceptable impulses such as aggression or sexual energy.
Reaction formation	Expressing the opposite impulse to the socially unacceptable impulse being experienced and which is threatening to the ego	A person goes out of their way to be friendly to a work colleague they actually dislike intensely.

SOURCE: ADAPTED FROM BARKWAY, 2013; BURGER, 2011; RANA & UPTON, 2013

The neo-Freudians

As with many ideas, evolution is not only inevitable but desirable. Carl Jung (1875–1961) and Alfred Adler (1870–1937) developed psychoanalytic theories that disagreed with important aspects of Freud's work. There was less emphasis on biological drives such as sex and aggression and a much greater emphasis on social relationships.

Another person who developed his ideas from Freud's original theories was Erik Erikson (1902–94; **Figure 2.2**). Emerging from his initial training within the psychodynamic orientation, Erikson developed a number of ideas that contributed to the ongoing development of the psychodynamic approach.

Erikson theorised that there are eight psychosocial stages in human development. Erikson was influenced by the ideas of Freud. However, instead of seeing a rigid series of stages that all people go through and with ongoing development stopping at adolescence, Erikson's ideas focused on a series of life conflicts or tasks that were faced, and addressed, by people at different ages. Erikson was particularly interested in the development of identity. He saw each stage as characterised by a different conflict that must be resolved by the individual. When the environment makes new demands on people, the conflicts arise. The individual can respond to this crisis in an adaptive (confidence) or maladaptive (feelings of failure) way. If a person does not successfully achieve the required task they will experience challenges in achieving subsequent task phases and they will need to resolve the earlier stage at some point in the future. The eight stages that Erikson identified should not be viewed as strictly linear, but as a framework that conceptualises a person as able to move back and forth as challenges are met and crises overcome, leading to further development (Hoffnung et al., 2013; McLeod, 2013). The eight development stages are outlined in **Table 2.3**.

Harry Stack Sullivan (1892–1949)

Within the psychodynamic perspective, a number of theorists veered away from traditional Freudian ideas and focused more strongly on how interpersonal interactions between people influenced personality development (Cervone & Pervin, 2013), which was in line with the developments of Freudian theory proposed by Alfred Adler (Corey, 2017). Harry Stack Sullivan was one of those theorists, and argued that the emotional experiences from infancy were not biologically driven

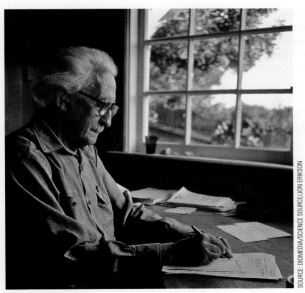

SOURCE: DIOMEDIA/SCIENCE SOURCE/JON ERIKSON

FIGURE 2.2
Erik Erikson (1902–94)

TABLE 2.3
Erikson's developmental stages (some stages overlap)

ERIKSON'S DEVELOPMENTAL STAGES	AGE	DESCRIPTION
Stage 1: Oral-sensory	Birth to 18 months	Trust vs mistrust Children are dependent on parents for survival physically and emotionally Trust develops when an infant's physical and emotional needs are met in a consistent, predictable and emotionally safe way. If an infant receives insufficient, inconsistent care and poor emotional attachment, mistrust can develop.
Stage 2: Muscular-anal	1.5 to three years	Autonomy vs shame/doubt Autonomy is seen in the child's capacity to develop independence in skills such as toileting and feeding. Autonomy develops through mastery where the child is provided with opportunities to attempt a task and retry after failed attempts. Shame/guilt occurs through failed efforts to achieve tasks because caregivers do not provide opportunities or deride efforts to achieve them.
Stage 3: Locomotor	Three to six years	Initiative vs guilt Initiative develops through opportunities for the child to use their imagination, engage in play and ask questions. Caregivers actively promote and support these opportunities. When these conditions and opportunities are not provided, feelings of guilt can develop.
Stage 4: Latency	Six to 12 years	Industry vs inferiority A sense of industry is developed when children receive recognition from others such as parents and teachers in completing productive accomplishments. If the child receives repeated criticism, feelings of inferiority can be internalised.
Stage 5: Adolescence	13 to 18 years	Role identity vs role confusion The transition between childhood and early adulthood is where a child experiences physical, emotional and social developmental changes and expectations. This stage is centred on the question 'Who am I?'. If an adolescent is unsure about their identity and future pathway, role confusion can ensue.
Stage 6: Young adulthood	19 to 40 years	Intimacy vs isolation The stage where adults begin to share themselves with others and to experience feelings of caring for others. If a person does not experience this sense of caring, emotional and social isolation can ensue.
Stage 7: Middle adulthood	40 to 65 years	Generativity vs stagnation Generativity represents the capacity to share experiences, mentor and lead others to be active participants, contributors/leaders in society, particularly younger generations. When an individual remains focused on meeting their own needs and desires, they are seen to be stagnating.
Stage 8: Maturity	65 to death	Ego integrity vs despair Ego integrity represents the idea of a life *well lived*. The older person has a sense of self-respect through understanding they have lived a life that is ethically and socially responsible, they have recognised and owned both the positive aspects and mistakes made and still contribute their experience and wisdom to younger generations.

SOURCE: ADAPTED FROM COON, MITTERER & MARTINI, 2019; HTTP://FACULTYWEB.CORTLAND.EDU/ANDERSMD/ERIK/SUM.HTML

but were the results of interactions and relations with others. This will ultimately affect the view the child has of themselves, because a sense of self emerges as a result of interactions with others. Relationships with others during infancy, childhood and early adolescence are characterised by significant social relationships that will impact on the young person's developing sense of self (Cervone & Pervin, 2013).

Relevance of psychodynamic orientation to mental health nursing practice

Understanding Freud's ideas can help mental health nurses understand how the human psyche, especially the unconscious part of the human mind, impacts on everyday behaviour. Freud's theories also demonstrate how events in a person's childhood may influence their personality, even if they are not consciously aware of this. Understanding the role of defence mechanisms as the ego's way of managing internal conflict can provide mental health nurses with a means to understanding consumers' reactions to health problems they are experiencing. Examples of such reactions include anxiety and anger.

Anxiety, for instance, can be thought of as the consequence of the ego being unable to cope with the demands of the id and superego (Rana & Upton, 2013). As such, anxiety represents ego dysfunction.

Defence mechanisms provide a good description of behaviours that can be observed in Freud's work, which also highlighted the importance of childhood experiences in personality development. Erikson's stages of development provide a useful framework to understand people's responses to health events at different points in their lives. This enables collaborative strategies to be developed that are developmentally relevant to the individual (Halter, 2014).

Critique of the psychodynamic orientation

Various criticisms have been made about Freud's theories. A number of concepts are seen to be poorly defined and hard to measure, and therefore lacking in scientific rigour. The role of the environment also does not feature in his theories. Unlike humanistic theories, Freud's ideas do not account for personal choice or free will. Instead, they position a person as a passive responder to forces outside their control.

CASE **STUDY**

DEFENCE MECHANISMS IN PRACTICE

Samantha is a 46-year-old woman, married and with two school-age children. She has been married for 20 years to Jeff, who works in information technology. Three months ago Jeff was retrenched from his position with a large multinational computer company. Samantha, who has not worked full-time since her children were born, has been unable to increase her hours of employment at the local university due to budget restrictions. While they have a small amount of savings, she and Jeff are concerned about their capacity to meet mortgage repayments, school fees as well as daily living expenses for more than the next few months. One day in the shower, Samantha notices a lump in her right breast. She tells Jeff, who

says she must have it checked out. Samantha insists that there is nothing to worry about as there is no history of breast cancer in her family and she is too young to have such a condition. She refuses to get a mammogram and instead focuses on Jeff's search for work and looking for additional work herself.

Questions

1   What defence mechanism is Samantha using?
2   In what way could this defence mechanism be useful for Samantha at this time in her life?
3   What are the possible negative outcomes of continued use of this defence mechanism by Samantha?

THE BEHAVIOURAL/SOCIAL COGNITIVE ORIENTATION

Behaviourists are interested in how people learn. The **behavioural orientation** argues that a person's behaviour can be objectively observed and studied and that personality is determined by prior learning. This is distinctly different from the psychodynamic orientation, where the emphasis is on exploring the unconscious processes occurring in a person's mind. The behaviourist orientation stresses the importance of the environment in shaping behaviour. The key term in the behaviourist orientation is *conditioning*. Conditioning occurs in two ways. The first of these is the concept of **classical conditioning** developed by Russian physiologist Ivan Pavlov, who showed how animals could be made to respond to a stimulus when it was paired with an event that had previously produced the response.

The second type of conditioning is known as **operant conditioning**. Depending on the type of reinforcement a person receives, behaviours may be more, or less, likely to be repeated. It can be **positive reinforcement** or **negative reinforcement** – either form makes a certain behaviour more likely (Weiten, 2011). The behaviourist approach argues that conditioning allows behaviour to be changed (Coon & Mitterer, 2012).

Ivan Pavlov

Pavlov (1849–1936) was interested in the effect of the relationship between a stimulus and the response it produced. Pavlov discovered that dogs could learn to salivate (respond) to a non-food stimulus (bell or light) if the stimulus was simultaneously presented with food. This work led to the process of classical conditioning. Pavlov asked why the dogs salivated when there was no food present, but only the laboratory assistants (**Figure 2.3**). The four essential features of classical conditioning, as outlined in **Table 2.4**, are:

1   **unconditioned stimulus**
2   neutral stimulus
3   conditioning process
4   **conditioned response**.

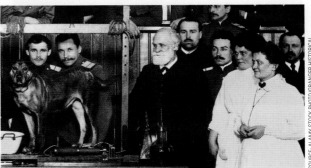

SOURCE: ALAMY STOCK PHOTO/GRANGER HISTORICAL PICTURE ARCHIVE

FIGURE 2.3
Pavlov's classical conditioning theory

TABLE 2.4
The essential features of classical conditioning

ESSENTIAL FEATURES OF CLASSICAL CONDITIONING	EXPLANATION	EXAMPLE
Unconditioned stimulus	A stimulus that produces an instinctive response. No learning is required	Unconditioned stimulus (food) and response (salivation) is instinctive and no learning is required
Neutral stimulus	A stimulus that does not cause an **unconditioned response**	Neutral stimulus (bell) that does not evoke salivation
Conditioning process	The unconditioned response becomes conditioned to the neutral stimulus (which is now referred to as the conditioned stimulus)	Conditioning process pairing neutral stimulus (bell) with unconditioned stimulus (food)
Conditioned response	The unconditioned response becomes conditioned to the neutral stimulus (which is now referred to as the conditioned stimulus)	**Conditioned stimulus** (neutral stimulus – bell) presented after conditioning process, which evoked a conditioned response (salivation) (Weiten, 2011).

John Watson (1878–1958; **Figure 2.4**) believed that to understand human behaviour it was necessary to understand how people learn. Building on the work of Pavlov, Watson argued that people are conditioned to respond to an event in more or less predictable ways (Bernstein et al., 2018; Burger, 2011). Maladaptive responses to events are viewed as the result of 'faulty conditioning'. In Watson's view, reconditioning was necessary to change these maladaptive responses.

Watson's 'Little Albert' experiment is a well-known example of classical conditioning and shows how condition responses are learned (Sigelman, Rider & De George-Walker, 2016). In this experiment, Watson elicited a fear of white rats in an 11-month-old infant, Albert. He achieved this by first eliciting a fear response (unconditioned response) from Albert whenever he made a loud noise (the unconditioned stimulus). He then introduced a white rat (conditioned stimulus) to Albert and whenever he did this he paired it with the loud noise. After several pairings, Albert displayed a fear response to the white rat in the absence of any loud noise (conditioned response).

SOURCE: CORBIS VIA GETTY IMAGES/HERITAGE IMAGE PARTNERSHIP LTD

FIGURE 2.4
J.B. Watson

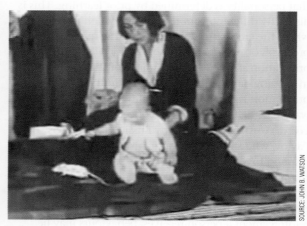

SOURCE: JOHN B. WATSON

FIGURE 2.5
Little Albert's classical condition experiment by J.B. Watson

B.F. Skinner

Developing his ideas from the work of Edward Thorndyke, B.F. Skinner (1904–90) believed that people do have such a thing as a mind (this was in direct contrast to Watson's position), but that it is simply more productive to study observable behaviour than internal mental events. Skinner's work was premised on the idea that the best way to understand human behaviour is to look at the causes of an action and its consequences. He called this approach *operant* *conditioning* (also known as instrumental conditioning), which involved the process of increasing or decreasing the likelihood that an individual will produce an active behaviour (an operant) as a result of interacting with the environment. Skinner's idea of reinforcement is central to operant conditioning. Reinforcement occurs when a stimulus increases the probability of a particular response that occurs in response to it (Upton, 2012). The process of reinforcement can be seen in **Figure 2.6**.

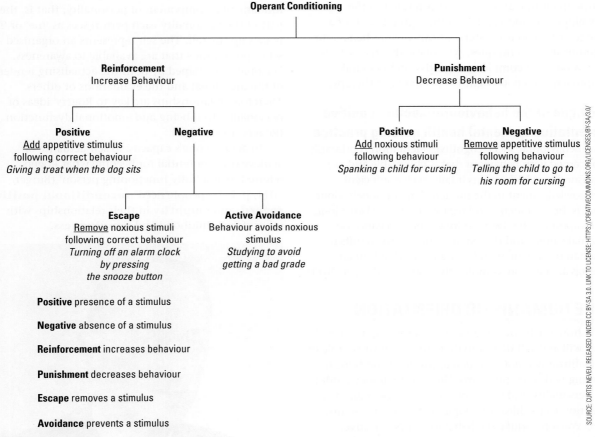

FIGURE 2.6
Operant conditioning and types of reinforcers

Albert Bandura

In contrast to the behaviourist position, which argues that internal events merely act as a go-between environment and behaviour, the *social cognitive orientation* posited that learning occurs by observing the behaviour of others, as well as by observing any environmental outcomes of the behaviour. Albert Bandura (1925–) argued that personality development occurred as a result of the individual's interaction within the environment and the individual's perception and thinking. **Self-efficacy** is the key to successful learning in Bandura's terms and is defined as the individual's belief that they can achieve a certain goal or master a particular situation (Corey, 2013). Bandura emphasised observational learning and modelling and coined the phrase '**reciprocal determinism**'.

Relevance of the behavioural/social cognitive orientation to mental health nursing practice

If you have tried to give up smoking and rewarded yourself with a treat for each day that you did not smoke, been given extra pocket money because you did an additional household task without being asked, or seen a parent in the supermarket ignore their child's crying for a sweet at the check-out, then you have used and/or seen others using principles of operant conditioning. In the context of mental health practice, operant conditioning has a number of applications; for example, it can be a way of understanding the development of phobias.

If a person finds themselves experiencing increasing anxiety when confronted with a particular object (e.g. a bird), any intervention that removes the object and leads to a reduction in anxiety will be more likely to be repeated if the individual is faced with the same situation again. Because of its emphasis on observation, the clear evidence for the behaviourist/social cognitive approach is provided through empirical research. This has led to the development and validation through research of a range of therapeutic interventions such as behaviour modification techniques, systematic desensitisation and a range of combined cognitive–behavioural approaches such as cognitive behavioural therapy.

Critique of the behavioural/social cognitive orientation to mental health nursing practice

The behavioural/social cognitive orientation is primarily concerned with behaviour that is observable and measurable, which means it fails to give sufficient acknowledgement to the human element of behaviour; that is, how thoughts and feelings influence behaviour. This approach has been critiqued for its reliance on animal studies and the extrapolation of the results to human behaviour, with the argument that human beings are far more complex than animals (Burger, 2011).

THE HUMANISTIC ORIENTATION

The humanistic perspective stresses the importance of free will and self-determination and the positive role of life-affirming emotions such as joy, love and hope in coping with life's problems. Humanistic understandings of personality and behaviour were seen by many as a reaction to the ideas of people such as Freud, Skinner and Watson. Unlike the behaviourist perspective, which was seen as too mechanistic and viewed people as having only a passive role in their development, and the psychodynamic approach that viewed people as victims of the unconscious, the humanistic perspective of personality and behaviour argues that people possess an innate capacity to develop and grow. The humanistic perspective is a more optimistic and person-oriented view, where a person cannot be reduced into component parts. Rather, humanistic theories look at people in a holistic sense and see people as unique in their humanness. Burger (2011) outlines four elements that are considered central to the humanistic orientation:

1 personal responsibility
2 being focused on the here and now
3 the concept of the phenomenology of a person
4 an emphasis on personal growth.

Carl Rogers

Perhaps one of the best-known exponents of the humanistic orientation is Carl Rogers (1902–87; **Figure 2.7**). Rogers' theory embodies the tenet of hope and an optimistic view of people. Central to his ideas was the belief that each person has the innate capacity to enjoy healthy relationships and positive creative growth. He referred to this as the 'actualising tendency' of people (Bernstein, Penner, Clarke-Stewart & Roy, 2013). In his theory of personality, Rogers identified the idea of **self-concept** (or self) as the fundamental component of personality; that is, the part of the personality each person sees as 'me' or 'I' makes up the self. The self represents an organised set of perceptions that are available to awareness. Personality is shaped by both the actualising tendency of the individual and the evaluations of others. Therefore, relationships are key to Rogers' ideas of personality, well-being and emotional dysfunction (Rogers, 1951, 1961).

To achieve one's capacity to self-actualise or achieve one's potential (or become what Rogers referred to as a 'fully functioning person' (Burger, 2011, p. 279), people need **unconditional positive regard**, and **empathy** in their relationships with others from childhood and **genuineness**.

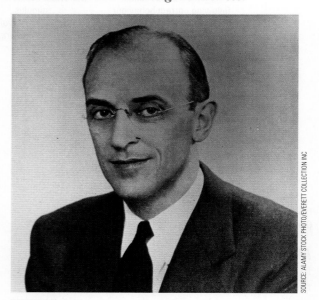

SOURCE: ALAMY STOCK PHOTO/EVERETT COLLECTION INC

FIGURE 2.7
Carl Rogers

Abraham Maslow

Abraham Maslow (1908–70) is another central figure in the development of the humanistic orientation. His research focused on 'self-actualising people' (Corey, 2013, p. 177). Maslow (1954, 1970) argued that a self-actualising person was different from someone who would be referred to as a 'normal person'. For Maslow, a self-actualising person was someone who possessed self-awareness, basic honesty, caring, and the ability to trust and be autonomous. Maslow described a range of other characteristics of a self-actualising person, including the capacity to welcome uncertainty in their lives, self-acceptance and acceptance of others not to live their lives according to the expectations of others, and possessing a sense of humour (Corey, 2013).

Maslow also proposed the concept of a **hierarchy of needs** through which people are motivated to fulfil basic needs before moving on to other needs. He believed that humans have an innate drive towards personal growth and strive for self-actualisation, which is the need to fulfil one's potential. In Maslow's view, this hierarchy of needs is systematic and higher needs will not be aroused until lower-order needs are fulfilled. A person with a healthy personality is self-actualised and pursues continuous personal growth (Corey, 2013; Weiten, 2011). Maslow's hierarchy of needs is represented in **Figure 2.8**.

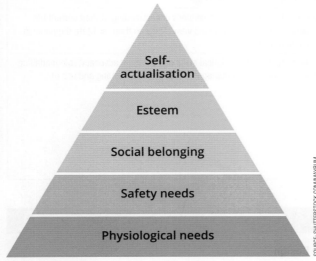

FIGURE 2.8
Maslow's hierarchy of needs

Relevance of the humanistic-orientation to mental health nursing practice

Rogers' ideas about the importance of the therapeutic relationship for successful counselling has resonated within mental health nursing education, practice and research for many years. Concepts such as unconditional positive regard and empathy are central to a person-centred focus of practice. Debate ensues regarding how mental health nurses should practise and whether it is possible to attempt to connect with and understand another person's world of which they may have no experience. However, to deny the importance of seeing the humanness of all people fails to acknowledge the inherent capacity of people to move forward in positive and productive ways.

Critique of the humanistic orientation

One of the main critiques of the humanistic orientation is the lack of scientific evidence for the concept of free will, a core concept of the approach (Burger, 2011). It is claimed that it is not possible to scientifically study free will. However, this argument implies that there is only one valid approach to studying human behaviour. Cervone and Pervin (2013) note that there are a variety of ways in which knowledge can be gained about human behaviour, of which humanistic views such as Rogers' is one. As you will read in Chapter 6, there are other ways in which to explore questions regarding human behaviour. A second criticism of the humanistic orientation is that because of its optimistic view of human nature, many of its ideas are over-simplistic and even naïve, and such ideas do not address the reality of emotional ill health, illness and antisocial behaviour.

THE USE OF PSYCHOLOGICAL AND SOCIOLOGICAL THEORIES OF PERSONALITY IN MENTAL HEALTH NURSING PRACTICE

In the preceding sections we have considered just a few of the major theoretical perspectives within psychology. Various nursing theorists have drawn from both psychology and sociology in order to understand human behaviour and how this influences the role of the mental health nurse.

Hildegard Peplau

While Florence Nightingale was the first nurse to document her ideas regarding health, illness and the role of nurses in health care generally, Hildegard Peplau (1909–99) was the first nurse to look specifically at the discipline of mental health nursing and is consequently viewed by many as the mother of mental health nursing. She was also the first nurse to draw on theories from other disciplines such as psychology; in particular, her work drew from the ideas of Harry Stack Sullivan and Abraham Maslow. Viewing mental health nursing as an essential therapeutic and interpersonal process, Peplau (1962) believed that the nurse–consumer relationship was the crux of mental health nursing. Through this relationship, the nurse uses themselves as the therapeutic instrument; that is, the nurse engages with consumers through a variety of psychosocial interventions to facilitate personal growth on the part of the consumer. This concept moved the idea of nursing practice from one of 'doing things' to people, to one of being with them. This changes the focus of working with a consumer from a passive relationship on their part to an active

SECTION 1

partnership and collaboration. Peplau (1962) also proposed that the therapeutic relationship passed through a number of phases, which evolved from the initial contact through to discharge. Peplau identified these phases as orientation, identification, exploitation and resolution (Peplau, 1991). In order to maximise their work with consumers, Peplau (1962) proposed that mental health nurses assume a variety of roles at different times, in response to the emerging needs of the consumer. These roles are outlined in **Table 2.5**.

TABLE 2.5
Peplau's nursing roles

PRIMARY ROLES	FEATURES OF EACH ROLE
Stranger role	Offering the consumer the same acceptance and courtesy that the nurse would to any stranger. The aim is to establish a safe interpersonal climate and build trust. The nurse must withhold any judgement, as when meeting as strangers both consumer and nurse are unknown to each other. This holds true even when the nurse has worked with a consumer previously. In the context of the current interpersonal context, they are again strangers
Resource role	Providing specific information (usually health related) that assists the consumer in their understanding of a particular issue.
Teacher role	Imparting information and using strategies to facilitate a consumer's learning. This can be either a formal or informal process.
Leader role	The mental health nurse assists the consumer to take up maximum responsibility for meeting their treatment goals in a mutually satisfying way.
Surrogate role	Serving as a substitute for another such as a parent or a sibling.
Counsellor role	The nurse uses the interpersonal process to facilitate the consumer's understanding of their current life circumstances and integrate this understanding into their world view. This can then facilitate the nurse in helping the consumer to make positive health choices.
Other roles, including: • technical expert • consultant • health teacher • observer/recorder • socialising agent • manager of the environment • mediator • researcher.	These roles incorporate activities related to education, clinical skills and practice, advocacy, role modelling educative, clinical skills and practice, advocacy, milieu management to promote healing and use of evidence to promote best practice.

SOURCE: HTTP://NURSESLABS.COM/HILDEGARD-PEPLAUS-INTERPERSONAL-RELATIONS-THEORY/

EVIDENCE-BASED PRACTICE

Applying Peplau's theory to mental health nursing practice

Title of study
Utilising Peplau's interpersonal approach to facilitate medication self-management for psychiatric patients

Authors
Judith M. Hochberger and Brenda Lingham

Background
Mental health nurses have a key role in promoting medication self-management as medication non-adherence can have a major impact on consumer well-being, treatment and outcomes. While many strategies have been identified to promote consumers self-managing medications, there is a lack of conceptual and evidence-based practice to support this. This discussion paper explored utilising Peplau's interpersonal approach to promote consumer adherence and medication usage, including self-administration of psychotropic medications.

Design
A critical literature review incorporating exploration of a critique of the nurse's role in promoting self-management of medication utilising Peplau's interpersonal theory with a recovery-oriented model of mental health nursing practice was undertaken.

Conclusions
Peplau's interpersonal theory provides a way for mental health nurses to integrate interpersonal communication skills and education to promote best outcomes with consumers in relation to medication self-management.

Implications
Mental health nurses must be encouraged to focus on how an effective therapeutic relationship contributes to consumer health outcomes.

SOURCE: HOCHBERGER, J.M. & LINGHAM, B. (2017). UTILIZING PEPLAU'S INTERPERSONAL APPROACH TO FACILITATE MEDICATION SELF-MANAGEMENT FOR PSYCHIATRIC PATIENTS. *ARCHIVES OF PSYCHIATRIC NURSING*, 31(1), 122–4. DOI:HTTPS://DOI.ORG/10.1016/J.APNU.2016.08.006

Phil Barker

Based on substantive clinical research, Phil Barker together with Poppy Buchanan Barker and others developed a second conceptual framework that describes the intended role of the mental health nurse. This model is known as the Tidal Model (Barker, Reynolds & Stevenson, 1997; Barker, Jackson & Stevenson, 1999). The key principles of this interdisciplinary model are active collaboration, person-centred care plans, multidisciplinary work and narrative-based interventions. The model focuses on the individual's human response to their illness rather than finding a cure *per se*, and is therefore grounded in the concepts of individual empowerment and humanistic concepts of humanness. The Tidal Model argues that the core requirement of mental health nursing is the need for mental health nurses to have a high level of empathy in order to 'know' what consumers need at any given point in their illness. This represents a continual and reciprocal process of the mental health nurse and consumer getting to know and re-know each other as the relationship evolves and the needs of the consumer change. Mental health nurses achieve this by moving between three interrelated domains (Barker, Jackson & Stevenson, 1999), which refer to the degree and depth to which the mental health nurse engages with consumers. The Tidal Model recognises that mental illness is a complex phenomenon and the idea of recovery is closely aligned with caring, as opposed to curing. This approach conceptualises the individual as living with a mental health condition and therefore managing symptoms as part of their life. Health is not seen in terms of merely the absence of symptoms, but as living a positive life in the presence of symptoms. Recovery is developing an identity that encompasses all parts of an individual's experience of wellness and illness (Helm, 2003) and involves metaphorically reducing the 'dis' from disease. Recovery is discussed in greater detail in Chapter 21.

RELEVANCE OF PSYCHOLOGICAL AND/OR NURSING THEORIES TO NURSING PRACTICE

Mental health nursing practice is founded on evidence from a range of sources. In this chapter, you have been briefly introduced to some of the major ideas from psychology and nursing that consider human behaviour and the factors that impact on it. The different ideas can complement and contradict each other. They can also reflect a very Westernised view of people and human behaviour.

A critique of these theories has been provided in order for you to reflect on how you might see these ideas applied to practice and what might be the benefits and issues of the various approaches. One theoretical perspective is not necessarily more appropriate than any other perspective. All the theories introduced in this chapter help nurses to understand the range of factors that can impact on a person's health and well-being. Rather than limiting practice to the choice of one theoretical view, this allows mental health nurses to integrate their understanding.

REFLECTION ON LEARNING FROM PRACTICE

As you have explored in this chapter, there are a number of theoretical frameworks that underpin mental health nursing practice. The type of role a mental health nurse may take on when a person is first admitted to an acute mental health facility may incorporate the stranger, surrogate and clinical practice role.

A mental health nurse working within a community-based setting may incorporate a more distinct counselling and/or educative role. But it is essential to remember that the mental health nurse will incorporate any number or combination of roles into the therapeutic role, based on the individual needs of the person.

Listening to the stories of people and understanding their unique, human response to their illness experience is the beginning of the healing journey.

Theoretical perspectives such as psychoanalytic theories can help the mental health nurse understand responses such as anxiety. Carl Rogers' ideas help the mental health nurse to understand and work with consumers to promote hope and support a person's capacity to build meaningful connections and live a meaningful life.

CHAPTER RESOURCES

SUMMARY

- The terms health, mental health, human behaviour and personality are broadly defined terms that have encompassed different views across time, cultures and understandings of people's place in the world.
- Biomedical theories of personality and human behaviours focus on the clustering of signs and symptoms resulting from an imbalance of physiological processes.
- The core assumption of the psychodynamic orientation is that abnormal behaviour reflects unconscious conflicts within the person.
- The behavioural orientation argues that a person's behaviour can be objectively observed and studied, and that personality is determined by prior learning. This is in contrast to the social cognitive orientation, which posited that learning occurs by observing the behaviour of others, as well as by observing any environmental outcomes of the behaviour.

- The humanistic perspective stresses the importance of free will and self-determination and the positive role of life-affirming emotions such as joy, love and hope in coping with life's problems. Humanistic understandings of personality and behaviour were seen by many as a reaction to psychodynamic and behavioural/social-cognitive theories.
- A variety of nursing theorists have drawn from both psychology and sociology in order to understand human behaviour and how this influences the role of the mental health nurse. Key nursing theorists who have contributed to mental health nursing practice are Hildegard Peplau and Phil Barker.
- Mental health nurses are able to use a variety of theoretical perspectives to inform their practice. This creates opportunities for individualised, recovery-oriented practice that demonstrates collaboration and partnership with consumers.

REVIEW QUESTIONS

1 What are defence mechanisms?
2 How does Maslow describe his theory of human needs?
3 How does Erikson describe his theory of human development?
4 In Pavlov's original work with dogs, the bell was the:
   a Unconditioned stimulus
   b Unconditioned response
   c Conditioned stimulus
   d Conditioned response
5 Julie has decided to give up smoking. Each week she puts asides the money she would have spent on cigarettes into a separate account. After two months, Julie realises she has saved nearly $1000. As a result, she continues to put this amount of money away as a weekly deposit. In

12 months she has enough money saved for a holiday. Julie's behaviour is the result of:
   a Negative reinforcement
   b Extinction
   c Positive reinforcement
   d Punishment
6 The humanistic orientation to personality understands the individual in terms of:
   a How they learn
   b The unconscious
   c Neurochemical changes in the brain
   d Self-concept
7 Discuss the following statement: Empathy is the primary ingredient for any helping relationship.

CRITICAL THINKING

1 What factors would a mental health nurse take into account when considering which theoretical perspective might help them to understand a consumer's behaviour?
2 Jennifer has been receiving chemotherapy as part of her breast cancer treatment. The nurse notes that when her husband attends the appointment with her there is very little conversation between them. Whenever Ivan tries to speak with Jennifer she turns her head and will not look at him. The nurse asks Ivan privately if everything is okay between him and Jennifer. Ivan becomes visibly distressed and explains that Jennifer refuses to talk about the cancer diagnosis and treatment.

They are sleeping in separate rooms and she will not let him see her undressed. 'I just want to be there for her… but she's locking me out', Ivan states. 'I have no-one I can speak to.' Using a psychodynamic perspective, how could the nurse understand Jennifer's current behaviour?
3 Are the factors contributing to mental health as described by Frisch and Frisch (2006) on page 17 still relevant in 2021?
4 Using Erikson's theory, identify what factors impact on a person's development over the course of their life.
5 How can the mental health nurse apply Bandura's concept of self-efficacy to support consumers in medication self-management?

USEFUL WEBSITES

- Approaches to Psychology – the humanistic approach: https://www.ryerson.ca/~glassman/humanist.html
- Australian Psychological Society: https://www.psychology.org.au

- Hildegard Peplau's interpersonal relations theory: https://nurseslabs.com/hildegard-peplaus-interpersonal-relations-theory

REFLECT ON THIS

Experiences of mental health during COVID-19

What is mental health and how have people experienced mental health during the COVID-19 pandemic? In this chapter, you have explored various theories that consider how people understand health and health behaviour choices. The COVID-19 pandemic has brought many challenges to peoples' mental health and well-being. Listen to the following podcast from the Black Dog Institute: https://www.blackdoginstitute.org.au/education-services/podcasts/being-well-podcast

In this podcast, you will hear from three people as they describe their experiences during the pandemic and the ways in which they have managed their mental health.

1   Do any of their points resonate with you?

2   What have you learned about the ways in which they define their mental health and how they have gone about managing their well-being during this time?

3   How can you incorporate these ideas into your own definition of mental health? As a nurse, how might your definition of mental health impact on your practice?

Theories of personality provide explanations for how people understand health and the subsequent impact on their health and health behaviour.

Read the article by Galderisi et al. (2015), who argue for a new definition of mental health that is broader and more inclusive than that proposed by the WHO. What aspects of the podcast link to these ideas? Note some examples and reflect on how they impact on your own definition of mental health.

REFERENCES

Barker, P., Jackson, S. & Stevenson, C. (1999). The need for psychiatric nursing: Towards a multidimensional theory of caring. *Nursing Inquiry*, 6, 103–11.

Barker, P.J., Reynolds, W. & Stevenson, C. (1997). The human science basis of psychiatric nursing: Theory and practice. *Journal of Advanced Nursing*, 25(4), 660–7.

Barkway, P. (2013). *Psychology for Health Professionals* (2nd edn). Marrickville: Elsevier.

Bernstein, D.A., Pooley, J.A., Cohen, L., Gouldthorp, B., Provost, S.C. & Cranney, J. (2018). *Psychology* (2nd Australian and New Zealand edn). South Melbourne: Cengage Learning.

Burger, J.M. (2011). *Personality*. Boston, MA: Wadsworth, Cengage Learning.

Cervone, D. & Pervin, L. (2013). *Personality: Theory and Research* (12th edn), Hoboken, NJ: Wiley.

Coon, D. & Mitterer, J.O. (2012). *Psychology: Modules for Active Learning* (12th edn). Belmont, CA: Wadsworth, Cengage Learning.

Coon, D., Mitterer, J. & Martini, T. (2019). *Introduction to Psychology: Gateways to Mind and Behavior* (15th edn). Boston, MA: Cengage Learning.

Corey, G. (2013). *Theory and Practice of Counselling and Psychotherapy* (9th edn). Boston, MA: Brooks/Cole, Cengage Learning.

Corey, G. (2017). *Theory and Practice of Counselling and Psychotherapy* (10th edn). South Melbourne: Cengage Learning.

Galderisi, S., Heinz, A., Kastrup, M., Beezhold, J. & Sartorius, N. (2015). Toward a new definition of mental health. *World Psychiatry*, 14(2), 231–3. doi: 10.1002/wps.20231

Forchuk, C. (1994). The orientation phase of the nurse–client relationship: Testing Peplau's theory. *Journal of Advanced Nursing*, 20(3), 532–7.

Frisch, N.C. & Frisch, L.E. (2006). *Psychiatric Mental Health Nursing* (3rd edn). Clifton Park, NY: Thomson/Delmar Learning.

Halter, M.J. (2014). *Varcarolis' Foundations of Psychiatric Mental Health Nursing. A Clinical Approach* (7th edn). St Louis, MI: Elsevier Saunders.

Helm, A. (2009). Recovery and reclamation: A pilgrimage in understanding who and what we are. In P. Barker (ed.), *Psychiatric and Mental Health Nursing. The Craft of Caring* (2nd edn, pp. 58–65). London: Hodder Arnold.

Hochberger, J.M. & Lingham, B. (2017). Utilizing Peplau's interpersonal approach to facilitate medication self-management for psychiatric patients. *Archives of Psychiatric Nursing*, 31(1), 122–4. doi:https://doi.org/10.1016/j.apnu.2016.08.006

Hoffnung, M., Hoffnung, R.J., Seifert, K.L., Burton Smith, R., Hine, A., Ward, L. & Pause, C. (2013). *Lifespan Development. A Chronological Approach* (2nd Australasian edn). Milton: John Wiley and Sons.

Hogan, A.J. (2019). Social and medical models of disability and mental health: Evolution and renewal. CMAJ, 7 January, 191:E16-8. doi: 10.1503/cmaj.181008

Maslow, A. (1954). *Motivation and Personality*. New York: Harper and Row.

Maslow, A. (1970). *Motivation and Personality* (2nd edn). New York: Harper and Row.

McLeod, S.A. (2013). Erik Erikson. Retrieved from http://www.simplypsychology.org/Erik-Erikson.html

Norman, I. & Ryrie, I. (2009). The art and science of mental health nursing: Reconciliation of two traditions in the cause of public health. *International Journal of Nursing Studies*, 46(12), 1537–40.

Nye, R.A. (2003). The evolution of the concept of medicalization in the late twentieth century. *Journal of the History of Behavioral Sciences*, 32(2), 115–29.

Peplau, H.E. (1962). Interpersonal techniques: The crux of psychiatric nursing. *American Journal of Nursing*, 62(6), 50–4.

Peplau, H.E. (1991). *Interpersonal Relations in Nursing: A Conceptual Frame of Reference for Psychodynamic Nursing*. New York: Springer Publishing Company.

Pickersgill, M.D. (2014). Debating DSM-5: Diagnosis and the sociology of critique. *Journal of Medical Ethics*, 40(8), 521–25. https://doi.org/10.1136/medethics-2013-101762

Rana, D. & Upton, D. (2013). *Psychology for Nurses*. London: Routledge.

Rogers, C. (1951). *Client-Centered Therapy*. Boston, MA: Houghton Mifflin.

Rogers, C. (1961). *On Becoming a Person. A Therapist's View of Psychotherapy*. Boston, MA: Houghton Mifflin.

Sigelman, C.K., Rider, E.A. & De George-Walker, L. (2016). *Life Span Human Development*, 2nd Australian and New Zealand edn. South Melbourne: Cengage Learning Australia.

Upton, D. (2012). *Introducing Psychology for Nurses and Healthcare Professionals*. Harlow: Pearson.

Weiten, W. (2011). *Psychology Themes & Variations (*8th edn). Las Vegas, NV: Wadsworth Cengage Learning.

World Health Organization. (WHO). (1946). Preamble to the Constitution of the World Health Organization as adopted by the International Health Conference, New York, 19–22 June, 1946; signed 22 July 1946 by the representatives of 61 States (Official Records of the World Health Organization, no. 2, p. 100) and entered into force on 7 April 1948.

CHAPTER 3

ETHICS, LAW AND MENTAL HEALTH NURSING PRACTICE

Terry Froggatt and Alison Hansen

LEARNING OUTCOMES

Upon completion of this chapter, you should be able to:

3.1 Understand the context of mental health legislation in Australia

3.2 Understand the facilitation of care and treatment of people with a mental health condition across different legislative jurisdictions

3.3 Consider the significance of recent developments in the legislative focus on recovery

3.4 Identify the ethical frameworks of practice for nurses and identify potential dilemmas and tensions

3.5 Understand and appreciate compulsory care and treatment from a consumer perspective

LEARNING FROM PRACTICE

The first time I was admitted to a mental health unit, I remember feeling terrified and alone. It was something I hadn't experienced before and I had no idea what was happening.

I had a previous history of depression and had been receiving treatment in the community by my GP. I stopped taking my medication because I was putting on weight. This caused me to spiral out of control. I stayed in bed all day, didn't eat and didn't drink. All I wanted to do was sleep. Then sleep wasn't enough. I felt empty and wanted to die. When I was 21, I was admitted to hospital as a compulsory patient after I attempted to take my own life.

I was transferred from the emergency department to the mental health unit. I wasn't told how long I would be there or that I wasn't allowed to leave. All I remember being told was that I was a risk to myself and therefore required immediate treatment.

I felt like I had lost control of my life and had no choices. I was told when I had to get up, when to eat and when I had to go to bed. When I refused the medication they tried to give me, they (the nurses) told me I had to have it and that I wasn't allowed to refuse. I still wanted to die and it felt like this was the only thing I had control over.

After four weeks of being in hospital, I still had thoughts of suicide. The doctors said I was showing little response to medication and suggested electroconvulsive therapy (ECT). I remember screaming when they told me this. I was even more terrified. I was told to calm down, and that this was now the best option for my recovery.

I received a course of six ECT treatments. I think at the third, I was starting to feel different…better. Although I can now say it helped…lifesaving, it was a scary experience. I was eventually discharged, but still on a community treatment order (CTO) and had to receive treatment in the community. If I stopped, I would be taken back to hospital. Over time, I have worked with my GP to find a medication that helps and doesn't have as many side effects. I still have thoughts of suicide, but I'm working through it.

Lydia, 28, consumer of mental health services

Describe the responsibilities of the mental health nurse in this scenario. Should legislation have the power to force treatment for people who are a risk to themselves? Should legislation take away the person's right to make their own decisions? How may the nurse support Lydia in this scenario?

INTRODUCTION

Historically, mental health care legislation was motivated by the aim of enforcing mandatory treatment, with a perception that individuals within the mental health care system were unable to make rational decisions themselves. This generated a system that, despite the very best of intentions, was often punitive and took away an individual's rights to make important decisions about their own health care. Over time, there has been increasing community demand for the 'consumer voice' within mental health care, and mental health legislation. In order to understand how the mental health care system operates in Australia, it is important to develop an understanding of the legal and ethical frameworks underpinning such practices. This chapter discusses contemporary mental health legislation, including the provision of compulsory care and treatment. You will note that some of the terminology around persons experiencing a mental health condition is varied. This is because most mental health legislation still uses the term 'patient'. In this chapter, we use 'patient', 'consumer' and 'person with a lived experience'.

CONTEXT OF MENTAL HEALTH LEGISLATION IN AUSTRALIA

The legislation that regulates the care of people with a mental health condition is enacted at the state and territory levels of government in Australia. Each state and territory has a Mental Health Act that applies to a specific jurisdiction. These Acts reflect society's expectations for governments to uphold the common rights and responsibilities of their citizens.

Ethics are a set of principles that provide the basis for moral and humane behaviour of individuals, organisations and governments. Ethics in health care are usually based on four bioethical constructs: autonomy, non-maleficence, beneficence and justice.

Although Mental Health Acts and ethical principles underpin the care of people with a mental health condition in Australia, there are other legal and policy mechanisms and standards that govern and regulate such important matters as: workplace health and safety, negligence, professional registration and practice, pharmaceuticals and complaints. This chapter will articulate these dimensions and implications for people with a mental health condition.

State and territory–Commonwealth legislative framework

The Australian legal system originates in the British legal system and is based on other Commonwealth countries – for example, New Zealand, Canada and the United Kingdom – and is sometimes referred to as 'common law' (MHCC, 2015a). The two sources of law in Australia are legislative law and common (or judge-made) law. Legislative law describes legislation that is passed by parliaments at the state and federal levels. Common law describes laws that are a result of judicial decisions based on cases that have been brought before the courts.

There are a number of key features within the Australian legal system:

- separation of the institutions responsible for law making and interpretation (parliaments and the courts)
- adversarial process whereby evidence for a case is brought before the court by two parties (rather than inquisitorial)
- natural justice ensures court proceedings are conducted fairly and without prejudice
- the ability of judges to make law based on previous decisions of courts (doctrine of precedent), when a gap exists in current law
- the presumption of innocence whereby a person is considered innocent until proven guilty (Forrester & Griffiths, 2011).

The Australian Parliament has the responsibility for progressing law through parliament, which is referred to as a Bill. Once a Bill is passed, it becomes an Act of Parliament. Once an Act has been passed, it becomes part of Australian legislation.

Mental health legislation in Australia is enacted by governments at the state/territory level. The Mental Health Act in each state/territory jurisdiction is intended to balance consumer rights and the need for treatment, while recognising the important role played by the carers and family members of people with a mental health condition. The legislation is usually designed to enable a person with a mental health problem to receive treatment and make their own decisions about their treatment, as well as facilitate treatment and provide support for those without the capacity to make their own decision, and who require treatment for their own safety and the safety of others.

Consideration of a person's decision-making capacity

The common law respects the right that all adults must be presumed to have capacity. Contemporary mental health legislation now requires a mental health service to demonstrate that a consumer *does not* have capacity to make decisions. Older mental health acts, however, may still have wording which requires a *consumer* to prove that they have capacity. The onus varies between the service provider and the consumer in such legislation. It is important to note that capacity is not an absolute, and a consumer's capacity may vary from day to day, depending on their condition. Where capacity is contested at law, the **burden of proof** lies with the person asserting the incapacity (see, for example, *Masterman-Lister v Brutton & Co* [2003] 3 All ER 162, 169; *L v Human Rights and Equal Opportunity Commission* (2006) 233 ALR 432). **Mental capacity** is a multidimensional construct that is central to an individual's ability to make autonomous decisions. The legal meaning of 'capacity' and approaches to assessing capacity vary across jurisdictions. In Australia, there is no uniform standard for capacity, which has led to significant variations across jurisdictions. For example, in Victoria there are a number of standards, 'including that the person must be not able to make reasonable judgements or understand the nature and effect of a document' (*Guardianship and Administration Act 1986* (Vic.)) (ALRC, n.d.). In New South Wales, 'the standard is where a person is totally or partially incapable of managing his or her person' (*Guardianship Act 1987* (NSW)) (ALRC, n.d.). However, there are elements that are generally applied across all Mental Health Acts in order to determine a person's capacity to make a decision. These are:

- ability to understand information related to the decision
- ability to retain information related to the decision
- ability to use and weigh the information to make the decision
- ability to communicate the decision (RANZCP, 2017).

In practice, registered nurses must seek to protect and advocate for the rights of people under their care. This may sometimes involve challenging the decisions made by others. The registered nurse is required to have a good working knowledge of the legislation relevant to their practice (Neilson, 2005). There are many situations that may be confronting for nurses and will require careful consideration of the legal position and ethical dimensions of providing care.

A **tort** is created by common law and describes legal wrongs committed by a person against another (ALRC, 2015). Tort law in Australia is the part of common law that deals with matters such as assault, battery, false imprisonment and negligence. This law provides for a remedy and provides compensation or damages.

Tort of assault

The tort of assault involves a person intentionally causing fear in another with unwanted contact. The threat does not need to involve physical contact, nor does it need to be an explicit threat (Forrester & Griffiths, 2011). For example, in a mental health setting it is an assault when a nurse threatens to place the person in seclusion if they do not comply with the nurse's direction. It is important to note that if the person believes they will be touched against their wishes and the person has not provided consent, the health professional can be at risk of assault. Consent is discussed further in this chapter.

Tort of battery

While assault involves the threat of physical contact, the tort of battery involves actual physical contact with another person without consent (Forrester & Griffiths, 2011). The physical contact needs to be intentional, and the person does not need to be aware that the physical contact occurred (e.g. the person was asleep) to be a battery.

Tort of false imprisonment

False imprisonment occurs when a person's freedom of movement has been totally restricted, with or without physical contact (Forrester & Griffiths, 2011). The person does not need to be aware that their freedom of movement has been restricted, and that false imprisonment has occurred. An example of this in health care is the use of heavy blankets placed across a consumer and tucked under the mattress to restrict the person's movement. It is important to note that the use of restrictive interventions could be an example of false imprisonment if it is done without consent and appropriate authorisation as outlined in the relevant Mental Health Act. Therefore, it is important that the mental health nurse understands the seriousness of false imprisonment and the issues and challenges associated with the use of restrictive interventions. This will be discussed further in this chapter.

Tort of negligence

Negligence is the civil action in which a patient sustains an injury as a result of an act or an omission to act, by a health professional or health care provider (Forrester & Griffiths, 2011). For negligence to be found to have occurred, the following four elements must be proven:

1 The patient was owed a duty of care (by the health professional).
2 The health professional breached or failed in their duty of care.
3 The breach or failure of the health professional's duty caused the patient's injury.
4 The patient's injury was foreseeable as a result of the health professional's action.

Due to their professional relationships with their patients, nurses would be seen to have a duty of care to patients, as does their employer (i.e. a hospital authority or health department). Standards of care for nurses are regulated by the Australian Health Practitioner Regulation Agency (AHPRA). Damage may be perceived as physical or psychological.

CASE STUDY

THE NURSE'S DUTY OF CARE

Peter is a new registered nurse in the dementia ward of the residential aged care facility where you work. A number of residents have said how 'grumpy' and 'rough' he is with them, but you have never seen him do anything untoward. This morning, Peter was showering George in room 12. You realised he had forgotten to take the towels with him, so you went to the room to give them to him. As you entered the room, the shower door was partially open, and you saw Peter punch George in the abdomen. Horrified, you retreated.

Questions

1   As a registered nurse, what is your duty of care towards George? What are your responsibilities as a registered nurse if you see something like this?
2   Consider the legislation you have read. Has Peter broken any laws?
3   Consider the Code of Conduct for Nurses in Australia. Discuss five points from the Code of Conduct where Peter's behaviour or actions contravene the code. You can download a copy of the code at http://www.nursingmidwiferyboard.gov.au

LEGISLATION FACILITATING CARE AND TREATMENT OF PEOPLE WITH A MENTAL HEALTH CONDITION

Mental health legislation has been scrutinised by mental health advocates and reformers over several decades. Seeking to balance individual freedoms with concerns for personal and societal safety and security is a constant challenge for communities, health professionals, legislators and governments in all states and territories. Based upon the principle of 'the least restrictive' laws and practices, the various state and territory Mental Health Acts prescribe and define: **voluntary treatment, involuntary treatment** and **detention** in a mental health facility, and **community treatment orders (CTOs)**. Mental health legislation typically provides for detention and treatment in hospital and for compulsory treatment in the community in the form of a CTO (O'Brien, 2014).

The Queensland *Mental Health Act 2016*, for example, articulates the powers, role and responsibilities of the authorised mental health practitioner in the assessment, admission and treatment of persons deemed to have a mental health condition. Similarly, the Northern Territory *Mental Health and Related Services Act 2016* provides for the care, treatment and protection of people with a mental health condition while at the same time protecting their civil rights. Interestingly, this legislation specifically defines a person who is considered to have a mental illness and exclusion criteria for those who do not. Too often a person is assumed to have a mental health condition as a precursor to an assessment, so it is important for the clinician to adopt a non-judgemental attitude rather than assume a person has a mental illness before a thorough and comprehensive assessment has been conducted.

Voluntary admission and treatment

A person can be admitted to hospital and receive treatment as a voluntary patient. A voluntary patient is free to leave the hospital or refuse treatment whenever they wish to do so.

Involuntary admission and treatment

A compulsory patient is a person who has been assessed by a mental health professional and put on a compulsory treatment order. They can be detained for a specified period and receive treatment against their wishes while they are in hospital; that is, involuntary admission and treatment. In Victoria, for example, treatment orders can only be made by the **Mental Health Tribunal** and only if a person meets defined criteria:

1   A person has a diagnosed mental illness.
2   Because the person has a mental illness, they are deemed to need immediate treatment to prevent:
    –   serious deterioration
    –   serious harm to themselves or other persons.
3   The person will receive immediate treatment.
4   There are no less restrictive means, reasonably available, for the person to get the treatment available.

Electroconvulsive therapy

The use of electroconvulsive therapy (ECT) can be controversial and is invasive. As a result, its use is regulated by Mental Health Acts in most Australian states and territories when used for a person receiving involuntary treatment (RANZCP, 2017). See also the discussion of ECT as a therapeutic treatment in Chapter 10.

ECT is a procedure performed under general anaesthetic and involves a small electric current being passed through the brain in order to induce a seizure. Treatment usually occurs several times a week, until a course of nine to 12 treatments has been reached, depending on the relevant state/territory criteria (RANZCP, 2017). It is most often used for people experiencing severe depression and those who are acutely suicidal. It can also be useful for people who cannot take medication due to side effects, or in those who may not be able to wait for a therapeutic response from medication (e.g. who pose a significant harm to themselves as a result of suicidal ideation, or who are experiencing catatonic depression and refusing to eat or drink (MHCC, 2015b).

Each Australian state and territory has different requirements for when ECT can used. Commonly, the Mental Health Acts state that at least two medical practitioners (one of whom must be a psychiatrist) must issue a certificate of opinion outlining the person's clinical condition, treatment history and alternative treatments (MHCC, 2015b). Where persons are unable to provide informed consent for ECT and the person's treating team want to proceed with the administration of ECT, an application for administration can be heard by the state or territory's relevant tribunal (RANZCP, 2017). For example, in Victoria the authorised psychiatrist must apply for approval from the Mental Health Tribunal. In this case, the Tribunal must be satisfied 1) that a person does not have capacity to give informed consent and 2) there is no less restrictive alternative treatment available.

The NSW *Mental Health Act 2007*, s. 89 states:

> Electro convulsive therapy may be administered only in the following circumstances:
>
> (a) to a person other than an involuntary patient or a person who is under the age of 16 years, if the person meets the requirements for informed consent to the treatment and medical certification set out in this Division,
>
> (b) to an involuntary patient or a person who is under the age of 16 years, after an ECT determination by the Tribunal at an ECT inquiry.

Some Acts make provision for emergency situations (i.e. life-threatening). The NT *Mental Health and Related Services Act 2016*, s. 66, for example, states:

> Electroconvulsive therapy may be performed on a person who is an involuntary patient where 2 authorised psychiatric practitioners are satisfied that it is immediately necessary:
>
> (a) to save the person's life; or
>
> (b) to prevent the person suffering serious mental or physical deterioration; or
>
> (c) to relieve severe distress.

The evidence base concerning the efficacy and safety of the use of ECT has been proven (Chakrabarti, Grover & Rajagopal, 2010). The effectiveness of ECT is high for those who have been found to be resistant to antidepressant medications, and has been noted to be unequalled by antidepressant medication and other treatments for depression (Rasmussen et al., 2007).

Although safe and effective, ECT is associated with several adverse side effects (Gregory-Roberts, Naismith, Cullen & Hickie, 2010), many of which are short term, and include headache, nausea and confusion (Andrade, Arumugham & Thirthalli, 2016). Amnesia has also been reported as a side effect; it has been suggested that there is no effect on long-term memory or intelligence, but memory loss has been reported as a significant problem for people who have received ECT treatment (Happell et al., 2008).

Despite the recorded benefits of ECT, its use continues to attract criticism, with much of the negative perceptions stemming from historical views portrayed in movies such as *One Flew Over the Cuckoo's Nest* (1975). As these historical perspectives can influence a person's view of ECT, it is important that the nurse is able to provide support and adequate information about the procedure. Nurses involved with ECT need to be able to provide consumers and their families with balanced information about the benefits and risks, and what can be expected both before and after the procedure (Cleary & Horsfall, 2014).

More generally, nurses need to provide care usual to that of any procedure where a person receives a general anaesthetic – for example, ensuring the person does not eat or drink prior to the procedure, maintaining physical observations as required and providing appropriate anaesthetic post-care.

Community treatment orders

Community treatment orders (CTOs) are used to provide compulsory treatment in the community. Most commonly, the person will have been in hospital under compulsory care, and the CTO is a condition of their discharge from the hospital. CTOs are considered by those who use them to provide for the least restrictive treatment, with the idea being that treatment in the community, even under legislation, is less restrictive than treatment in a hospital setting.

Seclusion and restraint

The use of restrictive interventions (seclusion and **restraint**) are used within mental health settings as a last resort, in order to prevent imminent or serious harm or injury to the consumer, or another person. Seclusion has been defined as the confinement of a person to an area, day or night, where it is not within the person's own control to leave (AIHW, 2018). A seclusion room has the windows and or doors locked from the *outside*, and as such, the person is unable to leave the room. Restraint has been defined as the physical or mechanical restriction of a person's freedom of movement (AIHW, 2018). Emotional restraint has also been recognised as occurring in the mental health care system and occurs when the person has been conditioned in a way that has resulted in a loss of confidence and fear associated with expressing their own views (Collins, 2008, cited in NMHCCF, 2009). Each state and territory Mental Health Act differs as to when seclusion and restraint can be used and for how long, who can authorise use, and who is to be notified when seclusion or restraint occurs (RANZCP, 2017).

The use of seclusion and restraint are justified on the legal basis of common-law; **duty of care** is owed to the patient, other patients, visitors and staff, in order to prevent imminent harm (MHCC, 2015b). The duty of care must be reasonable and proportionate in relation to the risks the person may pose to themselves or others (MHCC, 2015b).

Despite restrictive interventions being lawful, their use has raised a number of concerns regarding the rights of those who experience seclusion and/or restraint, as well as for clinicians who work within mental health settings. These concerns are not new, nor frivolous (see NSW Ministry of Health, 2017). In 1993, the Australian Human Rights Commission released its *Report of the National Inquiry into the Human Rights of People with Mental Illness* (the Burdekin Report), and made a number of recommendations on the use of seclusion as a last resort for treatment (Burdekin, 1993). This was followed by a number of other reports being released, highlighting the need to address the use of restrictive interventions and providing recommendations to ensure a national approach for reducing the use of seclusion and restraint, and reducing harm associated with their use. From 2007–09, the National Mental Health Seclusion and Restraint Project (known as the Beacon Project) aimed to reduce, and where possible eliminate, the use of seclusion (Melbourne Social Equity Unit, 2014. This project had some success; however, challenges remain and the impact of the project has not been sustained (NSW Ministry of Health, 2017).

All jurisdictions in Australia have continued to explore ways to reduce or in some instances eliminate the use of seclusion and restraint in mental health practice. The National Mental Health Commission (NMHC) has made significant progress in influencing the trajectory away from the use of seclusion and restraint. One of ten key recommendations made by the NMHC in 2012 was to 'reduce the use of involuntary practices and work to eliminate seclusion and restraint' (NMHC, 2012, p. 13). This remains a focus of mental health services globally,

as the negative impacts of seclusion and restraint are pronounced and their use has negative impacts on those who experience these restrictive interventions. The use of seclusion and restraint is controversial and potentially dangerous (Huckshorn, 2004) and has been described as a practice that contributes to avoidable harm (Newton et al., 2017). Seclusion and restraint are associated with both physical and psychological harm, not only to persons with mental illness, but also to staff (Duxbury, 2015, cited in NSW Ministry of Health, 2017). The literature suggests that patients largely perceive seclusion to be a negative event (Van Der Merwe et al., 2013). Consumers who experience seclusion often report feeling dehumanised, stripped of their autonomy, and lacking dignity and human rights (NSW Ministry of Health, 2017). The use of seclusion also impacts on carers and families. A carer described her daughter's experience of being secluded and restrained as a child and adolescent: 'The nightmares and trauma from these experiences continue to affect her every day, both mentally and physically' (NSW Ministry of Health, 2017, p. 22). In the past, clinicians have justified seclusion and restraint on the grounds that their use was therapeutic (NSW Ministry of Health, 2017; Van Der Merwe et al., 2013). However, there is now seen to be little benefit or therapeutic value for either the person or their treatment (Turner & Mooney, 2016). Mental health services, and clinicians who work within these services, are faced with ethical and practical challenges to safeguard the human rights of service users (Mayers, Keet, Winkler & Flisher, 2010). Many mental health services across Australia continue to actively reduce the use of seclusion by focusing on less restrictive ways to manage risk and reduce the risk of trauma associated with the use of restrictive interventions. For example, in New South Wales, health policy provides directives for use of seclusion and restraint. This policy has a focus on reducing, and where possible eliminating the use of seclusion and restraint and includes a number of principles to inform practice that focuses on the protection of human rights, safety for the person and staff and the involvement of the person's primary carer (MHCC, 2015b).

The Australian College of Mental Health Nurses (ACMHN) is involved in seclusion reduction and has developed a position statement to assist nurses in developing and maintaining best practice in this area. The position states that there is little credible research supporting the value of seclusion or restraint (ACMHN, 2016). On the other hand, research does exist that indicates there are very real alternatives to seclusion and restraint and that nurses must become familiar with best practice strategies and practices which reduce or eliminate their use.

Consent

Informed consent

Informed consent is a voluntary agreement with an action proposed by another. As a general rule, consent must be obtained from a person by a health professional prior to any treatment, procedure or intervention. Informed consent is defined by a number of elements that the patient needs to demonstrate. For consent to be valid, the following four elements must be considered:

1 Consent must be given freely and without coercion.
2 The consent provided must cover the procedure.
3 Consent must be informed (the health professional seeking consent must provide the person with relevant information).
4 The person must have the 'capacity' to consent (Forrester & Griffiths, 2011).

An adult said to have 'capacity' to consent must have met all four of these elements for their consent to be considered valid. At times, an adult may not have the capacity to consent – for example, when a person does not have the mental capacity, or is significantly affected by drugs or alcohol. Children are not able to provide consent for a treatment or procedure, and as a general rule a parent or legal guardian can provide consent. Legislation in Australia differs between jurisdictions as to the age when a person is considered to be a child or a young person, and at what age consent is valid at law (Forrester & Griffiths, 2011). Given the differences between states and territories in determining the age of consent in a young person, it is important too for nurses to consider local legislation when working with people under the age of 18 years. There are times where consent is not required (e.g. in an emergency or when treatment has been approved by a mental health tribunal).

CASE **STUDY**

ADMINISTRATION OF MEDICATIONS

Evan, who is 16 years old, has been admitted to a local mental health unit following an incident at his parents' home. Evan seemed convinced that there was someone in the ceiling listening to his thoughts, and whispering to him that he was 'under surveillance' and that he would shortly be arrested. Evan's parents had noticed a gradual deterioration in Evan's mental state over the past few months. They thought perhaps it was just a 'teenager thing' and that it would pass. They explained that Evan had been staying out late, avoiding his friends and when at home spent extended periods in his room. They had heard Evan speaking to someone when he was alone and his mobile phone was not with him.

Elisha is a nursing student on clinical placement from the local university's school of nursing. The nurse in charge of the unit has asked Elisha to give Evan some medication to 'settle him down'. Elisha has recently studied psychotropic medication administration and the Mental Health Act is one of her course subjects at the university. She feels 'out of her depth' with this request and wonders what she should do.

Questions

1 Would you encourage Elisha to just 'go ahead' and give the medication as requested?
2 Would you encourage Elisha to ask the nurse in charge some questions?
3 Would you ask Evan if he wished to take the medication and, if he refused, tell him that he could be made to take it even without his consent?
4 What is the legal position in this situation?

It is critically important for nurses to be aware of a person's legal status at all times. This may be determined by checking with the nurse in charge or examining the person's medical file. Coercion should not be used as a therapeutic strategy; understanding why, and explaining the benefits as well as the potential side effects of a proposed medication or treatment demonstrate a balanced approach that tends to improve the therapeutic relationship. Ultimately, however, a person who is detained under a treatment or community order may be forced to take medication against their will. It is important to consider the impacts of 'forcing' medication on a consumer, and how this relates to our understanding of trauma-informed care (discussed in Chapter 21). A consumer's reasons for medication refusal should not be trivialised, and the treating team needs to consider the impacts on the therapeutic relationship when forcing the issue.

Medication

Medication is widely used in the treatment of mental health conditions. Registered nurses are required to be competent and knowledgeable about medications and the regulations that govern their use.

A person who is admitted as a voluntary/ compulsory patient will often receive medication at the discretion of the treating team. The treating team will decide what medication will be prescribed, as well as the dose and frequency. This should be discussed with the person and the person's carer/s where appropriate. It is important that consent is sought from the person in relation to their treatment when possible. There are times when consent may be difficult to obtain (e.g. involuntary admission); however, we should always attempt to obtain consent. The person should still be fully informed about the medication that is being prescribed.

The role of the nurse concerning medication includes not only administration, but also documentation and monitoring of medication, as well as providing the person with information pertaining to their medication and providing support to manage their medication. When giving medication to an **involuntary patient**, the nurse may:

- administer medication as prescribed (e.g. oral administration by tablet, capsule, wafer or syrup, or by intramuscular administration)
- ensure prescribed medication is taken (reasonable force may be used where a person is resistive).

However, a nurse is not permitted to administer medication:

- in excess of the prescribed dose or that is inappropriate for a condition or diagnosis
- that does not comply with the relevant state or territory Mental Health Act.

Medication administration legislation is universal and covered by a plethora of laws, regulations, standards and guidelines. Nurses should be familiar with the regulations and standards that specifically pertain to their place of practice.

Sedation

Sedative medications may be used to assist a person's behaviour when they are a risk to themselves or to others (MHCC, 2015b), but are not used as a therapeutic treatment. The overuse of sedation can be referred to as chemical restraint. Definitions of chemical restraint are largely inconsistent across Australian states and territories, with only some Mental Health Acts clearly outlining a definition of use (RANZCP, 2017). Generally, the overuse of sedation as a chemical restraint is not supported within mental health services. Its use to control behaviour is controversial and has been described as being highly coercive and having significant effects on a person (Muir-Cochrane & Gerace, 2017).

Sedative medications may be a part of the treatment plan to manage symptoms of mental illness for some people. In some jurisdictions, where sedation is used as a part of a person's treatment plan, this is not considered chemical restraint (MHCC, 2015b). In such situations, the use of sedative medications must be justified, reasonable and the risk of associated harm considered (MHCC, 2015b). For many hospital services, the provision of certain types of sedative medicines are only permitted to be administered in certain areas of a hospital. For example, in some hospitals the sedative midazolam is only able to be

administered in an emergency department, where resuscitation equipment is readily available, and the person can be monitored for serious, adverse reactions.

Treatments that are prohibited

Under the NSW Mental Health Act, certain treatments are *not allowed* to be given to any patient in New South Wales. There are heavy civil penalties, including potentially disciplinary penalties, and criminal penalties related to the use of prohibited mental health treatments. Deep sleep therapy, insulin coma therapy and psychosurgery are prohibited under the NSW Act, for example. It is therefore important that nurses are aware of the mental health legislation relevant to their location.

MENTAL HEALTH CONDITIONS, OFFENDING AND THE LAW

Western society has overwhelmingly adopted the stigmatising belief that people with a mental health condition are dangerous, and that their behaviour poses a threat to others. The reality is, however, that people with a mental health condition are more likely to be *victims* of crime, rather than perpetrators. Despite this, in times of psychiatric crises, people with a mental health condition may be charged with a criminal offence. The legal system in Australia has provisions for people who have committed a crime and found to be mentally unwell at the time of their offence and therefore not criminally responsible for their actions. Mental impairment as outlined in the *Criminal Code Act 1995*, s. 7.3, states 'a person is not criminally responsible for an offence if, at the time of carrying out the conduct constituting the offence, the person was suffering from a mental impairment' (Commonwealth Consolidated Acts, n.d.).

Where a person's competence at the time of an offence is presented, psychiatrists and/or other health professionals may be required to write reports for the court, following an examination of the person. The court will then determine whether the person meets the grounds for mental impairment, and whether they will be found not guilty as a result of their mental impairment at the time of the offence.

Where a person is found not guilty by reason of mental impairment, they may be required to undertake treatment and rehabilitation in a forensic hospital, or may be placed on an order in the community. Forensic mental health is discussed further in Chapter 24.

A focus on recovery

A recent focus of legislation enshrines the concept of recovery and the important role of consumers and their carers in decisions regarding care and treatment. Most of the state and territory Mental Health Acts have been revised and amended over recent years. This has been largely a response to issues raised by consumers, carers, clinicians and other stakeholders throughout a significant consultation process (Tasmanian Government, 2015).

Perkins and colleagues (2012) describe recovery as a personal journey of discovery. It involves a person making sense of, and finding meaning in, what has happened; becoming an expert in their own self-care, 'building a new sense of self and purpose in life' by discovering their own resourcefulness and possibilities, and using these, and the resources available to them, to pursue their aspirations and goals (Perkins et al., 2012).

Patricia Deegan, a well-known person with a lived experience of mental illness and mental health advocate, writes that mental health recovery is:

> a process, a way of life, an attitude, and a way of approaching the day's challenges. It is not a perfectly linear process. At times our course is erratic, we falter, slide back, regroup and start again… The need is to meet the challenge of disability and to re-establish a new and valued sense of integrity and purpose within and beyond the limits of the disability; the aspiration is to live, work and love in a community in which one makes a significant contribution. (Flourish Australia, 2016)

The South Australia *Mental Health Act 2009* is recovery-focused in its intent and introduces the concept of CTOs while 'providing protections' of the freedom and legal rights of mentally ill persons (Government of South Australia, 2009). We discuss recovery in more detail in Chapter 21.

Similarly, the NT *Mental Health and Related Services Act 2016* provides for the care, treatment and protection of people with a mental illness while at the same time protecting their civil rights. This legislation specifically defines a person who is considered to have a mental illness and defines exclusion criteria for those considered not to have a mental illness.

Queensland enacted a new Mental Health Act in 2016 (Queensland Government, 2016). This Act reflects changing community and individual attitudes towards people with a mental health condition and their care. In particular, the Act regulates the use of mechanical restraint, seclusion, physical restraint and other practices (s. 24). The Act also acknowledges the role of a nominated support person, family, carers and other support persons. It articulates the powers, role and responsibilities of the authorised mental health practitioner in the assessment, admission and transfer of persons deemed to have a mental health condition. Much of the Act focuses upon the forensic provisions and the role of the psychiatrist, as opposed to other contemporary mental health legislation that tends to emphasise the autonomy and recovery of persons with a mental health condition. Nominated support persons are included in the legislation and according to the Act must be notified of significant events (s. 287 (2)) and included in decisions about the person's treatment and care (s. 291 [b]).

In New South Wales, the *Mental Health Amendment (Statutory Review) Act 2014* changed the term 'primary carer' to 'designated carer', and this allows a person who is a close friend or relative who has regular contact with and an interest in the care of the person with a mental health condition to be recognised as a carer. Those persons who are Aboriginal or Torres Strait Islander and have a 'relative' who has regular contact and interest in their care can include that person who is part of the extended family or kin according to the indigenous kinship system of the person's culture (MHCC, 2015c).

Clearly, the direction of mental health in the future points towards less paternalistic and controlling systems for people who have a lived experience of a mental health condition. However, the legislation can only do so much. Nurses' attitudes and behaviour towards mental health and people with a lived experience of a mental health condition are critical factors in supporting the rights of people to attain full citizenship and wholesome lives.

LEGAL AND ETHICAL DIMENSIONS OF PRACTICE FOR NURSES

Ethics can be described as moral principles that influence a person's behaviour. In nursing, ethics influences the way in which health professionals engage in decision-making processes, based on their view of what is considered to be right or wrong (Bennett & Bennett, 2011). Ethical decision-making requires people to approach a situation with the motivation and desire to determine what is required and act accordingly (Beauchamp & Childress, 2013). Thus, the way in which a person acts is based on the person's own morals. Decision-making in nursing care must be informed, and guided by reason, justification and argument (Beauchamp & Childress, 2013). This will allow the nurse to make a decision that supports the best action.

The ethics of health care are centred around moral philosophies that frame the way that we make decisions, justify our actions and demonstrate our humanity. Nurses are bound by codes of conduct that govern their practice. In Australia, the Nursing and Midwifery Board of Australia (NMBA) undertakes functions as set by the *Health Practitioner Regulation National Law* (the National Law), as in force in each state and territory.

The code of conduct for nurses articulates the legal requirements, professional behaviour and conduct expectations for all nurses regardless of what area they may practice in (NMBA, 2018). The code is consistent with the National Law, but is not a substitute for the National Law or other relevant legislation. The National Law always takes precedence.

Essentially, the code is divided into four domains:
1 practise legally
2 practise safely, effectively and collaboratively
3 act with professional integrity
4 promote health and well-being.

Each of these domains includes subcategories and statements that underpin the values, principles, obligations and behaviour expected of nurses (NMBA, 2018). The code also includes a glossary of terms which clarifies the meanings of the terms used in the code. The code is freely available by visiting the AHPRA website (https://www.ahpra.gov.au).

Ethical frameworks

An ethical framework for nursing practice is based on four sound ethical principles: autonomy, beneficence, non-maleficence and justice (Beauchamp & Childress, 2013). **Autonomy** refers to the respect that is shown by practitioners towards people's decisions and choices (Beauchamp & Childress, 2013; Bennett & Bennett, 2011). Respecting a person's autonomy in a mental health context involves the nurse supporting the person to make decisions about their care where possible and without coercion, and ensuring that the person is involved in their care and treatment at all stages. This includes respecting a person's decision even when in the nurse's opinion it may not be the right decision. **Beneficence** requires the practitioner to prevent evil or harm happening to people and **non-maleficence** obliges the practitioner to avoid inflicting evil or harm (Beauchamp & Childress, 2013; Bennett & Bennett, 2011). In a mental health context, this would involve the nurse ensuring that their actions support the person and do not intentionally put the person at risk and/or cause harm. Given what we know about mental health practice, there are times when a nurse's actions may have the potential for unintentional harm (e.g. use of seclusion). The nurse therefore needs to ensure that interventions are in place to reduce associated risk and/or harm, and that benefits outweigh risks. Intentional harm is not acceptable. Following such ethical principles, it can be argued that **justice** is achieved by creating an encounter that supports fairness, equality and non-discrimination towards people with mental health conditions.

The International Council of Nurses (ICN) Code of Ethics for nurses came into effect for all nurses in Australia in March 2018. The ICN Code has four principal elements that outline ethical conduct standards expected for nurses. These elements are:
1 nurses and people
2 nurses and practice

3 nurses and the profession
4 nurses and co-workers (ICN, 2012).

Element one recognises the nurse's responsibility to provide care to the individual, family and community that is respectful of their human rights, values, customs and spiritual beliefs. In doing this, the nurse must ensure information provided is accurate, sufficient, timely and culturally appropriate (ICN, 2012). This element also highlights the nurse's responsibility for initiating and supporting action to meet the needs of the public and, in particular, vulnerable populations, while advocating for equity and social justice in health care.

Element two describes the practice responsibilities of nurses, including the maintenance of standards of personal conduct, accountability and competence. This element highlights the responsibility of nurses to strive to foster and maintain a culture that promotes ethical behaviour (ICN, 2012).

Element three focuses on the role of nurses in assessing and implementing acceptable standards of practice, management, research and education (ICN, 2012). This is imperative to nursing practice, as nurses must always use the best available evidence to underpin all decision-making. This requires nurses to stay up to date in their area of practice to ensure positive outcomes for individuals and the community.

Finally, element four recognises the importance of collaborative and respectful relationships with colleagues, which may require nurses to act as a safeguard when individuals are at risk from a co-worker (ICN, 2012).

Underpinning all these elements is the responsibility nurses have to themselves, colleagues, individuals and families, and the public, to ensure that the professional standard of nursing remains high for the benefit of all.

The nursing profession recognises the universal human rights of people and the moral responsibility to safeguard the inherent dignity and equal worth of everyone (United Nations, 1978).

Nurses often find themselves conflicted by the very nature of their work, no more so than when required to carry out practices that directly affect a person's rights and freedoms. This is evident in mental health when compulsory assessment and treatment is required.

Compulsory assessment and treatment is considered to be controversial as it can involve:
1 restrictions on a consumer's right to legal representation
2 removal of a consumer's autonomy and freedom
3 limiting the treatment setting to an in-patient facility
4 providing a least restrictive environment for the consumer.

CASE **STUDY**

AN ETHICAL DILEMMA

Michael is a 45-year-old man who lives alone in the community. Anne and Mark are community mental health nurses who visit Michael in his home on a frequent basis to provide him with support and ensure he is adherent with his medication regimen. Michael has concerns regarding the medication, specifically that he is well and sees no reason why he should take it. Anne and Mark inform Michael that to cease taking prescribed medication is not advisable. Michael becomes upset and asks them to leave.

Questions

1 What is the ethical dilemma facing Anne and Mark?
2 Does Michael have the right to refuse to take prescribed medication?
3 Do Anne and Mark have to leave when Michael asks them?

COMPULSORY CARE AND TREATMENT FROM A CONSUMER PERSPECTIVE

In Australia, the human rights of people with a mental health condition have received increasing attention during the past two decades, more recently prompted in part by new obligations under the UN Convention on the Rights of Persons with Disabilities (UNCRPD) (UNHCHR, 2006; McSherry & Wilson, 2011). Enshrined in the Convention is the human right for individuals to not be subjected to medical treatment without full, free and informed consent (Bell, 2003; Quinn, 2011).

Like all Australian citizens, people with mental health conditions have inalienable human rights (UN General Assembly, 1948). Further guarantee of human rights for consumers has been enshrined within the UNCRPD. The document defines persons with disabilities as those who have long-term physical, mental, intellectual or sensory impairments that, in interaction with various barriers, may hinder their full and effective participation in society on an equal basis with others. The UNCRPD's purpose is to:

> Promote, protect and ensure the full and equal enjoyment of all human rights and fundamental freedoms by all persons with disabilities, and to promote respect for their inherent dignity (Article 1). (United Nations, 2006, p. 4)

Although these declarations, principles and guidelines have no binding legal effect, they provide the moral force for practical guidance to governments to incorporate these within their statutes and protocols (GNHRE, 2006). In their review of Australian legislation, Callaghan and Ryan (2012) discussed how changes to the Victorian and Tasmanian legislation attempted to give effect to the UNCRPD by replacing the dangerousness standard with a competency standard. Mental competency is a broader definition that may or may not include acts of dangerousness.

The five most frequently cited ethical issues reported in a study by Johnstone, Da Costa and Turale (2004) were:

1 protecting patients' rights and human dignity
2 providing care with possible risk to nurse's own health (e.g. TB, HIV, violence)
3 respecting/not respecting informed consent to treatment
4 staffing patterns that limit patient access to nursing care
5 use/non-use of physical/chemical restraints.

In considering ethical dilemmas involving patients' rights, dignity and autonomy, nurses must use established principles in reaching fair decisions. These principles include consideration of the:

- patient's autonomy
- patient's degree of competence
- responsibilities and accountabilities of the nurse
- risk factors associated with the patient's condition
- implications of detention and restrictions on movement.

Nurses working in mental health face daily dilemmas concerning autonomy versus paternalistic care. Assessing competence can be multifactorial and dynamic. The responsibility and accountability of nurses continues to increase. Risk-averse systems may directly conflict with patients' aspirations for recovery and empowerment. Maintaining trust and a therapeutic relationship, even when required to restrict a person's movement, is sometimes paradoxical and appears dichotomous to nurses. However, compassionate, ethical and caring nurses can manage these dilemmas with their patients and experience the unparalleled satisfaction and knowledge that their education, skills and competence have made a positive difference to a person's life.

REFLECTION ON LEARNING FROM PRACTICE

Lydia's experience is not unlike that of others when admitted to a mental health unit under the Mental Health Act. While the Mental Health Act aims to support people with a mental health condition who require treatment, it can be a stigmatising and scary experience for consumers. The challenging aspect of this is for mental health nurses to balance legislation whilst maximising choice, promoting safety and supporting consumers in their recovery.

Mental health nurses need to be aware of their professional, legal and ethical responsibilities in providing and supporting care for people with a mental illness. It is the responsibility of the nurse to ensure that care and treatment provided is supportive of the person's human rights, and inclusive of their and their primary carer/'s wishes.

CHAPTER RESOURCES

SUMMARY

- This chapter has explored the legal and ethical contexts for nurses working in the field of mental health in the context of mental health legislation in Australia.
- Mental health legislation in various jurisdictions of Australia is varied. However, commonalities lie in the preservation of dignity, upholding duty of care, and providing mental health care that is in a least restrictive environment.
- Contemporary ethical and legal frameworks facilitate recovery and promote autonomous decision making with carer input.

- Law and ethics apply in the context of nursing in Australia and all nurses working in health care need to be familiar with local Mental Health Acts and other relevant legislation.
- Of supreme importance are the issues of informed consent and involuntary or compulsory treatment, and the mental health nurse should adopt a consumer perspective.

REVIEW QUESTIONS

1   Choose the statement that best defines the difference between law and ethics:
    a   Ethics dictates behaviour, but law does not
    b   Law is 'prescriptive' and ethics is 'guiding'
    c   Ethics is based on law
    d   A person can be punished for breaching ethics
2   Where there is an actual or perceived conflict between the code of conduct for nurses and the law:
    a   The code takes precedence
    b   The law takes precedence
    c   The conflict is settled with consideration to the code and the law
    d   The conflict is decided by the Nursing and Midwifery Board of Australia
3   The following requirements are necessary for all patient consent:
    a   The consent must be voluntary, specific to the intervention/treatment, informed and the person must have capacity
    b   The consent does not need to be voluntary as long as the person has the legal capacity

    c   The consent can be considered valid if obtained through coercion as long as it is in the best interest of the patient
    d   The consent must be voluntary, cover any intervention/ treatment during admission, be informed and the person must have capacity
4   Each state and territory Mental Health Act is based on the principle that the person:
    a   Appears to be mentally ill
    b   Should be detained immediately for their safety and the safety of others
    c   Treatment is of the least restrictive type possible
    d   Must be admitted to hospital as an involuntary patient
5   Electroconvulsive therapy (ECT) is often used for those who are 'treatment resistant'. Common side effects include:
    a   Site irritation (such as burning), confusion and headache
    b   Short-term memory loss, confusion and headache
    c   Long-term memory loss, confusion and headache
    d   Nausea, vomiting and diarrhoea

CRITICAL THINKING

1 Australia's legal system requires health care clinicians to operate within a 'least restrictive' framework. Discuss where this approach is evident in the legislation.

2 What must a person be able to do to show they have capacity to make decisions?

3 What are the four elements that must be demonstrated to prove a case of negligence under the law of torts?

4 What is the difference between 'voluntary' and 'involuntary' treatment in the context of mental health legislation in your state or territory?

5 What does the mental health legislation in your state or territory stipulate about 'recovery'?

6 What are the four principles of bioethics?

USEFUL WEBSITES

- Australian Health Practitioner Regulation Agency (AHPRA): https://www.ahpra.gov.au
- Human Rights Commission: https://www.humanrights.gov.au
- Nursing and Midwifery Board Australia: https://www.nursingmidwiferyboard.gov.au
- United Nations Convention on the Rights of Persons with Disabilities: https://www.un.org/development/desa/disabilities/convention-on-the-rights-of-persons-with-disabilities.html

REFLECT ON THIS

Your mental health clinical placement

Undertaking clinical placement is an exciting experience, but it can also pose challenges for students. You may have undertaken a general nursing placement already, where you probably worked with consumers who were accepting of treatment and actively engaged in their healthcare. As this chapter has highlighted, a mental health placement may be different to this (however, no less rewarding). You may encounter people who refuse treatment or who are unable to give informed consent, but are very distressed and unwell.

1 Reflect upon what you would like to achieve on your mental health clinical placement. Now include some goals that will improve the mental health outcomes for people in your care.

2 What are some of the ethical and legal challenges that you think are faced by mental health nurses?

3 Discuss the pros and cons of enforcing treatment for people with mental illness. Do you think the pros always outweigh the cons? Can you think of an example or situation where they may not?

REFERENCES

Andrade, A., Arumugham, S.S. & Thirthalli, J. (2016). Adverse effects of electroconvulsive therapy. *Psychiatric Clinics of North America*, 39(3), 513–30.

Australian College of Mental Health Nurses (ACMHN). (2016). *Seclusion and Restraint Position Statement*. Retrieved from http://www.acmhn.org/images/stories/FINAL_Seclusion_and_Restraint_Position_Statement_-_August_2016.pdf.

Australian Institute of Health and Welfare (AIHW). (2018). Mental health services in Australia. Retrieved from https://www.aihw.gov.au/reports/mental-health-services/mental-health-services-in-australia/report-contents/restrictive-practices/seclusion.

Australian Law Reform Commission (ALRC). (n.d.). Equality, capacity and disability in Commonwealth laws. Retrieved from https://www.alrc.gov.au/publications/equality-capacity-and-disability-commonwealth-laws/capacity-and-decision-making. © Commonwealth of Australia. Australian Law Reform Commission (n.d.). Equality, capacity and disability in Commonwealth laws.

Australian Law Reform Commission (ALRC). (2015). *Traditional Rights and Freedoms Encroachments by Commonwealth Laws (ALRC Interim Report 127)*. Retrieved from https://www.alrc.gov.au/publications/what-tort.

Beauchamp, T.I. & Childress, J.F. (2013). *Principles of Biomedical Ethics*. New York: Oxford University Press.

Bell, C. (2003). *Peace Agreements and Human Rights*. New York: Oxford University Press.

Bennett, B. & Bennett, A. (2011). Law, ethics and mental health nursing. In K.L. Edward, L. Munro, A. Robbins & A. Welch (eds), *Mental Health Nursing: Dimensions of praxis* (pp. 88–120) South Melbourne: Oxford University Press.

Burdekin, B. (1993). *Report of the National Inquiry into the Human Rights of People with Mental Illness.* Sydney: Australian Human Rights Commission.

Callaghan, S. & Ryan, C.J. (2012). Rising to the human rights challenge in compulsory treatment – new approaches to mental health law in Australia. *Australian and New Zealand Journal of Psychiatry*, 46(7), 611–20. doi:10.1177/0004867412438872

Chakrabarti, S., Grover, S. & Rajagopal, R. (2010). Electroconvulsive therapy: A review of knowledge, experience and attitudes of patients concerning the treatment. *World Journal of Biological Psychiatry*, 11(3), 525–37.

Cleary, M. & Horsfall, J. (2014). Electroconvulsive therapy: Issues for mental health nurses to consider. *Issues in Mental Health Nursing*, 35(1), 73–6.

Commonwealth Consolidated Acts (n.d.). *Criminal Code Act 1995*. © Sourced from the Federal Register of Legislation on January 8, 2019. Criminal Code Act 1995. Retrieved from https://www.legislation.gov.au/Details/C2019C00003. For the latest information on Australian Government law please go to https://www.legislation.gov.au. Released under CC BY 4.0. Link to license: https://creativecommons.org/licenses/by/4.0/.

Flourish Australia. (2016). Road to recovery. Retrieved from https://www.flourishaustralia.org.au/road-recovery-0.

Forrester, K. & Griffiths, D. (2011). *Essentials of Law for Health Professionals* (3rd edn). Chatswood: Elsevier.

Global Network for the Study of Human Rights and the Environment (GNHRE). (2006). *International Council on Human Rights Policy (ICHRP)*. Retrieved from https://gnhre.org/partners/non-governmental-organisations/international-council-for-human-rights-policy.

Government of South Australia. (2009). *Mental Health Act 2009*. Retrieved from https://www.legislation.sa.gov.au/LZ/C/A/MENTAL%20HEALTH%20ACT%202009.aspx

Gregory-Roberts, E.M., Naismith, S.L., Cullen, K.M. & Hickie. I.B. (2010). Electroconvulsive therapy-induced persistent retrograde amnesia: Could it be minimised by ketamine or other pharmacological approaches? *Journal of Affective Disorders*, 126(1), 39–45.

Guardianship and Administration Act 1986 (Vic.). Retrieved from http://www8.austlii.edu.au/cgi-bin/viewdb/au/legis/vic/consol_act/gaaa1986304.

Happell, B., Cowin, L., Roper, C., Foster, K. & McMaster, R. (2008). *Introducing Mental Health Nursing*. Crows Nest: Allen &Unwin.

Huckshorn, K.A. (2004). Reducing seclusion and restraint use in mental health settings: Core strategies for prevention. *Journal of Psychosocial Nursing*, 42(9), 22–33.

International Council of Nurses (ICN). (2012). *The ICN Code of Ethics for Nurses*. Geneva: ICN. Retrieved from https://www.icn.ch/sites/default/files/inline-files/2012_ICN_Codeofethicsfornurses_%20eng.pdf.

Johnstone, M.-J., Da Costa, C. & Turale, S. (2004). Registered and enrolled nurses: Experiences of ethical issues in nursing practice. *Australian Journal of Advanced Nursing*, 22(1), 31–7.

L v Human Rights and Equal Opportunity Commission (2006) 233 ALR 432.

Masterman-Lister v Brutton & Co [2003] 3 All ER 162, 169.

Mayers, P., Keet, N., Winkler, G. & Flisher, A.J. (2010). Mental health service users' perceptions and experiences of sedation, seclusion and restraint. *International Journal of Social Psychiatry*, 56, 60–73.

McSherry, B. & Wilson, K. (2011). Detention and treatment down under: Human rights and mental health laws in Australia and New Zealand. *Medical Law Review*, 19(4), 548–80. doi:10.1093/medlaw/fwr024

Melbourne Social Equity Unit. (2014). *Seclusion and Restraint Project: Report*. Melbourne: University of Melbourne. Retrieved from https://socialequity.unimelb.edu.au/__data/assets/pdf_file/0017/2004722/Seclusion-and-Restraint-report.PDF.

Mental Health Act 2007 (NSW). Retrieved from https://www.legislation.nsw.gov.au/inforce/bb9dde66-bc52-ea95-89d4-8a3c5dd9507b/2007-8.pdf.

Mental Health and Related Services Act 2016 (NT). Retrieved from https://legislation.nt.gov.au/Legislation/MENTAL-HEALTH-AND-RELATED-SERVICES-ACT.

Mental Health Coordinating Council (MHCC). (2015a). *The Mental Health Rights Manual: An Online Guide to the Legal and Human Rights of People Navigating the Mental Health and Human Service Systems in NSW* (4th edn). Chapter 2 Section A: The legal framework. Retrieved from http://mhrm.mhcc.org.au/chapter-2/2a.aspx.

Mental Health Coordinating Council (MHCC). (2015b). *The Mental Health Rights Manual: An Online Guide to the Legal and Human Rights of People Navigating the Mental Health and Human Service Systems in NSW* (4th edn). Chapter 4 Section D: Compulsory treatment in hospital under the *Mental Health Act 2007* (NSW). Retrieved from http://mhrm.mhcc.org.au/chapter-4/4d.aspx.

Mental Health Coordinating Council (MHCC). (2015c). *The Mental Health Rights Manual: An Online Guide to the Legal and Human Rights of People Navigating the Mental Health and Human Service Systems in NSW* (4th edn). Chapter 9 Section A. Carers of people with mental health conditions – overview. Retrieved from http://mhrm.mhcc.org.au/chapter-9/9a.aspx.

Muir-Cochrane, E. & Gerace, A. (2017). The trouble with chemical restraint. *International Journal of Mental Health Nursing*, 26(S1), 28.

National Mental Health Commission (NMHC). (2012). *A Contributing Life: the 2012 National Report Card on Mental Health and Suicide Prevention*. Canberra: NMHC. Retrieved from http://www.mentalhealthcommission.gov.au/media/39270/NMHC_ReportCard_Enhanced.pdf. © National Mental Health Commission (NMHC).

National Mental Health Consumer and Carer Forum (NMHCCF). (2009). *Ending Seclusion and Restraint in Australian Mental Health Services*. Retrieved from: https://nmhccf.org.au/sites/default/files/docs/seclusion_restraint.pdf.

Neilson, G. (2005). The role of mental health legislation. *Canadian Journal of Psychiatry*, 50(11): S1.

Newton, J.R., Bosanac, P., Copolov, D., Hopwood, M., Keks, N., Paoletti, N., Tiller, J. & Castle, D. (2017). Targeting zero: Implications for public psychiatric services. *Australian and New Zealand Journal of Psychiatry*, 51(6), 560–2.

New South Wales Government. (2007). *NSW Mental Health Act 2007*, s. 89. https://www.legislation.nsw.gov.au/inforce/bb9dde66-bc52 ea95-89d4-8a3c5dd9507b/2007-8.pdf. © New South Wales Government. NSW legislation.

New South Wales Ministry of Health. (2017). *Review of Seclusion, Restraint and Observation of Consumers with a Mental Illness in NSW Health Facilities*. Sydney: NSW Ministry of Health. Retrieved from https://www.health.nsw.gov.au/patients/mentalhealth/Documents/report-seclusion-restraint-observation.pdf. For current information go to www.health.nsw.gov.au. Released under CC BY 4.0. Link to license: https://creativecommons.org/licenses/by/4.0/.

Northern Territory Government. (2016). *Northern Territory Mental Health and Related Services Act 2016*. s. 66. Retrieved from https://legislation.nt.gov.au/Legislation/MENTAL-HEALTH-AND-RELATED-SERVICES-ACT. © Northern Territory Government.

Nursing and Midwifery Board of Australia (NMBA). (2018). *Code of Conduct for Nurses*. Retrieved from www.nursingmidwiferyboard.gov.au/Codes-Guidelines-Statements/Professional-standards.aspx.

O'Brien A.J. (2014). Community treatment orders in New Zealand: Regional variability and international comparisons. *Australas Psychiatry* 22(4), 352–6. doi: 10.1177/1039856214531080

Perkins, R., Repper, J., Rinaldi, R. & Brown, H. (2012). Briefing: Recovery colleges. Centre for Mental Health Briefing Paper. Retrieved from: http://personcentredcare.health.org.uk/resources/briefing-recovery-colleges.

Queensland Government. (2016). *Mental Health Act 2016*. Retrieved from https://www.health.qld.gov.au/clinical-practice/guidelines-procedures/clinical-staff/mental-health/act.

Rasmussen, K.G., Mueller, M., Knapp, R.G., Husain, M.M., Rummans, T.A., Sampson, S.M. & Kellner, C.H. (2007). Antidepressant medication treatment failure does not predict lower remission with ECT for major depressive disorder: A report from the consortium for research in electroconvulsive therapy. *Journal of Clinical Psychiatry*, 68(11), 1701–6.

Royal Australian and New Zealand College of Psychiatrists (RANZCP). (2017). RANZCP mental health legislation – comparative tables as at 30 June 2017. Retrieved from https://www.ranzcp.org/Files/Resources/Mental-health-legislation-tables/Mental-Health-Acts-Comparative-Tables-all.aspx.

Tasmanian Government. (2015). *Consultation Feedback*. Department of Health and Human Services, Statewide Mental Health Services. Retrieved from https://www.dhhs.tas.gov.au/mentalhealth/rethink_mental_health_project/rethink_mental_health_project_-_supporting_documentation/review_report_

contents_page/introduction/summary/consultation_feedback/consultation_feedback.

Turner, K.V. & Mooney, P. (2016). A comparison of seclusion rates between intellectual disability and non-intellectual disability services: The effect of gender and diagnosis. *Journal of Forensic Psychiatry & Psychology*, 27(2), 265–80.

United Nations. (1948). *Universal Declaration of Human Rights*. Paris: UN General Assembly. Retrieved from https://www.refworld.org/docid/3ae6b3712c.html.

United Nations. (1978). *United National Yearbook on Human Rights*. New York: United Nations General Assembly.

United Nations. (2006). *Convention on the Rights of Persons with Disabilities*. New York: United Nations. Retrieved from http://www.un.org/disabilities/documents/convention/convoptprot-e.pdf.

Van Der Merwe, M., Muir-Cochrane. E., Jones, J., Tziggili, M. & Bowers, L. (2013). Improving seclusion practice: Implications of a review of staff and patient views. *Journal of Psychiatric and Mental Health Nursing*, 20(3), 203–15.

CHAPTER 4

TREATMENT MODALITIES UTILISED IN CONTEMPORARY MENTAL HEALTH SERVICE DELIVERY

Louise Alexander and Gylo (Julie) Hercelinskyj

LEARNING OUTCOMES

Upon completion of this chapter, you should be able to:

4.1 Review the pharmacological interventions used in contemporary mental health service delivery

4.2 Explore a range of psychosocial interventions used in contemporary mental health service

4.3 Understand the principles of motivational interviewing

4.4 Identify the key elements of mindfulness-based interventions

4.5 Identify the key elements of cognitive behavioural therapies

4.6 Identify the key elements of rational emotive behaviour therapy

4.7 Identify the key elements of dialectical behaviour therapy

4.8 Consider the usefulness of structured problem solving in therapeutic interventions

4.9 Understand the importance of psychoeducation in therapeutic interventions

---

LEARNING FROM PRACTICE

Jodie, 32 years old, was admitted to the mother baby unit 12 weeks after the birth of her first child. Jodie ran a successful small recruitment business and had been with her partner for seven years. When I met with Jodie for the first time, she explained that parenthood had been such a shock for her. She was a successful business woman, but she couldn't get a small infant to sleep.

Her confidence in being a parent was 'shot' and was impacting on her bonding with the baby and her relationship with her partner. She had no appetite, could not sleep and overall felt 'useless'. Sitting there with her, I observed a woman who looked exhausted, spoke with an increasingly tremulous voice and appeared on the verge of crying. Using the skills I had developed when working with other mothers who have been under stress, I leant forward, looked at Jodi and said, 'I can see you're exhausted and you would not have come in if things weren't desperate. What do you want to achieve during this admission?' Jodie looked at me and thought…

Ellie, Perinatal Mental Health Nurse

The mental health nurse used a range of strategies in this interaction. These encompass both broad therapeutic engagement skills as well as some strategies based on specific psychosocial approaches to practice. What clinical observations would have influenced the response made by the mental health nurse? What skills can you identify in this interaction?

INTRODUCTION

Consumers have access to a range of treatment and management options in contemporary mental health service delivery. While medications will often form a crucial component of a management plan, it is important to understand the range of options available to consumers. From psychosocial interventions through to the use of psychotropic medications, the aim of any treatment option is to provide the consumer with an individualised approach to addressing their health concerns, maximising quality of life and contributing as one component of their recovery journey. As members of the multidisciplinary team, mental health nurses have an important role to play in working collaboratively with consumers when they make choices regarding management options and providing support and education to consumers and relevant others. This requires that mental health nurses understand the various treatment and management options available. This chapter focuses on pharmacological interventions, psychosocial interventions and the mental health nurse's role in implementing these interventions. The physical intervention of electroconvulsive therapy and transcranial magnetic therapy is addressed in Chapter 10.

PHARMACOLOGICAL INTERVENTIONS

Treatment modalities in contemporary mental health practice encompass both biological and psychosocial interventions. Choosing which treatment options will work best is a collaborative decision, with the consumer central to the process. Some consumers will argue they do not find medication the best option for them while others believe it is an important element of their overall treatment plan. Before you consider the various groups of pharmacological agents in this section, we review some essential features of the central nervous system that are involved in the transmission and uptake of different medications.

Neurotransmitters

Neurotransmitters are responsible for the relay of signals between the neurones in the brain. Neurotransmitters play a pivotal role in physiological functions, and without them humans would not survive. They tell the brain when to breathe, the heart when to beat and control other such vital functions. There are two distinct types of neurotransmitter: inhibitory and excitatory. Inhibitory transmitters help the brain to calm, while excitatory transmitters help to stimulate the brain.

Dopamine

Dopamine is an integral excitatory neurotransmitter in the brain (**Figure 4.1**). Alterations in dopamine can affect concentration and focus and it is associated with attention deficit/hyperactivity disorder (see Chapter 15). Parkinson's disease is a movement condition that is the result of too little dopamine in the brain. The 'dopamine hypothesis' attempts to explain the biological aetiology of schizophrenia by theorising that there is a disproportionate activity of dopamine in the brain of people with schizophrenia (Adams & Urban, 2013). One of the rationales for this theory is the effect first generation antipsychotics and illicit drugs targeting dopamine have on behaviour. First generation antipsychotics (such as haloperidol) are effective on positive symptoms (e.g. hallucinations) because they block dopamine (which is understood to be highly active in people with schizophrenia). Illicit drugs such as speed can *cause* psychosis in some people and are known to increase concentrations of dopamine in the brain.

Serotonin

The inhibitory neurotransmitter **serotonin** is responsible for stabilising moods, regulating sleep, sexual functioning, aiding in digestion and regulating anxiety (**Figure 4.2**). Serotonin is responsible for happy moods and feeling depressed and, as such, antidepressant medications act on this neurotransmitter in the brain. Suicide and impulsive behaviours are also understood to be regulated by serotonin (Adams & Urban, 2013). Depression, bipolar disorder and anxiety are understood to stem from

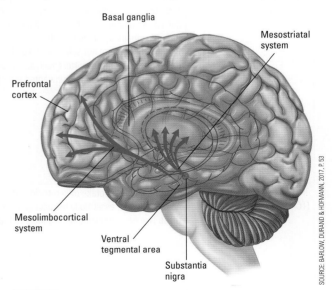

Basal ganglia

Mesostriatal system

Prefrontal cortex

Mesolimbocortical system

Ventral tegmental area

Substantia nigra

SOURCE: BARLOW, DURAND & HOFMANN, 2017, P. 53

FIGURE 4.1
Two major dopamine pathways in the brain

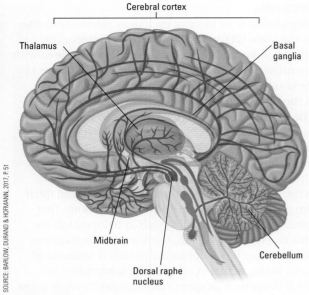

Cerebral cortex

Thalamus

Basal ganglia

Midbrain

Cerebellum

Dorsal raphe nucleus

SOURCE: BARLOW, DURAND & HOFMANN, 2017, P. 51

FIGURE 4.2
Major serotonin pathways in the brain

lowered levels of serotonin. Antidepressants allow serotonin to be used more efficiently by the brain, thus causing the improved mood associated with serotonin. They block the brain from reabsorbing the serotonin, thus allowing it to remain in the brain, doing what it is intended to do. Modern antidepressants such as selective serotonin reuptake inhibitors (SSRIs) are selective in the neurotransmitters that they affect, and as such cause fewer side effects than older medications like monoamine oxidase inhibitors (MAOIs; see Chapter 10).

Psychotropic medications

This section explores some of the intrusive interventions such as the administration of psychotropic medications. To understand more complex adherence issues with psychotropic medications, refer to the chapter for the condition you are exploring (e.g. for schizophrenia, see Chapter 8).

Antidepressants

The first antidepressants were developed in the 1950s and since that time there have been some major advancements in the development of psychotropic medications. There are four different classes of antidepressants, with differing mechanisms: monoamine oxidase inhibitors, tricyclic antidepressants, selective reuptake inhibitors, and serotonin and norepinephrine reuptake inhibitors. **Table 4.1** explores the different types of antidepressants and their mechanisms, while more details about individual antidepressants can be found in Chapter 10.

TABLE 4.1
Types of antidepressants and their mechanisms

TYPE OF ANTIDEPRESSANT	ACTION	COMMON SIDE EFFECTS AND PRECAUTIONS
Monoamine oxidase inhibitors (MAOIs)	MAOIs block monoamine oxidase, an enzyme responsible for breaking down neurotransmitters such as serotonin in the brain. By blocking reuptake, more serotonin is able to be utilised. Because MAOIs are not selective, they also break down other neurotransmitters such as dopamine and norepinephrine, resulting in unwanted effects and side effects.	Side effects: • gastrointestinal (GI) upset • dry mouth • headache • insomnia • dizziness • skin reactions. Precautions: • Interact with foods such as aged cheese, fermented foods, beer and soy products. • Strict adherence to diet necessary and failure to adhere can be dangerous. • MAOIs also interact with many medications including analgesics, herbal replacements and cold medicines.
Tricyclic antidepressants (TCAs)	TCAs block the reuptake of serotonin and norepinephrine, essentially increasing the amount of these two neurotransmitters available to the brain.	Side effects: • constipation • increased body temperature • dry mouth, nose • urinary retention • memory impairment. Precautions: • Can be highly lethal in overdose.

TYPE OF ANTIDEPRESSANT	ACTION	COMMON SIDE EFFECTS AND PRECAUTIONS
Selective serotonin reuptake inhibitors (SSRIs)	SSRIs increase the level of serotonin in the brain by preventing reabsorption or reuptake. This increases the amount of serotonin available to the brain and improves mood and decreases anxiety.	Side effects: • dry mouth • drowsiness • sexual dysfunction • GI upset.
Serotonin and norepinephrine reuptake inhibitors (SNRIs)	SNRIs are potent inhibitors of serotonin and norepinephrine and prevent their reuptake in the brain. They act in the same manner as SSRIs; however, they have the additional benefit of affecting norepinephrine too.	Side effects: • nausea • sweating • sexual dysfunction.

SOURCE: ADAPTED FROM ADAMS & URBAN, 2013; MCKENNA & MIRKOV, 2013

Antipsychotics

The first antipsychotic medications were developed in the 1950s. Antipsychotics became increasingly more effective at relieving psychosis, and this was partly responsible for the deinstitutionalisation of people with mental illness from institutions across the world in the 1980–90s. Antipsychotics continue to be developed with the aim of reducing the side effects that play a significant role in non-adherence. Chapter 8 extensively covers the different kinds of antipsychotics.

Long-acting depot intramuscular injectable medications

Long-acting intramuscular injectable medications (or LAIs) are an effective strategy for managing psychotic illness in individuals who:
- have poor insight into their condition and refuse to take oral medications
- prefer to take medication infrequently
- are non-adherent to treatment
- forget to take medication regularly, resulting in intermittent adherence and poor symptom control.

LAIs are essentially 2–4 weeks' worth of medication, injected into a large muscle, which is slowly released over the period until the next dose is due. Some of the fundamental issues with LAIs are the loss of control for a consumer who disagrees with their diagnosis experiences, and the impact this can have on the development and retention of a therapeutic relationship with mental health clinicians. While LAIs may make sense to clinicians and appear to be 'humanitarian' in their relief of perceived suffering from mental illness, consumers often feel distressed, controlled and angry at having yet another decision taken away from them. For these reasons, LAIs should only be used as a last resort. **Table 8.6** in Chapter 8 covers the range of LAIs for use to treat schizophrenia, bipolar disorder and psychosis.

Impact of side effects

There are many adverse side effects from psychotropic medications and it is very important for the clinician to consider this when administering such medications. Unwanted side effects are one of the major reasons behind non-adherence to antipsychotic medications. This is a complex issue and the clinician needs to consider the impact that distressing side effects such as movement disorders or sexual dysfunction has on consumers. For example, consider a consumer who has schizophrenia. He frequently hears voices and his psychiatrist has steadily increased his medication over the past few months in an effort to alleviate these hallucinations. Now the consumer no longer hears voices, but the increase in medication has resulted in considerable distressing side effects such as significant weight gain, which has led to self-esteem and confidence issues, in addition to physical health concerns such as hypertension. This is a good example of where symptom amelioration has resulted in intolerable side effects and significant **iatrogenic** illness. This consumer may say that he was happier when psychotic, because he was not obese and was able to play football. Similarly, sexual dysfunction, which is common to many antidepressants and some antipsychotics, may cause significant relationship issues for consumers that are worse than their initial illness.

Special consideration of medication use during pregnancy and breastfeeding

Many mental health conditions are diagnosed during the peak reproductive years – for example, bipolar disorder and depression. Left untreated, mental illness can pose a significant threat to the woman, unborn child, infant and family as a whole. For example, depression that is not identified and/or untreated can pose a high risk. Therefore, in supporting the pregnant woman it is essential that the multidisciplinary team understands and considers the use of the psychotropic medications during the **perinatal period**, extending from the antenatal period through to the postnatal period and includes breastfeeding considerations.

CASE **STUDY**

MEDICATION MANAGEMENT DURING THE PERINATAL PERIOD

You are on clinical placement in the perinatal unit and working with the mental health nurse on this team. You have the opportunity to meet a consumer who is expecting her first child when she attends her scheduled appointment. Nula is 33 years of age. This is a planned pregnancy and Nula and her husband have a number of supports in place, including her parents who will help care for the baby when it is born. Nula has a diagnosis of a mental health condition that they have been managing with medications for the past 12 years. She is on a tapered dose of her medication and is keen to breastfeed her baby. They are under the care of the perinatal mental health team, which also includes the psychiatrist, a midwife, the obstetrician and general practitioner (GP).

Questions

1 What education is important to provide to Nula regarding breastfeeding and taking antidepressant medications?
2 Lithium is a mood stabiliser and is said to have teratogenic properties. What does this term mean?
3 What are the risks to the developing foetus if a pregnant woman continues to take lithium during her pregnancy?

Table 4.2 outlines two examples of psychotropic medications that have specific considerations for use in the perinatal period.

PSYCHOSOCIAL INTERVENTIONS

How often have you heard someone say (or even said yourself), 'I wish I could stop smoking', 'I've tried cutting back on my drinking but haven't had any success' or 'I self-harm because I don't know how else to deal with these emotions'? Statements such as these (and there are many more similar statements that you will hear in the course of your work with consumers) all reflect a desire to change a particular behaviour. However, changing or modifying a behaviour is not always straightforward and people often find they try several times before change is successful. Simply having the knowledge that behaviour change is required is not sufficient to produce that change or maintain change over the longer term. Translating knowledge into specific, observable behaviour change is influenced by a range of factors. These factors include **values**, **attitudes**, **beliefs**, motivation and external factors. In order for behaviour change to be successful, the individual must develop a new set of understandings and practical and interpersonal skills.

The remainder of this chapter looks at a range of approaches that can be used by people who are seeking to change some aspect of their behaviour. Where relevant, the theoretical framework underpinning each approach is also reviewed to help you understand the concepts of each approach and the strategies involved.

MOTIVATIONAL INTERVIEWING

Motivational interviewing is a person-focused directive counselling approach that aims to help a person engage in behaviour change. It does this by increasing the individual's motivation to change by helping the person reconcile the tension between their ambivalence towards, and their desire for change. The primary goal of motivational interviewing is to assist a person to implement changes in specific behaviours by helping them

TABLE 4.2
Psychotropic medications with specific considerations for use in perinatal period

DRUG GROUP AND EXAMPLE	CONSIDERATIONS DURING THE PERINATAL PERIOD INCLUDING BREAST FEEDING
Mood stabilisers (lithium)	Category D drug Lithium is not administered during the first trimester, which makes it difficult for unplanned pregnancies. Appropriate psychoeducation for women on lithium who are in child-bearing years is very important. The most common malformations are cardiovascular, particularly Ebstein's anomaly of the tricuspid valves. Use of lithium during pregnancy requires the lowest dose possible and strict monitoring of serum levels throughout the perinatal period.
Antipsychotics (clozapine)	Category C drug While there is conflicting evidence regarding the use of antipsychotics, generally case reports have noted adverse effects (e.g. metabolic complication, gestational diabetes, increased plasma levels of clozapine in the neonate and poor pregnancy outcomes). Due to significant side effects, clozapine is not recommended for use in pregnancy.

SOURCE: ADAPTED FROM THERAPEUTIC GOODS ADMINISTRATION, 2017

to identify the discrepancy between their current behaviour(s) and future goals, work through any resistance to change and support them as they implement change.

Motivational interviewing is based on the trans-theoretical model of change developed by Prochaska and DiClemente in the late 1970s. Its original application included the areas of smoking cessation, dietary changes, exercise and activity promotion, management of anxiety and panic disorders (Prochaska & Velicer, 1997; Taylor et al., 2006). Contemporary applications of this approach are seen in the areas of treatment adherence and substance use management. The trans-theoretical model is also referred to as the stages of change model. It is one of the most commonly applied psychological models in practice. The model proposes that change progresses through a number of stages. Relapse can occur at any time and the individual can revert to any stage. The strengths of the model are that it enables people to develop an understanding of where they are in terms of their behaviour change journey and what interventions can be used. The model is heavily focused on decision-making and making intentional change. The six stages of the trans-theoretical model are precontemplation, preparation, action,

maintenance, relapse and termination. **Table 4.3** outlines each of these stages and their meaning, along with examples of specific interventions.

Figure 4.3 shows the connection between various stages of the stages of change model. Importantly, it illustrates the major actions and challenges of each stage, that the stages of change model is not linear and that a person will move between stages at different times.

The five principles of motivational interviewing

Table 4.4 reviews the five fundamental principles of motivational interviewing. Rana and Upton (2013, p. 243), refer to these principles and the conditions for change.

Resistance (in contemporary terms, this is referred to as maintaining sustain talk) is a key term in motivational interviewing. In the context of motivational interviewing, resistance is seen in the behaviour of the consumer and refers to statements/behaviours around not wishing to engage in the behaviour change. Andrews et al. (2013) identify that resistance often reflects a conflict between the stage of change at which a consumer is currently and the counsellor's communication style. Resistance can be verbal or non-verbal and in the context of motivational interviewing is something the

TABLE 4.3
Stages of the trans-theoretical model

STAGE	DETAILS	EXAMPLE STATEMENTS FOR SMOKING
Precontemplation	A person is often unaware that certain behaviour is problematic, and there is no intention to take any action to change behaviour in the next six months.	'I don't have a problem. I can stop smoking any time I want.'
Contemplation	A person will be actively considering implementing changes to the desired behaviour. They recognise the change and have considered the benefits as well as negative aspects of changing behaviour. However, even with this consideration they may still feel ambivalent towards changing their behaviour.	'I am not enjoying this any more, maybe this isn't any good for me.'
Preparation	In this stage, a person begins to take small specific steps towards implementing a change in their behaviour. They have decided to change their behaviour in the next 30 days and believe that the intended behaviour change will result in a positive change.	'That's it, I'm sick of not being able to breathe after a cigarette. I'm quitting!'
Action	A person has implemented behaviour change and is actively working towards maintaining it. The action phase is recognised by specific strategies that modify problematic behaviour or adopt new healthy behaviours.	'I have bought the patches and stopped going outside with my work colleagues who smoke. I'm actually doing something!'
Maintenance	A person has sustained the changing behaviour for more than six months. Behaviour is geared towards preventing relapse.	'I haven't smoked for two years.'
Relapse	*	

*While relapse is not an actual stage in the trans-theoretical model, it can occur at any stage of the model. Relapse is seen when a person recommences the behaviour they are seeking to change (e.g. 'I thought I could have a cigarette every now and then. I'm back to smoking 15 cigarettes a day.')

SOURCE: ADAPTED FROM ANDREWS ET AL., 2013; RANA & UPTON, 2013; RESNICOW & MCMASTER, 2012

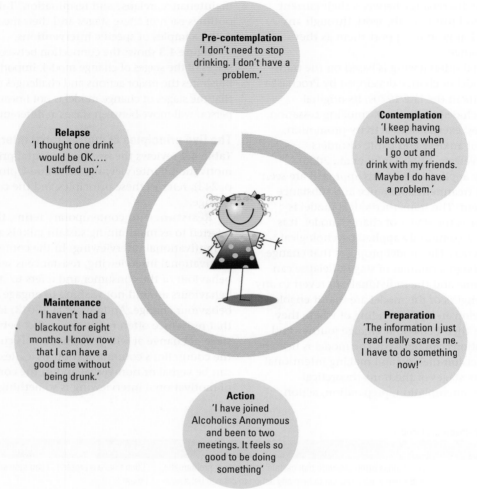

Pre-contemplation
'I don't need to stop drinking. I don't have a problem.'

Contemplation
'I keep having blackouts when I go out and drink with my friends. Maybe I do have a problem.'

Relapse
'I thought one drink would be OK.... I stuffed up.'

Preparation
'The information I just read really scares me. I have to do something now!'

Maintenance
'I haven't had a blackout for eight months. I know now that I can have a good time without being drunk.'

Action
'I have joined Alcoholics Anonymous and been to two meetings. It feels so good to be doing something'

FIGURE 4.3
Stages of change model

TABLE 4.4
Five principles of motivational interviewing

PRINCIPLE	EXPLANATION
Express empathy	• Empathy is expressed through effective listening skills and the understanding by the counsellor that **ambivalence** is normal.
Develop discrepancy	• The consumer rather than the clinician/counsellor should present the arguments for change. • Change is motivated when the consumer recognises a discrepancy between their present behaviour and their personal goals.
Avoid arguing	• Confrontation by the counsellor will only lead to increased resistance from the consumer to change.
Roll with resistance (in contemporary terms, this is referred to as maintaining sustain talk)	• The role of the clinician/counsellor is to reduce resistance. • If resistance increases, the clinician/counsellor needs to be able to utilise different strategies. • The consumer's objections do not demand a response. • The consumer finds their own answers and solutions.
Support self-efficacy	• A consumer's belief in the possibility of change is a motivator. • The counsellor's belief in the consumer's ability to change is a motivator. • The consumer is responsible for choosing and carrying out change.

SOURCE: RANA & UPTON, 2013

TREATMENT MODALITIES UTILISED IN CONTEMPORARY MENTAL HEALTH SERVICE DELIVERY **55**

clinician must expect as part of the change process that a person can experience. It often reflects great ambivalence. Maintaining a non-judgemental and respectful approach to the consumer is essential. Resistance that is not resolved contributes to less successful outcomes in terms of behaviour change.

Behaviours that can indicate resistance include arguing, interrupting, ignoring and denial. For example, arguments could involve the clinician challenging or discounting the ideas and views of the consumer. The clinician who constantly talks over the consumer is more likely to experience resistance from them; when someone feels they are not being paid attention to or are being side-tracked during the conversation, they are less likely to engage in the change process. Particular behaviours that represent denial can include disagreement, making excuses, minimising the issue, being pessimistic or unwilling to change. Motivational strategies include:

1 giving advice about specific behaviours
2 assisting consumers to access relevant supports
3 providing choice and encouragement to change rather than demanding change
4 increasing the desirability of making a change by helping the consumer work through their ambivalence
5 practising empathy
6 providing feedback

7 clarifying goals
8 actively helping (Rana & Upton, 2013).

The *how to* of motivational interviewing involves using a range of strategies. Effective communication is key in implementing the process of motivational interviewing. In the first instance, it is essential that the clinician establishes a rapport with the consumer. For the consumer to move forward and implement behavioural change, they have to trust the clinician. Consistency, unconditional positive regard and genuineness are all crucial in establishing trust and rapport. Another key element of the *how to* of motivational interviewing is working collaboratively to an agenda. Setting small achievable goals and prioritising them is more likely to achieve positive outcomes than trying to change multiple behaviours at the same time. Other specific tasks include identifying ambivalence and addressing resistance (Miller & Rollnick, 1991).

Application of motivational interviewing to practice

Motivational interviewing is utilised in a variety of clinical applications. These include smoking cessation, weight loss, as a strategy to promote adherence to medication regimens and, in particular, working with consumers who experience substance-use problems. **Table 4.5** and **Figure 4.4** show a cycle of change and interventions for a consumer experiencing substance abuse disorder (SUD).

TABLE 4.5
Cycle of change and interventions for consumers experiencing SUD

STAGE OF CHANGE	INDICATIONS	EVIDENCE	GOALS	INTERVENTIONS
Pre-contemplative: resistance to recognise or modify problem	The consumer feels coerced into attending a service or health professional and does not recognise their problem or is not really interested in changing their behaviour.	'I don't have a problem.' 'I'm here because my parents/partner/friends/ court want me or order me to come.'	To facilitate consideration that there is a substance use problem. To reduce the harms associated with substance use behaviour.	Raising awareness: • Use opportunities of engagement to raise awareness of SUD. • Take opportunities to introduce education about SUD. • Use harm minimisation strategies to reduce harm associated with substance use. • Provide education, support and resources for carers/family/ friends of consumer with SUD. • Continue with education and harm minimisation.

STAGE OF CHANGE	INDICATIONS	EVIDENCE	GOALS	INTERVENTIONS
Contemplative: serious consideration of problem resolution	The consumer becomes aware of the impact of their substance use, and the benefits for change; however, is not ready to make a commitment to take action.	'I love getting high but I'm getting sick of the comedowns.' 'I'm weighing up the pros and cons.'	To facilitate the development of awareness of problematic substance use. To identify potential at-risk themes or deviations in mental state related to the development of insight into substance use behaviour.	Resolve ambivalence and help to choose change: • Facilitate development of insight into risks versus benefits of substance use. This may include modelling setting short-term goals that foster small rewards to reinforce benefit; e.g. projecting money saved from reduced use that can be spent on other things the client values that build upon protective factors. • Identify themes of guilt, shame or hopelessness as insight develops into substance use behaviour as these may indicate an increase in risk and require additional supportive measures.
Preparation: early stirrings of action stage	The consumer is intending or preparing to take action.	'I want to cut down on how much I'm taking.' 'I'm drinking two less stubbies or I start drinking after lunch instead of before lunch.'	To encourage and support the person to commit to change.	Help identify appropriate change strategies: • Explore goal for substance use: abstinence or controlled use. • Facilitate development of insight into triggers for substance use, identify and develop alternative coping strategies to reduced substance use. • Identify social supports.
Action: modification of the target behaviour with significant overt efforts to change	The consumer is engaging in action to reduce or stop their substance use.	'I am really working hard to change.'	To facilitate and support an action plan incorporating relapse prevention.	Help implement change strategies and learn to eliminate potential for lapse and/or relapse: • May involve medically supervised detox and rehabilitation program. • Formulate support post-rehabilitation and may involve outreach, regular specialists appointments, peer support groups, Alcoholics Anonymous, Narcotics Anonymous, involvement of identified support people, incorporation of activities such as physical exercise, work, hobbies. • Review and monitoring of treatment goals and strategies.
Maintenance: stabilising behaviour change and avoiding relapse	The consumer is successful in reducing or stopping their substance use. This phase incorporates the formulation of important lapse and relapse strategies.	'I need to have regular appointments so that I stay on track.' 'My family/work, etc. are really stressful and I'm concerned that these may trigger me to use.'	To support ongoing change and development and modification of relapse prevention.	Develop new skills for maintaining recovery: • Facilitate insight and reflection of SUD patterns of use and associated behaviours. This will involve skill building to avoid lapses, preventing lapses becoming relapses and reducing the negative consequences of relapse.

SOURCE: ANDREWS ET AL., 2013, PP. 296–8; BRAY, KOWALCHUK & WATERS, N.D., SLIDE 4; O'DONNELL & GOLDING, N.D.; PROCHASKA, DICLEMENTE & NORCROSS, 1992, PP. 1103–4

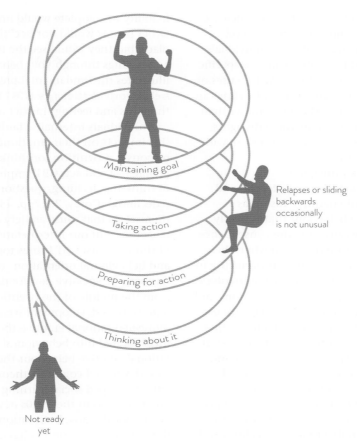

FIGURE 4.4
Moving through the cycle of change

MINDFULNESS-BASED INTERVENTIONS

Mindfulness is a self-awareness intervention that has been adapted from Buddhist mindfulness meditation. It is focused on the principle of being aware of an event in the present moment (psychologically, emotionally and physically), rather than reflecting back on it. This is done with a non-judgemental, non-reactive and accepting attitude. Mindfulness training is used by people to reduce stress and improve personal health and well-being.

Meditation is the most effective way in which to develop mindfulness skills. Meditation involves techniques that focus on awareness of one's own physical and emotional responses by developing concentration, clarity and calmness. Mindfulness training can be practised as a discrete entity, but it is also being increasingly incorporated into a number of therapeutic approaches. Several commonly utilised mindfulness approaches are outlined below.

Mindfulness-integrated cognitive behaviour therapy

The mindfulness-integrated cognitive behaviour therapy (MiCBT) approach combines a range of techniques for mindfulness training together with principles of cognitive behaviour therapy (CBT). Cayoun (2014), describes a four-stage process for MiCBT.

1 In stage one, a person learns the skills of mindfulness.
2 In stage two, a person applies the skills they have learned to their everyday lives to address feelings of discomfort.
3 In stage three, a person develops more effective interpersonal communication skills that they can use in emotionally challenging interactions.
4 In stage four, a person learns about self-care and caring for others in their daily lives.

Recent work by Sizoo and Kuiper (2017) suggests that both CBT and mindfulness-based stress reduction activities show promise as strategies for reducing anxiety and depression in adults with a diagnosis of autism spectrum disorder. They also suggest that MiCBT may provide a cohesive integration of these discrete approaches that could be researched further.

Acceptance and commitment therapy

Acceptance and commitment therapy (ACT) focuses on learning skills to help a person accept what is outside of their personal control and commit to action that enriches their lives. Attempts to control experiences such as anxiety will often be ineffective and increase the experience of distress and emotional turmoil. ACT also focuses on strategies that assist individuals to identify the values and translate them into specific achievable goals (Forman et al., 2007). ACT focuses on understanding that negative emotions and feelings are part of the human experience. Therefore, rather than either attempting to avoid or battle these thoughts, mindfulness techniques can help a person work with their thoughts in the here and now.

ACT is founded on six principles:

1 *Cognitive fusion/defusion:* Hayes, Pistorello and Levin (2012) represent cognitive fusion as thinking that leads to behaviour that is overly rigid and restricted because it is the consequence of repetitive negative thinking even when there are other positive events and aspects occurring in the individual's life. Cognitive defusion involves a process of considering how our perceptions and thoughts are represented in the language we use and are not set in stone. It is an objective rather than reactive process that helps a person to start understanding their experiences, thoughts and feelings in other ways. This helps to lessen the impact of negative thoughts as a person can begin to think differently about events and experiences.

2 *Expansion and acceptance:* This is the process of recognising uncomfortable thoughts, feelings and physical sensations and learning techniques to manage them rather than denying or trying to avoid them.

3 *Contact and connection with the present moment.*

4 *The observing self.*

5 *Values clarification:* the process of clarifying what is most important.

6 *Committed action* (AIPC, 2014; Harris, 2006; Hayes, Pistorello & Levin, 2012).

ACT has been utilised in working with consumers who experience anxiety and depression, chronic pain and anger management (Batten, 2011; Hayes, Pistorello & Levin, 2012). For example, using the principles outlined above, an ACT therapist would work with a consumer who is experiencing negative thoughts about their self-worth to assist them to develop psychological flexibility in terms of how they respond to their thoughts and feelings, being able to tolerate distressing/negative thoughts, develop skills to be present in the here and now and increase their openness to experience.

COGNITIVE BEHAVIOURAL THERAPY

Imagine you worked for several months to improve your fitness level in order to participate in a community marathon. Yet on the day of the marathon, you found that you could not finish the race because the route was much steeper than you had trained for. Your thoughts about this race and your inability to complete would impact on your feelings. Other people would not 'see' this process taking place; but they would see the impact of your thoughts and feelings through your behaviour. This example illustrates the fundamental premise of **cognitive behavioural therapy (CBT)** – that is, your thoughts and feelings impact on your behaviour.

Individuals internalise faulty thinking, and this impacts on their emotional and behavioural responses. Cognition (or thinking) governs how people feel and act. CBT emphasises 'the role of thinking, deciding, questioning, doing and redeciding' (Corey, 2017, p. 432). It is not events themselves that cause anxiety and maladaptive responses, but our interpretations and expectations of those events. CBT brings together the cognitive and behavioural orientations of psychology. There has been progressive development of CBT approaches from the middle of the twentieth century. Key figures in its development were Albert Ellis, who pioneered rational emotive therapy, which he later incorporated into behavioural strategies and renamed rational emotive behaviour therapy; Aaron Beck, who developed cognitive theory; Albert Bandura, who developed social learning theory; and Marsha Linehan, who in the 1990s developed dialectical behaviour therapy. Both rational emotive behaviour therapy and dialectical behaviour therapy are explored in more detail later in this chapter.

Based on the idea that therapy is an active learning process, CBT is educational and collaborative – it stresses the importance of learning new skills, ways of thinking about events and developing alternative coping strategies to more successfully manage stress (Corey, 2017). Behaviour theory maintains that behaviour is acquired, maintained and changed by conditioning and reinforcement. The behavioural component of CBT emphasises interventions that are focused on *doing* something, not merely talking (Frew & Spiegler, 2012). Activities such as keeping diaries and doing homework tasks are clear examples of the behavioural component of CBT.

The cognitive component of CBT maintains that irrational beliefs can distort reality, result in illogical evaluations (of self, others and the world), and may cause widespread harm (stop people achieving goals, distressing emotional surges, harmful behaviours); that is, behaviour is controlled by our thoughts.

CBT works on the premise that maladaptive responses result from cognitive distortions (positive or negative). Modifying thoughts (by cognitions and behavioural techniques) can improve emotional (feelings) and behaviour problems as people learn that not all negative emotions are wrong and not all positive emotions are functional.

Examples of common cognitive distortions are shown in **Table 4.6**.

TABLE 4.6
Common cognitive distortions

COGNITIVE DISTORTION	DEFINITION	EXAMPLE
Overgeneralisation	When a person decides that based on the outcome of one event/situation/interaction the same outcome is going to happen each time that event/situation/interaction takes place.	'All people from that country are like that.'
Personalisation	Believing that all outcomes are directly attributable to something the individual has done or said.	'If this doesn't work for us, it must be something I have done wrong.'
Dichotomous thinking	All or nothing thinking or thinking in black and white terms. The individual thinks in terms of something being good or bad/right or wrong.	'If I don't follow the exact process step by step and get it absolutely perfect, then I am a failure.'
Catastrophising	Thinking of the worst possible outcome.	'I know you don't think it much to worry about, but this is the end of everything.'
Perfectionism	Thinking that if everything is not perfect, then the individual has failed.	'If this isn't 100% successful then I failed and I'm useless.'
Pessimism	The automatic presumption that things will not work out or be successful.	'Nothing I do ever works out. I give up.'
Jumping to conclusions	Thinking that others will react, or are reacting, negatively without evidence to support that thought.	'People are always looking at me when I try to say something at meetings. They think I don't know what I'm talking about.'

SOURCE: ADAPTED FROM BERNSTEIN ET AL., 2018; CHOUDHURY, 2013; COREY, 2017; ELLIS & JOFFE ELLIS, 2011

CBT has been widely applied in clinical practice to the treatment of depression, anxiety, interpersonal relationships, substance use and phobias, and in assertiveness training.

Aaron Beck's cognitive theory

Corey (2017) credits Aaron Beck as being a major contributor to the development of **cognitive theory (CT)**, which was based on empirical research and developed at the same time as Ellis was developing rational emotive behaviour therapy. Research focused on the use of cognitive theory in treating consumers with depression. Ongoing work by therapists who have adopted Beck's ideas use cognitive therapy in their work with people experiencing panic disorder phobias and post-traumatic stress disorder. Beck describes that a person who is depressed experiences cognitive distortions (such as those described in **Table 4.4**), which impact their interpretation of life events in a negative way. The key term developed in Beck's early work is the **negative cognitive triad**, which involves three components. The first component relates to a negative view of oneself which is characterised by the person being overly critical about themselves. The second component represents a negative view of their personal world and, finally, an inability to view a hopeful or positive future (Corey, 2017). Beck also recognised that depression did not result just from disrupted cognitive processes, but that biological, environmental and biochemical processes

could contribute to its development. However, what maintained a person's experience of depression was this negative triad, regardless of the cause of the depression. This early work has been developed and expanded over half a century. As a result, Beck has developed a generic cognitive model that is based on a series of principles. These principles include: the way in which an individual responds to a situation or problems using their normal coping strategies in an exaggerated or disproportionate way; the use of distorted thinking patterns; beliefs that specifically reinforce the person's emotional or psychological distress; and the concept that when a person changes their beliefs, they begin the process of change in their emotional responses and behaviours (Beck & Haigh, 2014).

Cognitive therapy is an active insight–focused therapy and has a strong educational component. Therapy focuses on assisting consumers to understand 'the links between their thoughts, behaviours, emotions, physical responses, and situations' (Greenberger & Padesky, 2016, cited in Corey, 2017, p. 284).

The process of cognitive therapy has three main steps:

1 The person identifies the dysfunctional thinking.
2 The counsellor assists the person to examine and weigh the evidence for and against the dysfunctional thoughts that have been identified. The strategies of Socratic dialogue with the

counsellor, completing homework, collecting information on assumptions they have made, and forming alternative interpretations are various strategies used.

3 The counsellor acts as a guide and facilitates the person's developing insight regarding the dysfunctional thinking patterns and the way they feel and behave (adapted from Corey, 2017).

Beck, who was born in 1921, has continued to write as recently as 2016. Beck and Bredemeier (2016) proposed that depression is an individual's attempt or adjustment to conserve energy after the perceived loss of an important factor in their life such as a personal relationship or significant personal possession. The individual's capacity to reduce the negative impact of that loss is unsuccessful. This definition shows how Beck and colleagues continue to recognise that depression can be a response to a variety of factors and go on to present a unified model of depression.

RATIONAL EMOTIVE BEHAVIOUR THERAPY

Rational emotive behaviour therapy (REBT) is an action-oriented approach to emotional growth that emphasises an individual's capacity for creating their emotions; the ability to change and overcome the past by focusing on the present; and the power to choose and implement satisfying alternatives to their current patterns of behaving.

Key concepts of REBT

The central idea underpinning REBT is that people develop irrational beliefs from others as children and take these beliefs forward into their own lives and relationships with others as adults (Corey, 2017). Ellis says there are three basic irrational beliefs that people internalise. Ellis developed his original ideas in relation to irrational beliefs that people internalise. These irrational beliefs are characterised by thinking that is over-exaggerated, catastrophising, judgemental of self and/or others, demanding, and that leads to negative emotional responses. Some examples include the beliefs that a person must be perfect at everything they do and how they should be treated by others (Ellis & Joffe Ellis, 2011).

REBT was developed by Albert Ellis and uses what Ellis termed the ABC and ABCDE framework (Ellis & Joffe Ellis, 2011). The letter A stands for the activating event or situation, B refers to the individual's beliefs about those events and C refers to the cognitive emotional or behavioural consequences of all the beliefs the individual holds. The framework is designed to show the interrelationship between these components. **Figure 4.5** illustrates the ABC framework.

As part of the therapeutic process, D comes after C. D refers to disputing the irrational beliefs, which involves detecting, debating and discriminating them. Following this, the person is encouraged to develop a new belief system that is more effective; this is referred to as E. Taken together, **Figure 4.6** illustrates the complete ABCDE framework.

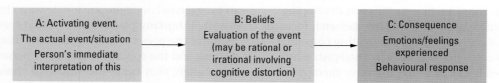

The person's emotional and behavioural response will be dependent on the extent to which their beliefs about the activating event are rational or irrational.

FIGURE 4.5
The ABC framework

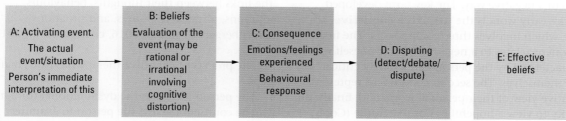

FIGURE 4.6
The ABCDE framework

As with all cognitive behavioural therapies, the therapeutic process for REBT is a collaborative one and the counsellor is responsible for facilitating the client's recognition of irrational versus rational thoughts and their relationship or connection to realistic or unrealistic goals, and to learn how to change their thinking patterns and subsequently their behaviour. Another key role of the counsellor is to facilitate the person's journey towards self-acceptance, acceptance of others and acceptance of life as it is (Ellis & Joffe Ellis, 2011). Techniques such as homework tasks (reading, written assignments such as journal writing) and experiential activities form the link between therapy sessions. Clients bring their completed 'homework' to review with their therapist. Thoughts and actions that can be used to replace current ineffective patterns of behaviour can be identified and taken away to practice.

DIALECTICAL BEHAVIOUR THERAPY

Dialectical behaviour therapy (DBT) was originally developed by therapists working with people who had a diagnosis of borderline personality disorder. Developed by Marsha Linehan in the late 1980s and 1990s (Linehan, 1993a), dialectical thinking is a cornerstone concept that refers to the individual's ability to find the balance between conflicting feelings and behaviours that they are experiencing (Cormier, Nurius & Osborn, 2009).

DBT was developed from what Pederson (2015, p. 27) identifies as a 'biosocial theory that emotional dysregulation transacts with invalidating environments'. DBT is strongly influenced by behavioural and cognitive behavioural therapies. From a behavioural perspective, DBT focuses on identifying antecedents – that is, the events preceding behaviours and triggers or prompting events for those behaviours. The therapist and consumer will also analyse the consequences that follow those behaviours both in terms of the immediate reactions as well as the longer-term repercussions that increase the likelihood (reinforce) that those behaviours will be repeated (Pederson, 2015).

DBT also draws heavily on CBT in that the therapist and consumer will also analyse the internal processes occurring during interactions and in various situations experienced by the consumer. However, DBT has a stronger emphasis on the emotions the person experiences, as opposed to CBT where there is a greater emphasis on the person's thinking patterns and interpretations of an event or interactions (Marra, 2005).

DBT shares an action-oriented problem-solving and educative focus similar to behavioural therapy and CBT. Key processes that demonstrate this are contingency management, systematic skills training from behavioural therapy and self-monitoring from CBT.

DBT is a structured process and includes the application of four core skills:
1   core mindfulness skills
2   interpersonal effectiveness skills
3   emotion regulation skills
4   distress tolerance skills (Linehan, 1993b).

Core mindfulness skills focus on learning skills of mindfulness. This is described as being able to observe, describe and participate in interactions as well as focusing on internal processes such as thoughts and emotions and learning to do this without labelling these experiences as 'good' or 'bad'. Rather, they are seen as experiences that have happened or are happening. The goal is to promote feelings of self-acceptance and learning to not avoid uncomfortable or negative thoughts, emotions or experiences (Keng, Smoski & Robins, 2011; Linehan, 1993b).

Emotion regulation skills include observing and describing:
1   the event prompting a particular emotion
2   how one (cognitively) interprets it
3   how one (subconsciously) experiences it (including autonomic nervous system response)
4   the behaviours that express it
5   how it affects functioning (Linehan, 1993b, p. 84).

Interpersonal effectiveness looks at practising and using assertive communication skills in interactions with others, while promoting distress tolerance skills assists the individual to develop ways of responding to stress that are less harmful than the coping strategies they may be using.

The following case study outlines how mental health nurses trained in DBT might work with consumers in the area of emotional regulation.

CASE **STUDY**

DIALECTICAL BEHAVIOUR THERAPY

Sylvia is 24 years old. She is attending an appointment with her case manager. Sylvia has experienced a series of relationship problems. She has been in several relationships which she describes as being wonderful to begin with, but she always feels she is going to be let down, and in the end each relationship ended with a great deal of drama.

Sylvia feels she has invested so much in each relationship and is 'over the moon' when they start, but then inevitably things 'go bad…I realise it won't be the happy ending…we start fighting, they say I am a slut the way I flirt with other men and I just want to curl up and die…It wasn't meant to be like this. I want to reach out to my family but we end up fighting, so I just stay away. I lock myself away emotionally and the only way I can cope is to cut myself… they never understand and it ends then.'

Sylvia's case manager has completed training in dialectical behaviour therapy. She explains the process of this approach and believes it may help Sylvia to manage her emotions, particularly negative ones. Sylvia agrees to 'give it a go'.

Questions

1   The case manager speaks with Sylvia regarding the strong emotions that she experiences and how often the emotions impact on Sylvia's behaviour. How could the case manager explain the process of emotional regulation?

2   Sylvia has previously used self-harm when unable to cope with strong negative emotions. In learning distress tolerance skills, what other strategies could Sylvia use if she feels she needs to use self-harming behaviour when experiencing strong negative emotions?

3   What challenges do you feel the nurse may experience when working with Sylvia on developing her skills in managing negative emotions? What support resources and strategies would assist the nurse?

SAFETY FIRST

WORKING WITHIN SCOPE OF PRACTICE

Safe nursing practice in mental health requires that nurses work within their scope of practice. This is stipulated as part of the requirements for registration by nurses through the code of ethics, professional standards and professional conduct. Mental health nurses are not therapists or counsellors. They use their knowledge of the principles of psychosocial approaches to inform their practice, but they do not practise as therapists, which requires specific training, education and supervision. An example of this is that nurse practitioners with this specialist education and training may employ such therapeutic interventions as part of their role. These professional standards and the relevant legislation also determine the registered nurse's responsibilities and accountability in relation to the administration of medications.

STRUCTURED PROBLEM SOLVING

Structured problem solving (also referred to as problem-solving therapy) is a practical approach to helping people identify and implement strategies to deal with everyday issues. Andrews et al. (2013) identify a six-step structured problem-solving process. These steps are:

- Step 1: identify the problem.
- Step 2: brainstorm possible solutions.

- Step 3: evaluate each solution.
- Step 4: choose the optimal solution.
- Step 5: develop and implement a plan of action.
- Step 6: evaluate the effectiveness of the chosen solution.

Structured problem solving has been applied in working with consumers who are experiencing anxiety and depression. It is a collaborative process that sits well within recovery-oriented practice. Pierce (2012) states that it is a practical, effective and easily learned process. It is underpinned by social problem-solving theory, which posits three major concepts: problem solving, the actual problem and the solution (D'Zurilla & Goldfried, 1971; D'Zurilla, Nezu & Maydeu-Olivares, 2004). Problem solving is described as the process a person goes through to develop a solution to a problem. The problem is viewed as any issue that interferes with living and needs to be resolved. The problem may be a practical or interpersonal one. The solution is the specific response implemented after the person has engaged in the problem-solving process (D'Zurilla, Nezu & Maydeu-Olivares, 2004). Another important distinction in this theory is between problem solving and solution implementation. Problem solving is a cognitive process of finding possible solutions to a specific problem, whereas solution implementation refers to the skills used to implement the solutions (D'Zurilla, Nezu & Maydeu-Olivares, 2004). This distinction can be seen in the six-step process outlined above, where steps one to four are concerned with the problem-solving process and steps five and six relate specifically to the implementation and evaluation of the chosen solution.

It is important that people develop confidence in using a problem-solving approach. Therefore, it is essential to begin working with issues or concerns that a person is more likely to achieve success in resolving, and building their sense of self-efficacy as they begin to tackle problematic issues.

Figure 4.7 provides an example of the structured problem-solving process.

PSYCHOEDUCATION

Your journey towards becoming a registered nurse involves provision of sound, evidence-based education. The need for this type of education is no less important for consumers with a diagnosis of a mental health condition. When you understand the principles underpinning a particular clinical intervention, you are more likely to implement that clinical skill with confidence and maintain practice on an ongoing basis. When a consumer understands their illness and the various treatment options available

to them, they are more likely to feel confident in following the strategies that they have developed with the multidisciplinary team. **Psychoeducation** involves information and education that focus on the consumer's knowledge and understanding and strategies for managing their condition (Lefley, 2009). It involves information and education about a mental health condition, signs and symptoms, and treatment options available. But for the psychoeducation to be truly part of recovery-oriented practice, it must be a collaborative process between the consumer *and must* involve their active participation and contribution. For example, what does a consumer really know about their mental health condition? What strategies have they used previously that have been effective?

Mental health nurses have a role to play in providing psychoeducation in a recovery-oriented framework. This includes an advocacy role, education regarding home care and strategies, and supporting consumers as they develop their own personal health and well-being plans.

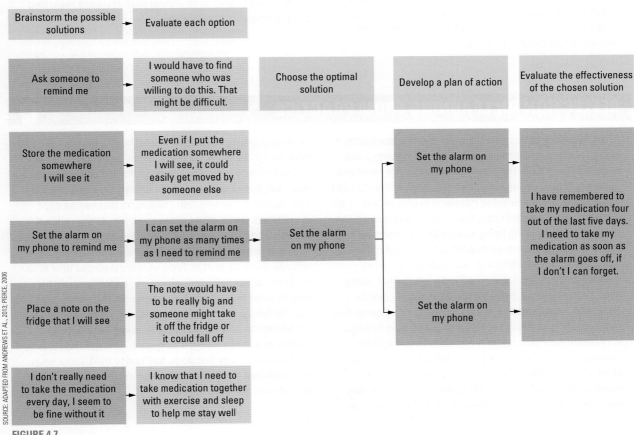

SOURCE: ADAPTED FROM ANDREWS ET AL., 2013; PIERCE, 2006

FIGURE 4.7
The structured problem-solving process

SECTION 1

EVIDENCE-BASED PRACTICE

Anti-psychotic medication side effects

Title of study

Living with antipsychotic medication side effects: The experience of Australian mental health consumers

Authors

Paul Morrison, Tom Meehan and Norman Jay Stomski

Background

While mental health consumers experience benefits from taking prescribed antipsychotic medications, people who take the prescribed medications can still experience a relapse episode. However, the relapse rates for consumers with a diagnosis of schizophrenia who do not take prescribed antipsychotic medication is even higher. Previous research indicates that the experience of side effects is a primary reason for non-adherence to prescribed antipsychotic medication. Therefore, it is essential for mental health nurses to understand consumers' experience of side effects from antipsychotic medications in order to collaborate management strategies with consumers.

Design

A phenomenological study was undertaken to understand the lived experience of side effects resulting from taking antipsychotic medication. Semi-structured interviews were held with ten consumer participants which were audio-taped and transcribed for analysis.

Results

Three major themes emerged relating to the impact of side effects, attitudes towards medications and side effects, and coping strategies to manage medication side effects.

Conclusions

Consumer participants described the high levels of sedation experienced from taking antipsychotic medication and the impact this had on their quality of life. Yet they did not complain about the side effects and, in some instances, were resigned to living with side effects if this led to a reduction in unpleasant and unwanted symptoms. When consumer participants did cease taking antipsychotic medication, it was often related to what the authors describe as 'dysphoric reactions' (p. 259); this was an intermittent occurrence. Self-help strategies by consumer participants to manage the side effects involved changing the dosage of the medication, using other forms of medication, using self-help strategies, personal support and ceasing their antipsychotic medication to relieve the side effects.

Implications

Nurses have a pivotal role in supporting consumers to enable them to take more control over decisions regarding their antipsychotic medication.

SOURCE: MORRISON, P., MEEHAN, T. & STOMSKI, N.J. (2015). LIVING WITH ANTIPSYCHOTIC MEDICATION SIDE EFFECTS: THE EXPERIENCE OF AUSTRALIAN MENTAL HEALTH CONSUMERS. *INTERNATIONAL JOURNAL OF MENTAL HEALTH NURSING*, 24(3), 253–61. DOI:10.1111/INM.12110

REFLECTION ON LEARNING FROM PRACTICE

At the beginning of this chapter, a perinatal mental health nurse reflected on their experience of working with Jodie. In the following days, the perinatal mental health nurse and Jodie spent time talking about the magnitude of the changes Jodie had experienced in her transition to parenthood. Jodie was also working with the psychologist. As a student, it can be scary contemplating being so direct with a consumer. However, as you have seen throughout this chapter, the many and varied psychosocial approaches used when working with consumers such as Jodie will involve asking such questions. Consumers will usually respond well to direct and open questions. In fact, for many consumers, their family and friends (while well-meaning) may have attempted to minimise their distress, or themselves became upset hearing that their loved one is not coping. One of the roles of the mental health nurse is to develop a rapport where expression of emotions, distress and feelings is welcome, and where this process enables the consumer to develop an understanding about their mental health and the need for help. One of the many ways the mental health team can aid in a consumer's recovery is through the use of medication. However, this chapter has also explored a number of other approaches to working with consumers that can be used in conjunction with medications or as standalone options. In Jodie's case, the perinatal mental health nurse used cognitive behavioural principles to provide feedback and positive reinforcement to Jodie as she developed new skills in caring for her baby and gaining more confidence in her role. Several days into Jodie's admission, she commented that the most powerful thing anyone had asked her during her admission was when the nurse asked her what she wanted to achieve from the admission. This question was the first opportunity that Jodie had had to think about what was important for her and made her feel that she mattered as a person, not just a mother.

CHAPTER RESOURCES

SUMMARY

- Pharmacological interventions are primary strategies used to help consumers manage symptoms of mental illness.
- Psychosocial interventions utilise a range of cognitive, behavioural and interpersonal strategies to help consumers identify issues, develop an understanding of factors contributing to these issues and strategies for addressing and/or managing them more effectively.
- Motivational interviewing comprises five principles that underpin its development and practice. These principles are: expressing empathy, rolling with resistance, developing discrepancy, avoiding argumentation and supporting self-efficacy.
- Mindfulness-based therapy is a useful way to help people reduce stress and improve personal health and well-being through meditation mindfulness training.
- CBT brings together the cognitive and behavioural orientations of psychology. There is an emphasis on cognition, decisions and consequences. It is not an event itself that creates anxiety and maladaptive responses, but a person's interpretations and expectations of that event.
- The key elements of rational emotive behaviour therapy are described in the ABCDE framework.
- Dialectical behaviour therapy aims to enhance a person's capacity to deal with the difficulties they experience in managing their emotional responses to interactions and events. The key elements are: core mindfulness skills, emotional regulation, distress tolerance skills and interpersonal effectiveness.
- Structured problem solving is an easily understood practical approach to assisting consumers to identify issues impacting their daily lives and creating and implementing practical and achievable solutions.
- Psychoeducation is a key role of the mental health nurse in supporting consumers and families to understand and be empowered to manage their lives.

REVIEW QUESTIONS

1   The ABC framework developed by Albert Ellis shows the relationship between:
  a   A personal emotion experienced after an event, the resulting behaviour and their thoughts about it
  b   A person's interpretation of an event, their feelings towards it, and other people's reactions to the event
  c   The behaviour of other people in an event, the person's beliefs about that behaviour and emotional consequences they experience
  d   The event, the person's beliefs about the event and the emotional cognitive or behavioural to the event

2   Emily's family think she drinks too much and are worried about it. When they confront Emily, she says she knows she has a problem but doesn't know what to do about it. According to the trans-theoretical model of change, which stage is Emily at?
  a   Contemplation
  b   Preparation
  c   Precontemplation
  d   Action

3   In the trans-theoretical model of change, the action stage refers to:
  a   Taking small steps towards implementing a change
  b   Talking to friends and family about why they are going to make a change
  c   Implementing the strategies to change their behaviour
  d   Looking at what actions other people had taken and incorporating these into their behaviour change

4   Motivational interviewing is comprised of five principles. These include expressing empathy, rolling with resistance and avoiding argumentation. The other two principles are:
  a   Rolling with the punches and developing a plan
  b   Supporting the counsellor's suggestions and rolling with the punches
  c   Developing discrepancy and supporting the counsellor's suggestions
  d   Developing discrepancy and supporting self-efficacy

5   Construct a table and list the similarities and differences between rational emotive behaviour therapy and cognitive therapy.

6   You are asked to explain structured problem-solving to your fellow students. Choose a problem that many people experience in daily life (e.g. difficulty speaking in front of people). Using the six-step structured problem-solving format, outline the details of each step.

7   Consider the following questions:
- Have you ever decided that you wanted to change a certain behaviour?
- What reasons or factors influenced your decision to make that change?
- What factors helped you to make that change?
- Were there any barriers to making that change?
- How long did you maintain the change in behaviour?
  a   Using the trans-theoretical model, can you identify the feelings and behaviours you experienced at each stage?
  b   If you were to use this model in the future with the same behaviour, what would you do differently?

8   What psychoeducation would the mental health nurse provide to a consumer commencing antidepressants?

CRITICAL THINKING

1   What are the risks associated with using psychotropic medication during the perinatal period? What factors would the perinatal mental health team need to take into consideration?

2   What is the rationale for having a large number of health professionals on a mental team such as that which is supporting a pregnant woman with a history of mental illness?

3   A consumer has recently commenced on a medication with a known side effect of weight gain. The consumer has been told it is important to eat sensibly and exercise regularly. How could the mental health nurse use their understanding of the transtheoretical model of change to support a consumer to increase their level of exercise?

REFLECT ON THIS

Mindfulness-based stress reduction
Use the key term 'mindfulness-based stress reduction' to find journal papers on this topic.

1   What are current applications of mindfulness-based stress reduction in clinical practice?

2   What other treatment modalities might be useful in supporting people to develop and maintain resilience and emotional well-being during a time of crisis such as the COVID-19 pandemic?

Review the literature on two additional approaches outlined in this chapter, and consider the following questions.

3   How easy is it to access these various interventions?

4   What are the strengths and limitations of the approaches you have researched?

5   What knowledge, skills and attitudes does a mental health nurse need in order to implement one of these therapeutic approaches? What training is required?

6   Are these approaches within the scope of practice of different disciplines, such as nursing, paramedicine or psychology?

7   What is the role of consumers in promoting understanding of these therapeutic approaches to the community?

REFERENCES

Adams, M.P. & Urban, C.Q. (2013). *Pharmacology. Connections to Practice* (2nd edn). Boston, MA: Pearson Education.

Andrews, G., Dean, K., Genderson, M., Hunt, C., Mitchell, P., Sachdev, P. & Trollor, J. (2013). *Management of Mental Disorders* (5th edn). Sydney: School of Psychiatry, University of NSW.

Australian Institute of Professional Counsellors (AIPC). (2014). Six principles of acceptance and commitment therapy. Retrieved from http://www.aipc.net.au/articles/six-principles-of-acceptance-and-commitment-therapy.

Barlow, D., Durand, M. & Hofmann, S. (2017). *Abnormal Psychology: An Integrative Approach* (8th edn). South Melbourne: Cengage.

Batten, S. (2011). *Essentials of Acceptance and Commitment Therapy.* Thousand Oaks, CA: Sage Publications.

Beck, A.T. & Bredemeier, K. (2016). A unified model of depression. *Clinical Psychological Science*, 4(4), 596–619. doi:10.1177/2167702616628523

Beck, A.T. & Haigh, E.A.P. (2014). Advances in cognitive theory and therapy: The generic cognitive model. *Annual Review of Clinical Psychology*,10(1), 1–24. doi:10.1146/annurev-clinpsy-032813-153734

Bernstein, D.A., Pooley, J.A., Cohen, L., Goulthorp, B., Provost, S. & Cranney, J. (2018). *Psychology* (Australian & New Zealand 2nd edn). South Melbourne: Cengage Learning.

Bray, J., Kowalchuk, A. & Waters, V. (n.d.). *Brief Intervention Stages of Change and Motivational Interviewing.* InSight SBIRT Residency Training Program. Retrieved from https://bluepeteraustralia.files.wordpress.com/2012/12/stages-of-change1.pdf.

Cayoun, B.A. (2014). *Mindfulness-integrated CBT for Well-being and Personal Growth: Four Steps to Enhance Inner Calm, Self-Confidence and Relationships.* Hoboken, NJ: Wiley.

Choudhury, K. (2013). *Managing Workplace Stress the Cognitive Behavioural Way.* Springer India.

Corey, G. (2017). *Theory and Practice of Counseling and Psychotherapy* (10th edn). South Melbourne: Cengage Learning.

Cormier, S., Nurius, P.S. & Osborn, C.J. (2009). *Interviewing and Change Strategies for Helpers. Fundamental Skills and Cognitive-behavioural Interventions* (6th edn).Belmont, CA: Brooks Cole, Cengage Learning.

D'Zurilla, T.J. & Goldfried, M.R. (1971). Problem solving and behavior modification. *Journal of Abnormal Psychology*, 78(1), 107–26. doi:10.1037/h0031360

D'Zurilla, T.J., Nezu, A.M. & Maydeu-Olivares, A. (2004). Social problem solving: Theory and assessment. In E.C. Chang, T.J. D'Zurilla & L.J. Sanna (eds), *Social Problem Solving: Theory, Research, and Training* (pp. 11–27). Washington, DC: American Psychological Association.

Ellis, A. & Joffe Ellis, D. (2011). *Rational Emotive Behavior Therapy* (1st edn). Washington, DC: American Psychological Association.

Forman, E.M., Herbert, J.D., Moitra, E., Yeomans, P.D. & Geller, P.A. (2007). A randomised controlled trial of acceptance and commitment therapy for anxiety and depression. *Behaviour Modification*, 31(6), 772–99.

Frew, J. & Spiegler, M.D. (2012). *Contemporary Psychotherapies for a Diverse World: First Revised Edition.* Florence: Taylor and Francis.

Greenberger, D. & Padesky, C. (2016). *Mind over Mood: Change how you feel by changing the way you think*. New York, NY: The Guilford Press.

Harris, R. (2006). Embracing your demons: An overview of acceptance and commitment therapy. *Psychotherapy in Australia*, 12(4), 70–6. Retrieved from https://www.actmindfully.com.au/upimages/ Dr_Russ_Harris_-_A_Non-technical_Overview_of_ACT.pdf.

Hayes, S.C., Pistorello, J. & Levin, M.E. (2012). Acceptance and commitment therapy as a unified model of behavior change. *The Counseling Psychologist*, 40(7), 976–1002. doi:10.1177/0011000012460836

Jagers. J.L. (n.d). Change: Where am I? Retrieved from https:// leejagers.wordpress.com/2008/03/14/change-where-am-i.

Keng, S.L., Smoski, M.J. & Robins, C.J. (2011). Effects of mindfulness on psychological health: A review of empirical studies. *Clinical Psychology Review*, 31(6), 1041–56. doi:10.1016/j.cpr.2011.04.006

Lefley, H.P. (2009). *Family Psychoeducation for Serious Mental Illness*. New York; NY: Oxford University Press.

Linehan, M.M. (1993a). *Cognitive-behavioral Treatment of Borderline Personality Disorder*. New York: Guilford Press.

Linehan, M.M. (1993b). *Skills Training Manual for Treating Borderline Personality Disorder*. New York: Guilford Press.

Marra, T. (2005). *Dialectical Behavioral Therapy in Private Practice: A Practical and Comprehensive Guide*. Oakland, CA: New Harbinger Publications, Inc.

McKenna, L. & Mirkov, S. (2014). *McKenna & Mirkov's Drug Handbook for Nursing and Midwifery* (7th edn). Sydney: Lippincott Williams & Wilkins.

Miller, W.R. & Rollnick, S. (1991). *Motivational Interviewing: Preparing People to Change Addictive Behavior*. New York: Guilford Press.

Morrison, P., Meehan, T. & Stomski, N.J. (2015). Living with antipsychotic medication side-effects: The experience of Australian mental health consumers. *International Journal of Mental Health Nursing*, 24(3), 253–61. doi:10.1111/inm.12110 wall boy

O'Donnell, D. & Golding, J. (n.d.). *The Stages of Change Model, and Treatment Planning*. Retrieved from https://docplayer.net/2805564-David-o-donnell-james-golding.html.

Pederson, L.D. (2015). *Dialectical Behavior Therapy: A Contemporary Guide for Practitioners*. Somerset: John Wiley & Sons.

Pierce, D. (2012). Problem solving therapy: Use and effectiveness in general practice. *Australian Family Physician*, 41, 676–9.

Prochaska, J.O., DiClemente, C.C. & Norcross, J.C. (1992). In search of how people change. Applications to addictive behaviors. *American Psychologist*, 47(9), 1102–14. doi:10.1037/0003-066X.47.9.1102

Prochaska, J. & Velicer, W.F. (1997). The transtheoretical model of health behavior change. *American Journal of Health Promotion*, 12(1) 38–48. doi:10.4278/0890-1171-12.1.38

Rana, D. & Upton, D. (2013). *Psychology for Nurses*. London: Routledge.

Resnicow, K. & McMaster, F. (2012). Motivational interviewing: Moving from why to how with autonomy support. *International Journal of Behavioral Nutrition and Physical Activity*, 9, 19. doi:10.1186/1479-5868-9-19

Sizoo, B.B. & Kuiper, E. (2017). Cognitive behavioural therapy and mindfulness based stress reduction may be equally effective in reducing anxiety and depression in adults with autism spectrum disorders. *Research in Developmental Disabilities*, 64, 47–55. doi:10.1016/j.ridd.2017.03.004

Taylor, D., Bury, M., Campling, N., Carter, S., Garfield, N., Newbould, J. & Rennie, T. (2006). *A Review of the Use of the Health Belief Model (HBM), the Theory of Planned Behaviour (TPB) and the Transtheoretical Model (TTM) to Study and Predict Health Behaviour Change*. London: The Department of Practice and Policy, School of Pharmacy, University of London.

Therapeutic Goods Administration. (2017). *Prescribing Medicines in Pregnancy Database*. Retrieved from https://www.tga.gov.au/ prescribing-medicines-pregnancy-database.

CHAPTER 5

MENTAL HEALTH NURSING AS A THERAPEUTIC PROCESS

Gylo (Julie) Hercelinskyj

LEARNING OUTCOMES

Upon completion of this chapter, you should be able to:

5.1 Explain the centrality of interpersonal communication in mental health nursing as a therapeutic process

5.2 Explore the core elements of the communication process

5.3 Understand the fundamental skills of effective communication

5.4 Understand the elements of the therapeutic relationship as a helping relationship

5.5 Appreciate the importance of therapeutic use of self and engagement from the consumer's and carer's perspectives

5.6 Explain the development of the therapeutic relationship using Egan's helping model

5.7 Explore the application of the therapeutic relationship to specific clinical contexts, such as resistance/aggression and medication adherence

---

LEARNING FROM PRACTICE

My adrenaline runs, leaving a bitter taste in my mouth. My heart races; the body's fight or flight responses kick in, my hands begin to shake. Every sense is heightened. Do I run? Do I stay?

This is the feeling I get every time there is a code grey on my unit. But I'm happy I still get these responses…these *human* responses, because to not get them is to become desensitised to violence and I don't want that. Anger is nothing to be blasé about.

Over the years, it gets easier. I start to see the signs before the consumer escalates to the point where they project their anger onto others. It's not always predictable, but knowing the signs helps me to have some sense of control in what is such an unpredictable environment.

People say, 'How could you work in a place like that?' But they don't see that so often the driver of violence is fear…a loss of control…distress… and I can relate to these feelings

because I try to imagine what I would feel and what I would do if it were me.

I've worked in both eras: the one where seclusion was punitive, and now where we utilise strategies built on therapeutic processes. I much prefer to work in this era. I hope that the nurses of the future prefer to work in their era.

Adele, mental health nurse, with 20 years' experience

The mental health nurse in this vignette has described a number of common feelings experienced by nurses working in environments where emotions can run high. While utilising medication has an important place in mental health care, what do you think are some of the other skills the mental health nurse can use when engaging with consumers who are distressed? Why would adopting 'talk therapy' be superior to using only medications for some consumers?

INTRODUCTION

Chapter 2 explored some of the major psychological theories explaining human thinking and behaviour. Importantly, the chapter concluded with a look at how two nursing theorists have applied some of these ideas specifically to mental health nursing practice. Mental health nurses translate this understanding of human personality, emotion and behaviour through their interactions with consumers and carers. But, as part of the mental health team, exactly what type of interactions do mental health nurses engage in? Are they the types of interactions they would have with friends or family? If not, in what way(s) do they differ? Why is it important that they are different? What qualities, values, knowledge and skills do nurses require to work effectively and collaboratively with consumers and carers?

In this chapter, we look at the specific ways in which nurses use their knowledge and understanding of mental health and mental illness in their interactions with consumers and carers, enabling them to work collaboratively and therapeutically with people.

We first explore the knowledge, values and skills that mental health nurses utilise to work in a therapeutic context with consumers and carers. However, it is not enough to simply know or understand this knowledge and these skills – it is also important to 'see' how this understanding is central to the role of the mental health nurse through its application to a range of contexts. This chapter also considers the issues related to challenges in therapeutic practice for consumers, carers and mental health nurses.

INTERPERSONAL COMMUNICATION WITHIN THE NURSE–CONSUMER RELATIONSHIP

The core of mental health nursing practice is therapeutic engagement, with a particular interest in and strong emphasis on **communication** within the nurse–consumer relationship.

Communication allows the nurse to engage with consumers and their families and work collaboratively in meeting their health-related needs. It is the foundation on which nurses build the collegial relationships with peers and colleagues that are vital to effective health outcomes for consumers and their families.

In its broadest sense, communication refers to the messages that are sent and received between people. But the process itself is more involved than this brief description implies. For instance, who is involved in communicating? How many people can

communicate at any one time? In which direction do messages travel between people? How is a message understood and responded to? What increases the likelihood of successful communication or unsuccessful communication? Are there different types of communication? Why do people communicate?

On an everyday basis, communication allows us to get things done, such as arranging appointments, giving information to someone, or achieving goals by doing well in an interview or an exam. The inability to communicate can make it difficult to successfully realise these types of needs and goals.

In the context of mental health nursing practice, and for the remainder of this chapter, the focus will be on **interpersonal communication**. Interpersonal communication occurs at a level where we exchange information about ourselves, our experiences, and our thoughts and feelings with another person. It is a level of communication that deals with personal matters.

Why we communicate

People communicate for a variety of reasons: to share ideas, feelings and thoughts and to satisfy emtional and physical needs. Interpersonal communication is the way in which people learn about themselves. Our sense of identity develops from our interactions with others. We come to know ourselves based on how we interact with and react to others, and their reaction to us. This idea of interactions is key to interpersonal communication. The very nature of interpersonal communication is a reciprocal process where the people involved are interdependent during the communication cycle (Adler, Rosenfeld & Proctor, 2013). Interpersonal communication is fundamentally about the relationship between people, and the way in which we communicate with each other, and what we communicate about will reflect the type of relationship we have with another person. This is important because how and why we communicate with consumers and carers is very different to how we communicate with friends or family. Yet, both are relationships characterised by interpersonal communication.

Interpersonal communication consists of different yet interrelated messages. These messages are verbal, vocal and non-verbal. Verbal messages relate to the words that we use. Non-verbal messages are all about the way in which we behave. The words we use, in combination with our body posture, facial expression and eye contact, send a message during interpersonal communication. It is important to also mention the vocal quality of interpersonal communication. When we speak, our words carry a certain tone of voice – for example, we may emphasise some words more than others, we may speak quite fast or slowly or even punctuate our words with utterances such as sighs, and 'um' or 'ahh'. The vocal aspect of verbal communication represents the emotional tone, our physical health and our thought processes.

CORE ELEMENTS OF THE COMMUNICATION PROCESS

Communication is a reciprocal process, and the best way to understand the elements involved in interpersonal communication is to imagine it as a circular process. However, this is not a closed circle, as some of the elements involved in communicating have the potential to disrupt and/or enhance the process. **Table 5.1** identifies a range of elements that are involved in interpersonal communication.

These elements can also be represented visually, as shown in **Figure 5.1**.

EFFECTIVE COMMUNICATION SKILLS

Students often say, 'I am a really good listener. I talk to people all the time.' However, good communication skills involve more than simply talking to (or at) someone. In order to be good communicators, we must first be good listeners. Having heard the information we have been given, and made sense of, we can then respond. So while 'talking' is without doubt part of the process, we also need to listen. To develop an effective therapeutic relationship with consumers, carers and family, mental health nurses must have a robust set of communication skills to use.

TABLE 5.1
Elements of the communication process

ELEMENT IN THE COMMUNICATION PROCESS	EXPLANATION
Sender/receiver and receiver/sender	All people involved in interpersonal communication will take on both the role of sender (initiating communication by transmitting a message) and receiver (taking in the message, making sense of it and then sending a response back).
Message(s)	A series of signals sent to the receiver. The receiver takes these signals in through any one or more of the senses. For example, you walk past a person in the street and you notice (visual sense) that they look dishevelled and unkempt and as you get closer you smell (olfactory sense) a strong body odour. From this, you may make a judgement as to how well this person is caring for themselves.
Encoding	Producing a message through verbal or written means.
Decoding	Understanding the message received. This is done when we listen to what someone has said or we read a blog post, letter or email.
Feedback message	Sending a message back to the receiver. This message will reveal the extent to which you have understood the message, your own feeling(s) and reaction to it. Without feedback, the sender is unable to adapt, revise, restate or even retract their original message. For example, when a teacher does not receive any feedback from their class, it is more difficult for them to gauge the level of understanding and appropriately modify their original message or move forward with the learning activity.
Feedforward message	Information the sender provides before transmitting a message. For example, asking someone to sit down because you need to tell them something.
Noise	Noise can be external – the sounds around us from other people's conversations, comments to us and/or the activities people are engaged in. Noise can also be internal –that is, our thoughts, the internal self-talk that we engage in. Noise has the potential to influence the way in which we understand things through potential distortion of the message. This distortion will impact on how we filter communication from others, make judgements about what we consider important, and ultimately the degree to which we understand the message being transmitted.
Cultural context	Culture impacts on the way in which individuals, groups and communities interact with each other, their expectations regarding, and experience of, communication. Culture will impact on the social, gender and occupational roles of people and this will be reflected in the way in which people communicate and interact with others. Culture is not only related to ethnicity. Culture is also seen in the organisational context in which the mental health nurse works and even between different health disciplines.
Ethics	Effective and person-centred communication is ethical. Ethical communication is respectful, and bound by professional and ethical standards of practice.

SOURCE: ADAPTED FROM DEVITO, 2013; THOMPSON, 2011.

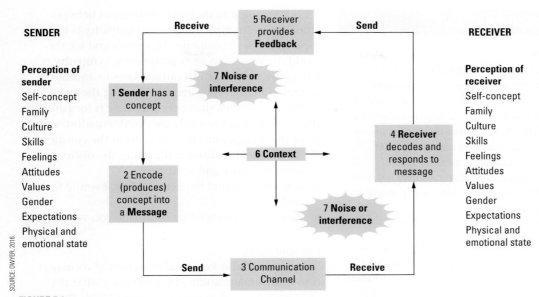

SOURCE: DWYER, 2016.

FIGURE 5.1
Elements of the communication process

Listening

Listening involves paying attention (or being attuned to) the whole message a person is sending. This means not just the verbal but also the non-verbal and vocal elements of communication. Non-verbal communication takes place physically through features such as our height, observed general level of fitness or even our weight. Posture, body movements, facial expressions, respiratory rate, general appearance and how close they stand to another person are just a few ways a consumer will communicate non-verbally with the mental health nurse.

It is also important to recognise how our own non-verbal communication impacts on the interaction with clients. We communicate non-verbally through the same channels as consumers, carers and their families. This highlights the reciprocal nature of interpersonal communication and the importance of developing self-awareness.

Egan (2014) uses the acronym SOLER to highlight some of the important skills that demonstrate being focused towards and paying attention to what another person is saying.

1   Facing the person *squarely*. This is the basic posture of involvement. It says: 'I am available to you'. The idea is to position yourself in a way that conveys the message that you are involved. If facing a person directly is a little too threatening or uncomfortable for them, a slightly angled position may be more effective. The key point is to sit in a way that shows your commitment to listening.

2   Maintaining an *open posture*. By doing this, you are adopting an open non-defensive posture.

3   *Leaning*. Inclining a little towards the other person can help to maximise the idea of involvement. But you also need to be sensitive to cultural and gender differences, as some people may find this uncomfortable. Take your cues from the other person.

4   Maintaining good *eye contact*. This means natural eye contact, not staring, but also not keeping your head down or staring into space.

5   Remaining relatively *relaxed*. This conveys the message that you feel 'at home' with the other person. It can also help to make the other person relax.

A sixth consideration is *vocal qualities* and *verbal tracking skills*. Tension can be heard verbally through increased rate of speech, increased volume and the way in which we keep pace with our responses to a person's message.

Observation skills

Think of observation skills as helping you to paint a picture of the consumer you are working with in terms of what you have observed about that person. Being observant of a person's communication means considering those non-verbal and physical aspects of their behaviour and interaction. For example, what is a person's posture like? Are they breathing rapidly? Do they look pale? Is their face flushed?

Having set yourself up physically to listen, you are now poised to do the work of listening. Listening as part of therapeutic communication is an active process, which is why you will often hear it referred to as 'active listening'. Listening in this context is vastly

CULTURAL CONSIDERATIONS

Respecting differences

Communication is a culturally sensitive process and care must be taken to be aware of and sensitive to cultural differences. While steady eye contact may be acceptable within some cultural groups, it can be very uncomfortable for other people. Mental health nurses must communicate in a culturally respectful, competent and safe manner. This means learning about another culture's values, beliefs and health care practices. Cultural safety requires that the mental health nurse behaves in a way that never alienates or humiliates another person.

different to hearing, partially listening or not listening at all. Egan describes effective listening as 'empathic listening' (2014, p. 82); that is, listening underpinned by empathy as a value. This is focused listening where the mental health nurse listens to the experiences, thoughts, behaviour and mood communicated by a consumer. This involves all aspects of the consumer's communication – verbal, non-verbal and vocal. The following skills represent key strategies to help you listen empathically.

Understanding and responding

There are a number of ways in which mental health nurses can respond to concerns and issues that consumers identify. But before you can respond, you need to understand what is being communicated to you. Understanding is crucial to working effectively with consumers and it is the mental health nurse's responsibility to utilise the necessary skills to establish understanding. Remember, however, that your understanding is only tentative until it is confirmed or negated by the consumer. You are seeking shared understanding, not your interpretation of what the consumer is sharing with you.

Understanding through empathy

Burnard (2005) viewed empathy as the capacity of the health professional to 'enter the perceptual world of another person' (p. 103). Empathy is both an attitude and a skill. As a skill, empathy enables the mental health nurse to demonstrate their understanding of the experience and the feelings underlying the experience. This requires the use of clear communication between the mental health nurse and consumer. When the mental health nurse demonstrates empathy, they have shown their capacity to enter into the consumer's world and get a feeling for what this world is like, as well as looking at the world through the other person's eyes or perspective. But this understanding is meaningless unless the mental health nurse can communicate their understanding of that person's feelings, experiences and behaviours back to them.

It is essential to make the distinction between empathy and sympathy. Whereas empathy is the capacity to be in someone else's shoes and see the world or event from their perspective, sympathy is where the mental health nurse relates to another person as though they are experiencing the event themselves. In this situation, the nurse is focusing on their own feelings towards the event/situation, which takes the therapeutic focus away from the consumer.

The following example illustrates the distinction between empathy and sympathy:

- *Sympathy:* 'If that happened to me, I would feel really angry.'
- *Empathy:* 'I can see that this made you very angry.'

Paraphrasing

Paraphrasing (also known as reflection of content) is to share understanding by rephrasing what the consumer has said in your own words. Note that the key word here is rephrase *not* restate, that is to acknowledge and summarise what is significant in the consumer's communication.

Paraphrasing demonstrates your intention to understand more fully, to share your tentative understanding with the person and seeking to ensure it is correct. It acknowledges what a person has said and demonstrates that you have listened. Effective paraphrasing enables the mental health nurse to give a clear message of what has been said.

When paraphrasing, we are attempting to produce a response that is interchangeable with what the client has said. We do this by rearranging the consumer's communication into a different order. This provides the opportunity for both the consumer and nurse to work on the information provided. Paraphrasing can also be used to provide feedback to the consumer, which again demonstrates listening and understanding of the core message being given.

An effective paraphrase neither adds to nor detracts from what the consumer has said. It is usually stated in a tentative manner, awaiting feedback on its accuracy.

Seeking clarification

We seek clarification whenever we are unsure about what a consumer is saying. Clarifying statements might include:

- 'I'm not sure I follow you...'
- 'Run that by me again...'
- 'I'm not certain what you mean...'

Stein-Parbury (2013) makes the point that when we request clarification, we are taking the responsibility for not understanding on ourselves. It is a request for more information or an example, so as to receive a clearer message. It is not meant to put the consumer on the defensive whereby they feel the need to justify themselves.

Reflection of feelings

Reflection of feelings relates to the mirroring of feelings expressed by another person. We attempt to rephrase indirect feelings in other words, verbalising what the other person has implied. We are all aware of our feelings to some extent and most of us are able to combine verbal, non-verbal and sensations to label these feelings. Accurately reflecting feelings allows consumers to feel that they have been heard. **Table 5.2** identifies several ways in which feelings can be shown.

TABLE 5.2
How a person may express feelings

REFLECTING FEELINGS	SIGNS
Physiological responses	Sweating, blushing, tears, goose bumps
Body language	The way a person sits, stands, gestures, etc.
Vocal qualities	A person's tone of voice, pitch, volume, pace of speech
Indirectly	Feelings can be inferred, such as 'You're not happy about being here, are you?'
Directly	Directly describing our feelings (e.g. 'I feel…')

The first task is to find a word that not only accurately describes the feeling, but also describes that feeling at the right intensity. This skill increases as your vocabulary of feeling words increases. It is not necessary to use the word 'feel' in every reflection you make. The aim is to integrate this skill into your overall style of responding.

Summarising

When we utilise the skill of summarising, we are putting together our understanding of what has been discussed. It is a brief and concise collection of paraphrases and feeling reflections that are accurately connected. Summarising allows us to check our understanding by verbalising it. It is most often used to bring an interaction to a close. (It is important to allow a consumer sufficient time to respond to this summary – do not rush.) Summarising is also useful when we want to rearrange the content of a message to give a new perspective on the information. It is also useful when we are losing touch with a consumer's story.

Probing skills

Egan (2014, p. 136) describes the skill of probing as a 'nudge'. When we probe through such skills as verbal and non-verbal prompting and asking questions, we are gently nudging someone to consider the issue they have identified more deeply, in a new way or to reaffirm their thoughts and feelings. The consumer remains at the centre of the therapeutic relationship and decision-making process.

Prompting

A prompt is a short verbal or non-verbal encouragement to confirm to the consumer that you are listening and to encourage them to keep talking. Non-verbal prompts can include any behaviour that shows interest and invites further conversation, such as leaning forward slightly when someone is talking or nodding in agreement. Verbal prompts are when phrases such as 'Go on', 'I see' or 'Okay' are intentionally and purposefully used to encourage further conversation.

Probing through questions

Questions can help consumers to explore, clarify and understand their feelings and thoughts. It assists the nurse in identifying what issues are facing a person and in gaining further information (Adler et al., 2013; Nelson-Jones, 1992).

Effective use of questions is a complicated communication skill. How helpful questions are depends on the degree of empathy established in the therapeutic interpersonal relationship and will determine how willing a person is to respond to questions. We can use questions as a way of demonstrating our genuineness and acceptance of the person. Questions that build on information already given are particularly useful. A second factor relates to how much control we wish to keep. The type of questions we ask will influence how much control a person feels they have over the direction the interaction is taking. Finally, questions need to be seen as relevant by the consumer. Only by viewing issues from the consumer's perspective can we ask questions that are relevant rather than appearing to hold an interrogation.

Purpose of questions

There are several reasons why asking questions is an important communication tool. These include encouraging the consumer to share their thoughts, hopes and/or concerns with us, to assist in clarifying our understanding, to explore specific topics in greater depth, to share information and to enable the consumer to explore possible options to the issues they are facing (Adler et al., 2013).

The open/closed continuum

Open questions are those questions that require more than just a 'yes' or 'no' response. These questions encourage the consumer to reflect and elaborate on their responses. Closed questions are those usually answered with a 'yes', 'no' or a minimal response. They control the direction of the conversation and limit the amount of information that can be shared.

Closed questions are useful when we need to obtain specific information, such as certain components of an admission (e.g. demographic data, information about past admissions and so forth) or when a consumer is particularly anxious and having difficulty focusing their thoughts on a broad, open question. However, too many closed questions can make an interaction seem like an interrogation.

The opening word and its effect

The opening word chosen in a conversation can influence the focus of the response. Consider the following words in **Table 5.3**.

TABLE 5.3
The opening word of questions

WORD CHOSEN	IMPLICATION
What	Implies that we are searching for facts.
How	Usually relates to questions that ask for feeling responses.
Why	Usually suggests we are searching for reasons or explanations.
When	Usually refers to a period of time.
Where	Focuses the consumer's response on location.
Would/could	Encourage an open focus to the interaction and enable the consumer to make a decision regarding their participation in the interaction.

SOURCE: AUSTRALIAN INSTITUTE OF PROFESSIONAL COUNSELLORS, N.D.

A guide to open questions

When issues are spelled out in terms of the person's experiences, feelings and behaviours, the issues become clearer. For example, questions could focus on:

- *experience:* what happened?
- *behaviour:* what did you do?
- *feeling:* how did it feel?
- *here and now:* how do you feel now?

SAFETY FIRST

DON'T JUST FOCUS ON THE PROBLEM!
In the context of the therapeutic relationship, it can be easy to think that mental health nurses only listen to problems. But this is not the case. Practising within a recovery-oriented framework means listening for the consumer's strengths, what worked previously, what their hopes are, and not just what they feel went wrong. By listening within this framework, mental health nurses help to promote a sense of hope, self-determination and empowerment in consumers and their families/carers.

THE THERAPEUTIC RELATIONSHIP

How do mental health nurses take ideas about communication and translate them into their work with consumers and carers? They achieve this through the **therapeutic relationship**. This relationship is a specific one and encompasses the use of specific knowledge (interpersonal communication), values

and skills. As described previously, interpersonal communication is the cornerstone of the therapeutic relationship.

The therapeutic relationship is a specific type of helping relationship. It is a relationship where the mental health nurse or clinician engages therapeutically with the consumer or carer to assist them to identify, plan and evaluate strategies to meet their health-related needs or objectives. Effective therapeutic relationships start with attitudes and values that promote trust and understanding between the mental health nurse and the individual. We consider the core values that promote effective therapeutic engagement.

Respect

The foundation of an effective therapeutic relationship is respect. Respect can be a difficult concept to define, but it is seen in the way that we interact with others: 'Respect is constructed and demonstrated in the interaction' (Candlin, 2011, p. 63). Respect is demonstrated verbally and non-verbally through such behaviours as being genuine, being non-judgemental, being competent in your role, keeping the consumer's health-related needs in focus and doing no harm (Egan, 2014).

Empathy

Empathy can be described as both a value that underpins the therapeutic relationship and a communication skill that is seen in the mental health nurse's interactions with consumers, family members and carers. As a value, empathy is related to developing the capacity to sense and acknowledge the feelings of another person. It is the ability to understand the consumer from their viewpoint (Egan, 2014). We consider empathy as a specific communication skill later in the chapter.

Unconditional positive regard

From a humanistic perspective, unconditional positive regard is central to developing and maintaining a positive therapeutic relationship. The capacity to value and respect another person regardless of how they behave is the essential feature of unconditional positive regard. It also is demonstrated through ongoing support and encouragement. In order to do this, DeVito (2016) believes we must listen without judgement, yet critically. This is a complex idea: How can we listen without judgement, but critically, and how can this be done in practice? This difficult concept is explored in the following sections.

Conditions of worth and the fully functioning person

Carl Rogers identified two important concepts as part of his person-centred theory (Rogers, 1951, p.196). In Chapter 2, the humanistic tendency towards growth and development was identified. According to Rogers, however, this growth could be thwarted by interactions with others in our environment. This means a person's sense of self-worth is influenced by the conditions placed on them by other people. The statement, 'If you do not pass I will not be happy with you', is an example of how conditions of worth can be communicated to a person (Joseph & Linley, 2012).

The idea of the fully functioning person states that when a person receives unconditional positive regard from others then they are more likely to experience positive feelings of self-worth and personal growth. The person who is fully functioning is viewed as being psychologically well-adjusted, congruent (i.e. harmonious) and open to experience; that is, according to Rogers a fully functioning person continues to grow and develop (Rogers, 1959, cited in Kirschenbaum & Henderson, 1990).

In practice, the idea of unconditional positive regard is seen in the mental health nurse's capacity to be open to listening to and accepting the validity of what a consumer is telling them, suspending judgement. It does not mean the nurse agrees with the consumer. Webb (2011) explains unconditional positive regard as a way of understanding a person's behaviour as a coping strategy that may or may not have been successful. Specific strategies that can be helpful in demonstrating unconditional positive regard are:

- asking the consumer to talk more about what was occurring at the time to impact their behaviour
- not passing judgement on behaviour or asking how other people may have felt
- being congruent and authentic in your verbal and non-verbal communication
- collaborating with the consumer in adopting different self-care strategies, based on the understanding that a person's behaviour may result from not coping.

THERAPEUTIC USE OF SELF

In the health care environment, health care clinicians use many tools to assist in their role of working with health care consumers. These tools may be low technology, such as a sphygmomanometer, or high technology such as magnetic resonance imaging (MRI). In mental health, the role of the mental health nurse is a unique one. While the therapeutic relationship and therapeutic engagement are fundamental parts of all nurses' roles, in mental health they are core to what nurses do. We use ourselves intentionally as part of the therapeutic process to develop a collaborative partnership with consumers, their families and carers to facilitate their recovery journey. This, in essence, is what is meant

by 'therapeutic use of self', a term first put forward by Joyce Travelbee in 1971. Therapeutic use of self incorporates how the mental health nurse uses personal strengths, previous experience in working with consumers, knowledge of human behaviour and interpersonal communication to collaborate in a purposeful, therapeutic and goal-directed manner with consumers, carers and families.

To use yourself as a therapeutic agent, there is a range of knowledge and skills that you begin to acquire as a student and that you build on for the rest of your professional career.

Self-awareness

One person cannot understand another if they first do not understand themselves. What this means is that in order to understand another person, we have to understand how we are being perceived and understood by them (Miller & Nambiar-Greenwood, 2011). Therefore, in the context of working therapeutically with consumers, we must be aware of how our communication is being received and understood, what picture or image we present to them by the way we dress, the language we use, and so on. This is what is referred to as self-awareness, the self-knowledge that a person develops about their strengths and limitations. This is particularly important where a mental health nurse has encountered experiences they have not resolved (e.g. witnessing a traumatic event in their personal lives) that makes it difficult for them to work effectively with consumers who have experienced trauma. Self-awareness is important because it enables us to be respectful, authentic, congruent and open with clients. When we know and understand ourselves, we are less likely to 'hide' behind a professional mask and more likely to interact with clients in a therapeutic partnership manner.

Two tools that are useful for developing self-awareness are the Johari window (Luft, 1969, cited in DeVito, 2013 ; Shamoa-Nir, 2017) and the self-awareness development tool (Jack &Miller, 2008).

Self-awareness is well explained by the model of the four selves (the Johari window). The Johari window has four quadrants, each representing a somewhat different self, as shown in **Figure 5.2**.

While this diagram suggests that each quadrant is discrete and distinct from the others, the four quadrants are interactive and interdependent.

Building on the Johari window concept, Jack and Miller (2008) created a framework for developing self-awareness in relation to practice. This framework has three phases: the now, transition and regroup phases (Jack & Miller, 2008). The framework is a developmental tool that enables the user to develop greater understanding and insight into their current

	Known to self	**Not known to self**
Known to others	**OPEN SELF** All that I know about myself and that I wish to share with others and also what others already know about me; e.g. my name, age, relationship status, hobbies. *THE SMALLER THE OPEN SELF THE LESS EFFECTIVE THE COMMUNICATION.*	**BLIND SELF** The blind self represents all those things about me that others know or are aware of but that I am unaware of; e.g. friends tell me that I avoid confrontation but I have never been aware of this.
Not known to others	**HIDDEN SELF** This quadrant comprises all the information that I know about myself but that I choose to keep hidden from others. The size of this window will change in relation to the various people in my life; e.g. I will share more with close friends than I do with some work colleagues. The more I share with others, the smaller this window becomes and the more I learn about myself.	**UNKNOWN SELF** The unknown self represents truths about ourselves that neither we nor others know about.

SOURCE: LUFT, 1969, CITED IN DEVITO, 2013

FIGURE 5.2
The Johari window: a model of self-awareness

TABLE 5.4
The self-awareness development tool

THE NOW STAGE	THE TRANSITION STAGE	THE REGROUP STAGE
Where you are in the moment, what you know about the situation or event, how you feel about it, what have been your usual ways of responding and what has led to your wish to transform your practice in this context. For example, does this situation/event make you feel uncomfortable, how does this impact on the way you behave and how would you like to respond?	Reflecting on what you already know about yourself. This includes current strengths and limitations, and asking what knowledge and/or skills do you need to develop? What support will you need to make this change?	Increased self-awareness is developing based on these new understandings. What new understandings and knowledge have you developed about yourself and the situation? How has this changed the way you think, feel and behave in this context?
CORRELATION OF THE SELF-AWARENESS TOOL WITH THE JOHARI WINDOW		
The 'now stage' can correspond to the quadrant of the Johari window. This is because the way in which you understand and experience an event, identify a learning need and/or require additional support through your learning will represent which quadrant is more open than others. For example, you receive feedback that you are not assertive in group situations. You know you do not like speaking in group situations, but did not share this with anyone else.	This transition stage equates with decreasing the hidden quadrant of the Johari window and increasing the size of the open window. This is achieved through open dialogue with a clinical educator, mentor or lecturer. This can be both exciting and challenging!	This regroup stage equates to decreasing the size of the unknown window. This occurs because you are learning more about yourself and how you have developed in your practice as well as how much more you will learn as your self-development continues.

SOURCE: JACK & MILLER, 2008

practice to enable continued professional growth based on new understandings. The three phases are presented in **Table 5.4**. The corresponding quadrants of the Johari window are included to show the correlation between these two concepts.

Using the environment (milieu) as part of the therapeutic process

So far in this chapter, we have emphasised the importance of effective communication as an interpersonal activity. This communication occurs within the context of the consumer's environment. Key to this is the idea that the environment is those aspects of the person's world they find themselves in and surrounded by. Considering this idea in the context of therapeutic communication enables us to see how the environment in a much broader sense can be part of the therapeutic process.

Environment can therefore be thought of as the internal (emotional, psychosocial and cultural) and external (physical) contexts of a consumer who is receiving health care. Bettelheim first coined the term 'milieu therapy' in 1948. Subsequent work by Maxwell Jones and others in 1953 saw the introduction of the therapeutic community that established the groundwork for milieu therapy and the nurse's role in this therapeutic approach. The concept of the therapeutic milieu can be a challenging one to grasp. It sets up the idea that people, setting, structure and the emotional climate of treatment are all important in healing and the recovery journey. One contemporary program that incorporates the idea of the importance of the physical environment in the therapeutic process is the Safewards model developed in the United Kingdom (Bowers et al., 2014).

DEVELOPING, MAINTAINING AND TERMINATING THERAPEUTIC RELATIONSHIPS

Any relationship goes through various phases or stages. There is always a beginning, a middle and an end. This is also the case in the context of the therapeutic relationship. One way to outline the phases of the therapeutic relationship is described in **Table 5.5**.

A second way in which to consider the therapeutic relationship is Egan's (2014) helping model, known as the problem management and opportunity-development approach to helping. This model incorporates all of the stages that are central to the helping process, in an approach that conceptualises what Egan describes as the helping relationship and consists of three stages and one action (or implementation) stage. Stage 1 relates to helping the person explore their concerns. Stage 2 consists of helping the person to determine what future they want (outcome) and set goals to achieve this (known as problem-managing). The third stage consists of assisting the person to develop plans to achieve their goals. The implementation stage occurs when plans are put into actions, using the strategies identified and developed previously. This process is best represented in what Egan (2014) refers to as the three key problem-management questions, as shown in **Figure 5.3**.

Consumer and carer attitudes towards therapeutic engagement

If effective therapeutic communication occurs within the partnership between the mental health nurse and consumer, then it is imperative that the consumer's views on what constitutes effective communication, and their experiences and attitudes towards it, are heard and central to any discussion.

In 2008, Gilburt, Rose and Slade highlighted that consumers viewed communication as being crucial to their experience of a positive admission. Three specific activities which contributed to this were listening, talking and understanding. Staff needed to be seen to be approachable and engage with consumers in order for communication to take place. Listening was highly regarded and described as a characteristic of being human. In addition, listeners who were open, non-judgemental and not patronising were valued by consumers. Trust was also viewed as essential to the positive experience of being admitted to an acute stay unit. Listening, talking and understanding are central to a positive therapeutic relationship whether a consumer is in hospital or working with a case manager in the community. This will make

TABLE 5.5
Phases of the therapeutic relationship

PHASE	FEATURES OF EACH PHASE
Orientation phase	This is where the mental health nurse and the consumer meet for the first time. Common questions that the consumer will have at this time are: 'What do I know about this person?', 'Can I trust them?', 'Are they knowledgeable and competent?' and 'What do I feel comfortable sharing with them?' Mental health nurses come to this phase asking questions such as: 'What concerns does the consumer have at this time?', 'How can I collaborate effectively with them?' and 'What knowledge and skills do I have in this area?'
Working or action phase	Health-related issues are identified and strategies to manage them are implemented during this phase. Consumer and nurse build on strengths, resources and supports for the consumer as well as identifying what additional strategies might be required. Ongoing reflection, evaluation and modification of plans take place during this phase.
Termination or moving on	This phase considers how effective the implemented strategies have been. Collaborative planning for the future is conducted. This will include goals, resources and supports.

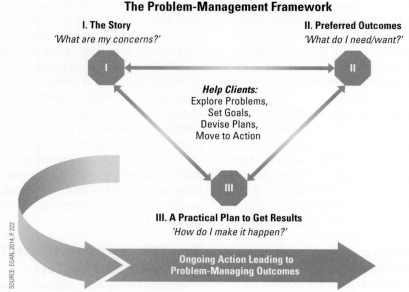

The Problem-Management Framework

I. The Story
'What are my concerns?'

II. Preferred Outcomes
'What do I need/want?'

Help Clients:
Explore Problems,
Set Goals,
Devise Plans,
Move to Action

III. A Practical Plan to Get Results
'How do I make it happen?'

**Ongoing Action Leading to
Problem-Managing Outcomes**

SOURCE: EGAN, 2014, P. 222

FIGURE 5.3
The problem management process

a difference to their experience of receiving mental health care (Gilburt, Rose & Slade, 2008). It suggests that the nurse–consumer relationship is dynamic and evolving, with consumers accepting and valuing varying degrees of direction from staff. There is a tension between the need to feel safe and protected and the autonomy-limiting practices that may sometimes be employed to achieve this.

Recent work by Molin, Graneheim and Lindgren (2016) also supports the view that the quality of interactions between consumers and clinicians influences the experience of receiving mental health care. Key attributes that consumer participants in this study identified related to the way they were treated by staff, feeling as though they were being listened to and how an absence of interaction led to consumers feeling invisible. The idea of clinicians using the professional role to distance themselves from consumers was also raised as an issue. Believing that it was the clinician's responsibility to initiate therapeutic relations, building trust, seeing best practice being implemented and sharing the decision-making responsibilities regarding their treatment were seen as core to their experience of good care practices.

The research reported here demonstrates that mental health nurses can and should work in a way that involves a range of interventions, but that their use is grounded in effective therapeutic engagement between themselves and the consumer. Existing research also highlights the importance that consumers place on the therapeutic relationship, with communication, trust and respect being highly valued.

Factors impacting on the therapeutic process

In an ideal world, people's interactions would take place in an emotionally safe environment with freedom to express ideas, opinions and feelings knowing that they will be understood, and that communication will be clear, culturally respectful, without bias and reciprocal. We would expect this type of communication to be our experience in our professional lives with colleagues and, importantly, consumers and their families' carers. However, the reality of people's professional and personal interactions is not always so clear-cut. People may be reluctant to disclose their thoughts and feelings or speak about aspects of themselves that they are uncomfortable about. The therapeutic relationship is influenced by many factors, making it dynamic, not static. Two significant factors are transference and countertransference.

Transference

Chapter 2 outlined Freud's theory of personality development. Freud developed the idea of **transference** as being the process where a person transfers their feelings from important people (usually from childhood) onto a therapist or mental health nurse. Evans (2007) explains that transference represents a person's fundamental ways of relating to those they love, fundamental ways that repeat throughout one's life. According to Freud, this is an unconscious process; and this has significant implications for the ongoing effectiveness of the therapeutic relationship between the mental health nurse and consumer. A transference reaction can be either positive or negative and is not limited to the relationship between the therapist and the client, as in Freud's original thinking. Transference can occur in any context where one person is seeking assistance, mentoring or coaching from someone considered to be an expert in the knowledge or skill sought or required (Weiten, 2017).

To recognise a transference reaction, begin by considering the intensity of the consumer's response to you. This may be either an extremely negative or angry response or an overly admiring or even adoring response. When we begin to recognise these disproportionately intense responses as possible transference reactions, it is more likely that we can address them in an appropriately professional manner rather than becoming defensive and taking the situation personally. Transference reactions that are not recognised and addressed can potentially limit the growth in the development of positive interactions for the consumer.

Countertransference occurs because of the therapist's emotional response to the person with whom they are working. This countertransference reaction can result in a 'distorted perception of the consumer's behaviour' (Corey & Corey, 2007, p. 67). A mental health nurse's experience of countertransference can have a significant impact on the therapeutic relationship with the consumer. It can lead to over- or under-engagement with the consumer, both of which are detrimental to an effective collaboration and partnership between the mental health nurse and consumer. It is essential that the mental health nurse constantly evaluates their part in the therapeutic relationship and how their reactions to consumer's comments or behaviours can impact on the consumer's recovery journey.

Similarly, countertransference can be recognised by the mental health nurse's response to a consumer that is inappropriately intense. Self-awareness and reflection are essential skills and processes that mental health nurses must develop and use in order to recognise and manage such an occurrence.

Professional responsibilities in the therapeutic relationship

A therapeutic relationship is not a social friendship. As part of a consumer's recovery journey, the therapeutic relationship is a professional relationship in which the mental health nurse integrates their knowledge, values and skills in collaboration with the consumer to identify health-related concerns and work towards identifying the supports, activities, information and education a consumer may require to meet their needs.

It is the mental health nurse's responsibility to implement and maintain appropriate professional boundaries in their work with consumers and families/carers/significant others. Professional boundaries are essential, as mental health nurses engage with people in situations involving personal and/or close contact (NMBA, 2018). This creates a power differential between the nurse and consumers and others. In order to engage and work safely with consumers, mental health nurses must ensure appropriate professional boundaries are in place. This starts with the knowledge that working therapeutically with consumers and others involves a clear start and end point to the therapeutic relationship. Professional boundaries are one aspect of behaving with professional integrity (NMBA, 2018).

SAFETY FIRST

HOW DOES A NURSE MAINTAIN PROFESSIONAL BOUNDARIES IN THE THERAPEUTIC RELATIONSHIP?
Think of professional boundaries as being like a fence. The fence signifies the area in which you can move. It is clearly defined. Professional boundaries define the area of your practice, what your role is and what you can do. If you step past the boundary of the fence, you have violated that boundary and stepped into someone else's territory. Therefore, mental health nurses must:

- have a clear understanding of their role, responsibilities and accountability within the therapeutic relationship
- understand that there is an inherent power imbalance between nurses and the consumers and families with whom they work
- avoid potential conflicts, particularly with people who they may have a social relationship with outside of their professional role. This is particularly important when living and working in regional, rural or remote areas
- recognise that it is the nurse's professional responsibility to establish and maintain professional boundaries
- utilise active reflection and learning to promote ongoing understanding and maintaining of professional boundaries.

Clinical supervision as active reflection

Clinical supervision is a structured critical reflective process in which the clinician reflects on events and issues occurring in their practice with a more senior clinician who is trained to provide clinical supervision. Engaging in clinical supervision aims to help nurses develop increasing self-awareness in their understanding of their practice and work with consumers, families and colleagues. In Australia, the use of clinical supervision is supported by professional organisations such as the Australian College of Mental Health Nurses and the Australian College of Nurses. Clinical supervision is also used in other professions such as psychology, social work and counselling. Clinical supervision can be done on an individual basis or in group sessions. It promotes understanding and self-awareness of practice, the nurse's professional role and responsibilities, maintaining professional boundaries, and working through challenging clinical and/or interprofessional situations. Clinical supervision is not performance management, professional supervision or education. For example, as part of the clinical supervision process, a mental health nurse may identify a learning need, but this would then be addressed outside of the context of clinical supervision. Features such as regular meetings, clear goals and objectives, and confidentiality are central to the success of clinical supervision.

Self-disclosure

Self-disclosure in mental health nursing occurs when a mental health nurse purposefully shares personal aspects of themselves with therapeutic intent. There are, however, varying views on the usefulness of self-disclosure. Benefits that have been identified include modelling appropriate behaviour, normalising experiences, enhancing the therapeutic relationship by increasing trust and decreasing role distancing (Ashmore & Banks, 2002), and this is identified as common practice (Henretty & Levitt, 2010). However, other authors have identified that there are risks associated with the use of self-disclosure. These risks include overburdening consumers, the divergent reactions that consumers can have to nurse self-disclosure, increasing confusion about the mental health nurse's role, decreased trust and feelings of safety (Hanson, 2007). Recent work by Unhjem, Vatne and Hem (2018), which explored what information mental health nurses disclose and their reasons for these self disclosures, identified that nurses working in mental health use self-disclosure for a variety of reasons that pertain largely to enhancing the effectiveness of the therapeutic relationship. Topics of self-disclosure were related to themes of family, life events such as the loss of a valued pet, interests and activities, and identity. Decisions about what to disclose focused on disclosures that were viewed as being helpful and encouraging, normalising a consumer's experience, modelling coping behaviours and promoting increased understanding of the consumer's experiences (Unhjem et al., 2018).

THE APPLICATION OF THERAPEUTIC COMMUNICATION QUALITIES AND SKILLS IN THE CLINICAL CONTEXT

The preceding discussion introduced the core elements of therapeutic communication. Communicating therapeutically with consumers and families takes place within the context of the collaborative relationship and is the foundation upon which the mental health nurse bases their practice.

SAFETY FIRST

A GUIDE TO SELF-DISCLOSURE

The decision to use self-disclosure as a therapeutic communication strategy is a debated topic in mental health. However, the benefits of using self-disclosure cannot be guaranteed, and the decision must be based on a case-by-case assessment and clinical judgement.

Self-disclosure must be used appropriately for the benefit of the consumer and not the mental health nurse's own personal concerns and/or issues. Other factors that must be considered include:

1 The content of the self-disclosure (is it appropriate to the conversations?).
2 Is it the appropriate time to use self-disclosure?
3 Does the consumer's current level of wellness/illness in terms of their diagnosis impact on how they might understand and interpret the self-disclosure?
4 How often is the nurse using self-disclosure? Is it too often?
5 What are reasons for the disclosure?

SOURCE: UNHJEM ET AL., 2018.

Health care consumers and their families who are seeking or being required to receive mental health care under a compulsory treatment order are often facing an unknown journey. It should not be unexpected that this can lead to feelings of anxiety, trepidation or fear even when they are seeking care options voluntarily. Nurses, paramedics and other health care staff are at the forefront of these moments, whether they are in an emergency department or the community. Any clinical context can be stressful and unpredictable (Victorian Auditor-General, 2015).

Workplace aggression

Workplace aggression is a serious issue both nationally and internationally. Chapman, Styles, Perry and Combs (2010) surveyed registered nurses in Western Australia. Their findings indicated that 75% of those surveyed experienced workplace violence in the previous 12 months. Farrell, Shafiei and Salmon (2010) reported that over 50% of registered nurses surveyed had experienced some form of workplace aggression. Of this, 36% of aggressive incidents involved health care consumers and 32% of incidents of workplace aggression were experienced as bullying by managers and supervisors. Hills, Joyce and Humphreys (2012) also report that 70.6% of medical practitioners surveyed had experienced verbal or written aggression and over 32% had experienced physical aggression in the preceding 12 months. Nurses working in mental health and emergency departments (ED) are identified as a high-risk group for experiencing verbal or physical aggression (Chapman et al., 2010). Yet many incidents of occupational violence are unreported. Reasons for this include the belief that occupational violence is an inherent part of the job, poor reporting systems and lack of organisational support and follow-up (Chapman et al., 2010).

This small snapshot of workplace violence highlights the challenge of clearly defining what constitutes aggression and violence in the workplace. For the purposes of this text, we use the following definition from the Victorian Government's 2011 policy on preventing occupational violence. In its policy framework, including principles for managing weapons in Victorian health services, the Department of Health defines occupational violence as: 'Any incident where an employee is abused, threatened or assaulted in circumstances arising out of, or in the course of, their employment' (Department of Health, 2011, p. 8). The following sections outline factors that may lead to

aggression, and indicate how the therapeutic relationship might be applied to manage these situations.

Aetiology and factors leading to aggression

All people can become angry. It is a human response to feeling threatened, fearful or powerless. But not everyone behaves aggressively. Authors such as Okey (1992), Anderson and Bushman (2002), and Seto, Charette and Nicholls (2018) have argued that aggression is the result of the interactions of a range of biological, environmental and interpersonal factors. This holistic view moves away from a reductionist view of aggression as being simply biological, environmental or interpersonal. The 'Safety first' boxes review a range of factors that can increase the risk of aggressive behaviour, and provide points on how to interact with an angry person.

SAFETY FIRST

PREDICTING RISK OF AGGRESSION

There are a range of biological, environmental and inter-personal factors that can increase the risk of aggression in the clinical setting.

1 Biological:
 – illicit drug use (this is a significant factor, and substance intoxication is a higher risk factor for violence than a mental health condition)
 – gender (male)
 – age
 – diagnosis (e.g. schizophrenia)
 – substance misuse (e.g. methamphetamine).
2 Environmental:
 – consumer overcrowding
 – peak times such as staff handover when staff are less visible and available to interact with consumers
 – staff rigidness
 – staffing profiles – young, petite females who are inexperienced – increases likelihood of assault (van der Zwan, Davies, Andrews & Brooks, 2011)
 – staff inability to manage demanding patients promptly due to stress and overcrowding often results in reactive management techniques
 – staff react to violence, rather than proactively work to prevent it occurring
 – medication administration
 – restraint
 – care provision.
3 Interpersonal:
 – limitation of consumer freedoms
 – consumer–consumer provocation
 – previous positive history for violence
 – involuntary (compulsory) admission
 – staff assaults – young male, with schizophrenia, presenting to ED in high demand times – more prominent in assault data
 – previous positive history of aggressive behaviour.

SOURCE: ADAPTED FROM DEPARTMENT OF HEALTH, 2013

SAFETY FIRST

INTERACTING WITH AGGRESSIVE CONSUMERS

When interacting with a person who is angry, you must be mindful of your safety and the safety of others, including the angry individual.

SAFETY OF THE MENTAL HEALTH NURSE:

- Keep a safe distance from the aggressive person.
- Do not approach someone by surprise.
- Do not place yourself in a corner, or in a room without an exit.
- Approach the person with other staff.
- Be clear about what is unacceptable behaviour.
- Tell staff where you are going and what you are doing.
- Duress or call for help when feeling unsafe.
- Be mindful of objects in the vicinity of the client – chairs, tables, televisions, DVD players, electrical appliances.

SAFETY OF OTHERS:

- Others may congregate to see what is happening or can attempt to become involved by defending the agitated consumer's cause, or by defending nursing staff – either way, this exacerbates the situation.
- Greater numbers of people can result in difficulty defusing a situation and potentially interferes with the consumer's privacy during an incident.
- Direct others to their rooms or outside, or ask a colleague to set up a distracting activity.

In the event that physical restraint is necessary, look for signs and symptoms of positional asphyxia including the consumer saying they cannot breathe, gurgling/gasping sounds indicating compromised airway, cyanosis, increased panic, prolonged resistance or sudden tranquillity. Risk factors for this include obesity, pre-existing medical conditions, pressure on abdomen and psychosis.

SOURCE: ADAPTED FROM BARNETT, STIRLING & PANDYAN, 2012; PATERSON & BRADLEY, 2010 IN DUXBURY, AIKEN & DALE, 2011; VICTORIA POLICE, 2012

Applying therapeutic communication skills with a person who is angry and at increased risk of aggressive behaviour

As stated previously, a person does not suddenly become aggressive. A high level of consumer interaction is essential to creating a therapeutic environment. This equates to getting out of the office and interacting, observing and intervening. Collaborative interactions encourage the consumer to take responsibility for their outcomes. More effective problem-solving and solutions to issues are developed through collaboration. Positive role modelling by the mental health nurse, the use of community meetings, offering alternatives such as sitting somewhere quiet, the use of PRN medication and positive interactions with staff are a few ways in which mental health nurses and consumers can promote a non-violent culture within an acute care environment.

The mental health nurse's effective use of foundation and advanced communication skills is essential to reduce increased tension and the frustration being expressed by a person at risk of behaving aggressively. This process is referred to as defusion. **De-escalation** is the use of more advanced assertive communication skills to therapeutically connect with a person (Duperouzel, 2008; Finfgeld-Connett, 2009). Defusion and de-escalation are outlined in **Table 5.6**.

Use of restrictive interventions

Restraint and seclusion are designated through legislation in Australia as restrictive interventions. A restrictive intervention is one that restricts an individual's capacity to modify behaviour, and restrict movement within their environment for the individual's safety and the safety of others. While there is no consistent definition used across all Australian states and territories, there are common themes that can be seen in each definition. **Table 5.7** provides some examples.

TABLE 5.6
Defusion and de-escalation skills

VERBAL SKILLS	NON-VERBAL SKILLS	VOCAL SKILLS
Identify expectations: Identifying the person's expectations while being respectful and empathetic can help you understand what is troubling them. Avoid ultimatums. *Identify needs:* Many instances of aggression occur because a person's needs are not being met, they feel helpless and/or disempowered. It is essential that the person knows that you will support them in this as much as you can, without making promises that you cannot keep. *Actively listen:* Seek to understand. Pay attention, focus on clarifying and understanding by identifying the content and emotional response(s) the person is communicating (e.g. 'You feel angry because you've had to wait longer than expected'), check that you have understood what the person has said – if you haven't, they will usually tell you (e.g. 'It's not that I had to wait, they just don't show you any respect'). *Use plain and direct language:* A person who is emotionally aroused cannot absorb as much information as a calm person, so keep communication short and use simple words. *Set limits:* An assertive response is to set the limit and then explain the reason for the limit, perhaps with some negotiation or alternative option around meeting the person's needs (e.g. 'I'm sorry, you can't smoke here because smoking is banned inside the hospital, but you can go outside to smoke').	*Maintain a calm presence and pay attention:* Your behaviour will calm the person as much, if not more, than the words you say. When someone is emotionally aroused, they can feel out of control. Having a calming presence and being attentive can help the person to feel that someone is there to help them regain control. It is harder to maintain feelings of anger when a person feels they are being listened to. *Be aware of your non-verbal behaviour:* Do not copy the aggressive behaviour or postures back to the person as this is more likely to increase arousal. *If possible, increase personal space:* Give the person more rather than less personal space – at least two arm lengths away – and avoid touching them. *Maintain an open and relaxed posture:* This means adopting a non-threatening posture by keeping your hands open and relaxed by your sides and your face slightly forward. Do not fold your arms, keep your hands behind your back, on your hips or in your pockets. *Maintain appropriate eye contact:* It is important to avoid staring but use broken eye contact, remembering cultural appropriateness (e.g. direct eye contact with Aboriginal and/or Torres Strait Islander people may be considered culturally inappropriate or threatening). *Stay calm:* Take slow, deep breaths, use positive self-talk (e.g. saying to yourself, 'Stay calm, stay positive'). Remember to blink, as when we are emotionally aroused, we can forget to do this, which increases the likelihood of staring.	Taking note of the vocal element of your communication interactions with consumers can reduce anger and aggression Consider your: • tone of voice – try to keep your tone calm and loud enough for them to hear if they are shouting over the top of you • rate of speech – try to speak slowly and clearly so that you will be easily understood. When someone is emotionally upset and agitated it can be difficult for them to keep up with what you are saying.

SOURCE: ADAPTED FROM NEW SOUTH WALES, DEPARTMENT OF EDUCATION AND TRAINING, 2008

CASE **STUDY**

ANTHONY'S APPOINTMENT

I went to my appointment as usual. Since my discharge I had been having appointments every few weeks with Jenna, my case worker. Only this day when I went to the desk, I noticed how noisy the waiting room was with people crowding around the reception desk, people yelling and phones ringing. When it came to my turn to speak, I was told that I had missed my appointment and Jenna couldn't see me. The person at reception said they were booked out and if I couldn't be on time, that was too bad and I would have to wait till the next available time. But I was sure I had the right time and I said so. Fumbling in my pockets for the card with the appointment date, she told me to 'go away and think about my rudeness'. Who was this person? I hadn't seen them before. In fact she was the one who was acting like a bitch towards me! Where was Jenna? When I tried to explain what I was doing she crossed her arms and almost yelled that if I didn't move away from the desk she would call security. I could feel myself starting to shake, my face feeling hotter and hotter and clenching and unclenching my fists. I was trying so hard to keep control and I knew if I didn't move I might do something I'd regret. Just then Jenna came through the door and I saw her. I don't know what it

was she saw or heard, but she came straight over and said, 'Hi Anthony, I'm glad you made it.' Looking at the person behind the desk, she asked, 'All good here?' 'He was late for his appointment and you have no gaps, it's his fault.' 'I was trying to look for my appointment card Jenna. But she threatened to get security if I didn't go. She wouldn't even let me find the card to show her! Bitch!!' Now I was really getting worked up and yelling so everyone was staring at me like I had shit on my face or something. Looking at me calmly, Jenna said, 'Anthony I have some time in 20 minutes, so we can have a quick catch-up if you'd like. Is that OK with you?' She didn't crowd me. She gave me some space, but I knew she was watching me and listening. Suddenly I felt like a balloon which had too much air in it being deflated. 'Sounds like a plan,' I replied, my voice still trembling.

Questions

1   Using the biological, environmental and interactional framework, what factors can you identify that are relevant to Anthony's response to the interaction on his arrival at the community health clinic?

2   What skills did the case manager, Jenna, use to help calm the situation?

REFLECT ON THIS

In 2015, Bowers and colleagues published a paper titled 'Reducing conflict and containment rates on acute psychiatric wards: The Safewards cluster randomised controlled trial'. In this study, they explored mental health staff's work to avert or minimise harm from any patient's behaviour that might threaten safety, and especially the efficacy of those interventions.

Collaborating with 31 staff and patients, who were randomly selected from inpatient wards at 15 different hospitals, the results indicated that wards in the experimental condition group had a reduced rate of conflict and containment events compared with the control intervention group. The authors' conclusions argued that simple interventions that aim to improve staff relationships with patients can reduce the frequency of conflict and containment.

In 2020, the pioneering work of mental health practitioner Geoffrey Brennan was featured in the *Journal of Mental Health Practice* (Cole, 2020). Mr Brennan has been

involved in the development of 10 interventions central to the Safewards model. These include mutual expectations, soft words, positive language, bad news mitigation, mutual help meetings, reassurance and discharge messages. Read this short paper, which can be accessed via your university's library:

Bowers, L., James, K., Quirk, A., Simpson, A., Stewart, D. & Hodsoll, J. (2015). Reducing conflict and containment rates on acute psychiatric wards: The Safewards cluster randomised controlled trial. *International Journal of Nursing Studies*, 52(9), 1412–22.

Reflect on the following questions:

1   What examples of positive language have you heard staff use when speaking with consumers?

2   What information is available to consumers that can help them and staff build therapeutic relationships?

3   How does the Safewards model promote recovery-oriented practice?

The use of restraint and seclusion is only permitted under specific conditions and there are stringent requirements regarding its implementation and reporting. These requirements include authorisation, recording and reporting requirements, regular

observations and communication, and meeting the human rights of the individual in relation to nutrition, hydration and elimination. This is covered in detail in Chapter 3. However, if we consider the concept of a restrictive intervention more broadly, then restraint can

TABLE 5.7
Selected definitions of restrictive interventions

STATE	RESTRAINT	SECLUSION
Mental Health Act 2014 (Vic.)	Bodily restraint 'means a form of physical or mechanical restraint that prevents a person having free movement of his or her limbs, but does not include the use of furniture (including beds with cot sides and chairs with tables fitted on their arms) that restricts the person's ability to get off the furniture' (p. 2).	'the sole confinement of a person to a room or any other enclosed space from which it is not within the control of the person confined to leave' (p. 12).
Queensland Mental Health Act 2016 (Qld)	'…restraint of the person by the use of a mechanical appliance, approved under section 162B, preventing the free movement of the person's body or a limb of the person' (p. 104). 'Physical restraint, of a patient, is the use by a person of his or her body to restrict the patient's movement' (p. 215). Physical restraint is identified under use of force (p. 417).	'…the confinement of the patient at any time of the day or night alone in a room or area from which free exit is prevented' (p. 207).

SOURCE: QUEENSLAND GOVERNMENT, 2016; VICTORIAN CONSOLIDATED LEGISLATION, 2014

also be achieved chemically. While the use of chemical restraint is identified under the sections referring to medical treatment in the Victoria and Queensland legislation, it is not included in the sections under restraint. Nurses will see chemical restraint used in clinical areas such as ED as well as in mental health units. Like restraint, the use of seclusion is strictly monitored under state and territory legislation.

In working to reduce the use of such restrictive interventions, it is essential that therapeutic environments foster non-coercive/trauma-informed, person-centred and recovery-oriented practice as the core element of the therapeutic relationship between mental health nurses, consumers and carers. Before a judgement to use either physical or chemical forms of restraint and/or seclusion is made, health care staff should ask themselves the following questions:

- What is the rationale for physically restraining, sedating/medicating a consumer?
- Is the decision being made for the consumer's benefit, the clinical staff or other consumers? Is this a good enough reason?
- What other less restrictive interventions have been implemented prior to this decision?
- Has the consumer been involved in the decision-making process?

Splitting

Splitting is viewed as a behaviour in which a person will try to meet their needs by asking different staff for the same thing until their request is met. It is often viewed as manipulative behaviour. A potentially more damaging type of behaviour that may mimic splitting on the mental health ward is often seen in consumers with borderline personality disorder (see Chapter 12). This behaviour presents as fluctuations between idealisation and devaluation. For example, Jenny is a consumer on the acute mental health unit. Jenny asks her contact nurse, Ivy, to let her access the kitchen after hours and she obliges. Jenny states, 'you're the best nurse here!' (idealisation). Later, Jenny wants someone to sit with her and play a game, but Ivy is about to leave for the night

so she says she cannot. Jenny becomes enraged and says, 'you're such a stupid cow, I hate you!' (devaluation). Clearly this can result in frustration for staff, but also a potential to create a rift in the multidisciplinary team. While professionalism dictates that nurses must not judge the behaviour or the person, some staff may respond by seeing the consumer as likable and others will dislike the consumer.

Possible indicators of staff splitting may include:

- diagnostic uncertainty with contradictory evaluation of the consumer
- groups of staff members becoming isolated from each other (cliques)
- staff breaks are dominated by discussion of a specific consumer
- blurring of staff–consumer boundaries
- 'good' and 'bad' nurses make accusations about each other.

The types of consumer interactions that may lead to an increase in staff splitting include:

- blaming and accusing others
- constant comparison of staff members with each other
- distorting or giving only partial descriptions of interactions with other staff members
- not dealing directly with the disputed staff person.

Limit setting is considered an effective strategy for addressing splitting behaviour. A person uses splitting behaviour in an effort to meet their needs based on their current understanding and knowledge. The primary purpose of limit setting is educative. It must never be used as punishment. Limit setting provides clear structure and boundaries that aim to promote security as well as encouraging the consumer to assume responsibility for their behaviour. Successfully utilised, limit setting can assist a consumer to feel more in control of their actions and reduce feelings of being judged negatively by others (Maguire, Daffern & Martin, 2013). It requires clear assertive communication on the part of the nurse, together with a respectful non-judgemental attitude.

CLINICAL **OBSERVATIONS**

Responding to splitting behaviour

Engage with the consumer in a consistent and collaborative exploration of their emotions, behaviour and its approach (Kraft & Goin, 2006; Swift, 2009).

- The specific behaviour that is unacceptable needs to be clearly identified and the reason why it is unacceptable explained.
- Identify reasonable consequences that are direct, specific and consistent. Consequences must be within your scope of practice, organisational policies and procedures, and meet legislative, ethical and best practice requirements.
- Differentiate between the consumer and their behaviour.
- Acknowledge and positively reinforce behaviour that meets limits.
- Implement consequences if required.
- Do not set too many limits. This creates the potential for a power struggle and undermines the therapeutic relationship you are trying to establish and maintain. Setting limits is aimed at increasing self-esteem, as a person experiences success for positive behaviour rather than failure.
- Awareness of your own feelings/responses is essential. Debriefing/supervision is important to help you manage your own responses and build your confidence in using this strategy.

Medication adherence

Adherence or concordance are technical terms that relate to whether a person has taken a prescribed course of medication, followed a program of exercise, or made dietary changes according to the prescriber's instructions on a medication. The terms used to describe a decision to not complete a course of medication are '**non-adherence**' or 'non-concordance'. 'Non-compliance' is also a term that is used, although this term is considered outdated as it implies the consumer is a passive recipient of orders from a health professional. Just as we may make a choice not to continue taking a prescribed course of medication, people with a lived experience of a mental health condition will also make choices about what medications, diets and/or exercise programs they may or may not adhere to.

The literature shows that non-adherence to medication used in the treatment of people with a lived experience of mental health disorders such as a major depressive disorder or schizophrenia can result in increased rates of relapse, hospital admissions and emergency department presentations, and increased severity of symptoms. Importantly, overall *relapse rates are lower for mental health consumers who adhere to medication regimens* (Ho et al., 2016; Morrison, Meehan & Stomski, 2015). **Table 5.8** identifies some of the factors that facilitate or restrict adherence.

Psychoeducation provides the consumer and their family/carers with a conceptual and practical

CLINICAL **OBSERVATIONS**

Non-adherence makes sense to the individual

On the surface when you are unwell and go to see your local GP, you may leave the appointment with a prescription for a medication. You take this to the pharmacist, start the course of medication as prescribed and then after three or four days find you have missed several doses. What might your reaction be? Do you restart the medications and finish the course, or not? If you start them, you might ask someone to remind you for the first day as you get back into the routine of taking the correct number of daily doses. Maybe you have started feeling a little unwell and think that finishing the course would be a wise choice. There are also a variety of reasons why you might not restart these medications. Perhaps you are feeling better and see no reason to restart. Perhaps you have experienced some side effects such as nausea and are unhappy about restarting the course of medications. Or perhaps you do not think you really need to take them as you did not believe you were that unwell to begin with. The take-home message in this example is that you made a choice *not* to continue taking the prescribed course of medications. You have not adhered to the prescribed medication regimen.

TABLE 5.8
Factors facilitating or restricting adherence

FACTORS FACILITATING ADHERENCE	FACTORS RESTRICTING ADHERENCE
- Social supports - Involvement in the treatment planning process - Education about the medication effects and side effects meaning the consumer is prepared for them - Choice - Collaboration and partnership as part of the team	- The experience of side effects particularly when they are not anticipated - Symptoms of illness - Paternalistic attitudes of health care professionals

approach to illness and treatment, and increases satisfaction with treatment and adherence. The goals of psychoeducation include:

- providing information and knowledge (e.g. understanding about a particular mental health condition such as the causes, triggers, impact and management of depression)
- developing understanding and facilitating consumer's use of a treatment option (e.g. using medications such as antidepressants or treatment options such as electroconvulsive therapy)
- collaborating with consumers and families to promote recovery-oriented practice.

Psychoeducation can take place formally or informally, on an individual or group basis and can be delivered in a variety of formats. The key to the effectiveness of psychoeducation depends on several factors. These include:

- the consumer/family's readiness to learn
- the way the topic is organised for learning
- the degree to which the consumer/family are involved in the learning process
- previous experiences in learning (either positive or negative)
- the extent to which a consumer believes they need to learn the particular information.

Examples of different types of psychoeducational programs include relapse prevention programs, health and well-being education, medication education, family support and education programs and stress management techniques.

SAFETY FIRST

DON'T JUST FOCUS ON THE PROBLEM!

In the context of the therapeutic relationship, it can be easy to think that mental health nurses only listen for problems. But this is not the case. Practising within a recovery-oriented framework means that you listen for the consumer's strengths, what worked for them previously and what their hopes are — not just what they feel went wrong. It is by listening within this framework that mental health nurses help to promote a sense of hope, self-determination and empowerment within consumers.

REFLECTION ON LEARNING FROM PRACTICE

After reading this chapter, it should be evident that there are a number of effective actions the mental health nurse can adopt that occur either outside the realm of, or as an adjunct to, pharmacological therapy. The development and maintenance of therapeutic rapport is essential in mental health nursing, and adopting a holistic approach to care utilising psychological approaches to engagement has been proven to be effective.

When considering what approach to utilise when engaging with someone who is distressed, it is important to consider the holistic needs of the consumer, and ensure that legal and ethical principles covered in Chapter 3, are also applied. While the mental health unit can be a confronting place for students and clinicians, it is also important to consider the distress such environments can cause consumers living within them. When the nurse considers all of these factors, they promote an environment that is both physically and psychologically safe.

CHAPTER RESOURCES

SUMMARY

- Utilising effective interpersonal communication skills is central to best practice in mental health nursing and recovery-oriented practice.
- Core elements of interpersonal communication involve the message and feedback message between the sender and receiver.
- Communicating effectively with consumers, families and carers involves the use of a range of verbal and non-verbal communication skills.
- Effective use of interpersonal communication skills requires the mental health nurse to integrate their attitudes, professional values and skills and use themselves with therapeutic intent in collaboration with consumers, families and carers.

- The therapeutic relationship is a professional relationship that proceeds through a number of phases. It is a collaborative endeavour. The mental health nurse is responsible for initiating, maintaining and ending the therapeutic relationship and must maintain appropriate professional boundaries at all times.
- The therapeutic relationship goes through a number of phases: orientation; working or action; termination and moving on. Another way of understanding this relationship is with Egan's helping model.
- Nurses will interact with consumers in a variety of contexts. Some of these interactions will be emotionally challenging for both the consumer and the nurse. Understanding contributing factors and implementing person-centred strategies to understand issues and address them are paramount.

REVIEW QUESTIONS

1 The skill of paraphrasing involves the nurse:
   a Restating what the consumer has told them
   b Rephrasing what the consumer has said in their own words
   c Providing a collection of summary statements
   d Interpreting the consumer's feelings
2 The key attitudes required to facilitate an effective therapeutic relationship are:
   a Respect, empathy, unconditional positive regard
   b Respect, sympathy, unconditional positive regard
   c Respect, empathy, conditional regard
   d Purpose, respect, empathy
3 Paul is working in a community mental health facility with adolescents. Paul is being persistently asked by one adolescent if he is gay. Paul does not answer this question, stating it is not relevant to their working together. What quadrant of the Johari window model is Paul using?
   a Open
   b Unknown
   c Hidden
   d Fake
4 You are about to meet Nuala, a 28-year-old woman attending her first outpatient appointment and long acting injection since her discharge from hospital three weeks ago. How would you use your understanding of the orientation phase of the therapeutic relationship to prepare for this appointment?
5 Mary is a 32-year-old woman who was diagnosed three years earlier with major depressive disorder. She has been unemployed for 18 months. Her relationship with her partner Ingrid is strained and she is worried about how she can get her life 'back on track'. Using Egan's helping model, outline the major features of each phase a counsellor would use in working with Mary.
6 List a minimum of four biological, environmental and interpersonal risk factors for aggression.
7 The skills involved in defusion and de-escalation of aggression are categorised into three groups. These groups are:
   a Verbal, para-verbal and physical
   b Verbal, non-verbal and physical
   c Vocal, non-verbal and physical
   d Verbal, non-verbal and vocal

CRITICAL THINKING

1 Consider the terms 'abuse', 'threaten' and 'assault' in the context of aggression. What does each of these terms mean?
2 In understanding each of these terms, is it possible to identify different forms of occupational violence? What are they?
3 Read the following statements and then consider the questions:
   ■ 'When I was restrained, it was the culmination of escalated situations based on my feeling totally without choices, and not in control at all. [However], it became a "war of words", all about who had the power. I was restrained and forcibly injected. I did not speak to anyone for the next two days, and developing any sort of trusting relationship was seriously delayed' – Tom Lane (2002, cited in National Executive Training Institute (NETI) (2005).
   ■ 'The first time I helped with a restraint, a four-point restraint, I walked out of the room in tears because it was one of the most horrible things I had ever seen' – Female Direct Care National Executive Training Institute (NETI) (2005).

   a Is the use of chemical restraint for the provision of care aimed to improve the underlying condition or to modify behaviour?
   b What are the potential impacts of trauma on the consumer?
   c How might the use of restraint and seclusion impact on the therapeutic relationship?
4 Psychoeducation is considered a primary intervention to work with consumers who do not or are reluctant to adhere to prescribed medications. What other types of therapeutic approaches might be useful strategies to utilise?
5 Why is the use of self-disclosure such a contentious issue in mental health nursing? Why is it important to address the factors identified in the 'Safety first' box (page 80) before using self-disclosure? In groups or with another person, discuss what would be some appropriate topics that mental health nurses might self-disclose. What would be inappropriate topics to self-disclose? What are your reasons for these choices? What does the literature say?

USEFUL WEBSITES

- AUSMED provides a number of resources for nurses working across a range of clinical contexts. This information sheet has some useful broad ideas relating to communicating with people receiving health care: https://www.ausmed.com/articles/communicating-with-patients
- Black Dog Institute has an interesting fact sheet on positive psychology. Ideas related to unconditional positive regard

inform this approach to working with people: https://www.blackdoginstitute.org.au/docs/default-source/factsheets/positivepsychology.pdf?sfvrsn=2
- Nursing and Midwifery Board of Australia: http://www.nursingmidwiferyboard.gov.au/Codes-Guidelines-Statements/Professional-standards.aspx

REFLECT ON THIS

Communicating on COVID-19

There has been a huge amount of information and discussion related to COVID-19, vaccination protocols and take-up of immunisation in the community. Debates about these issues have been published across multiple platforms, whether mainstream media (print, digital, etc.) or social media, blogs and vlogs (Twitter, Facebook, YouTube, etc.).

In relation to this wealth of information, consider the following questions:

1   How effectively do you believe this information has been disseminated and received in culturally diverse communities? What might be the challenges in delivering the key messages to these communities?

2   How can health professionals work with communities to deliver health education and information effectively?

3   Reflect on your own knowledge and skills in developing health education and working collaboratively with consumers.

    a   How prepared are you to take on this aspect of your role?

    b   What support/education might assist you in developing your skills and confidence?

REFERENCES

Adler, R.B., Rosenfeld, L.B. & Proctor II, R.F. (2013). *Interplay: The Process of Interpersonal Communication* (12th edn). New York: Oxford University Press.

Anderson, C.A. & Bushman, B.J. (2002). Human aggression. *Annual Review of Psychology*, 53(1), 27–51. doi:10.1146/annurev.psych.53.100901.135231

Ashmore, R. & Banks, D. (2002). Mental health nursing. Self-disclosure in adult and mental health nursing students. *British Journal of Nursing*, 11(3), 172–7. https://doi.org/10.12968/bjon.2002.11.3.10065

Australian Institute of Professional Counsellors (AIPC). (n.d.). *Counselling Micro Skills*. Retrieved from http://www.aipc.net.au/student_bonuses/Counselling%20Micro%20Skills.pdf.

Barnett, R., Stirling, C. & Pandyan, A.D. (2012). A review of the scientific literature related to adverse impact of physical restraint: Gaining a clearer understanding of the physiological factors involved in cases of restraint-related death. *Medicine, Science and the Law*, 52, 137–42. doi:10.1258/msl.2011.011101

Bettelheim, B. (1948). A therapeutic milieu, *American Journal of Orthopsychiatry*, 18(2), 191–206. Retrieved from https://onlinelibrary.wiley.com/doi/pdf/10.1111/j.1939-0025.1948.tb05078.x.

Bowers, L., Alexander, J., Bilgin, H., Botha, M., Dack, C., James, K., Jarrett, M., Jeffery, D., Nijman, H., Owiti, J.A., Papadopoulos, C., Ross, J., Wright, S. & Stewart, D. (2014). Safewards: Evidence and appraisal. *Journal of Psychiatric Mental Health Nursing*, 21, 354–64. https://doi-org.ezproxy2.acu.edu.au/10.1111/jpm.12085

Bowers, L., James, K., Quirk, A., Simpson, A., Stewart, D. & Hodsoll, J. (2015). Reducing conflict and containment rates on acute psychiatric wards: The Safewards cluster randomised controlled trial. *International Journal of Nursing Studies*, 52(9), 1412–22.

Burnard, P. (2005). *Counselling Skills for Health Professionals* (4th edn). Cheltenham, UK: Stanley Thornes.

Candlin, S. (2011). *Therapeutic Communication. A Lifespan Approach*. Frenchs Forest, NSW: Pearson Education Australia.

Chapman, R., Styles, I., Perry, L. & Combs, S. (2010). Examining the characteristics of workplace violence in one non-tertiary hospital. *Journal of Clinical Nursing*, 19, 479–88. doi:10.1111/j.1365.2702.2009.02952.x

Cole, E. (2020). Transforming mental health nursing practice with Safewards. *Mental Health Practice*, 23(6), 10–12. doi:10.7748/mhp.23.6.10.s4

Corey, M. & Corey, G. (2007). *Becoming a Helper* (5th edn). Belmont, CA: Thomson.

Department of Health. (2011). *Preventing Occupational Violence: A Policy Framework Including Principles for Managing Weapons in Victorian Health Services*. Melbourne: Victorian Government. © State of Victoria 2018. Victorian Government. Retrieved from: http://www.health.vic.gov.au/__data/assets/pdf_file/0006/680937/Preventing-occupational-violence.pdf. p. 8.

Department of Health. (2013). Reducing restrictive interventions: Literature review and document analysis. © Copyright, State of Victoria. Retrieved from https://www2.health.vic.gov.au/about/publications/researchandreports/reducing-restrictive-interventions-literature-review-2013.

DeVito, J.A. (2013). *The Interpersonal Communication Book* (13th edn). Boston, MA: Pearson.

DeVito, J.A. (2016). *The Interpersonal Communication Book* (14th edn). Boston, MA: Pearson.

Duperouzel, H. (2008). It's OK for people to feel angry. The exemplary management of imminent aggression. *Journal of Intellectual Disabilities*, 12(4), 295–307. doi:10.1177/1744629508100495

Duxbury, J., Aiken., F. & Dale, C. (2011). Deaths in custody: The role of restraint. *Journal of Learning Disabilities and Offending Behaviour*, 2(4), 178–89. doi:10.1108/20420921111207873

Dwyer, J. (2016). *The Business Communication Handbook* (10th edn). South Melbourne: Cengage.

Egan, G. (2014). *The Skilled Helper: A Problem-management and Opportunity-development Approach to Helping* (10th edn). Belmont, CA: Brooks/Cole, Cengage Learning.

Evans, A.M. (2007). Transference in the nurse–patient relationship. *Journal of Psychiatric and Mental Health Nursing*, 14(2), 189–95. doi:10.1111/j.1365.2850.2007.01062.x

Farrell, G.A., Shafiei, T. & Salmon, P. (2010). Facing up to 'challenging behaviour': A model for training in staff–client interaction. *Journal of Advanced Nursing*, 66(7), 1644–55. doi:10.1111/j.1365.2648.2010.05340.x

Finfgeld-Connett, D. (2009). Model of therapeutic and non-therapeutic responses to patient aggression. *Issues in Mental Health Nursing*, 30(9), 530–7. doi:10.1080/01612840902722120

Gilburt, H., Rose, D. & Slade, M. (2008). The importance of relationships in mental health care. A qualitative study of service users' experiences of psychiatric hospital admission in the UK. *BMC Health Services Research*, 8(92). Retrieved from: http://www.biomedcentral.com/1472-6963/8/92.

Hanson, J. (2007). Should your lips be zipped? How therapist self-disclosure and non-disclosure affects clients. *Counselling & Psychotherapy Research*, 5(2), 96–104. https://doi.org/10.1080/17441690500226658

Henretty, J.R. & Levitt, H.M. (2010). The role of therapist self-disclosure in psychotherapy: A qualitative review. *Clinical Psychology Review*, 30(1), 63–77. https://doi.org/10.1016/j.cpr.2009.09.004

Hills, D.J., Joyce, C.M. & Humphreys, J.S. (2012). A national study of workplace aggression in Australian clinical medical practice. *Medical Journal of Australia*, 197(6), 336–40, doi:10.5694/mja12.10444

Ho, S.C., Chong, H.Y., Chaiyakunapruk, N., Tangiisuran, B. & Jacob, S.A. (2016). Clinical and economic impact of non-adherence to antidepressants in major depressive disorder: A systematic review. *Journal of Affective Disorders*, 193, 1–10. doi:https://doi.org/10.1016/j.jad.2015.12.029

Jack, K. & Miller, E. (2008). Exploring self-awareness in mental health practice. *Mental Health Practice*, 12(3), 31–5.

Jones, A.C. (2005). Transference, counter-transference and repetition: some implications for nursing practice. *Journal of Clinical Nursing*, 14(10), 1177–84.

Jones, M. (1953). *The Therapeutic Community: A New Treatment Method in Psychiatry*. New York: Basic Books.

Joseph, S. & Linley, P.A. (2012). Positive therapy: A positive psychological theory of therapeutic practice. In P. Linley & S. Joseph (eds), *Positive Psychology in Practice* (pp. 354–70). Hoboken, NJ: John Wiley & Sons.

Kirschenbaum, H. & Henderson, V.L. (1990). *The Carl Rogers Reader*. London: Constable.

Kraft Goin, M. (2006). Borderline personality disorder: Splitting countertransference. *Psychiatric Times*, 15(11), 25 August. Retrieved from https://www.psychiatrictimes.com/view/borderline-personality-disorder-splitting-countertransference

Luft, J. (1969). *Of Human Interaction*. Palo Alto, CA: National Press Books.

Maguire, T., Daffern, M. & Martin, T. (2014). Exploring nurses' and patients' perspectives of limit setting in a forensic mental health setting. *International Journal of Mental Health Nursing*, 23(2), 153–60. https://doi.org/10.1111/inm.12034

Miller, E. & Nambiar-Greenwood, G. (2011). The nurse–patient relationship. In L. Webb (ed.), *Nursing: Communication Skills in Practice* (pp. 20–32). Oxford: Oxford University Press.

Molin, J., Graneheim, U.H. & Lindgren, B. (2016). Quality of interactions influences everyday life in psychiatric inpatient care-patients' perspectives. *International Journal of Qualitative Studies on Health and Well-being*, 11. doi:http://dx.doi.org/10.3402/qhw.v11.29897

Morrison, P., Meehan, T. & Stomski, N.J. (2015). Living with antipsychotic medication side-effects: The experience of Australian mental health consumers. *International Journal of Mental Health Nursing*, 24(3), 253–61. doi:10.1111/inm.12110

National Executive Training Institute (NETI). (2005). *Training Curriculum for Reduction of Seclusion and Restraint. Draft Curriculum Manual.* Alexandria, VA: National Association of State Mental Health Program Directors (NASMHPD), National Technical Assistance Center for State Mental Health Planning (NTAC).

Nelson-Jones, R. (1992). *Lifeskills Helping: A Textbook of Practical Counselling and Helping Skills*. Sydney: Holt, Rinehart & Winston.

New South Wales Department of Education and Training. (2008). Use communication strategies to de-escalate conflict: https://sielearning.tafensw.edu.au/MCS/9362/Sterilisation%20disk%203/lo/7380/7380_00.htm.

Nursing and Midwifery Board of Australia (NMBA). (2018). *Code of Conduct for Nurses*. Retrieved from www.nursingmidwiferyboard.gov.au/Codes-Guidelines-Statements/Professional-standards.aspx.

Okey, J. (1992). Human aggression: The etiology of individual differences. *Journal of Humanistic Psychology*, 32(1), 51. doi:10.1177/0022167892321005

Queensland Government. (2016). *Queensland Mental Health Act 2016.* Retrieved from http://classic.austlii.edu.au/cgi-bin/download.cgi/cgi-bin/download.cgi/download/au/legis/qld/consol_act/mha2016128.pdf.

Rogers, C. (1951). *Client-Centered Therapy*. Boston, MA: Houghton Mifflin.

Rogers, C. (1961). *On Becoming a Person. A Therapist's View of Psychotherapy*. Boston, MA: Houghton Mifflin.

Seto, M.C., Charette, Y., Nicholls, T.L. & Crocker, A. G. (2018). Individual, service, and neighborhood predictors of aggression among persons with mental disorders. *Criminal Justice and Behavior*, 45(7), 929–48. https://doi.org/10.1177/0093854818765047

Shamoa-Nir, L. (2017). The window becomes a mirror: The use of the Johari window model to evaluate stereotypes in intergroup dialogue in Israel. *Israel Affairs*, 23(4), 727–46. https://doi.org/10.1080/13537121.2017.1333737

Stein-Parbury, J. (2013). *Patient and Person: Developing Interpersonal Skills in Nursing* (5th edn). Sydney: Elsevier.

Stone, T., McMillan, M., Hazelton, M. & Clayton, E.H. (2011). Wounding words: Swearing and verbal aggression in an inpatient setting. *Perspectives in Psychiatric Care*, 47(4), 194–203. doi:10.1111/j.1744-6163.2010.00295.x

Swift, E. (2009). The efficacy of treatments for borderline personality disorder. *Mental Health Practice* (through 2013), 13(4), 30–3. Retrieved from https://www.proquest.com/scholarly-journals/efficacy-treatments-borderline-personality/docview/217213328/se-2?accountid=8194

The Lancet. (2013). Editorial: Facing up to restraint in mental health units. *The Lancet*, 382(9891), 480. doi:http://dx.doi.org.ezproxy2.acu.edu.au/10.1016/S0140-6736(13)61697-9

Thomas, L. (2017). Nursing children and young people: What mental health training is required? *British Journal of Nursing*, 26(4), 234–7. doi:10.12968/bjon.2017.26.4.234

Thompson, N. (2011). *Effective Communication. A Guide for the People Professions* (2nd edn). London: Palgrave Macmillan.

Travelbee, J. (1971). *Interpersonal Aspects of Nursing* (2nd edn). Philadelphia, PA: F.A. Davis.

Unhjem, J., Vatne, S. & Hem, M. (2018). Transforming nurse–patient relationships: A qualitative study of nurse self-disclosure in mental health care. *Journal of Clinical Nursing*, 27(5.6), E798–E807. https://doi.org10.1111/jocn.14191

van der Zwan, R., Davies, L., Andrews, D. & Brooks, A. (2011). Aggression and violence in the ED: Issues associated with the implementation of restraint and seclusion. *Health Promotion Journal of Australia*, 22(2), 124–7. doi:10.1071/HE11124

Victoria Police. (2012). *Positional/Restraint Asphyxia (Version 1.0)*. Retrieved from http://www.police.vic.gov.au/retrievemedia.asp?media_id=79880.

Victorian Auditor-General. (2015). *Occupational Violence Against Healthcare Workers. Victorian Auditor-General's Report*. Melbourne: Victorian Government Printer. Retrieved from https://www.audit.vic.gov.au/sites/default/files/2017-07/20150506-Occ-Violence.pdf.

Victorian Consolidated Legislation. (2014). *Victorian Mental Health Act*. Retrieved from http://www.astss.org.au/wp-content/uploads/2016/01/14-026aa-authorised.pdf.

Webb, L. (2011). *Nursing: Communication Skills in Practice*. Oxford: Oxford University Press.

Weiten, W. (2017). Psychology. *Themes and Variations*, 3rd edn. Boston, MA: Cengage Learning.

CHAPTER 6

USING EVIDENCE TO GUIDE MENTAL HEALTH NURSING PRACTICE

Brian Phillips

LEARNING OUTCOMES

Upon completion of this chapter, you should be able to:

6.1 Understand the significance of evidence-based practice in nursing, including clinical reasoning and decision-making

6.2 Understand research sources, levels and types of research in order to implement evidence-based nursing practice

6.3 Understand how to critically appraise research evidence and have an awareness of critical appraisal tools

6.4 Apply research evidence in clinical practice strategies

6.5 Understand and use mental health routine outcome measures to inform individual clinical practice

LEARNING FROM PRACTICE

I am discussing Meryl's medication concerns with her as part of our agreed weekly home visits. We first met up a week ago following a discharge referral from the local hospital acute mental health unit. Meryl has been discharged on paroxetine 20 mg mane with supportive follow-up from our multidisciplinary primary health team and medical support from her local general practitioner. The discharge referral noted she has had two prior admissions subsequent to major depressive episodes. My current role is to provide twice-weekly home visits to monitor progress and support her engagement with the team during her recovery.

We are sitting at her kitchen table. Meryl is telling me about her past experiences of depression and the different therapies she has tried. I take particular note that she says her past medication 'hasn't worked' and goes on to state that, 'I've tried everything….' Now that she has been discharged home, she blames her current medications for 'putting on weight [and] …feeling ugly'. Meryl says that she wants to stop her medications and just continue therapy with our team psychologist.

Following my discussion with Meryl, I recheck the current evidence base about the clinical problem she has expressed and the alternatives she is considering. My health organisation has provided electronic access to eTG (Therapeutic Guidelines Ltd, 2016) and I am able to quickly establish the current best guidance on pharmacology and psychotherapy for depression. This includes a comprehensive discussion on the metabolic side effects Meryl was concerned with. On the next home visit to Meryl, I will have the best possible current information related to her choices. I can support her with an evidence-based nursing approach that is also sensitive to her concerns and preferences. Given that current guidance supports continuing antidepressant treatment for moderate or chronic depressive disorders (NICE, 2016), I have also informed myself further on metabolic side effects and given thought to the issue of weight gain that we might explore.

Aaron, community mental health nurse

Medication non-adherence is common among consumers with a mental health condition. Discuss the role of evidence-based research in the provision of information to consumers. Why is it important to consider Meryl's wishes in treatment?

INTRODUCTION

The term **evidence-based practice (EBP)** has become commonplace throughout clinical settings. Policy statements, clinical protocols and health care managers justify health care provision on the basis of evidence. Likewise, people who need nursing care for mental health problems are seeking evidence-based care; this means being assured of receiving the current best nursing care that is possible. Recently, the Nursing and Midwifery Board of Australia (NMBA, 2016) made it a regulatory requirement that evidence-based practice is used to assure the delivery of safe, quality nursing practice. This chapter discusses what 'evidence' is, where to find evidence for practice, how to know what is the 'best current evidence', and then integrate this as a practical part of clinical decision-making to ensure the best possible nursing care is being offered to consumers. Evidence-based practice applies to all contexts in which nursing care is provided. However, this chapter focuses on the particular issues related to mental health.

WHAT IS EVIDENCE-BASED PRACTICE?

Historically, nursing practice has been taught as an apprenticeship – that is, traditionally, beginner nurses were taught to provide care in a manner modelled by more senior nursing staff. While such approaches were thought to be the best practice at the time, and not all practice based on tradition was necessarily bad or detrimental, such approaches are inconsistent with evidence-based practice precisely because they were based on 'the way it has always been done' rather than evidence. Evidence based on research findings is regarded as the best available evidence for the provision of health care interventions.

The development of evidence-based nursing owes its origins to the work of Archie Cochrane (1909–88) and the acceptance of evidence-based medicine that followed. Cochrane was a medical researcher who challenged the state of health services in the United Kingdom and medicine more generally. He argued strongly that medical care must be based on research evidence that showed that treatment was not only effective, but also efficient (The Cochrane Collaboration, 2016). Cochrane argued that the most reliable scientific evidence to support treatment was the systematic review of randomised controlled trials. In response to Cochrane's work, the medical profession created the Cochrane Collaboration; now called the Cochrane Library (see http://www.cochranelibrary.com).

The nursing profession has progressively adopted an evidence-based nursing approach. In its recent revision of the *Registered Nurse Standards for Practice*, the NMBA's adoption of evidence-based practice has become the expected standard for nursing in Australia (NMBA, 2016). The Standards for Practice define evidence-based practice as 'accessing and making judgements to translate the best available evidence, which includes the most current, valid, and available research findings into practice' (p. 6). This definition makes clear that evidence-based practice is about how nurses come to make clinical decisions. Rather than doing what has always been done, nurses are now expected to have made an evidence-based decision. Underpinning an evidence-based decision is research evidence and a framework for translating outcomes of research into practice.

Evidence and clinical reasoning

Evidence-based nursing practice is not a formula or 'cookbook' approach to clinical decision-making. The above descriptions show that evidence is one (albeit, very significant) factor underpinning a complex decision-making process. The nurse is actively engaged in a process of carefully thinking through research evidence, and relating it to a decision about nursing care. This is a process that requires good thinking skills and an understanding of what needs to be considered when making a **clinical decision**.

Strauss, Glasziou, Richardson and Haynes (2011, p. 1) make it clear that practising in an evidence-based manner requires integrating at least three elements in the decision-making process:
1   clinical expertise
2   the best possible research evidence
3   the person's unique context and preferences.

The Institute for Johns Hopkins Nursing summarises this in its definition of evidence-based nursing:

> a problem-solving approach to clinical decision-making within a health care organization. It integrates the best scientific evidence with the best available experiential (patient and practitioner) evidence. EBP considers internal and external influences on practice and encourages critical thinking in the judicious application of such evidence to the care of individual patients, a patient population, or a system.

Source: Costa & Poe, 2012, cited in Dearholt & Dang, 2012, p.4

This kind of definition articulates the components of decision-making for evidence-based nursing practice. The clinical decision-making model by Russell and Gregory (2008) in **Figure 6.1** demonstrates the multiple factors that a nurse takes into consideration for effective clinical decision-making. Note that in addition to establishing the best research evidence (1), three other elements are necessary for an effective evidence-based clinical decision: (2) patient preferences and circumstances, (3) the judgement and expertise of the nurse, and (4) the opportunity and limits of the available resources.

Arriving at an evidence-based decision involves the clinical judgement and expertise of the nurse. The nurse brings to the decision-making process the knowledge and skills developed in their initial professional education and their background of clinical experience. As further experiences of applying knowledge and skills in practice are obtained and then reflected upon, clinical judgement is further developed and refined. With time, increased experience and critical reflection, clinical decisions are enhanced as the nurse gains in expertise.

The decision-making model in **Figure 6.1** clearly shows that a nursing decision includes considering the person. The person's experience, psychosocial (including cultural and spiritual) circumstances and personal wishes shape how the research evidence is ultimately utilised for the person's benefit. In this model of clinical decision-making, the person's situation and preferences sit alongside the other components that contribute to an agreed decision on the nursing care to be provided.

Ultimately, the clinical decision on the best course of action can become limited by the resources available. Resources can be the person's accommodation, their social environment, a ward environment, the funding available, or even the

geographical location such as remoteness or inner-city locations can change what is possible. While resources can create potential courses of action, at other times they can impose practical constraints where alternative courses of action need to be considered and negotiated with the person.

Clinical reasoning

For a nurse, good **clinical reasoning** means that all the components of each clinical decision are brought together in a logical, rigorous and reflective process (see **Figure 6.2**). Hence, clinical decision-making is inextricably linked to the quality of thinking involved. Levett-Jones and Hoffman (2013) state that clinical reasoning is a continuous, cyclical process. They argue that clinical reasoning is more than a careful, focused sequence of steps to arrive at an answer. Evaluation and reflection mean that each decision is also a point at which a nurse learns and gains from the experience. Critical thinking and reflection skills are applied with a willingness to keep the person central while examining for bias, stereotypes, stigma and preconceptions that can get in the way of good thinking.

In **Figure 6.2**, Levett-Jones and colleagues (2010) describe clinical reasoning as a circular process with eight stages: look, collect, process, decide, plan, act, evaluate and reflect. As a circular process, clinical reasoning does not have a distinct beginning or end – that is, evaluation and reflection should lead the nurse into considering the person again. While it is depicted as a sequence, Levett-Jones and Hoffman emphasise that the reality of clinical practice means that the different stages can become blurred and overlap, and the clinician might even move back and forth in the cycle as the situation and their thinking evolves.

Good thinking is developed over time and involves practice and experience – it is more than having a thorough and accurate knowledge of a subject, but is actively taking an ethical stance to value personal qualities such as inquisitiveness, precision and integrity (Levett-Jones, 2018). A useful strategy that nurses working in mental health settings frequently make use of is discussion with a critical friend or clinical supervision in which the task of the friend is to deliberately facilitate questioning and perspective-taking.

IMPLEMENTING EVIDENCE-BASED NURSING PRACTICE

Strauss et al. (2011) have highlighted that when we make a clinical decision from a position of certainty or 'knowing' what to do, we feel reassured and do not stop to question our knowledge or certainty. This can be a false reassurance and provide false comfort,

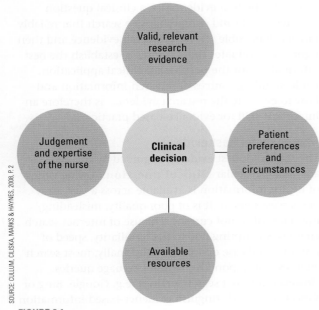

SOURCE: CULLUM, CILISKA, MARKS & HAYNES, 2008, P. 2

FIGURE 6.1
The components of an evidence-based nursing decision

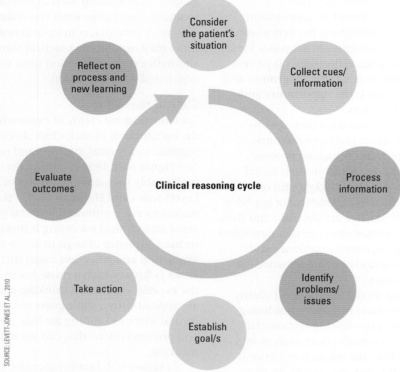

SOURCE: LEVETT-JONES ET AL. 2010

FIGURE 6.2
The clinical reasoning cycle

as we might have failed to check and recognise that our knowledge is no longer current. On the other hand, an experience of not knowing something may instead lead to avoiding such situations in the future. As time goes by, encountering situations of 'not-knowing' inevitably increase. Both situations have negative consequences for the clinician and the person needing nursing care. While it is necessary to remain competent, keeping up to date with changes in the research evidence can be a significant challenge for time-poor clinicians.

Strauss et al. (2011) describe two kinds of evidence-seeking behaviour with which clinicians can engage as 'pull' and 'push'. 'Pull' is a behaviour that relates to actively searching out the evidence and 'pulling' it to us in order to appraise it. For instance, when prompted to search for knowledge, we might access a library research database and search out information. On the other hand, 'push' evidence is evidence that finds us before we are aware of it. It refers to evidence that is sent to us; that is, it is 'pushed' out to us via email – and has become increasingly available with the arrival of dedicated evidence-based subscription services. Clinicians can organise dedicated evidence-based services to 'push' out clinical updates that are tightly focused on the topics nurses are interested in. This technique assures that we are alerted to evidence updates even before we are in a situation of needing assurance that evidence for our practice

is current. For example, *NURSING+* incorporates an email alert system for 'push' emails to alert the nurse to updates on their topic or clinical problem using a set of keyword filters to refine information relevant to the particular practice context such as mental health topics (see https://plus.mcmaster.ca/np).

Critical appraisal of research sources

To obtain the best evidence for a clinical question requires a wide and comprehensive search that reliably targets all possible relevant research evidence and then rigorously evaluates these studies to establish the best information for the purpose of clinical application. Understanding sources of research information and how to evaluate the research evidence, is therefore an important skill for evidence-based practice.

Searching for best evidence

The search for best evidence is guided by the need to answer a particular **clinical question**. A wide variety of health information is available across a vast array of sources; some of it is of poor quality, misleading, not relevant or not current. The use of internet search engines is tempting due to the familiarity, speed of response and ease of access. Additionally, most search engines will respond to natural language queries. However, internet search engines (e.g. Google, Bing or Yahoo!) do not distinguish evidence-based information from consumer-oriented, industry-sponsored testimonial or even fraudulent and misleading information. For example, a search for the phrase 'paroxetine side effects' produced 1.68 million results on Google and 44 400 results on Google Scholar. While Google Scholar produced very large numbers of results, this can be a false reassurance as the latest research may not yet be available to the search engine (see http://www.google.com/intl/en/scholar/inclusion.html). Research publications are not necessarily made available as open source material and are unable to be found by internet searching.

Research-evidence databases offer an effective and efficient approach for this purpose and access to these databases is increasingly made available within clinical settings. Nevertheless, careful preparation is needed for a database search to effectively meet the needs of a busy clinician. A database search must be broad enough to canvass the entire width of the available research yet be sufficiently specific so the user can be confident that the best available evidence has been located.

The immediate question prompted by a problem encountered in clinical practice is not usually in a form to effectively query an evidence-based database. Developing good questions helps to precisely and accurately state the clinical problem or issue, and makes the search effective and efficient. Asking good questions takes practice. Good questions are those that are searchable and answerable, but not all clinical questions are searchable or answerable. For instance, there might not be any research on the topic and so research databases do not yet hold any information. A question might not be searchable because of the way the question is constructed or because the terms used are everyday words rather than clinical terms used in the database indexing.

At least two types of questions can arise in clinical decision-making: background questions and foreground questions. **Background questions** are general clinical knowledge questions that aim to understand the issue in its broadest context. These kinds of questions seek to establish what is currently known about the clinical problem or issue. Background questions can frequently be answered in up-to-date textbooks. Background questions are commonly phrased as 'what', 'where' or 'when' questions (Stillwell, Fineout-Overholt, Melnyk & Williamson, 2010). A background question might be: 'What are the signs and symptoms of a major depressive episode?'

Foreground questions are specific questions that drive the search strategy and directly inform clinical practice decisions. These questions are best structured using the acronym PICO (Fineout-Overholt & Stillwell, 2011; Stillwell et al., 2010). Some writers add a 'T' (in order to include a time component into the question) into the structure; this is not included in the examples discussed here. **PICO** stands for:

P: the *patient*, *population*, *predicament* or *problem* is precisely defined.

I: specifies the *intervention* or issue of concern.

C: *comparison* intervention (if relevant). Identifying interventions to be excluded or compared helps to narrow down the results of the search so that the results have much greater relevance.

O: *outcomes* of clinical importance. Outcomes need to be specified and measurable.

Table 6.1 shows the search terms developed from an answerable clinical question using PICO. For instance, to help Meryl in the 'Learning from practice' vignette at the beginning of the chapter, the nurse may want to inform her of the current best evidence about her proposed action. To do this, Meryl's comments need to be reframed into an answerable question. Answerable questions establish the underlying issue or question in a crisp and precise sentence, as can be seen in **Table 6.1**.

TABLE 6.1
Example of search terms framed using PICO

Question: Is paroxetine effective for depression compared with psychological therapy alone?	
P: patient, population, predicament, or problem	Depression
I: intervention	Paroxetine, selective serotonin reuptake inhibitor (SSRI)
C: comparison intervention (if relevant)	Psychotherapy, cognitive therapy#
O: outcomes of clinical importance	#

= MIGHT NOT ALWAYS BE USED DEPENDING ON QUESTION.

Table 6.1 sets out the PICO into search terms that can be plugged into the query fields of a suitable database. In the first instance, using search engines and databases enabling a search focused on evidence-based practice is the best approach. Some databases, such as the Turning Research into Practice database (TRIPdatabase), provide a search facility specific to questions developed using PICO. Other databases, such as PubMed, provide search facilities that can limit results to the appropriate evidence level. A careful choice of search terms will also either broaden or narrow the search. Typically, database searches can produce a large number of varying research studies that may or may not be applicable, and further evaluation will be needed in the form of an appraisal before the research can be applied to the specific practice problem.

CASE **STUDY**

A NEW CLIENT

Tomas is a 19-year-old consumer recently diagnosed with schizophrenia and living with his mother. He has been unable to return to his study course or find work since dropping out of his VET course the previous semester. He is reluctant to accept the diagnosis and struggles to agree with a need to take his olanzapine. His mother has expressed worries that she 'cannot talk to him any more' and get him to take his medication. She says he is becoming worse and asks you what she should do. Tomas is a new client and it is not clear how to quickly develop medication adherence with Tomas and support his mother. You decide to locate and review the most current and best evidence to develop your response.

Questions

1   What background questions need to be answered in order to then develop the specific foreground question?
2   Develop a searchable and answerable foreground question using the PICO format to locate the highest level of evidence to inform your approach to help Tomas and his mother.

Levels and types of research evidence

Clinicians do not approach research evidence for the same purpose as that of a researcher. Researchers pose questions as research problems – frequently, for the purpose of discovery through hypothesis testing. From this perspective, researchers are interested in the best way to answer the research question. Instead, clinicians need to have confidence that they are utilising the best currently available evidence about the specific clinical problem impacting on their client. Therefore, the clinician asks questions of the current research evidence that best answers the clinical problem.

Clinicians seek to find the best possible answer to clinical questions from databases containing very large pools of research. To find the best possible current evidence, an understanding of how to classify the quality of research is needed. Research evidence is frequently depicted in a hierarchy, often called an 'evidence pyramid', where the top of the pyramid represents the highest level of research evidence available. The pyramid in **Figure 6.3** depicts six levels of research-based evidence. The best – or most trustworthy – evidence is at the top of the pyramid.

Any search for evidence for practice should start at the top of the pyramid. Clinicians should only move down the levels when the evidence is not available at a higher level. **Figure 6.3** is divided into two broad layers: filtered information and unfiltered information. *Filtered information* is sources of research evidence in which studies based on similar

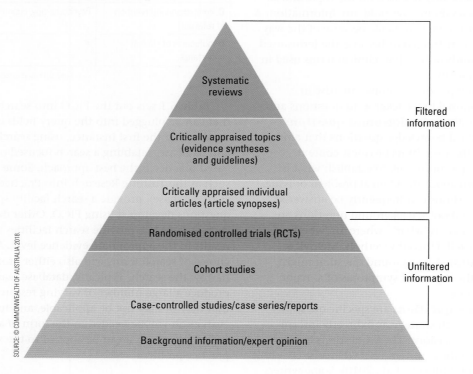

SOURCE: © COMMONWEALTH OF AUSTRALIA 2018.

FIGURE 6.3
Evidence pyramid

characteristics are brought together using systematic and structured appraisal methods. For this reason, filtered information is often referred to as filtered, or *pre-appraised* evidence. On the other hand, *unfiltered information* consists of sources of research evidence that is not yet critically appraised. If no pre-appraised evidence is available then unfiltered information needs to be considered. However, unfiltered information requires the clinician to undertake a wide search for applicable original research and then critically appraise the evidence using appropriate methods.

Filtered (pre-appraised) information

Filtered (pre-appraised) information is shown in **Figure 6.3** as having three main levels, with systematic reviews being the best source of evidence available. However, clinicians frequently face problems for which systematic reviews are not possible because the research is not available yet, not sufficiently developed, may not be applicable or the clinical problem is highly complex. For these reasons, clinical guidelines and evidence syntheses are highly valued.

Systematic reviews

McKibbon and Marks (2008, p. 32) define a **systematic review** as 'an article that poses a clinical question, uses predefined methods to search for studies that provide evidence to answer the question' and then applies a rigorous protocol to combine research results from original studies into a set of tables. Depending on the protocol, a variety of relevant metrics will be provided for the reader. One overall summary statistic of interest for clinicians is that of effect size (ES). An **effect size (ES)** is a way of measuring the predicted strength that an intervention or treatment will have on a specific outcome (Rice, 2009). Meta-analyses combine the ES across the selected studies to increase the probability of correctly detecting an accurate relationship between the intervention and the outcomes. A systematic review will describe how the ES was derived and provide a discussion to assist the reader to interpret the statistic used (Costa & Poe, 2012). It is the ability to combine results from multiple studies that makes the systematic review a powerful and highly valuable resource for clinicians. Where available, systematic reviews offer the best form of evidence to answer clinical questions about the effectiveness of clinical treatments.

Evidence-based (topic) syntheses and guidelines

Systematic reviews may not be the highest level of evidence available, so **topic syntheses** and **best practice or clinical guidelines** will also draw upon lower levels of research evidence when higher levels of research evidence do not yet exist. Because of rapidly

changing knowledge, guidelines need to be regularly updated. Clinicians need to note the currency of topic syntheses or guidelines. An expiry date is usually provided on clinical guidelines.

Clinical or best practice guidelines address clinical scenarios that are complex and there is a need to authoritatively draw together a large array of varied information for clinicians to rely upon with confidence – for example, best practice guidelines for schizophrenia (RANZCP, 2009). Current syntheses and guidelines are highly valued as a resource as they inform clinicians of the current state of knowledge for commonly occurring, complex or challenging clinical scenarios. A number of portals exist that enable a search for clinical guidelines; some examples are shown in **Table 6.2**.

TABLE 6.2
Examples of portals for clinical guidelines

GUIDELINES PORTAL	URL
Agency for Healthcare Research and Quality	https://www.ahrq.gov/gam/index.html
Australian Clinical Practice Guidelines	https://www.clinicalguidelines.gov.au
Electronic Therapeutic Guidelines (eTG)	https://tgldcdp.tg.org.au/etgcomplete
National Institute for Health and Care Excellence	https://www.nice.org.uk
National Institute for Health Research Dissemination Centre	https://discover.dc.nihr.ac.uk/portal/home (see 'Themed Reviews')
Nursing Reference Centre	Via the EBSCO database: https://www.ebsco.com/
Trip database	https://www.tripdatabase.com (search using 'guidelines' as the search type)
WHO Guidelines	http://www.who.int/publications/guidelines/mental_health/en

Article synopses

Article synopses are structured summaries that provide an appraisal of an individual research study or review (McKibbon & Marks, 2008, p. 32). Because they are single studies or reviews, they are not ranked as highly on the evidence pyramid. Nonetheless, synopses are valuable for keeping current with rapidly changing research evidence in a specific or specialised area of clinical practice for which the clinician needs to remain current with the leading edge of thinking in the specialty area. Subscription services have arisen to meet the need for clinicians to stay current. Research synopses can be obtained as a 'push' service via specialist subscription services. **Table 6.3** shows three examples useful for nurses working in mental health. For instance, *Evidence-Based Mental Health* is a service tailored to the needs of psychiatrists and

TABLE 6.3

Examples of evidence-based sources that enable 'push' alerts by subscription

PUBLICATION	URL
Evidence-Based Mental Health	http://ebmh.bmj.com
Evidence-Based Nursing	http://ebn.bmj.com
Worldviews on Evidence-Based Nursing	http://www.nursingsociety.org/learn-grow/publications/worldviews-on-evidence-based-nursing

TABLE 6.4

The hierarchy of evidence for intervention/treatment questions

I	Evidence from a systematic review or meta-analysis of all relevant RCTs
II	Evidence obtained from well-designed RCTs
III	Evidence obtained from well-designed controlled trials without randomisation
IV	Evidence from well-designed case-control and cohort studies
V	Evidence from systematic reviews of descriptive and qualitative studies
VI	Evidence from single descriptive or qualitative studies
VII	Evidence from the opinion of authorities and/or reports of expert committees

SOURCE: MELNYK & FINEOUT-OVERHOLT, 2011, P. 12

psychologists. *Evidence-Based Nursing* has the needs of nurses as the target audience, as does *Worldviews on Evidence-Based Nursing*. Each of these sources has topic filters to enable alerts to be tailored for particular topics or interests.

Unfiltered information

When evidence does not exist in a pre-appraised (or filtered) form, then locating relevant evidence by searching research databases is the next step. **Unfiltered information** can be at different levels in the research hierarchy, as shown in **Figure 6.3**, and undertaken with different levels of methodological rigour. For these reasons, the clinician will need to locate the research studies and undertake the critical appraisal.

To ensure the best evidence is located, database searching must be thorough and as wide as possible. Different databases incorporate different ranges of research journals to service different audiences. For instance, original research published in the *International Journal of Mental Health Nursing* is indexed in a number of databases including CINAHL and MEDLINE. CINAHL is an acronym for the Cumulative Index of Nursing and Allied Health Literature and indexes up to 5531 (depending on the subscription type) journals related to nursing and allied health disciplines (see https://health.ebsco.com). Similarly, MEDLINE indexes up to 5600 biomedical and health journals depending on the subscription product that has been purchased by the library. MEDLINE can also be searched via the freely available US National Library of Medicine PubMed site (see https://www.ncbi.nlm.nih.gov/pubmed). Given the very large volume of information available, knowledge of effective database searching is a necessary skill. Training on database searching, and framing good clinical questions using PICO, is freely available from most university libraries.

Different research designs are ranked at different levels (see **Table 6.4**) and different research designs best fit different kinds of clinical questions. The ranking shown in **Table 6.4** is a hierarchy for ranking research designs to inform questions about the effectiveness of treatment interventions. Systematic reviews or

meta-analyses are the best research designs for evidence about treatment effectiveness. The highest possible level should always be chosen. Some familiarity with research design will be needed in order to undertake critical appraisal of original research studies.

Randomised controlled trials

Randomised controlled trials (RCTs) are regarded as the 'gold standard' for establishing the efficacy for treatment or clinical intervention. The design of RCTs is the most rigorous means of determining a cause–effect relationship. This is due to the characteristics of experimental design of (1) *randomisation* of subjects to intervention groups, (2) a *control* group that serves as a comparison, and (3) *manipulation* of variables. These characteristics mean that clinicians can be confident of the cause–effect relationship between treatment and outcome rather than an alternative explanation.

Quasi-experimental designs

Cohort studies and **case-controlled studies** are two different forms of quasi-experimental designs. They are sometimes also referred to as observational studies. Like experimental designs, they seek to determine the relationship between variables and outcomes. However, because they lack randomisation, it is not possible to rule out unaccounted systematic influences that might affect the outcome. Quasi-experimental designs are used when it is not possible or it is unethical to manipulate the variables involved; instead, researchers utilise already existing groups and circumstances.

Non-experimental designs

Descriptive design is a form of non-experimental study. Rather than establishing a cause–effect relationship, the purpose is to study naturally occurring events and provide a precise and detailed description. In this kind of study, the researcher is seeking to describe a characteristic of a group or pattern of events. Descriptive research may be qualitative or quantitative; for instance, the Australian

Census is a statistical description of the national population every five years.

Qualitative research designs

Qualitative studies are a valuable asset to the evidence hierarchy when it comes to clinical decision-making involving questions of human meaning and subjective experience. Qualitative designs are highly diverse, arising out of different research traditions. Arguably, the qualitative approaches most common in nursing research are ethnography, grounded theory, phenomenology and hermeneutics. While there are overlapping methods for gathering data and management of data, the interpretation of human experience and meaning takes place through the different interpretive lenses depending on which of these approaches is being used.

Non-research-based evidence

Not all evidence is research-based. The available research evidence may not be applicable to the question being asked, or the research evidence simply does not yet exist for the practice question. The notion of 'best available evidence' therefore requires an appropriate consideration of non-research evidence. Non-research-based evidence includes expert opinion, theory, organisational experience, personal experience and consumer preference. As the lowest ranked level of evidence, Level VII evidence should be utilised cautiously with an awareness of the limitations.

Textbooks

Textbooks do not appear in the levels of evidence hierarchy. Nonetheless, textbooks do have a valuable place in a search for research evidence. Textbooks have a role to distil or consolidate fields of well-established research. McKibbon and Marks (2008, p. 31) argue that a recently published textbook is useful for addressing

> 'stable' information needs, that is, facts that seldom change, such as gross anatomy, basic principles and mechanisms, and specific disease characteristics [and] can also provide summaries of new or complex topics or discuss issues in the context of other related areas of knowledge.

Textbooks can therefore be good sources of evidence for background questions. The kinds of questions that might be asked of a textbook could be, for example: Where is the limbic system located? Or, what is a Mental State Examination?

CRITICAL APPRAISAL OF RESEARCH EVIDENCE

Having found a number of original research studies using a clinical question framed using PICO, there remains the need to critically appraise the results of the database search according to their strength, quality and applicability. Ultimately, the appraiser or appraisal team, seeks to establish the best currently available evidence for the clinical question. Cullum (2008) argues that in applying a **critical appraisal** to the research evidence, the researcher is attempting to make a judgement according to three broad questions:

1   Is the design and method likely to have led to a result that is trustworthy?
2   If so, is it relevant to the clinical practice issue?
3   What were the results?

These questions are applied in different ways depending on whether the research is quantitative or qualitative. Quantitative methods are designed to test theory and produce results that can be replicated and generalisable. **Quantitative research** uses well-established methods to determine measurable relationships between variables through **hypothesis testing**. While research studies are peer reviewed, this does not mean all published research is of the same quality. Hence, critical appraisal closely examines the study design, methods, results (in statistical format) and conclusions. In examining for quality and rigour, critical appraisal looks closely at reliability, validity and precision. Costa and Poe (2012, p. 102) define these three key concepts as follows:

> **Validity** is the extent to which the research measures what it is intended to measure and how well the findings approximate the truthfulness of the subject of interest.

> **Reliability** refers to the consistency or repeatability of measurement.

> **Precision** has to do with how to interpret statistical measures of central tendency and statistical significance … of populations and characteristics of populations.

Not all clinical questions are suited to being answered by research approaches that are designed using quantitative methods. For instance, mental health clinicians are frequently concerned to understand the meaning and experience of mental health issues and recovery. These kinds of concerns are best answered using qualitative research designs. Qualitative research is based on a highly diverse group of methodologies that seek to obtain an understanding of phenomena through inductive analysis. There are a number of different ways to describe or categorise qualitative research. Methodologies that tend to appear in nursing research fall into the following broad groupings:

- *Ethnography* involves the study of a social group's culture from the perspective of the person living the culture in order to produce a rich description of their lived experience. Techniques used can include participant observation, in-depth interviews and artefacts.

- *Grounded theory* seeks to generate theory about how people deal with situations. Collection of data uses some of the techniques from ethnography. Categories or concepts are derived (i.e. 'grounded') from within the data. Theorising is inductively developed through a process that systematically explains (theorises) the linkages or relationships between the categories or concepts.
- *Phenomenology* seeks to grasp the essential meaning of lived experiences through processes that explicitly recognise or 'bracket' the interpretive role of the researcher in the analysis. The specific approach taken depends on the philosophical stance being used by the researcher.
- *Hermeneutics* is a variety of interpretative approach that draws upon dialogue (conversational or textual) in order to understand meaning or experience. Hermeneutic interpretation emphasises a close or immersive engagement with language to reach (or co-create) an in-depth understanding or meaning.

Critical appraisal of qualitative research requires a different approach to that used for quantitative research. Unlike the scientific method of hypothesis testing, qualitative research approaches are underpinned by a different relationship between the research question, philosophical tradition, methods and analysis. Therefore, concepts of reliability, validity and precision are not valid for examining qualitative research approaches. Lincoln and Guba (1986) have instead proposed that the concept of rigour in qualitative research can be approximated through a concept of *trustworthiness*, the criteria of which are: credibility, transferability, dependability and confirmability. However, Lincoln and Guba also caution that even these concepts do not suit all qualitative approaches. Hence, an appraisal of qualitative research involves careful consideration of the fit between the research question, philosophy, methodology, methods and approach to interpretation.

Critical appraisal tools

More recently, **critical appraisal tools (CATs)** have been developed to assist in the rapid evaluation of original research studies. Featherstone et al. (2015) caution that rapid reviews using CATs do not serve the same purpose as a systematic review and should not be considered as a substitute for a systematic review. Nevertheless, reviews using CATs will assist a review team to bring together the relevant current research and provide a structure for the team to rigorously

evaluate the evidence. Clinical teams might use CATs to help develop evidence-based clinical protocols for a ward, or conduct a review of current nursing care to ensure best practice is being applied. The critical appraisal team will need a reasonable level of familiarity with different research designs, including knowledge of common statistics.

A CAT offers a structured process or framework to guide the appraiser through a rigorous process of selecting and appraising each of the research studies and evaluate the strengths and quality of different elements, such as the level of evidence in the literature review, design of the study, sampling methods, validity, reliability and precision.

A number of sources make CATs freely available. While not nursing-specific, the Critical Appraisal Skills Programme (CASP) website offers a list of CATs that can be downloaded and are free to use (Better Value Healthcare, 2018). Like similar websites, the CASP site offers CATs specific to different research designs. The Institute for Johns Hopkins Nursing offers a project model for critical appraisal using specific CATs for each type of research design (Dearholt & Dang, 2012). The Johns Hopkins model additionally offers a synthesis and recommendations tool to specifically guide translating the appraisal findings of the team into practical action recommendations.

A different approach to CAT is offered by the Joanna Briggs Institute (JBI; see http://joannabriggs. org). While JBI offer checklists for appraisal of different research designs, JBI COnNECT+ provides a portal for appraisers to conduct complete evidence-based practice projects and to begin developing and sharing a library of evidence-based resources for their health care organisation. A number of web-based tools are made available for different kinds of projects. In particular, nurses and students are stepped through the critical appraisal process and development of the final appraised product using RAPid.

TRANSLATING EVIDENCE INTO CLINICAL PRACTICE

Having the best available research evidence is necessary for informing the best possible care for someone needing nursing care. However, the best research evidence available (such as a systematic review) is likely to have been developed with a sample or with conditions that are not immediately applicable to the specific person's particular preference and context – that is, the conditions of the research study that produced the level of treatment effectiveness will vary from the reality of the clinical application of the evidence. A form of translating research evidence into practice is therefore necessary.

To translate research evidence into clinical practice, Rice (2013) suggests returning once again to the PICO acronym; this time, as a means of asking questions related to the specific clinical application, person, their preferences and situation (see **Table 6.5**). In doing so, the question structure must support an open negotiation with the person in which the best available evidence is a transparent element in the conversation about the clinical problem.

TABLE 6.5
PICO questions for clinical application

PICO	CLINICAL APPLICATION
Person's condition specificity	1 Is the person's condition or issue the same as that in the evidence-based literature?
	2 Are the characteristics of the current setting the same as that in the evidence-based literature?
Intervention effectiveness	3 How has the intervention been applied with this population?
	4 Are the risks and benefits of using the intervention known for this population?
Comparative/ alternative	5 Is there evidence showing that alternative interventions have better outcomes?
	6 Which alternatives have demonstrated less risks for this person?
Outcome	7 What is the level of satisfaction for the person and clinician?

SOURCE: ADAPTED FROM RICE, 2013, P. 218

Rice states that the clinician needs to ask a series of six questions:

1 Is the person's condition or issue the same as that in the evidence-based literature?
2 Are the characteristics of the current setting the same as that in the evidence-based literature?

If the differences between the characteristics of the evidence-based literature are too dissimilar to that of the person or their situation, then the expected evidence-based outcomes may not be achieved. Similarly, to determine if the intervention being considered may be effective for this specific person, the clinician needs to ask:

3 How has the intervention been applied to this population?
4 Are the risks and benefits of using the intervention known for this population?

Keeping the person's wishes and situation central to the conversation also means that implementing the evidence-based treatment or intervention is a shared decision-making process. This may lead to alternative treatments or interventions being considered. In this case, alternatives (also evidence-based) may need to prompt two further questions:

5 Is there evidence showing that alternative interventions have better outcomes?

6 Which alternatives have demonstrated less risk for this person?

As the process is one where evidence-based treatments or interventions may be modified to suit the specific circumstances and acceptability to the person, the final step is an evaluation of clinical outcomes. A seventh step is implemented:

7 What is the level of satisfaction for the person and clinician?

CULTURAL CONSIDERATIONS

The role of shared decision-making
Hulme (2010) has argued that research evidence frequently provides little guidance for the clinician to understand the applicability or acceptability of the evidence for particular ethnic groups. When it is not known if the best evidence fits with a person's cultural background, beliefs, values or preferences, then shared decision-making becomes a particularly important approach in negotiating a decision that is acceptable and respectful of cultural difference.

MENTAL HEALTH OUTCOME MEASURES

Routine outcome measures are well-established measures of change that have occurred for the consumer due to their receiving mental health care. A range of outcome measures has been established as part of the National Outcomes and Casemix Collection (NOCC) hosted by the Australian Mental Health Outcomes and Classification Network (AMHOCN; http://www.amhocn.org). Unlike rating scales that evaluate the impact of interventions on specific clinical signs and symptoms that the clinician is intending to treat, routine outcome measures evaluate the impact on the person's functioning in such areas as social activity, activities of daily living or general levels of emotional distress. By drawing upon a range of clinician and consumer-rated measures, this data can be used by multiple stakeholders for benchmarking and other quality improvement activities by teams and services. The measures listed in **Table 6.6** are the routine outcome measures collected by NOCC for adults. Routine outcome measures have been collected by public mental health services since 2003 and are used to support national and local service quality improvement activities (Coombs, Stapley & Pirkis, 2011). These measures can also be used to inform individual clinical practice; for example, repeated measures over the course of a person receiving care can show functional

TABLE 6.6
The NOOC measures for adults

INSTRUMENT	DESCRIPTION
Health of the Nation Outcomes Scales (HoNOS)	A 12-item clinician-rated instrument measuring behaviour, impairment, symptoms and social functioning. It can be considered as a general measure of symptom severity. There are variants of HoNOS for different age groups and settings.
Life Skills Profile (LSP-16)	A 16-item clinician-rated instrument. The LSP-16 assesses abilities with basic life skills. Its focus is on general functioning and adaptation to community living, rather than the person's clinical signs and symptoms.
Kessler (K-10+)	A 10-item self-report questionnaire intended to be a general measure of non-specific psychological distress and functioning related to nervousness, agitation, psychological fatigue and depression.
Behaviour and Symptom Identification Scale (BASIS-32)	A 32-item self-rated survey intended to measure changes in symptoms and functioning difficulties.
Mental Health Inventory (MHI-38)	The MHI-38 can be used for self-reporting or as a part of an interview. It is intended as a general measure of psychological distress and well-being.
Resource Utilisation Groups – Activities of Daily Living (RUG-ADL)	A clinician-rated scale designed for use in long-term care facilities for older people. The RUG-ADL measures a person's dependency and functional abilities such as bed mobility, toileting, transfer and eating.
Focus of Care (FoC)	A clinician-rated single item requiring the clinician to make a judgement about the person's primary goal of care from one of four options: acute; functional gain; intensive extended care; and maintenance.

SOURCE: ADAPTED FROM HTTP://WWW.AMHOCN.ORG

improvement, and use of routine outcome measures as part of clinician–consumer discussions about goals can facilitate engagement and collaboration.

A different set of outcome measures has been developed for community mental health organisations, to capture the lesser focus on clinically defined care and, instead, a greater focus on community participation, social inclusion and recovery (Australian Mental Health Oucomes and Classification Network & Community Mental Health Australia, 2015).

REFLECTION ON LEARNING FROM PRACTICE

This chapter has explored the need for evidence-based nursing practice in mental health for the benefit of both consumers and clinicians. When we use evidence to inform our decision-making, we add credibility to our practice and ensure that consumers have an opportunity to make informed choices that are realistic, and will have the best likely outcomes. The nurse in the Learning from practice vignette demonstrated how robust research into metabolic side effects ensured she could provide Meryl with the best options that were scientifically based, while being empathically considered.

CHAPTER RESOURCES

SUMMARY

- Evidence-based nursing care assures the highest quality of care and best outcomes and is an expected standard of care for registered nurses in Australia. Clinical decision-making is an active process involving clinical reasoning informed by the research evidence, the clinical expertise of the nurse, the available resources, and the client's preferences and situation. Locating evidence-based sources involves reframing clinical questions into a searchable question using the PICO format.

- Evidence for decision-making in clinical practice is arranged in a hierarchy. Systematic reviews of research evidence are the highest level of evidence. Unfiltered sources of evidence should only be used if filtered sources are not available. When filtered information is not available, unfiltered sources of research evidence, such as original research studies, need critical appraisal.

- Critical appraisal tools offer a rigorous and structured approach to rapidly appraise the research evidence.

- Applying best evidence requires consideration of the person's situation and context, including cultural background.
- Having the best available research evidence is necessary for informing the best possible care for someone needing nursing care. The PICO framework is useful as a means of asking questions related to the specific clinical application, person, their preferences and situation.

- Mental health outcome measures are routinely collected by public mental health providers. When used as repeated measures over a period of time, they can also be used to evaluate clinical practice in areas of functioning such as activities of daily living.

REVIEW QUESTIONS

1   Evidence-based nursing practice is best described as:
a   Accessing and using the best available research evidence to inform clinical decision-making about nursing care
b   Applying the most recent research study related to a clinical problem
c   Nursing care that is respectful of and responsive to the individual patient situation and preferences
d   Nursing care that is modelled on the practices and behaviour of senior clinicians

2   When a nurse is evaluating the relevance of a research-based study or report to support their clinical practice, which criteria should be applied?
a   Web search engine ranking
b   Advice of the senior nurse
c   Level of evidence
d   Statistical power

3   When a nurse keeps the person's wishes central to the conversation about implementing evidence-based nursing care, this is called:
a   Psychoeducation
b   Shared decision-making
c   Recovery-based practice
d   Goal setting

4   A systematic review must have all the following, except:
a   Documents criteria used to include or exclude research studies
b   Provides a discussion to assist in interpreting the review findings
c   Addresses a specific clinical question
d   A discussion of related published papers that sets out an argument or point of view

5   A nurse is asking a good foreground question when they:
a   Enter the clinical problem as key words in a web search engine
b   Reframe the clinical problem using a PICO question template
c   Ask a senior medical specialist about the clinical problem
d   Enter the clinical problem as key words in a research database search engine

6   A nurse is reading a recently published research study showing that a particular food group has a positive effect on mood disorders, and is considering if the study means that the nursing team should change their clinical practice.

What is the best step the nursing team should next undertake so that their practice is evidence-based?
a   Check that the study was approved by a human research ethics committee
b   Examine the research study to see if the results show a high level of statistical significance
c   Immediately change practice to recommend changing what clients with mood disorders eat
d   Undertake a rapid review of the article using a relevant critical appraisal tool from http://www.casp-uk.net

7   A nurse is translating research evidence into practice when:
a   they use the Life Skills Profile (LSP-16) to evaluate the community supported housing program
b   they conduct their own research study to test if a diversional therapy program decreases the use of psychotropic PRN medications on the ward
c   they are considering the suitability of the appraised evidence to the particular circumstances and preferences of the person, group or community
d   they enter a clinical supervision arrangement to reflect on their practice

8   Routine mental health outcome measures can be effectively used to:
a   Screen for medication side effects
b   Establish a benchmark for quality improvement activities
c   Assess for signs and symptoms of schizophrenia
d   Evaluate the nurse's clinical competence

9   An example of a 'background question' would be:
a   Does a 'suicide contract' reduce the risk of suicide?
b   Asking if there is a plan to take your own life?
c   How do men express hopelessness differently from women?
d   What are the risk factors for suicide?

10 Clinical reasoning is a process that is:
a   A cyclical process involving four steps: evidence, clinical expertise, resources and the person's preferences
b   A circular process involving eight steps: look, collect, process, decide, plan, act, evaluate and reflect
c   A sequential and recursive process of: engaging, focusing, evoking and planning
d   Set out in a statement with the parameters of population, intervention, comparison and outcomes

CRITICAL THINKING

1   In your recent interactions with a client, you observe behaviours that are not what you expected to see. You describe the observed behaviours later that day. In doing so, you realise that you do not know the meaning of the unexpected behaviours. As you are wanting to develop your evidence-based practice, discuss some of the actions you could now take.

2   An unfamiliar medication has been charted by the psychiatric registrar. It has caused you to think that you may not be keeping up with current changes to practice.

Discuss some of the ways in which you can routinely be alerted to changes in evidence-based practice specific to your clinical context.

3   Although you have provided information to a client, they decline the current best-practice approach. Discuss how to respond in order to ensure that your client receives the best evidence-based care.

REFLECT ON THIS

Using the Cochrane Library to research COVID-19
There is a great deal of attention being paid to the evidence underpinning our developing understanding of coronavirus and the COVID-19 pandemic. While our understanding continues to develop, the Cochrane Library has begun to present the latest evidence available in a number of areas related to COVID-19 through its special collection section: https://www.cochranelibrary.com/collections/doi/SC000045/full

Explore this section and choose one systematic review to read. Then answer the following questions.

1   Identify the review question and search strategy used by the reviewers. How did the reviewers evaluate credibility?

2   Did the reviewers provide assistance in translating the results into your own practice?

3   Read the synopsis of evidence article 'Educational interventions for patients receiving psychotropic medication' (Joanna Briggs Institute, 2007).
   a   Describe the type of evidence sources used by the authors.
   b   What comment was made about the quality of the research?
   c   Did the authors provide suggestions for translating the evidence into your own practice?

The full reference entry for the article referred to in question 3 can be found in the 'References' section at the end of this chapter.

REFERENCES

Australian Mental Health Outcomes and Classification Network, & Community Mental Health Australia. (2015). *Implementing Routine Outcome Measurement in Community Managed Organisations*. Retrieved from http://www.amhocn.org/sites/default/files/publication_files/implementing_routine_outcome_measurement_in_cmos.pdf.

Better Value Healthcare. (2018). Critical Appraisal Skills Programme. Retrieved from http://www.casp-uk.net.

Cochrane Library Special Collection. (2021). Retrieved from https://www.cochranelibrary.com/collections/doi/SC000047/fulll

Commonwealth of Australia. (2018). National Health and Medical Research Council. Released under CC BY 3.0 AU. Link to license: https://creativecommons.org/licenses/by/3.0/au/. © Commonwealth of Australia 2018.

Coombs, T., Stapley, K. & Pirkis, J. (2011). The multiple uses of routine mental health outcome measures in Australia and New Zealand: Experiences from the field. *Australasian Psychiatry*, 19(3), 247–53. doi:10.3109/10398562.2011.562507

Costa, L. & Poe, S.S. (2012). Evidence appraisal: Research. In S. Dearholt & D. Dang (eds), *Johns Hopkins Nursing Evidence-based Practice: Models and Guidelines* (2nd edn, pp. 83–124). Indianapolis, IN: Sigma Theta Tau International.

Cullum, N. (2008). Users' guides to the nursing literature: An introduction. In N. Cullum, D. Ciliska, R.B. Haynes & S. Marks (eds), *Evidence-based Nursing: An Introduction* (pp. 101–15). Oxford: Blackwell Publishing.

Cullum, N., Ciliska, D., Marks, S. & Haynes, R.B. (2008). An introduction to evidence-based nursing. In N. Cullum, D. Ciliska, R.B. Haynes & S. Marks (eds), *Evidence-based Nursing: An Introduction* (pp. 1–8). Oxford: Blackwell Publishing.

Dearholt, S. & Dang, D. (eds). (2012). *Johns Hopkins Nursing Evidence-based Practice: Models and Guidelines* (2nd edn). Indianapolis, IN: Sigma Theta Tau International.

Featherstone, R.M., Dryden, D.M., Foisy, M., Guise, J.-M., Mitchell, M.D., Paynter, R. A., … Hartling, L. (2015). Advancing knowledge of rapid reviews: An analysis of results, conclusions and recommendations from published review articles examining rapid reviews. *Systematic Reviews*, 4(1), 50. doi:10.1186/s13643-015-0040-4

Fineout-Overholt, E. & Stillwell, S.B. (2011). Asking compelling, clinical questions. In B.M. Melnyk & E. Fineout-Overholt (eds), *Evidence-based Practice in Nursing & Healthcare: A Guide to Best Practice* (2nd edn, pp. 25–39). Philadelphia, PA: Wolters Kluwer/Lippincott Williams & Wilkins Health.

Hulme, P.A. (2010). Cultural considerations in evidence-based practice. *Journal of Transcultural Nursing*, 21(3), 271–80. doi:10.1177/1043659609358782

Joanna Briggs Institute. (2007). Educational interventions for patients receiving psychotropic medication. *Nursing Standard*, 22(12), 40+. Retrieved from http://link.galegroup.com/apps/doc/A172905636/SPJ. SP16?u=nurscare&sid=SPJ.SP16&xid=9d2a0e10.

Levett-Jones, T. (2018). *Clinical Reasoning: Learning to Think Like a Nurse* (2nd edn). Melbourne: Pearson Australia.

Levett-Jones, T. & Hoffman, K. (2013). Clinical reasoning: What it is and why it matters. In T. Levett-Jones & K. Hoffman (eds), *Clinical Reasoning: Learning to Think Like a Nurse* (pp. 2–15). Melbourne: Pearson Australia.

Levett-Jones, T., Hoffman, K., Dempsey, J., Jeong, S.Y., Noble, D., Norton, C.A. & Hickey, N. (2010). The 'five rights' of clinical reasoning: An educational model to enhance nursing students' ability to identify and manage clinically 'at risk' patients. *Nurse Education Today*, 30(6), 515–20. doi:10.1016/j.nedt. 2009.10.020.

Lincoln, Y.S. & Guba, E.G. (1986). But is it rigorous? Trustworthiness and authenticity in naturalistic evaluation. *New Directions for Program Evaluation*, 1986(30), 73–84. doi:10.1002/ev.1427.

McKibbon, K.A. & Marks, S. (2008). Searching for the best evidence. Part 1: where to look. In N. Cullum, D. Ciliska, R.B. Haynes & S. Marks (eds), *Evidence-based Nursing: An Introduction* (pp. 30–6). Oxford: Blackwell Publishing.

Melnyk, B.M. & Fineout-Overholt, E. (2011). Making the case for evidence-based practice and cultivating a spirit of inquiry. In B.M. Melnyk & E. Fineout-Overholt (eds), *Evidence-based Practice in Nursing & Healthcare: A Guide to Best Practice* (2nd edn, pp. 3–24). Philadelphia, PA: Wolters Kluwer/Lippincott Williams & Wilkins Health.

National Institute for Health and Care Excellence (NICE). (2009). *Depression in Adults: Recognition and Management (NICE Clinical Guideline CG90)*. Retrieved from https://www.nice.org.uk/guidance/cg90.

Nursing and Midwifery Board of Australia (NMBA). (2016). *Registered Nurse Standards for Practice*. Melbourne: NMBA.

Rice, M.J. (2009). Effect size in psychiatric evidence-based practice care. *Journal of the American Psychiatric Nurses Association*, 15(2), 138–42.

Rice, M.J. (2013). Evidence-based practice: A model for clinical application. *Journal of the American Psychiatric Nurses Association*, 19(4), 217–21. doi:10.1177/1078390313495563

Royal Australian & New Zealand College of Psychiatrists (RANZCP). (2009). *Schizophrenia: Australian Treatment Guide for Consumers and Carers*. Retrieved from https://www.ranzcp.org/Files/Resources/ Publications/CPG/Australian_Versions/AUS_Schizophrenia-pdf.aspx.

Russell, C.K. & Gregory, D.M. (2008). Evaluation of qualitative research studies. In N. Cullum, D. Ciliska, R.B. Haynes & S. Marks (eds), *Evidence-based Nursing: An Introduction* (pp. 204–18). Oxford: Blackwell Publishing.

Stillwell, S.B., Fineout-Overholt, E., Melnyk, B.M. & Williamson, K.M. (2010). Asking the clinical question: A key step in evidence-based practice. *American Journal of Nursing*, 110(3), 58–61. doi:10.1097/01. NAJ.0000368959.11129.79.

Strauss, S.E., Glasziou, P., Richardson, W.S. & Haynes, R.B. (2011). *Evidence-based Medicine: How to Practice and Teach EBM* (4th edn). Edinburgh: Churchill Livingstone.

The Cochrane Collaboration. (2016). Cochrane. Retrieved from http://www.cochrane.org.

Therapeutic Guidelines Ltd. (2016). *eTG Complete*. Retrieved from http://online.tg.com.au.ezproxy.cdu.edu.au/ip.

SECTION 2

THE CLINICAL CONTEXT OF PRACTICE

Section 2 explores the clinical context of practice in mental health. The key approach taken in this section is to bring together the diagnostic criteria of each mental health condition described in the *Diagnostic and Statistical Manual of Mental Disorders* (DSM-5) with clinically recognisable signs and symptoms, which then progress to management, therapeutic interventions, with the consumers' and carers' experiences being central in this process. Chapter 7 provides the foundation for understanding each mental health condition. It explores assessment in mental health and helps the student nurse to develop their skills in assessing a person's mental health. This chapter introduces the principles and processes of modern diagnostic classification systems. Chapters 8 to 19 explore specific mental health conditions. You will gain knowledge regarding the aetiology, incidence, epidemiology, comorbidity, diagnostic criteria and clinical manifestation of each mental health condition, the likely clinical presentations, risk assessment, challenges with mental state examination, treatment and mental health nursing considerations; central to all chapters are the consumers' and carers' experiences, and recovery and relapse prevention.

CHAPTER **7**

ASSESSMENT AND DIAGNOSIS

Louise Alexander and Terry Froggatt

LEARNING OUTCOMES

Upon completion of this chapter, you should be able to:

7.1 Understand the context of practice of nursing assessment in mental health

7.2 Demonstrate an ability to formulate nursing assessment in mental health, including why and how mental health assessments are conducted

7.3 Develop an understanding of multiple comprehensive mental health assessment tools, including patient history, mini mental state examinations, alcohol and drug assessment, physical health assessment and strength-based assessment

7.4 Understand the principles and processes involved in using modern diagnostic classification systems in mental health assessment: the DSM-5 and the ICD-10

LEARNING FROM PRACTICE

The first time I did an MSE [mental state examination], I was so nervous! I was so worried about asking the wrong thing, or saying something that would trigger the consumer I was interviewing. In hindsight, now that I am a qualified mental health nurse, I realise that the consumer was just a person going through a really difficult time, and I had nothing to worry about. I also realised it is likely that no one had asked him about suicide before, but he probably wanted someone to talk to about his feelings. My buddy nurse was really helpful and I learned so much from watching her interact with consumers. It never looked like she was doing an interview; she was just having a conversation. She seemed to be able to ask any question and I think it was because of the tone she used, and how genuine she was. She really cared about the consumers she worked with and this came through in every interaction she had with them. I never wanted to be a mental health nurse, not for one second! But during my placement, I started to gain the impression that I could make a difference. I've been a mental health nurse now for three years and I don't regret a single moment.

Llewellyn, mental health nurse

Llewellyn's story is not an uncommon one. Many students who enter the mental health unit of their degree, do so with great trepidation and worry. Reflect on how you feel about your mental health placement? What are you most worried about, and what are you doing to combat this anxiety?

INTRODUCTION

The mental state examination (MSE) is central to mental health nurses' practice, in the same way that vital signs are a key component of assessment in the acute care context. The MSE provides a 'baseline' assessment at admission, enables clinicians to see changes over periods of time (such as per day or shift) and facilitates diagnosis. This chapter describes the different types of assessment used in mental health and is pivotal for understanding the context of the chapters in Sections 2 and 3.

THE CONTEXT OF PRACTICE

In the past, the term mental health was often misunderstood and generally interpreted as referring to mental illness. Today, mental health is considered a desirable quality and is more than the absence of illness. Mental health is in many instances perceived as a positive concept related to the social and emotional well-being of individuals and communities. It is now well accepted that mental health is influenced by a range of determinants, but that it generally relates to a person's overall well-being, their ability to cope with stress and sadness, the fulfilment of goals and potential, and a sense of connection with others.

The term 'social and emotional well-being' is becoming popular, and is preferred by some Aboriginal and Torres Strait Islander people as it reflects their more holistic view of health. Well-being is more than just wellness, which is often conceived as being free from illness; whereas, well-being is a much broader concept and pertains to a person's physical, emotional and social condition. Mental illnesses are usually diagnosed by a health professional and are determined by specific criteria. Mental illnesses encompass a wide variety of signs, symptoms, experiences and disorders. For example, mental illnesses can include mood disorders (such as depression, anxiety and bipolar disorder), psychotic disorders (such as schizophrenia), eating disorders and personality disorders. Serious and enduring mental illnesses generally refer to the most severe psychiatric disorders, including psychotic disorders (e.g. schizophrenia spectrum disorders and bipolar disorder).

A person's physical health relates to their body, or soma. There are many classifications of diseases, conditions and risk factors that can impact upon a person's emotional and social well-being. Some common ones are cardiovascular risk factors, such as high blood pressure, high cholesterol, unhealthy diet, overweight and obesity, tobacco use, physical inactivity, diabetes and family history, which can contribute to the development of cardiovascular disease (CVD) and overall cardiovascular risk.

Sometimes such conditions may be referred to as modifiable and non-modifiable risk factors.

The International Diabetes Federation (2018) defines metabolic syndrome as central obesity (defined as an increased waist circumference based on ethnicity-specific values or BMI >30 kg/m^2), as well as any two of either; raised triglycerides, reduced HDL cholesterol, raised blood glucose.

The Mental Health Commission of NSW's *Physical Health and Mental Wellbeing: Evidence Guide* (2016) also includes high blood pressure or raised fasting plasma glucose. These conditions may identify individuals at risk of future disease and research is being carried out to understand their predictive value.

Recovery and resilience

Recovery, as defined by people who have a lived experience of a mental health condition, means gaining and retaining hope, understanding one's abilities and disabilities, engagement in an active life, personal autonomy, social identity, meaning and purpose in life, and a positive sense of self. Recovery is not thought to be the same as being cured. Recovery refers to both internal conditions experienced by those who describe themselves as being in recovery, such as hope, healing, empowerment and connection, and external conditions that facilitate recovery – the implementation of human rights, a positive culture of healing, and recovery-oriented services. Developing the skills to work effectively with people with a mental health condition requires both knowledge and compassion. One of the most important skills you will need is the ability to effectively assess a person and identify their needs. Assisting people to recognise their strengths and ability to overcome adversity is an important aspect of **resilience**, as is teaching people the skills required to become more self-aware and mindful in their everyday lives. You will explore recovery and resilience in greater depth in Chapter 21.

ASSESSMENT IN MENTAL HEALTH

This chapter introduces the practice of assessment, why assessments are conducted, and how an assessment can fulfil several therapeutic aims. Increasingly, mental health care is becoming much less paternalistic. Partnering, sharing and empowering are some of the ways autonomy can be handed back to the person with a lived experience of a mental health condition – no more so than at their first point of contact with health professionals. Although inpatient care continues to be a major component of the mental health service system in Australia, there is also a focus upon primary care, early interventions and community support services, which you will explore later in this book. An important aspect of the assessment process is making decisions about the level of intervention required in the least restrictive environment. Being aware of the options available ensures that appropriate, safe and compassionate care is at the centre of the assessment process regardless of the circumstances in which it may be conducted.

There are several assessment tools used to conduct assessments in both a general and specific sense. Comprehensive assessment schema and instruments designed to determine if specific diagnostic criteria apply are explained in this chapter. Often these instruments are based upon principles that may be underpinned by legislative requirements, government and local policy, and ethical standards. Throughout the chapter, you are required to consider and reflect upon these important underpinnings, which are demonstrated in case studies and individual accounts of a person's lived experience. The terminology, definitions and content in this chapter relate to all the diagnostic chapters within this section. By reading this chapter first, more meaning will be derived from the content in the following chapters.

Why we should conduct a mental health assessment

There are several reasons why it is important to assess a person's mental health. The primary reason is to determine whether a person is experiencing biological, psychological or social distress, and the possible causes or reasons for this.

The elimination of physical causes is a critical factor when conducting a mental health assessment. You may recall from your previous nursing subjects that some physical (organic) conditions can manifest with mental health conditions. Conditions that affect the thyroid and tumours on the brain are well understood possible physical causes of a mental health condition. In many clinical settings, eliminating physical causes may include routine blood tests or other health screens.

Establishing that a person is cognitively impaired or displaying evidence of emotional or personality problems may indicate possible reasons for someone behaving in ways that are significantly different to their usual behaviour or character. We live in a social world; our well-being can be strongly influenced by what is known as the 'social determinants' of health. These factors are considered when conducting a mental health assessment. Issues such as housing, income, employment and economic status have been found to impact upon a person's mental health and well-being.

These factors are only a part of the mental health assessment process from a nurse's perspective. Often, the mental health assessment is the first opportunity for a nurse to develop a therapeutic relationship with the person being assessed and with their family or carer. This is a critical point in forming a

professional relationship, which can endure over time and be a major factor in a person's ultimately successful recovery journey. There are several processes available to nurses when conducting a mental health assessment. These processes are often formalised and involve important documented procedures that ensure accuracy, privacy, confidentiality and the collection of epidemiological data.

It has been argued that the mental health assessment process is more of an art than a science (Snowden, 2003). It is true that there are no definitive, evidence-based, scientifically sound tests for many of the conditions that people present with when being assessed. Nevertheless, there is much that we do know from research and the scientific evidence.

Four ways of knowing, and judgements about safety

Nurses gain their knowledge in four ways of knowing (Carper, 1978). These are:

1 *empirical knowing*: knowledge through facts, evidence and tests, etc.
2 *personal knowing, or tacit knowledge*: the things learned along life's journey
3 *aesthetic knowing*: is knowledge about creativity and beauty, the things that give sensory pleasure and satisfaction
4 *ethical knowing*: essentially, what is right and what is wrong in a moral sense.

When we use these ways of knowing in the assessment process, we will be more likely to form a more accurate and holistic picture of the person and their situation.

One other key aspect of the assessment process is making judgements concerning safety. Health professionals have a clear duty of care to provide measurable, high-quality and safe environments. The clinician becomes a skilled practitioner in the assessment of risk. This is particularly important when assessing a person's capacity for self-harm (non-suicidal self-injury) and/or suicide. All mental health assessments must include a measure-of-risk component.

How we conduct an assessment in mental health

Mental health professionals use a variety of assessment tools, instruments and processes to assist them in their assessment. Some of these are quite formal; for example, psychometric assessment instruments, which may use questionnaires or surveys (empirical). The *Diagnostic and Statistical Manual of Mental Disorders* (DSM-5; APA, 2013) and the International Classification System (ICD-10; WHO, 2004) have formalised classifications or categories with set criteria that describe the elements of a condition and a diagnosis that can be formed from these criteria. The MSE or its variants are commonly used in the mental health systems in most states and territories. The ways in which nurses conduct an assessment are very important.

The therapeutic relationship

The way that the nurse interacts with the person being assessed is critical. Some basic things to consider are outlined in **Table 7.1**. The concepts outlined in the table interlink the therapeutic relationship with the MSE.

Developing a professional therapeutic relationship is a powerful therapeutic tool. It will take time, patience and understanding for it to develop. When successful, this is possibly one of the greatest rewards in being an excellent practitioner.

TABLE 7.1

Basic concepts for developing a therapeutic relationship

CONCEPT	EXAMPLES
Greeting	Welcome the person with a smile, try to keep calm and confident. Ask the person how they prefer to be addressed – Mr, Mrs, Ms or first name or preferred name (e.g. Terence or Terry). Introduce yourself and/or others, your role and why you are conducting the interview. Wear a name tag or display your official identification. Indicate how you prefer to be addressed – Nurse, Doctor, first name, Mr, Mrs, Ms, etc.
Explaining	Explain what is happening now, what may happen next, and why. Explain where the person is and why they are there. Explain the purpose of the interview and why you are writing things down. Explain that this is an important element of their overall care and treatment plan.
Listening	Listen carefully to not only what the person is saying but how they say it – volume, tone and cadence. Give the person time to answer, and don't be afraid of periods of silence. Provide prompts if necessary but don't interrupt or finish sentences or words.
Reiterating	Say the important things the person has said back to them; e.g. 'Your children are aged 14, 16 and 19, is that right?'
Clarifying	When you do not clearly understand what the person is explaining, seek clarification. You might ask if they could say it in different words so that you may understand better.
Demonstrating empathy	Try to put yourself in the person's place. What did you feel like the last time you visited a health professional, had an interview for a job or met someone for the first time? How do you feel about answering questions, especially personal ones?
Caring	Show that you are attentive and that you care, be kind, be generous with your time. Attend to any of the person's immediate needs; are they too warm, too cold, thirsty, hungry or tired, for example? Do they need a break?
Privacy	Reassure the person that the service you are providing is governed by privacy legislation. Check that you are in a physical space that protects privacy. Use screens if the person's dignity could be compromised.
Confidentiality	Inform the person that the information you are collecting will only be used by the people designated to care for them. Explain that you work in a team environment and that team members (name some of them if possible) will use the assessment to formulate a care/treatment plan in consultation with themselves.
Developing trust	Probably the most important factor in developing a therapeutic relationship is trust. Don't be tempted to make promises that you will be unable to deliver. Be honest. Be truthful and demonstrate that when you say something, the person can rely upon it.
Assessing risk	Although by necessity intrusive, questions regarding a person's safety must form an essential part of the assessment interview. There are several ways in which this can be administered without necessarily undermining the fundamentals of a healthy therapeutic relationship.
Closing the interview	This is a time for the assessor to be reflective of the interview – reiterate any points that need to be clarified, explain what's likely to happen next, and ask if the person has any final comments or questions. Respectfully thank the person for their cooperation.

The mental health assessment process

Any assessment involves a process that contains several logical, sequential stages or steps. The following stages have been developed from current practice and evidence-based research (NICE, 2014). The following sample scripts may be useful when you are conducting a mental health assessment; it is also useful to practise these scripts with a peer or other willing person.

Environment

Environmental considerations are an important consideration when conducting a mental health assessment, and you should check that the environment is appropriate prior to commencement. For example: Is the location safe? Does the area have uncluttered and clearly marked exits? What is the room/place's temperature (e.g. too hot or too cold)? Is it indoor or outdoor? What are the privacy/confidentiality implications? Is the furniture comfortable, practical and safe? Can you offer the person a cold/hot drink? Is there a call/alarm device close at hand? Are others close by if there is an incident?

Explaining the process

You could use this sample content to structure an explanation of the process. You may say:

- As a member of your care/treatment team I would like to conduct an assessment so that we may better understand how we can assist you. Is that okay?

- During this assessment, if you begin to feel distressed, please let me know. We can take a break at any time, or if you are too distressed right now, I can return a little later.
- You should know that you must be provided with a statement of your rights and responsibilities (at this point you should provide the approved document, if it has not already been provided).
- Do you have any questions or concerns before we begin?
- I understand that you have come here today after the police brought you in. That can be very upsetting. They have given me some information about what happened, but I would really like to hear your version of events.

Note taking and recording

If you are taking notes, filling in a form or recording the interview, make sure the person understands why you are doing this. People who are feeling paranoid, frightened or suspicious may be further upset by someone taking notes of what they say. Allow time for the person to respond – be friendly, yet professional. Speak clearly and listen carefully. It is important to remember that an interview has a beginning, middle and end, and that as this interview may take considerable time, taking appropriate breaks may be necessary. Try to be conversational in your questioning rather than follow a 'script'.

COMPREHENSIVE MENTAL HEALTH ASSESSMENT

The comprehensive mental health assessment is an important tool in assessing and evaluating a person's mental health condition. The core features are:
- conversation
- signs and symptoms
- establishing a therapeutic alliance.

   The aim of the assessment is to bring together all of the facts and to formulate clear treatment goals and plans. The person and their family or carers should be encouraged to take part in this process. This process of assessment has been shown to strengthen engagement and is essential for the assessment to be effective. Through the process of engagement, a therapeutic alliance is more likely to develop. The therapeutic relationship is central to all stages of the continuum of care from assessment through to referral and follow-up. The key components of a comprehensive assessment include:
- history
- psychosocial/developmental and personal history
- mental state
- cognitive assessment
- substance use
- sexual history (including abuse)
- medical/biological – physical assessment
- risk.

History

When we consider a consumer's history, we are referring to the history of their present condition, psychiatric/mental health and medical history. We would consider substance use and abuse, social history and family history. A person's psychosocial/developmental history would include:
- their current living situation
- level of support
- where they grew up
- how they would describe their childhood
- whether there is a history of trauma
- sexual history
- level of education.
   A person's social history consists of their:
- current social situation
- family and work status
- socioeconomic position
- friends
- hobbies or interests.
   When discussing a person's family history, a genogram (a type of diagram, which is also explored in Chapter 22) is used to determine significant family relationships and/or events:
- Where does the person see themselves in relation to other family members?
- What is the quality of their family relationships or contact with family members?
- Do any of their family members have a history of a mental health condition?
- Is there a history of suicide in other family members?
- Has sexual abuse taken place?

THE MENTAL STATE EXAMINATION DEFINED

There are a number of different ways of remembering the MSE. The initialism 'BATOMIPJR' (Behaviour and appearance, Affect, Thought, Orientation, Mood, Insight, Perception, Judgement and Risk) is sometimes used to guide the interview. Another initialism – PAMS-GOT-JIMI – is also useful. This stands for Perception, Affect, Mood, Speech, General Appearance and Behaviour, Orientation, Thought Content and Form, Judgement, Insight, Memory and Intelligence. Students (and clinicians) often find it helpful to remember one of these acronyms to inform their interview and to record notes.

It is important to consider the MSE as a 'snapshot' of the individual on a particular day. Much in the way that a set of vital signs on admission can provide a baseline of physical health, the MSE on admission can provide clinicians with an understanding of the individual's current state. This is important, as over a period of time there may be changes or improvements. Consider a person who is sad, depressed and dishevelled. Once they commence treatment, we would hope to see an improvement and the MSE is a way of measuring this over time.

The following framework will be utilised throughout Section 2 of this book to help you understand commonalities of an MSE. While some variation will appear in some chapters, the initialism should be closely followed wherever relevant in your practice.

Behaviour and appearance

This section considers how the individual behaves and looks.

The observation of *behaviour* includes the non-verbal communication of the person being assessed, such as posture and body language (relaxed, rigid, tense, erect and closed). This also includes how amenable the individual is to being interviewed. Are they engaged, suspicious or reluctant, perhaps? People who are brought to hospital under duress are often very upset and may be angry and not wish to cooperate with the process. The degree of facial expression (eye contact – fixed, passive, intense) and motor activity (slowed, immobile, restless, clumsy, tremors, wringing hands, pacing) is also important.

Appearance is another measure that forms part of an MSE. It is important to avoid judgemental interpretations of appearance (e.g. the individual is not wearing clothes that are 'fashionable') and instead look for the appropriateness and presentation of hygiene and grooming. Is the person wearing clothing that is suitable for the climate (e.g. wearing multiple sweaters on a hot day) and is their attire neat, tidy and clean? Or are they dishevelled and unkempt? When someone has been avoiding cleaning their clothing or bathing they may emit an odour. We call this 'malodour' or 'malodorous' and it can be suggestive of the person's level of functioning.

Physical characteristics such as height, weight, hair style and colour, scars, tattoos and body markings are also important. If the person is 35 years old, for example, do they look their stated age or do they appear older?

Mood

Mood is a subjective experience best described as an internal state and is understood by the clinician through direct questioning. Because it is 'internal', we cannot assume a person's mood state; we must ask them. There are a number of ways we can ask a person about their mood; for example, 'Ben could you describe your mood for me today?' It is important to measure a person's mood, and we do so by asking them to rate their mood; for example, 'Ben on a scale of 1–10 where 1 is very depressed and 10 is happy and excited, how would you rate your mood?' The clinician should further explore the person's response; for example, 'Ben you said you were feeling great anguish. What do you mean when you say this?' People's understanding of concepts are different (even between clinicians) and therefore seeking clarification in the person's own words is very important. Mood states can fluctuate and we call this a **labile mood**. A labile (or unstable) mood is one that oscillates between mood states, such as feeling angry, tearful, happy and irritable (perhaps all in the space of one 10-minute conversation).

Assessment includes depth of mood, fluctuations in mood and intensity of mood. A mood may be described as depressed, despairing, irritable, anxious, angry, elevated, euphoric, empty, guilty or perplexed.

When we explore mood (some facilities will explore this under 'behaviour'), we must also explore *libido*, *appetite* and *sleep* patterns. Libido refers to an individual's interest in sex and intimacy and this can be affected in a variety of ways. People who are experiencing depression may lose sexual urges or desires, while individuals who are manic may experience a heightened sex drive. While you may feel embarrassed or uncomfortable asking questions about someone's sexual relationships, it is an important area to explore. When individuals are vulnerable and their decision-making processes are impaired, they may make choices which they later regret. Vulnerable sexual encounters may increase the risk of sexually transmitted infections and unplanned pregnancy. Choosing the correct time to explore this within an MSE is vital. After first discussing general interpersonal relationships with others, you may then ask about intimate relationships. You may consider asking, 'Sometimes when people are feeling depressed they find that intimacy with their partner is affected. Do you think this is something you can relate to?'

Much like libido affects sexual desires, mental health conditions may affect an individual's appetite. Volition or motivation to prepare meals may be impacted by a mood disorder. An individual may have noticed recent changes in their weight. Consider asking, 'Have you noticed that your clothes fit you differently more recently?' Individuals who are paranoid may think their food is contaminated and hence may have changes to their weight, and eating disorders can result in weight fluctuations (sometimes life-threatening) and appetite changes. It is important to consider the 'bigger picture' of a mental health condition; for example, safe storage and preparation of meals in a hygienic way may be affected by someone who has cut the power to their house due to paranoia.

Sleep is an important part of a healthy lifestyle, but many people experience difficulties with their sleeping patterns for a variety of reasons. Mood disorders can significantly disrupt sleeping patterns. Depression may result in an individual wanting to sleep all the time, or feeling tired all the time but not sleeping well. To the contrary, mania is a condition where a person needs little or no sleep, yet feels energetic and rested. Consumers who are paranoid may feel unable to sleep because they may feel the need to be 'on alert' all the time. When considering sleep hygiene, ask whether the consumer:

- has a bedtime routine (e.g. goes to bed at the same time, a warm bath/shower, etc.)
- wakes during the night
- has difficulty falling or staying asleep
- wakes frequently overnight
- requires very little sleep (yet feels energised)
- naps during the day
- uses sleep aids such as prescribed sleeping tablets (are they taken according to the prescription?)
- uses non-prescribed drugs to help sleep (e.g. illicit drugs or over-the-counter preparations)
- uses stimulants during the day to remain awake (e.g. over-the-counter preparations or illicit drugs)
- ruminates or thinks about things when trying to sleep
- avoids caffeine prior to bed
- wakes up to use the bathroom
- wakes up feeling rested

- only uses their bed for sleeping (rather than watching television, reading or using social media)
- gets enough exercise.

Affect

Affect is an objective assessment of the degree of emotional expression that a person exhibits. When we assess affect, we are establishing how harmonious a person's mood is with the way they present. As such, affect and mood are intimately related. Generally, we are looking for congruity or harmony between mood and affect; for example, when a person is describing something upsetting, do they actually *look* upset or are they smiling inappropriately? If they were smiling in such a way, this would be described as an *incongruent* affect. Similarly, if a person is laughing during a funeral, this would be known as an *inappropriate* affect.

Therefore, consider whether the person's affect is appropriate to the situation, consistent with their mood and congruent with their thoughts. Assessment of affect includes observing fluctuations and intensity.

There are a number of universally accepted terms when describing someone's affect. Some of the more common examples include normal, labile, restricted, flat and blunted. As mentioned earlier in relation to mood, labile is a term that is used to describe fluctuations in states. A **labile affect** may move between different affective states in a short period. A **normal affect** comprises reactive facial expressions that are harmonious with the situation. A **restricted affect** is one that has a mild narrowing in the expression of emotional intensity. A **blunted affect** is one that has a moderate restriction in emotional expression, while a **flat affect** is an absence of emotional expression.

Thought content

As it suggests, thought content is measured quite simply by what the person is saying, or telling you. Generally, thought content comprises *obsessions* and *compulsions*, *delusions*, and *suicidality* and *homicidality*. Obsessions are intrusive, and usually unwanted, thoughts, while compulsions are repetitive and ritualised behaviours. Suicide refers to the deliberate intent to die by self-directed methods. Suicide needs to be measured in terms of intent, plan, and access to means, lethality and preparation. When people are feeling suicidal, they may also experience homicidal thoughts where they plan to kill someone else (often their children) before they die by suicide. It is important that the clinician explores suicide and homicide intent, and this is explained in detail in Chapter 20.

The exploration of delusions is a fundamental aspect of exploring thought content. A **delusion** is a fixed, false belief that is held despite evidence to the contrary, and that is not shared by a majority of people. Delusions can be defined as either *bizarre* or *non-bizarre*. A bizarre delusion is something that falls outside the realms of possibility; for example, a man who believes that he is half human and half wolf and believes he can understand dog howling and barking as communication. This is quite simply impossible, and there should be little dispute as to whether or not it is possible. Non-bizarre delusions are harder to distinguish from probability; for example, a woman who believes that her husband is being unfaithful with the next-door neighbour, or the employee who believes other staff are plotting to have him fired. These situations are quite possible. The different types of delusion are listed in **Table 7.2**.

TABLE 7.2
Types of delusion

TYPE OF DELUSION	DEFINITION	EXAMPLES
Erotomanic	A fixed false belief where the individual believes that someone (usually of a higher status) is romantically attracted (or involved) with them.	A woman who believes that the US President is in love with her, and is planning on breaking the news to the world soon via a press conference.
Grandiose	An exaggerated, false belief of one's power, importance or worth.	A man with no medical training who takes a new idea to cure cancer to the CSIRO, and becomes irate when they refute his idea as nonsense.
Persecutory	A fixed, false belief that one is being persecuted, harassed or 'set up'.	A woman who attends her local police department claiming that her neighbour is making prank phone calls to her at work.
Somatic	A fixed, false belief that there is something physically/medically wrong, despite evidence to the contrary.	A woman who believes she is pregnant, but urine and blood pregnancy testing is negative.
Jealous	A fixed, false belief that a partner or spouse is unfaithful.	A woman who claims her husband is cheating on her with their daughter's best friend, despite repeated denial of this.
Nihilistic	A fixed, false belief that parts of the body (or the entire body) or world do not exist.	A man who believes that his heart is no longer beating, and that he is dead inside.
Religious	A fixed, false belief that has a spiritual or religious basis, but which is not a common belief shared by other people.	A woman who believes that she is Mother Teresa reincarnated and that she is able to perform miracles on people who are ill.
Referential	A fixed, false belief that unconnected events or occurrences hold special significance specific to them.	A man who believes that recent floods in Asia are a sign from God aimed specifically to let him know he can begin to enact the second stage of his 'grand financial plan'.

Part of the MSE in this section involves exploration of delusional content, and the following questions may assist in guiding the conversation:

- Do you ever feel that people are watching or following you?
- Do you ever feel that people wish to harm you?
- Why do you think you have been chosen?
- How do you feel about the police and other authority figures?
- Do you ever have amazing ideas that just come to you?
- You said your heart isn't beating, but you are sitting here talking to me. How can you explain this?

Thought process or form

Thought process or form differs from thought content in that it explores the manner in which thoughts are constructed, organised and expressed rather than the *content* of speech.

Thought process or form involves assessment of how a person is thinking and refers either to the act of thinking or the resulting ideas or arrangements of ideas that are expressed. When thoughts are 'normal', they are usually goal directed and sequential. **Table 7.3** outlines the variations to thought process.

Speech

Thoughts are expressed through speech and as such it is important to observe a consumer's speech. The speech component of the MSE involves an assessment of the *rate*, *volume*, *amount* and *tone*. It is also common to note the goal directedness of speech in this section of the MSE. **Table 7.4** outlines the variations in speech.

Orientation

This considers whether the person is orientated to the time (e.g. date, year), place (e.g. a hospital) or person (e.g. do they know who you are?). Impairments of orientation may indicate memory difficulties, confusion or intoxication. They must be taken seriously, as the person may have a physical cause for their disorientation; for example, a head injury or hypoglycaemia. Asking a person what they ate for breakfast or dinner may provide an insight into short-term memory without being too direct. Asking

TABLE 7.3
Variations to thought process

THOUGHT PROCESS OR FORM	DEFINITION	EXAMPLES
Circumstantiality	The over-inclusion of superfluous or irrelevant information that inhibits the person from making their point. It is important to note, the person does eventually get to the point.	Nurse: 'Jenny have you had a shower today?' Jenny: 'I slept in today. It's so much easier to sleep in when the weather is cold and I enjoy snuggling down into the doona. No matter how much of a rush I'm in, I just can't resist a sleep in! Then I end up spending less time eating my breakfast, but the thing is I like to take my time eating my breakfast. I don't always eat the same thing though, which I guess is part of the problem with my timings. I haven't had breakfast yet, but I have had a shower today.'
Clang associations or clanging	Words are chosen for their sound, rather than their meaning. Words usually rhyme or have a similar sound when pronounced.	Consumer: 'To be green and mean, but not to gleam or ream but to seem like a dream.'
Tangentiality	Is an initial appropriate response to a topic, but does not provide an answer and may continue to go off topic. The person essentially does not get back to the point.	Nurse: 'Jerry can you tell me where you were born?' Jerry: 'I think it would be nice to be born in a cold climate because I always find myself feeling warm. The best thing about the cold is snow, but I've only been to the snow a few times. I think it would be great to have a white Christmas though because turkey needs to be kept pretty warm.'
Flight of ideas	Accelerated or rapid speech and multiple associations that frequently change topics. This is often based on cogent (logical) ideas, but they are usually very superficially connected. Often understood to be a severe form of tangentiality.	A woman who begins discussing her pets, but quickly shifts to talking about cattle, pet insurance and lion poaching.
Loosening of associations (also known as derailment)	Unrelated, or seemingly unrelated ideas that rapidly change in such a way that they are almost impossible to follow or comprehend. The association between concepts is 'loosely' (or not) framed. The structure of sentences is grammatically correct, but they do not make sense. Loose associations differ from circumstantiality and tangentiality by severity and in that connections between thoughts are almost impossible to see.	Consumer: 'Janice plays with the remote controls, but she doesn't give credit to the chef in the southern states.'
Thought blocking	Sudden interruption in the train of thought resulting in silence/s.	Nurse: 'So Yen, your father tells me that you like playing soccer?' Yen: 'Yeah I've been playing soccer since I was…'
Neologism	The development of a new term or expression, or the marrying or joining of two existing words.	Consumer: 'One day I will be forgiven and I will enter the serpie dimension of forgiveness, which is just past purgatory'. (Serpie is a made-up term, developed by the consumer.) Consumer: 'Sometimes when my dog goes to lick my face, she gives me a snick; I don't know if she is going to bite, or lick me.' (Snick is the joining of 'snarl' and 'lick'.)
Perseveration	The repetition of a particular phrase or word in response to varied stimuli.	Nurse: 'Benny can you tell me when your mother is coming to visit?' Benny: 'Tee tee.' Nurse: 'How are you feeling today Benny?' Benny: 'Tee tee.'
Word salad	A mixture of indecipherable speech, words or phrases.	Consumer: 'Potatoes, like driven cars. Every cloud has a silver lining!'

questions about childhood may provide an insight into long-term memory.

Insight

Insight refers to the person's own perception of the nature of their current situation or difficulties, what might be causing them and why, and what might be done to resolve the situation. It may be described as lacking in insight (complete denial that anything is wrong), having poor insight (slight awareness), limited insight (aware of problem but unable to identify cause or future considerations) or good insight (emotionally aware of motives and feelings). For consumers with a psychotic illness, reality testing is important to assess.

TABLE 7.4
Variations in speech

SPEECH TERM	DEFINITION
General terms or quality	Presence of stutter, lisp, speech impediment, rhythm, accent and clarity.
Rate	Refers to the speed or how fast speech is. Terms such as pressured, rapid, slow may be used.
Volume	Relates to the loudness of speech. Terms such as normal, shouting, loud, whispering or soft may be used.
Amount or quantity	Speech may be abundant, absent, spontaneous, minimal, monosyllabic, talkative or voluminous. Speech may also be latent, with lengthy pauses between answers to questions, or in conversations.
Tone	Describes intonations of voice modulation; for example monotonous (monotone), decreased or normal.

Consider the following questions when assessing the consumer for insight:

- Can you tell me why you think you are here in the hospital?
- How would you feel about taking some medication to help you?
- Do you think there is anything that we can do to help you?
- Do you understand what type of ward this is in the hospital?
- Has your doctor or a friend perhaps suggested to you in the past that you may be experiencing a mental health issue?
- How do you explain these experiences that are happening to you?

Perception

Perceptual disturbances are common to psychotic mental health conditions and the exploration of perceptions includes assessment for presence of hallucinations, illusions, depersonalisation and derealisation. A *hallucination* is a false sensory experience that others do not experience. This experience occurs in the absence of stimuli that are in the external environment. Hallucinations affect the senses (sight, taste, touch, smell and hearing) and are of an internal origin. **Table 7.5** defines the different types of hallucinations and provides examples.

TABLE 7.5
Different types of hallucinations

HALLUCINATION	DEFINITION	EXAMPLES
Visual	Seeing a person or object that does not exist in the environment.	• A man who sees a spirit guide who leads him to safety. • A woman who sees the words 'you must die' written in blood on her bedroom wall.
Auditory	Hearing voices or sounds that do not exist in the environment but appear to be projections of inner thoughts and feelings.	• A man who hears his deceased wife telling him to come and join her in the afterlife. • A woman who hears a werewolf snarling and barking at her outside her house.
Olfactory	Smelling odours that are not present in the environment.	• A man who knows his colleagues are going to kill him because he can smell gas in his office. • A woman who can smell rotting flesh in her house because it is built on an ancient burial ground.
Gustatory	Tasting sensations that have no stimulus.	• A man who can taste poison in his coffee. • A woman whose food tastes 'off' because her local supermarket manager is trying to kill her with poison.
Tactile	Feeling strange sensations where no external objects stimulate such feelings.	• A man who can feel cockroaches trying to crawl out of his skin. • A woman who can feel the devil tickling her toes at night.
Somatic	A false sensation within the body.	• A man who can feel a pulsating cancerous growth inside his heart. • A woman who can feel a parasite in her intestines trying to burrow out.

Auditory and visual hallucinations are the most common experiences for people who experience symptoms of psychosis, and some of the following questions may assist in guiding the discussion:

- Have you ever been alone in a room and heard a voice (or seen someone) that you couldn't explain?
- I have worked with people in the past who were able to see things or hear things that other people couldn't. Is this something you can relate to?
- Do you ever hear/see things that other people can't?
- Do you think that you have special powers or abilities that others don't have?
- Some people I have worked with describe hearing voices. Have you heard voices?
- Have you ever seen something that you couldn't explain?
- I can see you are a little distracted now – is there someone else in this room besides you and I?

An **illusion** is a misinterpretation of a real stimulus – for example, a person who believes that a piece of fluff on the carpet is a spider, or that a shadow is a ghost. **Depersonalisation** is a feeling of unreality where a person may feel that parts, or all, of themselves, do not exist. **Derealisation** is a change in a person's sense of reality, where they may feel as if the world around them does not exist or that their surroundings have changed.

Judgement

Judgement is an individual's ability to apply previous learnings to current experiences and to apply logical reasoning in decision-making. Judgement is the person's capacity to make sound, reasoned and responsible decisions. Assessment considers the individual's likely behaviour in terms of impulsivity, social cognition, self-awareness and planning ability. Assessing capacity for judgement involves providing a real-life scenario against which to test decision-making,

such as asking, 'What would you do in a crowded room that started to fill with smoke'? Many clinicians choose to use examples from the consumer's background; for example exploring how they look after young children in their care, and their own ability to stay safe. This may also include determining engagement or participation in treatment, and while judgement and insight are often compared, they are not the same.

Risk

Assessing risk is an important concept in nursing. The safety of consumers, their families and health care workers needs to be factored into many aspects of nursing work. This is no more so than when assessing a person's mental health. Most health services have established protocols and procedures to assist mental health professionals to assess risk. High priority is given to the area of self-harm/non-suicidal self-injury and the potential for harm to others, including oneself and one's colleagues.

Risk assessment

When individuals are unwell, they may become more vulnerable and therefore may be exposed to a number of potential risk factors that can impede both their physical and mental health. While risk of self-harm/non-suicidal self-injury and suicide are common vulnerabilities in the mental health context, they are not the only ones.

Static and dynamic risk factors

Risk factors can be deemed *static* or *dynamic*. Static risk factors are those that are unchanged and include things such as past history, genetics, history of substance misuse, personality traits, diagnosis and biological factors (such as age, gender, etc.). Dynamic factors are those that are more fluid and susceptible to change. These include active substance misuse, environmental stressors and social issues (such as homelessness or conflict).

Risks may be broken down into three distinct sections: risk to self, risk *to* others and risk *by* others. **Table 7.6** outlines different types of risks.

Now that we have demonstrated that risk assessment within the mental health context is multifaceted, we look at suicide and self-harm/non-suicidal self-injury in more detail.

Risk factors for suicide and self-harm/non-suicidal self-injury

Health professionals are in a key position for identifying people at risk of suicide and preventing suicide. Not all health professionals work with consumers who are suicidal on a regular basis and therefore it can be challenging when a consumer

TABLE 7.6
Different types of risks

RISK CATEGORY	EXAMPLES
Risk to self	• Self-harm/non-suicidal self-injury • Suicide • Self-neglect • Reputation • Medication non-adherence • Substance misuse • Physical health condition (e.g. hypertension, epilepsy, diabetes, alcohol withdrawal, falls) • Legal issues related to offending behaviour • Financial status
Risk *to* others	• Interpersonal violence • Sexual assault/abuse • Harassment • Damage to property • Stalking
Risk *by* others	• Assault • Sexual exploitation or abuse • Financial exploitation or abuse • Verbal abuse

presents with suicide risk. The information in this section does not replace specialised training, but it may be a helpful guide. We also discuss suicide and self-harm/non-suicidal self-injury in Chapter 20.

The management of a person at risk of suicide requires the assessment of risk, followed by appropriate interventions to minimise any risk. In estimating the risk, health professionals need to consider those factors that elevate suicide risk and consider those factors that mitigate suicide risk. These risk and protective factors are also an important consideration in any management decisions.

Sometimes a person will clearly articulate suicidal ideation, while at other times the cues will be subtler – a person may describe feelings of hopelessness, depression, insomnia or express a desire for medication change. Health professionals must be alert for the cues and ready to ask the patient directly about suicide intent.

Risk factors for suicide may include:

- previous suicide attempt/s
- concurrent mental health conditions
- increasing substance misuse
- low social support/living alone
- male gender (three times more likely than females)
- expressing feelings of hopelessness.

Suicide risk assessment

When a thorough risk assessment is undertaken in a systematic way, it is more than a guess or intuition – it is a reasoned and structured clinical judgement.

- Be familiar with the concept of risk and the factors associated with increased risk.
- Establish rapport with the individual.
- Conduct and document a thorough risk assessment.
- Use clearly defined and commonly understood categories for defining levels of risk (e.g. nonexistent, mild, moderate, high and imminent).
- Recognise the need for ongoing monitoring of suicide risk, as risk fluctuates as circumstances change.

CASE **STUDY**

GENERAL APPEARANCE

Ethan is a 22-year-old consumer currently in the mental health unit. Ethan lives in the remote Pilbara region of Western Australia. For the past two years, he has been living with schizophrenia, which has resulted in significant issues to his functioning. He is no longer able to work or study, and his mother, Dana, is worried that despite treatment Ethan has 'only gotten worse'. Dana has noticed that Ethan has difficulty organising himself and attending to his personal hygiene. She finds this embarrassing, and it upsets her that people in the town talk about her son. Dana laments that a person's worth should be understood as more than what they look like and wants you to know that Ethan is a kind, caring and loving person.

When assessing someone's mental state, these issues in functioning may be evident in several domains.

Questions

1 Describe the ways in which Ethan's personal appearance may be affected by difficulties in organising himself. How might his mental illness interfere with his ability to take care of himself?
2 You ask to speak to Dana while Ethan is settling into his room. What corroborative information could you gather from Dana about Ethan's mental state?
3 Key in the word 'dishevelled' into the images option in the search engine of your computer. Select three images from your search and, using accurate and non-judgemental terminology, describe how the person looks.
4 Noticing Dana's continued distress about her son, you suggest that she might benefit from joining a support group. Research the carer support groups that are available in the Pilbara region.

Communicating with an emotionally distressed person can be difficult, but it is important to persist and gather the information required to estimate the risk, identify protective factors and determine the appropriate management.

Developing suicide risk assessment strategies

Suicide in Australia has been described as 'being at epidemic proportions'. Young people, the elderly, people in certain professions and members of the transgender, transexual, queer, intersex, asexual and more (LGBTQ(IA+)) community have been recognised as being particularly at risk (Rosenstreich, 2013). Much is being done to raise general awareness of this problem. Mental health professionals are often confronted by people who are without hope, and who may believe that taking their own life is the only way to end their suffering. Observation, developing trust and asking direct questions are important strategies in the mental health professional's 'tool box'. If you develop these skills well, and early in your career, they can save lives.

Mini mental state examination

A cognitive assessment uses tests to establish whether a person is orientated to time, place and person. This may include the **mini mental state examination (MMSE)** (Folstein, Folstein & McHugh, 1975), a commonly used set of questions for screening cognitive function. This examination is primarily used to determine:

- level of consciousness
- memory
- orientation
- concentration
- abstract thought
- judgement and insight.

The MMSE is not suitable for making a diagnosis but can be used to indicate the presence of cognitive impairment such as in a person with suspected dementia or following a head injury (Monroe & Carter, 2012). The MMSE is far more sensitive in detecting cognitive impairment than using informal questioning or an overall impression of a patient's orientation. The MMSE was originally distributed without cost, but the current copyright holder is Psychological Assessment Resources (PAR) which 'will not grant permission to include or reproduce an entire test or scale in any publication (including dissertations and theses) or on any website' (PAR, 2018). All users need to purchase the tests from PAR. The test takes only about 10 minutes but is limited because it will not detect subtle memory losses, particularly in well-educated patients. Note that:

- in interpreting test scores, allowance may have to be made for education and ethnicity
- the MMSE provides measures of orientation, registration (immediate memory), short-term memory (but not long-term memory) as well as language functioning
- the examination has been validated in several populations. Scores of 25–30 out of 30 are considered normal; the National Institute for Health and Care Excellence (NICE) classifies 21–24 as mild, 10–20 as moderate and <10 as severe impairment. The MMSE may not be an appropriate assessment if the patient has learning, linguistic/ communication or other disabilities (e.g. sensory impairments) (PAR, 2018).

Before administering the MMSE, it is important to ensure the consumer is comfortable and to establish a rapport. Praising success may help to maintain the rapport and is acceptable. However, persisting on items the patient finds difficult should be avoided. Be sensitive – the assessment may be quite overwhelming for the person and/or their relative or carer.

Alcohol and drug assessment

The use of alcohol and drugs (which are non-prescribed and may be licit or illicit) is common in people who present with a mental health condition. This is sometimes called comorbidity; that is, two significant health conditions presenting simultaneously. Each condition requires being assessed in a non-judgemental and objective way.

Alcohol and drug assessment is a specialised area of nursing practice. We cover this topic extensively in Chapter 14.

Physical health assessment

There is a reciprocal relationship between more severe and enduring mental health conditions and poor physical health, including cardiovascular disease and diabetes, and this is becoming increasingly clear. Consequently, the physical health care of people with severe and enduring mental illness has been identified as a serious public health challenge. The national survey, *People Living with Psychotic Illness 2010* (Commonwealth of Australia, 2011), found that physical health was one of the biggest challenges for one quarter of participants.

The life expectancy for people experiencing severe mental illness is reduced by 15 to 20 years (Colton & Manderscheid, 2006) – largely due to cardiovascular disease and cancer rather than suicide – and the gap appears to be widening (Lambert et al., 2017). Despite improvements in physical health and longevity in the general population through healthier lifestyle choices and medical advances, people who have a lived experience of a severe mental health condition have not shared in these benefits. They often experience economic and social marginalisation, including from health care professionals and systems, in addition to severe metabolic consequences from antipsychotic medication.

While steps have been taken to reduce the number of premature deaths, more needs to be done to ensure that people with an enduring mental health condition have the same life expectancy, and equal expectations of life, as those people who do not have such an experience. Significantly improving the physical health of mental health consumers is becoming a priority area for clinicians and policymakers, yet the practical steps needed to achieve this are less clear.

There are, however, some common themes evident in national (NMHC, 2018) and state mental health commission reports (State of Victoria, Department of Health and Human Services, 2017), including:

- integration – the need for a holistic, collaborative and coordinated approach
- addressing the side effects of antipsychotic medication
- education
- the need to overcome the physical/mental comorbidity that is typically experienced by consumers. Despite ongoing attempts to address the poor physical health of mental health consumers, much remains to be achieved.

The evidence for comprehensive lifestyle interventions to help improve the physical health of consumers living with severe mental illness is clear. There are excellent examples of proven strategies to improve access to physical health services, as well as health promotion, prevention and early intervention for people with coexisting mental and physical health issues.

Although there remain significant physical health issues for people with mental health conditions (e.g. anxiety, depression, eating disorders and traumatic stress disorders), a serious challenge exists for nurses in trying to improve the physical health for those consumers who have a lived experience of serious mental health issues, specifically bipolar affective disorder, schizophrenia and other psychotic illnesses.

There is substantial evidence in Australia and internationally that the risk factors for chronic physical disease are higher among people living with severe and enduring mental health issues than in the general population. The interrelationship between mental health issues and poor physical health is well established (RANZCP, 2015). For example, a 2015 review of 25 unique studies internationally found that people who have a diagnosis of schizophrenia are 2.5 times more likely to have diabetes compared with the general population (RANZCP, 2015). Similarly, high rates of, and risk for, metabolic syndrome have been documented in bipolar disorder, depression and other mental health conditions such as post-traumatic stress disorder. Specific to psychosis, the rate of metabolic syndrome is 32.5%, with rates of up to 60% observed in those with a longer duration of illness and use of antipsychotic medication (RANZCP, 2015).

The Australian Survey of High Impact Psychosis (SHIP) provides detailed information about the prevalence of metabolic comorbidities among Australians living with psychosis (RANZCP, 2015). Similar to data from other countries, the rate of metabolic syndrome was found to be 61% regardless of diagnostic group, while 66% identified as smokers (RANZCP, 2015). The percentage of those surveyed who met the threshold for individual items of metabolic syndrome included 84% with abdominal obesity, 58% with reduced HDL cholesterol, 56% with high triglycerides, 54% with elevated blood pressure and 35% with elevated fasting blood glucose levels. Physical activity levels were far lower in people who have a diagnosis of psychoses, and heavy alcohol use was more common compared with those in the general population (RANZCP, 2015).

Antipsychotic-induced weight gain

Antipsychotic-induced weight gain can affect more than 80% of people treated with antipsychotic medication, particularly younger consumers and those with limited previous use of antipsychotic medication (Maayan & Correll, 2010). Varying patterns of weight gain are observed with different medications and there is growing evidence that rapid changes in key metabolic measures are observed in healthy volunteers after even short-term exposure to some antipsychotics (Maayan & Correll, 2010).

Such evidence has seen the inclusion of revised treatment guidelines in *Medical Management in Early Psychosis: A Guide for Medical Practitioners* (Orygen, 2017). The guidelines recommend that olanzapine, the second-generation antipsychotic linked to the greatest weight gain and metabolic abnormalities, should be used only as a second-line treatment for those experiencing a first-episode psychosis.

A clinical algorithm pertaining to people who received a diagnosis of schizophrenia shows that they are 2.5 times more likely to have diabetes (Pillinger et al., 2017).

The Mental Health Commission of NSW's *Physical Health and Mental Wellbeing: Evidence Guide* (2016) has been endorsed by NSW Health and is available on its website (see https://nswmentalhealthcommission.com.au).

Principles regarding physical health monitoring and treatment

The Healthy Active Lives (HeAL) International Consensus Statement aims to reflect an international consensus on principles, processes and standards to combat the stigma, discrimination and prejudice that prevent young people experiencing psychosis from leading healthy active lives and to confront the perception that poor physical health is inevitable (HeAL, 2013).

The following excerpts from the declaration (HeAL, 2013, p. 3) indicate the intent of taking personal responsibility for one's well-being and the expectation that the person is assisted by their health professional.

> I, my family and my supporters, are respected, informed and helped to take responsibility for treatment decisions affecting my physical health.

> I expect both positive physical and mental health outcomes of my care to be equally valued and supported.

> From the start of my treatment and as a fundamental component of my health care, I am helped to minimize my risks of developing obesity, cardiovascular disease and diabetes.

A report in July 2015 by the Consumer Workforce – Partnership Dialogue Forum in Victoria acknowledged the contribution of medication-induced weight gain and poor physical health, and highlighted the need for organisation and sector incentives to deliver more treatment choices beyond medications (State of Victoria, Department of Health and Human Services, 2017). In Australia, 70% of antipsychotic medications are prescribed by general practitioners (Morrison, Raymond & Firipis, 2013).

The Royal College of Psychiatrists in the United Kingdom released a report in 2013 titled *Whole-person Care: From Rhetoric to Reality*. Aimed at achieving parity between mental and physical health, it argued that the mental health treatment gap was embedded and amounted to an abuse of basic human rights (Royal College of Psychiatrists, 2013). Australian data has also confirmed these apparent health disparities, demonstrating that people experiencing mental health conditions are a vulnerable, marginalised, stigmatised and, in many cases, discriminated-against population with extremely poor health outcomes, deserving of a greater level of physical health care (Royal College of Psychiatrists, 2013). It has also been shown that people experiencing severe mental health conditions are less likely to receive high-quality medical care than those without severe mental illness (Royal College of Psychiatrists, 2013) and to have higher mortality from cancer.

Keeping Body and Mind Together: Improving the Physical Health and Life Expectancy of People with Serious Mental Illness (published by the RANZCP in 2015), adds another voice to the call for broad cultural and structural reform. This report highlights the need for a high-level commitment to action from all levels of government, from within the health system, from mental health clinicians including psychiatrists, and from other health professionals (RANZCP, 2015).

The report lists several recommendations, including the incorporation of health promotion (e.g. smoking cessation programs) as a core element of service delivery within both inpatient and community mental health settings, and the delivery of screening and lifestyle interventions to prevent the development of chronic conditions. It highlights the need to create integrated pathways to care for people with more chronic health conditions and for drug therapy complemented by talking therapies, peer support and non-pharmacological treatments (RANZCP, 2015).

A focus on improving the physical health and well-being of mental health consumers is also evident at an international level. In 2013, the World Health Organization (WHO) published the *Mental Health Action Plan 2013–2020*, in which the concept of integrated and coordinated prevention across all ages, health promotion, rehabilitation care and support to meet both mental and physical health care needs was incorporated in a road map for global mental health.

The 2013 HeAL Declaration has been endorsed in many countries, including Australia, New Zealand, the United Kingdom, Canada, Italy, Norway, Japan and Singapore; and by several international associations, including the International Early Psychosis Association, European Psychiatric Association and WHO Collaborating Centre.

In 2013, Rethink Mental Illness, a national mental health charity in the United Kingdom, produced the Lethal Discrimination report (Rethink Mental Illness, 2013). This highlights the extent of problems in the United Kingdom and recommends actions for change within the National Health Service and at a governmental level. This report balances the challenges of reform with examples of innovation.

A scoping study by the Mental Health Co-ordinating Council in 2014 found that existing practices and physical health initiatives within the NSW community-managed organisations (CMO) sector broadly mirrored those reported in the peer-reviewed literature, with a growing number of NSW CMOs facilitating programs aimed at improving the physical health outcomes, despite higher rates of primary care attendance for consumers who have received a diagnosis of a mental health condition (Mental Health Coordinating Council, 2015).

Assessing the benefits of physical activity

People experiencing mental health issues spend less time being physically active, and more time being sedentary, compared with the general population (Mental Health Commission of NSW, 2016). The ideal physical activity program for consumers who experience a mental health condition is the one they are prepared to do, consistent with the message of 'move more and sit less' (Mental Health Commission of NSW, 2016). Motivating the general population to engage in regular physical activity presents considerable difficulties, all of which are compounded by the experience of a mental health condition, including poor motivation, access to exercise equipment, cost, knowledge and symptoms. Increasing the physical activity levels of people experiencing mental health issues is a realistic goal and should be a key target of any lifestyle intervention. Based on current evidence, recommendations for increasing physical activity include referral to, or engagement with, dedicated allied health clinicians with expertise in exercise prescription such as accredited exercise physiologists (AEP) or physiotherapists. This ensures that programs meet the basic principles of exercise prescription and reflect the best-practice guidelines incorporating progressive overload, aerobic and resistance components, and individualised sessions using established motivational strategies (Mental Health Commission of NSW, 2016).

Furthermore, the inclusion of dedicated exercise clinicians within the multidisciplinary mental health team allows for partnerships with the university sector and hence workforce development through clinical practicum opportunities.

A combination of supervised and group-based structured exercise sessions and physical activity counselling has been shown to be more effective than either strategy in isolation (Mental Health Commission of NSW, 2016). A combined approach also helps to ensure adherence, improves motivation and provides consumers with individualised education through established principles of self-management. Although this is resource-intensive, approaches that are not delivered face to face (e.g. via telephone) may not provide the same level of benefit.

Providing access to basic exercise equipment serves several purposes. First, it allows for comprehensive testing to monitor progress and evaluate goals. Second, it allows for supervised, face-to-face sessions to be conducted in a supportive environment and, third, it provides another means of engagement with mental health services, which improves outcomes (Mental Health Commission of NSW, 2016).

There is growing evidence that people experiencing mental health issues have poorer diets than the general population, due in part to increased hunger, cravings and faster eating as side effects of antipsychotic medication (Mental Health Commission of NSW, 2016). Dietary intake is a key modifiable risk factor that can be addressed by evidence-based lifestyle interventions. The principles of achieving this with consumers with severe mental health issues overlap substantially with those targeting physical activity.

APDs are the allied health clinicians who are best placed to provide the dietary aspects of lifestyle interventions to people experiencing severe mental health conditions (Mental Health Commission of NSW, 2016). The inclusion of dietitians in the multidisciplinary team also allows for partnerships with the university sector and the creation of clinical practicum opportunities for dietetic students and hence workforce development.

Individualised consultations, group education sessions, supermarket tours, cooking groups and budgeting guidance are components of effective dietetic interventions. Dietetic consultations focus on nutritional adequacy and on energy balance to prevent weight gain (Mental Health Commission of NSW, 2016). Consultations may also cover food quality, portion control, mindful eating, understanding nutrition labels, writing shopping lists, organising a healthy kitchen and general cooking skills.

The role of the nurse in the initial assessment and referral to other members of the multidisciplinary team is critical, and identifying physical as well as mental health problems are the responsibility of the assessor.

Strengths-based assessment

In the past, mental health assessments have tended to focus upon a person's problems and difficulties. Over more recent times, there has been a refocusing towards an assessment of a person's strengths, and this is known as strengths-based assessment. There are certain skills, strategies and techniques required to conduct this form of assessment, including:

- adopting open-ended questions and a style that lets a person describe their circumstances with no presumption of deficits
- assuming a person has some resources and capacity to address problems – the job of the assessor is to recognise and elicit these
- countering problem-based world views often held by people by looking for examples when a person demonstrates strengths or resourcefulness in the face of problems. For example, 'You have said you are homeless now, what skills or strategies do you use to make sure you have somewhere to sleep each night?'
- asking about when times are/were good, and exploring the circumstances and resources a person has and uses at these times
- using positive language in questions where possible.

By adopting a strengths-based assessment, the mental health nurse can collaborate with the consumer in reaching recovery outcomes that are positive as they draw on their existing strengths.

MODERN DIAGNOSTIC CLASSIFICATION SYSTEMS IN MENTAL HEALTH ASSESSMENT

The American Psychiatric Association's *Diagnostic and Statistical Manual of Mental Disorders* (DSM-5; APA, 2013) is an official system of classification that has a huge (perhaps excessive) influence on how everything works in the mental health world: who gets diagnosed, who gets treated, who pays for it, whether disability is appropriate and whether someone can be involuntarily admitted, released from legal responsibility or sue for damages (Hardiman & Xa in Kirk, 2005; Sadler, 2005; Schwartz & Wiggins, 2002). This system of classification will feature significantly in everyday practice in a mental health setting. There is a clear rationale for practitioners to become knowledgeable on this topic and it is of paramount importance that nurses not only have knowledge and insight about what classification is, but also how it is used.

DSM-5 and ICD-10

Mental health conditions (or illnesses) are currently diagnosed under two separate classification systems: one created by WHO, the International Classification of Diseases (ICD) (WHO, 2004), and the other developed by the American Psychiatric Association (APA), the DSM. Both classification systems are regularly reviewed and updated. The APA released the fifth edition of the DSM in 2013 and the future ICD edition, ICD-11, is at a critical juncture in its development, with revisions still to be made and implemented.

The structured classification of symptoms, as represented in the systems mentioned above, is considered necessary for a common understanding of diseases and illnesses that can be shared, not only within communities, cities and countries, but also globally (WHO, 2008).

Classification is also considered useful in identifying illnesses, providing education, designing and delivering treatment and for research and epidemiological purposes (Australian Government, 2012; Reed, 2010). The WHO's ICD diagnostic classification system is the global standard for health reporting and clinical applications (Reed, 2010; WHO, 2004). In addition, the psychiatric professions in many countries use the APA's DSM-5 (Ebert, 2008; Reed, 2010; Stein et al., 2010).

Use of diagnostic classifications can be problematic. In the absence of pathophysiological certainty, psychiatric diagnoses are socially constructed (Robertson & Walter, 2007; Wolff, 2007; Young, 2009). Therefore, the diagnostic classification of mental illness has inherent problems, such as being based on values rather than facts (Robertson & Walter, 2007; Stein et al., 2010). An example provided by Robertson and Walter (2007) is the diagnosis of acute delirium, which is a physical condition confirmable through tests, using validated measures. In comparison, a mental illness is diagnosed by considering patterns of behaviour (observed or not) that deviate from socially constructed norms.

Structured classification criteria, which are essentially statements set against socially constructed norms, are regarded by some authors as unreliable (Garb, 2005; Reed, 2010; Robertson & Walter, 2007; Stein et al., 2010).

The DSM system of classification as a guide

The DSM-5 provides the authoritative list of what are mental disorders (as they are described in the DSM). It is important to consider that the DSM-5 system of diagnosis is a guide, no more and no less. This is partly since operational definitions of mental health conditions have been elusive. Historically, mental health conditions have emerged from a practical necessity as opposed to having met an independent set of abstract and operationalised definitional criteria. Indeed, the concept of mental health conditions is so unclear, difficult to comprehend and diverse that it remains difficult to define (Frances & Widiger, 2012).

A multidisciplinary approach

The people who are chosen to develop the DSM-5 are thought to be experts because they have specialised in one or another psychiatric diagnosis. It is often said that such experts are often situated in research institutions as opposed to the 'real-world' clinical environment (Frances & Widiger, 2012). Experts are usually confident in their views; however, they may have little awareness of how little they know about issues in actual clinical practice, drug company marketing, resources allocation, health economics, forensic misuse and all the practical influences of a DSM-5. Experts are extremely valuable in the development of classification systems such as the DSM-5, but their opinions should always be considered along with much broader perspectives (Frances & Widiger, 2012).

We do, however, often see some common themes in the definition of mental health conditions; these are: distress, disability, dyscontrol and dysfunction (Bergner, 1997; Klein, 1999; Widiger & Sankis, 2000). Nevertheless, these themes are rather too imprecise and non-specific to be of operational value. Thus, the definition of mental health conditions has been somewhat elastic and has tended to follow practice rather than to guide it. Only six disorders were listed in the initial DSM in the mid-twentieth century; now there are close to three hundred. Despite these limitations, the definitions of individual mental health conditions contained in the DSM-5 achieves great practical utility. The DSM-5 is imperfect, but it is indispensable.

The DSM-5 is, as the title suggests, the fifth iteration of the manual. The first iteration was published in 1952 in the United States. Subsequent editions have always attracted controversy and debate. This tells us that there were and still are many challenges around the concept of mental health conditions. One clear example of how things change and evolve is the classification of homosexuality. In 1952, the APA listed homosexuality in the DSM as a sociopathic personality disturbance. A large-scale study of homosexuality in 1962 concluded 'homosexuality is a pathological hidden fear of the opposite sex caused by traumatic parent–child relationships' (Bieber, 1962). Therefore, it is important to keep in mind that classification systems often reflect the culture and values of the time in which they were constructed.

The case for making an accurate diagnosis

A crucial issue for clinical decision-making and research progress in mental health is the quality of diagnosis. Narrow et al. (2013) conducted research to measure the degree to which two practitioners could independently agree on the presence or absence of selected DSM-5 diagnosis when the same consumer was interviewed on separate occasions. They found that most diagnoses had a very good reliability (Narrow et al., 2013). This kind of research, although useful, begins with a premise that the classification system is valid in the first place, which we have seen is hotly disputed.

For some people, a diagnosis may be much more than a label; for example, for many the provision of services or compensation may depend upon having a mental health diagnosis (Woods, Walsh, Saksa & McGlashan, 2010).

In the absence of definitive scientific evidence, the diagnosis of a mental health condition is made following a series of interviews by a person qualified and empowered to make psychiatric diagnoses. During the interview process, an extensive set of questions is asked. Judgements are formed, based on the combination of observations, questions and subjective responses. The findings of the assessment, together with collateral information from family members and friends when available, are matched with diagnostic criteria from the chosen diagnostic tool (DSM-5 or ICD-10) and a diagnosis is given.

It is important to understand that psychiatric classification for an individual has significant implications that reach well beyond the boundaries of a single diagnostic act. The moment of diagnosis can be a relief and yet feel devastating. Relief comes from finally having an explanation for the experiences and difficulties, and devastation arises from receiving a label that shatters the person's sense of self, place in the world and view of the future, particularly in the case of diagnoses such as schizophrenia.

REFLECTION ON LEARNING FROM PRACTICE

Llewellyn's experiences as a student highlight the difficulties that many of us share around mental health conditions, and our concerns about the 'unknown'. As Llewellyn has shown, these concerns are often unfounded, and the best way of handling anxiety about an upcoming placement is to be familiar with the content.

The MSE is a complex series of assessments that help formulate a direction or pathway to treatment for people with mental illness. By understanding how to conduct the MSE, the nurse is able to identify disturbances in thinking and behaviour, and ensure that supportive and collaborative nursing care can be provided.

CHAPTER RESOURCES

SUMMARY

- The mental state assessment is a biopsychosocial tool used to gather information about a consumers situation.
- Physical and mental health are equally important for individuals and certain factors make people with mental health conditions more vulnerable to physical health issues such as metabolic syndrome.

- The Mental State Examination (MSE) is a 'snapshot' of an individual's mental health at the time of the assessment. There are static and dynamic risk factors, and risk assessment is more comprehensive than suicide and self-harm.
- The *Diagnostic and Statistical Manual of Mental Disorders* (DSM-5; APA, 2013) is considered the benchmark for diagnostics in Australia.

REVIEW QUESTIONS

1 The two major classification systems for diagnosing and classifying mental illness are:
  a DSM-5 and HoNOS
  b ICD-10 and DSM-5
  c HoNOS and CANFOR–S
  d CANFOR–S and ICD-10
2 Problems inherent in the diagnostic classification of mental illness are that:
  a Psychiatric diagnoses are socially constructed
  b Psychiatric diagnoses are not socially constructed

  c Psychiatric diagnoses are based on values rather than facts
  d a and c only
3 The structured classification of mental illness symptoms is considered useful:
  a For research and epidemiological purposes
  b In identifying illnesses and providing education
  c In designing and delivering treatment
  d All the above

CRITICAL THINKING

1 The mental state examination (MSE) is a formal assessment used in both diagnostics and ongoing assessment. How can the principles of a therapeutic relationship facilitate the process of obtaining information through an MSE?

2 What is the difference between mood and affect?

USEFUL WEBSITES

- Department of Health – Risk identification and management: https://ww2.health.wa.gov.au/~/media/Files/Corporate/general%20documents/Quality/PDF/WA%20Health%20Clinical%20Risk%20Management%20Guidelines.pdf

- VicHealth – Suicide risk assessment: https://www2.health.vic.gov.au/mental-health/practice-and-service-quality/safety/suicide-prevention-in-mental-health-services/suicide-risk-assessment

REFLECT ON THIS

A team effort

Undertaking a mental health assessment is a team effort and we seek the input of many clinicians within the multidisciplinary team (MDT) when compiling MSE information. Consider the members of the MDT who might have had involvement with someone who has an existing mental health issue.

1   What information would you gather from them in undertaking your assessment of a consumer?

Consider what you would ask the following MDT members:

■   psychologist
■   occupational therapist
■   psychiatrist
■   social worker
■   general practitioner.

2   Don't forget the important roles played by carers and family. What would you want to ask them?

REFERENCES

American Psychiatric Association (APA). (2013). *Diagnostic and Statistical Manual of Mental Disorders (DSM-5)* (5th edn). Washington, DC: APA.

Australian Government. (2012). *MHPOD: Classification of Mental Disorders*. Retrieved from https://www.mhpod.gov.au.

Bergner, R.M. (1997). What is psychopathology? And so what? *Clinical Psychology: Science and Practice*, 4(3), 235–48.

Bieber, I. (1962). *Homosexuality: A Psychoanalytic Study*. New York: Basic Books.

Carper, B.A. (1978). Fundamental patterns of knowing in nursing. *Advances in Nursing Science*, 1(1), 13–23.

Colton, C.W. & Manderscheid, R.W. (2006). Congruencies in increased mortality rates, years of potential life lost, and causes of death among public mental health clients in eight states. *Preventing Chronic Disease: Public Health Research, Practice, and Policy*, 3, 1–14.

Commonwealth of Australia. (2011). *People Living with Psychotic Illness in 2010: Report of the Second Australian National Survey*. Canberra: Australian Government. Retrieved from http://www.health.gov.au/internet/main/publishing.nsf/content/717137a2f9b9fcc2ca257bf0001c118f/$file/psych10.pdf.

Damegunta, S.R. & Gundugurti, P.R. (2017). A cross-sectional study to estimate cardiovascular risk factors in patients with bipolar disorder. *Indian Journal of Psychological Medicine*, 39(5), 634–40. doi:10.4103/IJPSYM.IJPSYM_369_17

Ebert, M.H. (2008). *Current Diagnosis & Treatment: Psychiatry*. New York: McGraw-Hill Medical.

Folstein, M.F., Folstein, S.E. & McHugh, P.R. (1975). 'Mini-Mental State': A practical method for grading the cognitive state of patients for the clinician. *Journal of Psychiatric Research*, 12, 189–98.

Frances, A.J. & Widiger, T. (2012). Psychiatric diagnosis: Lessons from the DSM-IV past and cautions for the DSM-5 future. *Annual Review of Clinical Psychology*, 8, 109–30.

Garb, H.N. (2005). Clinical judgment and decision making. *Annual Review of Clinical Psychology*, 1(1), 67–89.

HeAL. (2013). *Healthy Active Lives. Keeping the Body in Mind in Youth with Psychosis*. Retrieved from https://docs.wixstatic.com/ugd/3536bf_81c20d5af8e14e7b978d913f00a85397.pdf.

International Diabetes Federation. (2018). *Resources and Tools*. Retrieved from https://www.idf.org.

Kirk, S.A. (2005). *Mental Disorders in the Social Environment: Critical Perspectives*. New York: Columbia University Press.

Klein, D.F. (1999). Harmful dysfunction, disorder, disease, illness, and evolution. *Journal of Abnormal Psychology*, 108(3), 421–9.

Lambert, T.J.R., Reavley, N.J., Jorm, A.F. & Oakley Brown, M.A. (2017). Royal Australian and New Zealand College of Psychiatrists' expert consensus statement for the treatment, management and monitoring of physical health of people with enduring psychotic illness. *Australian and New Zealand Journal of Psychiatry*, 51(4), 322–37. doi:10.1177/0004867416686693

Maayan, L. & Correll, C.U. (2010). Management of antipsychotic-related weight gain. *Expert Review of Neurotherapeutics*, 10(7), 1175–1200. doi:10.1586/ern.10.85

Mental Health Commission of NSW. (2016). *Physical Health and Mental Wellbeing: Evidence Guide*. Sydney: Mental Health Commission of NSW. Retrieved from https://nswmentalhealthcommission.com.au/sites/default/files/publication-documents/Physical%20health%20and%20wellbeing%20-%20final%208%20Apr%202016%20WEB.pdf.

Mental Health Coordinating Council. (2015). *Working for Mental Health*. Sydney: Mental Health Coordinating Council.

Monroe, T. & Carter, M. (2012). Using the Folstein Mini Mental State Exam (MMSE) to explore methodological issues in cognitive aging research. *European Journal of Ageing*, 9(3), 265–74. Retrieved from https://www.ncbi.nlm.nih.gov/pmc/articles/PMC5547414.

Morrison, O., Raymond, C. & Firipis, M. (2013). Use of antipsychotics in children and adolescents: Report. Drug Utilisation Subcommittee (DUSC) of the Pharmaceutical Benefits Advisory Committee (PBAC).

Narrow, W.E., Clarke, D.E., Kuramoto, S.J., Kraemer, H.C., Kupfer, D.J., Greiner, L. & Regier, D.A. (2013). DSM-5 field trials in the United States and Canada, part III: Development and reliability testing of a cross-cutting symptom assessment for DSM-5. *American Journal of Psychiatry*, 170(1), 71–82.

National Institute for Health and Care Excellence (NICE). (2014). *Service User Experience in Adult Mental Health: Evidence Update May 2014*. National Institute for Health and Care Excellence.

National Mental Health Commission (NMHC). (2018). *Monitoring Mental Health and Suicide Prevention Reform: Fifth National Mental Health and Suicide Prevention Plan, 2018*. Sydney: NMHC. Retrieved from http://www.mentalhealthcommission.gov.au/media/250552/Fifth%20National%20Mental%20Health%20and%20Suicide%20Prevention%20Plan%202018%20Progress%20r....pdf.

Orygen (2017). *Medical Management in Early Psychosis: A Guide for Medical Practitioners*. Melbourne: Early Psychosis Prevention and Intervention Centre.

Pillinger, T., Beck, K., Gobjila, C., Donocik, J.G., Jauhar, S. & Howes, O.D. (2017). Impaired glucose homeostasis in first-episode schizophrenia: A systematic review and meta-analysis. *JAMA Psychiatry*, 74(3), 261–9. doi:10.1001/jamapsychiatry. 2016.3803

Psychological Assessment Resources (PAR). (2018). PAR website. https://www.parinc.com.

Reed, G.M. (2010). Toward ICD-11: Improving the clinical utility of WHO's International Classification of Mental Disorders. *Professional Psychology: Research and Practice*, 41(6), 457–64.

Rethink Mental Illness. (2013). *Lethal Discrimination*. London: Rethink Mental Illness. Retrieved from https://www.rethink.org/media/810988/Rethink%20Mental%20Illness%20-%20Lethal%20Discrimination.pdf.

Robertson, M. & Walter, G. (2007). The ethics of psychiatric diagnosis. *Psychiatric Annals*, 37(12), 792.

Rosenstreich, G. (2013). *LGBTI People: Mental Health and Suicide* (2nd edn). Sydney: National LGBTI Health Alliance. Retrieved from https://www.beyondblue.org.au/docs/default-source/default-document-library/bw0258-lgbti-mental-health-and-suicide-2013-2nd-edition.pdf?sfvrsn=2.

Royal Australian and New Zealand College of Psychiatrists (RANZCP). (2015). *Keeping Body and Mind Together: Improving the Physical Health and Life Expectancy of People with Serious Mental Illness*. Melbourne: RANZCP.

Royal College of Psychiatrists. (2013). *Whole-person Care: From Rhetoric to Reality*. London: Royal College of Psychiatrists.

Sadler, J.Z. (2005). *Values and Psychiatric Diagnosis*. Oxford: Oxford University Press.

Schwartz, M. & Wiggins, O. (2002). The hegemony of the DSMs. In J.Z. Sadler (ed.), *Descriptions and Prescriptions: Values, Mental Disorders and the DSM*. Baltimore, MD: Johns Hopkins University Press.

Snowden, L.R. (2003). Bias in mental health assessment and intervention: Theory and evidence. *American Journal of Public Health*, 93(2), 239–43.

State of Victoria, Department of Health and Human Services. (2017). *Victoria's Mental Health Services Annual Report 2016–2017. Summary*. Melbourne: Victorian Government.

Stein, D.J., Phillips, K.A., Bolton, D., Fulford, K.W.M., Sadler, J.Z. & Kendler, K.S. (2010). What is a mental/psychiatric disorder? From DSM-IV to DSM-V. *Psychological Medicine*, 40(11), 1759–65.

Widiger, T.A. & Sankis, L.M. (2000). Adult psychopathology: Issues and controversies. *Annual Review of Psychology*, 51(1), 377.

Wolff, N. (2007). The social construction of the cost of mental illness. *Evidence & Policy: A Journal of Research, Debate and Practice*, 3(1), 67–78.

Woods, S.W., Walsh, B.C., Saksa, J.R. & McGlashan, T.H. (2010). The case for including attenuated psychotic symptom in DSM-5 as a psychosis risk syndrome. *Schizophrenia Research*, 123(2/3), 199–207.

World Health Organization (WHO). (1993). *The ICD-10 Classification of Mental and Behavioural Disorders: Diagnostic Criteria for Research*. Geneva: WHO.

World Health Organization (WHO). (2004). *International Statistical Classification of Diseases and Related Health Problems* (10th rev.). Geneva: WHO.

World Health Organization (WHO). (2008). *Closing the Gap in a Generation: Health Equity through Action on the Social Determinants of Health: Final Report*. Geneva: WHO.

World Health Organization (WHO). (2013). *Mental Health Action Plan 2013–2020*. Geneva: WHO.

Young, E. (2009). Memoirs: Rewriting the social construction of mental illness. *Narrative Inquiry*, 19(1), 52–68.

SCHIZOPHRENIA SPECTRUM AND OTHER PSYCHOTIC DISORDERS

Louise Alexander

LEARNING OUTCOMES

Upon completion of this chapter, you should be able to:

8.1 Understand the aetiology and epidemiology of schizophrenia

8.2 Be aware of the diagnostic criteria for the clinical presentation of schizophrenia

8.3 Understand the intricacies of the mental state examination related to schizophrenia spectrum disorders, including assessment of risk

8.4 Identify the main antipsychotic treatments, including medication and non-pharmacological treatments

8.5 Appreciate the consumer's experience in the recovery process and describe the process of recovery and relapse for individuals experiencing schizophrenia

8.6 Understand other psychotic disorders

LEARNING FROM PRACTICE

I can't remember a time when I didn't feel different. Things for me started to get really hard when I was 14. I started to have issues with school and stopped spending time with my friends. When I was 21, I had what I was told was my first psychotic episode. I was so frightened and confused. I believed that certain songs had special hidden messages in them that only I could understand. Now when I look back on it, it seems so unreal. How could this have happened to me? I spent so much time listening to music, writing down certain lyrics trying to make connections to news events with them and not sleeping because of it.

I remember being in the supermarket…at this stage things were pretty bad for me, but I didn't realise what was happening wasn't real. It felt so real at the time! A song came on while I was in the supermarket and it was one of my 'special' songs. I must have looked so strange. I sat down in the stationery aisle opening up the packets of pens and paper so I could write the time, the name of the song, and how it all connected to news events at the time because this is what God was telling me to do. His voice was so clear and all-consuming. I knew I had to listen when I heard his voice. I know it sounds ridiculous, but unless you live it, you can never imagine how scary and consuming it is to be psychotic.

I was diagnosed with schizophrenia a few months after that incident. It took a long time for me to believe that I had a mental illness, even when I was 'well'. I've had three more episodes of psychosis since then, but haven't had one in three years now. This is the longest I have been well. While I know the medication keeps me well, sometimes I find it hard to take it and am tempted to skip a dose… Sometimes it's a daily struggle.

Tim, 33, living with schizophrenia

Consider the challenges Tim may face in trusting his experiences of reality since being diagnosed with schizophrenia. Do you think individuals like Tim who have schizophrenia may question the reality of their experiences and find it difficult to trust in their beliefs? How can the nurse help Tim overcome or manage this?

INTRODUCTION

The word 'schizophrenia' originates from the Modern Latin term *split* (schizo) *mind* (phrenos) and was coined by Swiss psychiatrist, Eugen Bleuler, in the early 1900s. Sadly, it is this very definition that often presents as the foundation for misunderstanding about this condition – that schizophrenia is a split personality. On the contrary, **schizophrenia** is more akin to a *disintegrating* personality; however for many the very term often conjures up images of danger and possible personal threat. This chapter explores schizophrenia and other such conditions that are associated with disturbances in *perception*, *thinking*, disordered motor *behaviour* and a cluster of symptoms referred to as *negative symptoms*. While conditions on the schizophrenia spectrum include schizotypal personality disorder, delusional disorder, schizophreniform disorder, schizoaffective disorder and brief psychotic disorder; none is as prominently known and yet misunderstood as that of schizophrenia.

Incidence

Studies exploring the incidence of schizophrenia have noted the condition affecting between 0.2–0.8% of the population at any given time, and there are some subtle differences in schizophrenia rates and outcomes. Higher rates of schizophrenia are seen in migrants, males and individuals raised in cities (Akdeniz, Tost & Meyer-Lindenberg, 2014; APA, 2013). If schizophrenia affects approximately 1% of the population, this means that in Australia, with a population of 25 million, approximately 250 000 people are experiencing schizophrenia, while worldwide, schizophrenia affects 75 million people. In New Zealand, with a population of approximately 4.7 million people, around 47 000 people are living with schizophrenia. In addition, there are slight differences between genders for both the course of the condition and the clinical manifestations.

AETIOLOGY

Considered one of the most serious mental illnesses (SMI), there are many theories as to the aetiology of schizophrenia. There is no one clear indicator, however, and the condition is considered multifactorial in nature, combining genetic, biological, psychological and environmental factors.

Genetic factors

While schizophrenia is thought to be considerably heritable, over half the individuals who have the condition do not have an immediate relative affected, indicating its complexity (Akdeniz, Tost & Meyer-Lindenberg, 2014). Genetic heritability factors are supported by studies which have explored the occurrence of schizophrenia in twins where a prevalence rate of monozygotic twin development of the condition is around 40–50% (Cunningham & Peters, 2014). Gene exploration has identified around 40 genes that are associated with schizophrenia; however, genome mapping continues and consequently this number will likely increase. Despite this, it is understood that schizophrenia in its inherited form is polygenic in nature. The likelihood of an individual developing schizophrenia if they have one parent with the condition is thought to be less than 10% (Australian Government Department of Health, 2007).

The relative risk of developing schizophrenia is dependent on a number of factors, as listed in **Table 8.1**. You can see that when explored in the context of hereditary, rates of schizophrenia are *much* higher (Gottesman, Munk Laursen, Bertelsen & Mortensen, 2010).

TABLE 8.1
Relative risk of schizophrenia

PARENTAL DIAGNOSIS	OCCURRENCE OF SCHIZOPHRENIA/BIPOLAR AFFECTIVE DISORDER IN OFFSPRING
Neither parent has schizophrenia	0.86%
One parent has schizophrenia	7%
Both parents have schizophrenia	27.3% (increases to 39.2% when including schizophrenia-related conditions)
One parent with schizophrenia, the other with bipolar disorder (BPAD)	15.6% (schizophrenia) 11.7% (BPAD)
Both parents either BPAD or schizophrenia – chances of offspring developing *any* mental health condition	67.5% (if parent has schizophrenia) 44.2% (if parent has BPAD)

Biological factors

The neurotransmitter dopamine is responsible for a number of functions, including the transmission of signals between cells, and can impact on cognitive functioning (Australian Government Department of Health, 2007). One theory about the development of schizophrenia involves the destruction of neurotransmitters during foetal development resulting in dysregulation of this important neurotransmitter (Antai-Otong, 2008).

Other biological theories of schizophrenia include structural anatomical changes to the brain (namely the amygdala and hippocampus), resulting in issues with memory and learning. In addition to this, it is theorised that perceptual and thinking disturbance (such as hallucinations and delusions) may originate from these damaged areas (Antai-Otong, 2008).

Individual factors

All individuals are unique, and that is what makes people interesting and diverse. However, there are some common personality traits that may be more prevalent in those people who have a diagnosis of schizophrenia. Negative affectivity is a personality trait associated with perceptions of the world as potentially threatening, challenging and worrying. In some studies, people who have a diagnosis of schizophrenia have scored highly in this area. In contrast, positive affectivity is demonstrated with higher levels of social engagement, happiness and self-assurance, and individuals who have a diagnosis of schizophrenia have scored low in this area, indicating a tendency towards social withdrawal (Horan, Blanchard, Clark & Green, 2008). An individual's temperament may also play a factor in the development of schizophrenia. Those with introverted or avoidant personalities appear to experience schizophrenia at rates higher than individuals who do not have these traits (Fresán et al., 2015). It is important to remember, however, that more than just one factor is associated with the development of schizophrenia, and therefore temperament alone is not causal; for example, consider the impact that having a negative affect may have on obtaining employment, developing and sustaining relationships and completing education. Anything that impacts these elements likely also has a flow-on effect that may contribute to the development of schizophrenia too, so isolating one factor and attributing 'blame' to it is very difficult.

Stress has been linked to many adverse health conditions and experiences, and schizophrenia does not appear to be any less vulnerable to this phenomenon than other conditions. Stress is known to exacerbate schizophrenia in individuals who have experienced the condition, including causing relapse (Kring, Johnson, Davison & Neale, 2012). When exploring relapse potential in an individual with a previous episode of schizophrenia, presence of psychological protective factors such as positive relationships with others and healthy coping mechanisms in times of stress are contributing factors in better outcomes.

Environmental factors

As with many conditions, the uterine environment is particularly important to foetal development, and schizophrenia is no different in potential issues that may affect this. Birth trauma and brain developmental issues have been linked to the development of schizophrenia, in addition to perinatal malnutrition and illness. Schizophrenia is more prevalent in individuals presenting with positive histories for childhood adversity (e.g. trauma, abuse and neglect), ethnic discrimination, *actual* lower social status and *perceived* lower social status (Akdeniz, Tost & Meyer-Lindenberg, 2014).

More recently, studies associating the season of birth have correlated with the development of schizophrenia; most certainly these incidences are enough to suggest more than an anomaly. Regardless of hemisphere, individuals born in late winter to early spring develop schizophrenia at a rate around 10% higher than those born outside this period. While there are a number of possible reasons for this, two of the more popular theories are the link between perinatal-influenza during early pregnancy, and vitamin D deficiencies (Schwartz, 2014). This is consistent with further studies that have identified that other perinatal-infections such as *Toxoplasma gondii* and rubella increase the likelihood of a child developing schizophrenia (Kring et al., 2012; Schwartz, 2014).

Cannabis use has been extensively studied as an influencing factor in worsening symptoms of schizophrenia, and more recently has been linked with the onset of schizophrenia, particularly in those individuals with genetic vulnerability (De Hert et al., 2010; Kring et al., 2012). Cannabis is an illegal substance that can have an hallucinogenic effect, and is known as a depressant drug. There is also significant research indicating the correlation between prevalence of cannabis use in individuals with schizophrenia and literature that supports the notion that cannabis results in worsening of the condition (De Hert et al., 2010).

Individuals born and raised in urban regions of a lower socioeconomic status (SES) are more likely to develop schizophrenia (Kring et al., 2012; Torrey & Yolken, 2014). While SES incorporates access to a larger number of factors, education, health care, neighbourhood and income are likely to be of noteworthy impact on rates of schizophrenia. When exploring SES as a *causative* factor in the development of schizophrenia, it is also necessary to consider the impacts that onset of the illness has on SES. The impacts on ability to climb the SES 'ladder' while experiencing the challenges associated with schizophrenia likely have significant consequences on earning, forming meaningful relationships, ability to secure safe housing and undertake any education necessary to maintain financial security. In this instance, low SES is a *result* of schizophrenia, not a cause. Alternatively, the impacts of low SES and its associated disadvantage may result in stress and vulnerability factors that result in the onset of the condition in susceptible and healthy individuals (Hur et al., 2015).

Social systems and availability of support persons also play roles in both the development and relapse of schizophrenia. Social connections are an incredibly important characteristic of human necessity. Lack of social connectedness is significant in relapse of schizophrenia, and studies have indicated that relapse is more likely to occur in the first 12 months after remission of an episode (Boyer et al., 2013). The benefit of having social connections with friendship and family groups is of paramount importance, and an absence of this is characteristic of poor outcomes for many mental health conditions (Akdeniz, Tost & Meyer-Lindenberg, 2014). Therefore, feeling connected with others and having a sense of social inclusion are important in preventing mental health conditions such as schizophrenia.

Cultural competence and manifestations

Schizophrenia is an indiscriminate condition affecting individuals regardless of culture or ethnicity. There are, however, a number of anomalies within some cultures and now we look at this further.

Aboriginal and Torres Strait Islander peoples

Since British colonisation of Australia, Aboriginal and Torres Strait Islander peoples have been introduced to many influences that have caused great destruction of their traditions and culture. This has resulted in serious trauma and there is research to suggest that this trauma is transgenerational, and still has significant impacts in these populations. Since the 1980s, Aboriginal and Torres Strait Islander peoples have demonstrated consistently higher rates of mental illness, culminating in extraordinarily high rates of suicide. Presentation of schizophrenia in Aboriginal and Torres Strait Islander peoples is likely to be described differently by both the family and the individual, in contrast to the Westernised notion of schizophrenia that is medically adopted in Australia. Carers and loved ones from specific communities may describe behaviour that is 'silly' (*Rama rama*) or use terms such as 'madness' (*Walpanalpa*) to describe behaviour that is deemed to deviate from cultural traditions (Mental Illness Fellowship of Australia, 2008). But it is important to note that even these

terms vary between communities. Aboriginal and Torres Strait Islander peoples have a strong connection to ancestry and the land, and it is not uncommon for them to discuss 'spirits'. Therefore, care and cultural sensitivity need to be taken when assessing mental state (see the 'Cultural considerations' box).

CULTURAL CONSIDERATIONS

What is cultural competence?

Health care is complex and the needs of all individuals receiving care need to be considered to ensure that the provision of such care is person-centred and holistic, taking into account their individual cultural needs. Cultural competence is the provision of health care that meets the diverse needs of people from a range of cultural backgrounds (Jeffreys, 2015). Cultural competence meets the language, cultural and social requirements of individuals, and is associated with improved health care outcomes.

In Australia, there are over 500 varied cultural groups making Australia a diverse, multicultural nation (Australian Government, 2017). While Indigenous people account for only a small percentage of Australia's population (2.4%), Indigenous Australians have poorer health outcomes, and care, attention and sensitivity should be at the forefront of every interaction. When working with Indigenous consumers, it is important to:

- determine the need for an Indigenous interpreter. English may be the consumer's second or third language
- ask the Indigenous consumer about any gender-specific or cultural practices that may affect their treatment
- avoid direct eye contact (as it may be considered rude)
- consider the use of silence (as silence is customary for many Indigenous cultures)
- be sensitive in gathering personal information — consumers may feel ashamed or embarrassed by their experiences and this will impact on their willingness to share information with you
- ask about dietary issues, including food beliefs and taboos
- consider involving family. Indigenous family ties are often very strong, and family play a pivotal role in caring for their loved one, making them feel safe and providing information to clinical staff about cultural norms.

Behaviours that *may* indicate schizophrenia include:

- disturbances of sleep (**insomnia** or sleeping outside of normal places)
- wandering (particularly at night)
- muttering to self

- migrating between communities regularly
- flouting taboos (such as saying the names of people who have died)
- anger and aggression
- hearing voices (Mental Illness Fellowship of Australia, 2008).

A number of significant social factors influence the rates of mental health conditions in Indigenous populations, but the most common are issues pertaining to lower SES, high unemployment rates, lower rates of education, use of illicit substances and higher rates of imprisonment, which all are compounded by issues associated with remoteness and accessibility to adequate health care. Indigenous mental health workers need to exercise cultural sensitivity, respect for values and be prepared to use non-traditional tools to evaluate a person's mental state (such as pictorial cards to describe mood states).

Migrants

Australia is a multicultural country with an abundance of cultural diversity. It appears that first- and second-generation migrants demonstrate rates of schizophrenia that are higher than other Australians. This elevated rate seems to occur around 10 years after settlement, indicating that necessity to migrate and issues with integration may be mitigating factors (Victorian Transcultural Mental Health, 2014).

Other issues when considering migrants and schizophrenia are:

- difficulties due to language barriers, resulting in misdiagnosis
- cultural and religious practices that may impact on diagnosis or experiences that are perceived to be psychotic in nature. For example, in some African countries, access to basic mental health care is limited to cities, and as such individuals' experiences of mental health care from rural areas may be severely limited to non-traditional medicine (Ventevogel, Jordans, Reis & de Jong, 2013). These experiences will likely impact on their experiences of mental health care in Australia
- a propensity to seek non-Western help for psychotic phenomena due to diversity in belief systems (e.g. seeking a witch doctor or clergy for a perceived 'possession')
- stigma associated with mental health conditions in many cultures resulting in fear and reluctance to seek help.

Comorbidity

Like many other mental health conditions, schizophrenia is associated with incidences of comorbidity with other conditions. In particular, conditions of substance misuse are most common

(namely tobacco use); however, anxiety disorders are also being diagnosed more frequently in those with schizophrenia (APA, 2013). In addition to these, there are also increasing rates of obsessive-compulsive disorder and panic disorder in persons who have a diagnosis of schizophrenia. Due to some similarities between schizotypal and paranoid personality disorders with schizophrenia, there is sometimes an affinity for either of these conditions to precede the development of schizophrenia too (APA, 2013). Issues associated with SES and resulting implications for physical health through poverty, access to health care and mental health literacy are also of concern.

Due to the sometimes catastrophic implications schizophrenia can have on an individual's life, resulting in global functioning issues, those experiencing the condition have a lower life expectancy. Higher rates of smoking and substance misuse noted within this population and resulting implications to health are seen. In addition, more deaths from both metastasised and primary cancers (but not higher *rates* of cancer) are also noted in populations with schizophrenia and SMI (Irwin, Henderson, Knight & Pirl, 2014). In fact, individuals with schizophrenia are almost two times more likely to die from cancer than those not experiencing a mental health condition. It is understood that this is likely a combination of causes such as lifestyle factors (obesity, smoking, etc.) and poor physical health resulting in inability to cope with cancer treatments such as surgery and chemotherapy, which are prescribed at lower rates in those with schizophrenia (Irwin et al., 2014). The notion of under-detection of cancers within this population, however, should not be dismissed, and raises serious concerns about medical assessment of, and illness detection in, those with a mental health condition.

Higher rates of cardiovascular disease and diabetes are thought to be directly related to the condition's treatment with atypical antipsychotics, which while treating illness symptoms well, have many adverse side effects such as appetite stimulation with resulting weight gain. This weight gain, in addition to plasma lipid changes, can result in a cluster of conditions known collectively as **metabolic syndrome** (or *MetSy*) (see **Table 8.7** later in the chapter). Metabolic syndrome is characterised by hypertension, increased waist circumference, elevated blood glucose and triglyceride elevation. Metabolic syndrome is discussed in more depth when we explore the side effects of antipsychotic therapy.

Clinical course

Schizophrenia can be separated into three distinct phases: the **prodrome**, **active phase** and the **residual phase**. Like many other mental health conditions, schizophrenia is thought to emerge in the late teens into early adulthood, with a first episode-age-onset for males of the early 20s, and for females in the late 20s, and again in the post-menopausal period (APA, 2013). While the development of the condition varies between individuals, it is usually gradual or attenuated with symptoms emerging as mild, and culminating in significant distress as the condition progresses. The prodrome is considered the early, emerging stage of schizophrenia, and may be likened to 'the warning' or a sub-threshold presentation where symptoms do not yet warrant a conclusive diagnosis. During the prodrome, the individual experiences subtle behavioural changes and diminishing functioning. This includes occupational, social, vocational and psychological functioning. When explored retrospectively (i.e. after diagnosis), the prodrome may create the picture of an individual who had many emerging signs of schizophrenia, but because they were mild, did not merit further investigation (Fleischhacker & Stolerman, 2014). The prodrome may last for a period of years, and because it usually occurs in adolescence and emerges during formative social and emotional developmental stages, it can have catastrophic impacts on an individual's life. The prodrome may include the emergence of symptoms listed in the 'Clinical observations' box.

CLINICAL **OBSERVATIONS**

Possible early symptoms of the prodrome
Possible early symptoms are:
- strange beliefs, perceptions or bodily sensations
- issues with maintaining concentration
- suspicious thoughts
- superstitious beliefs
- changes to affect
- emergence of mild negative symptoms
- social withdrawal.

Young people who are considered to have an ultra-high risk (UHR) of developing psychosis frequently present with these symptoms in an attenuated, and then increasing form. UHR indicators include the presence of mild psychotic symptoms; florid psychotic symptoms that spontaneously resolve; a first-degree relative with a diagnosis of a psychotic disorder or themselves having a schizotypal personality disorder; and substantial decline in functioning (Fleischhacker & Stolerman, 2014).

There are many schools of thinking regarding the prodrome of schizophrenia (including its very existence) and thus there are a number of theories as to how it should be best treated or managed. Some

researchers claim psychopharmacological management (with atypical antipsychotics) is warranted, while others believe psychological therapies are most effective. Some argue a combination of both is best. What we do know is that *any* intervention during this crucial period will be more beneficial than doing nothing at all (Orygen Youth Health, 2018).

The *active* phase of schizophrenia occurs after the prodrome and is characterised by psychosis. **Psychosis** is a generic term used to describe a series of acute symptoms; delusions, hallucinations and thought disorder, which as you will note are all characteristic of schizophrenia. During psychosis, the individual loses touch with reality and may exhibit strange or odd behaviours. For example, they may believe that someone is watching them in their house through electronic devices (television, radio, microwave, etc.), and as such, disconnect the power supply to their property. It is important to note that the individual may be frightened or distressed by these experiences and therefore require a degree of sensitivity and validation in rapport development with the nurse. The active phase is when the individual is most likely to require hospitalisation and as such come into contact with the mental health team. Left untreated, the active phase may go on for weeks or months.

Following the active phase (and with the addition of treatment) is the *residual* phase. This phase has often been described as resembling the prodromal phase. During this phase, the individual may withdraw, display a distorted affect (flat or blunted) and may demonstrate some odd or bizarre behaviour, but are no longer classified as psychotic. They may also experience issues with their concentration and display more negative symptoms. While the florid or psychotic symptoms have subsided, the individual may still experience some issues with odd beliefs. For example, while the individual no longer believes people are watching them through electronic devices, they may still be suspicious of people.

Prognosis

It is understood that the earlier an individual is diagnosed with schizophrenia, the more likely this is to be associated with a poorer outcome (APA, 2013). Given the peak development milestones and achievements of adolescence, this is not surprising. For example, issues with concentration in the prodrome period of emerging schizophrenia can have serious impacts on educational attainment with resulting influences on future employment (and thus housing, nutrition, etc.). Factors associated with favourable and unfavourable outcomes include the presence and/or absence of risk or protective factors (see **Table 8.2**).

TABLE 8.2
Possible outcomes of schizophrenia

POSITIVE OUTCOMES	NEGATIVE OUTCOMES
Onset of illness is acute	Onset of illness is gradual
Positive symptoms	Negative symptoms
Negative family history for schizophrenia	Positive family history for schizophrenia
Intact premorbid personality	Fractured premorbid personality
IQ average	IQ low
High SES	Low SES
Good social structures and networks	Socially isolated/few friends
No comorbidities	Comorbid alcohol and other drug (A&OD) use (or dually diagnosed)
Female	Male
Married	Single

SOURCE: FLEISCHHACKER & STOLERMAN, 2014

While schizophrenia is an SMI, with the right support and therapy there is the potential for recovery. About 20% of people diagnosed with schizophrenia experience long-term remission without further relapse. Of the remaining individuals with schizophrenia, 40% will experience recurrent illness and require some assistance with daily functioning. The remaining individuals are seriously impacted by their illness, require intensive assistance and are chronically impacted by symptoms of the disorder (Fleischhacker & Stolerman, 2014).

Schizophrenia and suicide

It is believed that around 50% of individuals with schizophrenia attempt suicide and people with schizophrenia constitute between 5–10% of all deaths from suicide in Australia (Schizophrenia Research Institute, 2014) at a rate about 12 times the national average (Schizophrenia Fellowship of NSW, 2008). People who have died by suicide or made a non-fatal attempt at suicide are more likely to do so in the residual phase when depressive symptoms may be more apparent, or when the individual is experiencing **command hallucinations**. Whatever the cause, suicide is devastating and preventable; Chapter 20 will explore this important topic in greater detail.

DIAGNOSTIC CRITERIA SCHIZOPHRENIA

In Chapter 7, we explored a number of diagnostic concepts that are a key feature of schizophrenia. The following diagnostic criteria identify the clinical presentation required to be diagnosed with schizophrenia.

DIAGNOSTIC CRITERIA

Schizophrenia

A Two (or more) of the following, each present for a significant portion of time during a 1-month period (or less if successfully treated). At least one of these must be (1), (2), or (3):
  1 Delusions
  2 Hallucinations
  3 Disorganized speech (e.g. frequent derailment or incoherence)
  4 Grossly disorganized or catatonic behavior
  5 Negative symptoms (i.e. diminished emotional expression or avolition).

B For a significant portion of the time since the onset of the disturbance, level of functioning in one or more major areas, such as work, interpersonal relations, or self-care, is markedly below the level achieved prior to the onset (or when the onset is in childhood or adolescence, there is failure to achieve expected level of interpersonal, academic, or occupational functioning).

C Continuous signs of the disturbance persist for at least 6 months. This 6-month period must include at least 1 month of symptoms (or less if successfully treated) that meet Criterion A (i.e., active-phase symptoms) and may include periods of prodromal or residual symptoms. During these prodromal or residual periods, the signs of the disturbance may be manifested by only negative symptoms or by two or more symptoms listed in Criterion A present in an attenuated form (e.g., odd beliefs, unusual perceptual experiences).

D Schizoaffective disorder and depressive or bipolar disorder with psychotic features have been ruled out because either 1) no major depressive or manic episodes have occurred concurrently with the active-phase symptoms, or 2) if mood episodes have occurred during active-phase symptoms, they have been present for a minority of the total duration of the active and residual periods of the illness.

E The disturbance is not attributable to the physiological effects of a substance (e.g., a drug of abuse, a medication) or another medical condition.

F If there is a history of autism spectrum disorder or a communication disorder of childhood onset, the additional diagnosis of schizophrenia is made only if prominent delusions or hallucinations, in addition to the other required symptoms of schizophrenia, are also present for at least 1 month (or less if successfully treated).

SOURCE: REPRINTED WITH PERMISSION FROM THE *DIAGNOSTIC AND STATISTICAL MANUAL OF MENTAL DISORDERS*, FIFTH EDITION, (COPYRIGHT ©2013). AMERICAN PSYCHIATRIC ASSOCIATION. ALL RIGHTS RESERVED.

Catatonia

You will notice that criterion 4 of schizophrenia includes what is called *catatonic* behaviour. **Catatonia** is characterised by extremes of activity or inactivity. These abnormal behaviours and activities can last for short or lengthy periods of time. For example, some individuals may be extremely active, moving continuously in activities that are unrelated to their environment; while others may be immobile, unresponsive or remain in a fixed position (which may appear uncomfortable). Other possible signs of catatonia include:

- grimacing
- stupor
- rigidity of posture or bizarre posturing
- fixed staring
- excessive movement or motor activity
- reduction in pain sensitivity which can result in harm to self through misadventure or intention
- echolalia
- mutism.

In individuals with catatonic schizophrenia (as it was formerly known), the catatonic symptoms are often more prevalent; however, it is important to note that other symptoms of psychosis such as delusions and hallucinations are still usually experienced by the individual. Physical illness or exhaustion may occur in individuals who are rigid or in fixed positions due to dehydration or malnutrition and as such they may require medical intervention. Fortunately, catatonia is relatively rare and responds well to antipsychotic medication and, in particular, electroconvulsive therapy (see Chapter 10).

Disorders of the schizophrenia spectrum

As mentioned previously, there are a number of conditions that fall within the spectrum of schizophrenia disorders. In this section we explore schizophreniform disorder and schizoaffective disorder.

Schizophreniform disorder

Schizophreniform disorder is a condition identical to schizophrenia in diagnostic criteria, differentiated only by the duration period. While schizophrenia is a condition present for at least six months (including one month of symptoms), schizophreniform disorder is present for *longer* than one month but *less* than six months (APA, 2013). This period includes the prodrome, and both active and residual symptoms (which were discussed earlier) within this six-month period and may include recovery. Over 65% of individuals presenting with schizophreniform disorder will go on to develop schizophrenia or schizoaffective disorder, while the remainder will maintain their original diagnosis (APA, 2013).

Schizoaffective disorder

Schizoaffective disorder is a complex condition where an individual experiences a period of disordered mood (either mania or depression) while simultaneously experiencing symptoms of schizophrenia (APA, 2013). **Table 8.3** demonstrates the condition's affective requirements, which need to align with the criteria of

schizophrenia. Diagnosis for this condition is based on the following criteria:

A. Continuous duration of illness where major mood episode (depressive or manic) occurs simultaneously with schizophrenia.

B. Delusions or hallucinations for 2 or more weeks in the absence of a major mood episode (depressive or manic) during the lifetime of the illness.

C. Symptoms that meet major mood episode are present for most of the time of the florid and residual portions of the disorder. (APA, 2013)

As can be seen in **Table 8.3**, schizoaffective disorder is a complex condition resulting in significant distress. An individual may be diagnosed with bipolar type (which like its namesake includes episodes of mania and depression) or depressive type (episodes of depression only). Due to the complexity of this condition and its affinity to present as other serious mental conditions, diagnosis is challenging and may occur over a number of years.

Schizoaffective disorder is not as common as schizophrenia. In fact, it is diagnosed about one-third as often as schizophrenia, affecting about 0.3% of the population (APA, 2013). Schizoaffective disorder is more common in females than in males and it is understood that this is likely due to the prevalence of depressive-type, which seems to impact women more frequently (APA, 2013).

Aetiological information pertaining to schizoaffective disorder is not as readily available as that which explores schizophrenia. As with many mental health conditions, first-degree relatives are considered at a higher risk of developing schizoaffective disorder, as are individuals who themselves have been diagnosed with schizophrenia. There are also links between other serious mental conditions such as bipolar disorder and potential to develop schizoaffective disorder (APA, 2013).

Positive symptoms

The term 'positive' symptom can be confusing for some people. The term is not meant to be taken in a literal sense. **Positive symptoms** are a collection of experiences that occur in schizophrenia. A helpful way of remembering positive symptoms is to consider they are experiences that appear in *addition* to 'normal' human characteristics and behaviours; that is, an individual has *additional* specific behaviours or characteristics (such as hallucinations). Traditionally, positive symptoms responded better to typical antipsychotic medications (such as chlorpromazine), but with the emergence of atypical medications (such as olanzapine), this is no longer the case.

DIAGNOSTIC CRITERIA

Schizoaffective Disorder

TABLE 8.3
Diagnostic criteria schizoaffective disorder

A.	An uninterrupted period of illness during which there is a major mood episode (major depressive or manic) concurrent with Criterion A of schizophrenia. **Note:** The major depressive episode must include Criterion A1: Depressed mood.
B.	Delusions or hallucinations for 2 or more weeks in the absence of a major mood episode (depressive or manic) during the lifetime duration of the illness.
C.	Symptoms that meet criteria for a major mood episode are present for the majority of the total duration of the active and residual portions of the illness.

D. The disturbance is not attributable to the effects of a substance (e.g., a drug of abuse, a medication) or another medical condition.

Specify whether:

Bipolar type: This subtype applies if a manic episode is part of the presentation. Major depressive episodes may also occur.

Depressive type: This subtype applies if only major depressive episodes are part of the presentation.

Specify if:

With catatonia

Specify if:

The following course specifiers are only to be used after a 1-year duration of the disorder and if they are not in contradiction to the diagnostic course criteria.

First episode, currently in acute episode: First manifestation of the disorder meeting the defining diagnostic symptom and time criteria. An acute episode is a time period in which the symptom criteria are fulfilled.

First episode, currently in partial remission: Partial remission is a time period during which an improvement after a previous episode is maintained and in which the defining criteria of the disorder are only partially fulfilled.

First episode, currently in full remission: Full remission is a period of time after a previous episode during which no disorder-specific symptoms are present.

Multiple episodes, currently in acute episode: Multiple episodes may be determined after a minimum of two episodes (i.e., after a first episode, a remission and a minimum of one relapse).

Multiple episodes, currently in partial remission

Multiple episodes, currently in full remission

Continuous: Symptoms fulfilling the diagnostic symptom criteria of the disorder are remaining for the majority of the illness course, with subthreshold symptom periods being very brief relative to the overall course.

Unspecified

Specify current severity:

Severity is rated by a quantitative assessment of the primary symptoms of psychosis, including delusions, hallucinations, disorganized speech, abnormal psychomotor behavior, and negative symptoms. Each of these symptoms may be rated for its current severity (most severe in the last 7 days) on a 5-point scale ranging from 0 (not present) to 4 (present and severe). (See Clinician-Rated Dimensions of Psychosis Symptom Severity in the chapter "Assessment Measures.")

Note: Diagnosis of schizoaffective disorder can be made without using this severity specifier.

Positive symptoms include:

- hallucinations
- delusions
- thought and speech disorder
- agitation and hostility
- movement disorders
- paranoia and suspicion.

Negative symptoms

Like its antonym, negative symptoms are not intended to be thought of as more detrimental. While negative symptoms comprise experiences seen commonly in affective disorders, they are known collectively as negative symptoms only to schizophrenia. **Negative symptoms** are a cluster of normal behaviours or abilities *removed* from an individual; for example, a person who no longer takes pleasure in activities they previously enjoyed (**anhedonia**) such as walking their dog, or has a flat affect.

Negative symptoms include:

- affective blunting
- anhedonia
- apathy
- **poverty of speech** and thought
- social withdrawal.

Cognitive symptoms

As it name suggests, the cognitive symptoms of schizophrenia impact on a person's understanding or awareness. **Cognitive symptoms** are common and occur in around 40–60% of individuals experiencing schizophrenia. While they may be a little harder to identify, cognitive testing can indicate that a person is experiencing cognitive symptoms such as issues with **executive functioning (EF)**. Because EF requires sustained and undivided attention, individuals experiencing difficulties with EF may exhibit issues with planning or implementing goals, problem-solving and undertaking goal-directed behaviours. Due to the nature of cognitive symptoms and their impact on such vast areas of an individual's life, a person can experience serious issues with maintaining employment and successfully undertaking activities of daily living.

Cognitive symptoms include:

- poor concentration
- issues with memory
- problems with executive functioning.

CLINICAL PRESENTATION AND THE MENTAL STATE EXAMINATION

In Chapter 7, we explored the process of assessment and diagnosis. This section explores assessment in the context of schizophrenia. There are an infinite possible number of clinical presentations for schizophrenia and no two cases are the same. In fact, individuals who experience a relapse of schizophrenia generally present with variations from previous episodes. There are,

however, a number of clinical presentations that *may* be more common than others. They include:

- religious delusions (including involvement of God and Satan)
- suspiciousness towards food, believing it to be poisoned resulting in refusal to eat food pre-packaged or not prepared by someone trustworthy
- concerns with technology (e.g. devices intruding on one's thoughts, such as television or radio)
- concern or involvement of worldwide, well-known institutions (such as the FBI, NASA, KGB)
- current or contemporary newsworthy issues (such as current political issues or major world events)
- concerns or suspicions about persons of authority (e.g. police).

While every individual presentation is different, there are a number of likely areas that warrant further exploration when interviewing an individual with a diagnosis of schizophrenia. **Table 8.4** outlines common obstacles and nursing interventions associated with the clinical presentation of schizophrenia.

TABLE 8.4
Common issues for individuals with schizophrenia on a mental health unit

CHALLENGES	NURSING INTERVENTION
Consumer is distracted	Providing a low-stimulus environment is very important. This may involve encouraging them to retreat to their bedroom, going to the unit's 'quiet room' or finding a quiet area outside. For an MSE, ensure you choose a quiet and low-stimulus room. This will help to prevent distraction from external sources, and also ensures the consumer's privacy is maintained.
Consumer actively responding to internal stimuli (hallucinations)	Experiencing hallucinations is a very distressing experience for most consumers. It is important for the nurse to validate this experience by acknowledging just how frightening this must be without concurring in their basis of reality. Try to distract the consumer by: • suggesting they listen to music through headphones • using a low-stimulus room • exercising or going for a walk • having a warm drink • relaxation techniques • distraction by playing a board game • engaging them in a conversation about their experiences • considering PRN medication (often anxiolytic or antipsychotic).
Arguments with other co-consumers on the mental health unit (MHU)	Sometimes disagreements may occur. This is a normal aspect of social interactions. It is important for the nurse to remember that hospitalisation is a traumatic and distressing time for most consumers, and coupled with poor insight, paranoia and issues with trust, this can make for volatile situations. When arguments occur: • ensure you are safe • try to establish the issue – it may be something simple that can be readily rectified • ensure other staff have a 'high profile' on the unit by discreetly remaining in the vicinity • separate people who are arguing, perhaps asking them to retreat to their room, or asking one of them to go outside • ensure privacy and confidentially are maintained (do not engage in a discussion about another consumer's mental health condition in an effort to defuse a situation) • ask other consumers to leave; it can be distressing for them to witness escalating behaviours and they may inadvertently become involved • consider the need for extra staff (or security) if the situation becomes unsafe • consider the need for PRN medication.

CHALLENGES	NURSING INTERVENTION
Limit setting	This can be a challenge for any health care clinician. It is important for behaviours that are challenging or unacceptable to be addressed. When individuals are unwell, they may behave out of character and the potential to damage their reputation is high. To set limits, consider the following: • Ask the consumer to wait five minutes, and ensure you do get back to them within that time. • Establish why behaviour is being challenging, as it may be something that can be easily rectified. • Reiterate the need to respect everyone on the unit. • In consultation with the consumer, develop a plan of realistic needs.
Refusal of medication	This is a common experience of the nurse on the MHU and may be triggered by a number of issues such as: • paranoia • mistrust of staff • previous experiences • poor insight • side effects • poor psychoeducation • loss of control or power. It is important that the nurse considers the reasons underlying the refusal in order to address it. When consumers are restrained for medication administration, it causes great distress and can have serious impacts on rapport. Consider the following when managing medication refusal: • Negotiate with the consumer by giving them options (e.g. 'You can have this medication in a tablet, liquid or injection form. Would you like five minutes to decide how you would like it?'). • Validate their distress (e.g. 'I can see that you are very angry about having this medication. It must be difficult to feel you have no say about what goes in your body'). • Use a clinician who has a rapport with the consumer. • Avoid authoritarian language. • Reflect on your non-verbal communication, including your body posture and distance from the consumer.
Consumer remains withdrawn and asocial	This is a common factor resulting from the negative symptoms of schizophrenia and can be a challenge for the clinician. The following strategies may assist: • Consider restrictions on time spent in isolation (e.g. in their bedroom). • Approach the consumer to play a game, do the crossword puzzle together, go for a walk, etc., and make this a daily occurrence. • Consider a management plan where the consumer agrees to spend more time trying to engage with others. • Encourage socialisation with co-consumers through ward activities such as an art group, relaxation group or current affairs group. • Remain present or have a high profile on the unit (rather than spending time in the office) equates to being approachable and readily available. • Using humour and/or finding common ground can be especially helpful.
Sleeping issues	Antipsychotic medications have a number of actions, and in the early stages of treatment sedation is one of the common effects. It is therefore important for the nurse to establish effective sleeping patterns that balance the consumer's need to rest with their need to engage with other forms of treatment and develop a routine. Promoting sleep hygiene is important. Consider the following helpful sleep-promoting techniques: • avoiding caffeine and/or nicotine (particularly in the evening) • developing sleeping rituals • completing a sleep diary • exercising • waking at the same time in the morning to develop a routine • eating healthily • ensuring the sleeping area is conducive to sleep • warm shower or bath before bed • relaxation techniques.

COMMONALITIES OF THE MSE: SCHIZOPHRENIA

General appearance and behaviour

An individual with schizophrenia *may* present with the following anomalies in their appearance and behaviour:

- dishevelled (due to disorganisation, issues with EF, decreased motivation due to negative symptoms, etc.)
- uncooperative with interview (due to poor **insight** into illness and belief in the need to require intervention) or suspiciousness and **paranoia**
- poor eye contact (due to negative symptoms) or intense eye contact (paranoia)
- movements or gestures may be overt and the individual may present as distracted.

Mood

Individuals with schizophrenia who are paranoid may be fearful, afraid or distressed. Individuals exhibiting significant negative symptoms may present as withdrawn or depressed. Due to suspiciousness, the individual may refuse to eat food that has not been prepared by a trustworthy person, so exploration of appetite is important. It is not uncommon for individuals who have a diagnosis of schizophrenia to disconnect the power to their home due to paranoia, and therefore storage of food items may become unhygienic and spoiled, rendering them unsafe for consumption. Exploration of libido is also important, and may indicate issues with trustworthiness or significant distractibility, rendering relationships difficult to maintain. Sleep may be impacted in times of stress or heightened paranoia, and therefore exploration of sleep patterns is essential.

Affect

In individuals who are experiencing increased negative symptoms of schizophrenia it is common to see affective blunting. This can range from restricted affect, where there is some distortion of emotional expression, to a flat affect, whereby emotional expression is absent. It is important to consider how congruent the affect is to the individual's mood. Are they smiling while discussing details of a perceived plot to kill them, for example?

Perception

The most common perceptual disturbances in schizophrenia are auditory and visual **hallucinations**.

Auditory hallucinations

Auditory hallucinations (such as hearing the voice of God) are commonly heard at a normal volume (although sometimes reported as whispering or yelling), in both ears, for periods longer than a few minutes and often make sense (i.e. are not nonsense). These voices for some individuals may be negative ('You are worthless, you should kill yourself') or positive in nature ('You are important and special; this is why you have been chosen'). Voices can be male or female (and less frequently, childlike), although McCarthy-Jones et al. (2014) note in their study exploring hallucinations that male voices were more common. While the individual may recognise the voice as someone who is known to them, unknown voices are just as common.

The following subtypes of auditory hallucinations are common in schizophrenia:

- command hallucinations ('Quickly! Turn off the TV, they can see you. Hurry!')
- running-commentary hallucinations on behaviour ('It is interesting that you have chosen a red pen to fill out your deposit slip today')
- multiple voices who converse to each about the individual or other things (male voice: 'He will never amount to anything, he will never measure up to our expectations'. Female voice: 'Exactly, he is so pathetic; he can't even get his hair right!')
- non-verbal auditory hallucinations (such as music, sounds, white noise, humming, running water, animal noises).

Visual hallucinations

Visual hallucinations are another common perceptual phenomenon of schizophrenia. Visual hallucinations commonly occur simultaneously alongside auditory hallucinations in over 80% of persons with schizophrenia (Waters et al., 2014). Visual hallucinations are often described as three-dimensional, solid, both colour and black and white, and can last for a few seconds or minutes. Typically, visual hallucinations may include images of people (including God, Satan, fairies, ghosts, etc.), animals, shadows or objects, and those of a distressing nature may include insects, blood or offensive writing (Waters et al., 2014).

Perceptual disturbances less commonly seen in schizophrenia include:

- olfactory hallucinations (e.g. smelling rotting food or gas)
- tactile hallucinations (e.g. feeling spiders crawling on skin)
- gustatory hallucinations (e.g. tasting 'poison' in food).

Thought

Content

Delusions are a diagnostic component of schizophrenia (and psychosis) and are therefore very common in the conversations of consumers who have a diagnosis of this condition. Thought content of an individual with schizophrenia may include delusions such as:

- paranoid delusions
- delusions (or ideas) of reference (often from the television or radio)
- **bizarre delusions** (a male consumer believes he is pregnant with the baby of Satan).

Obsessions in the context of schizophrenia are an area that has been receiving increased attention. Given there is a propensity for comorbid obsessive compulsive disorder (OCD) in persons experiencing schizophrenia, this may warrant further exploration in the MSE domain.

As mentioned previously, suicide is a serious issue with schizophrenia and therefore it is important to ensure that suicidal themes in conversation are adequately explored. It is important to be mindful to explore suicidality within the exploration of command hallucinations.

Form

Commonly one sees disorganisation of thoughts when assessing form of thought. Does the conversation make sense? Are you readily able to understand what the consumer is telling you, or does their thought pattern follow no logical, discernible path? Common thought form abnormalities seen in schizophrenia include:

- **loosening of associations** (ideas so poorly linked they lack logical connection)
- **tangentiality** (irrelevant or indirect responses to questions)
- **derailment** (illogical and loosely connected thoughts)
- **circumstantiality** (communication that is overly inclusive of irrelevant or superfluous information)
- **neologisms** (creation of new words that have no meaning to others)
- **word salad** (incomprehensible words and phrases expressed in unintelligible speech)
- **echolalia** (mimicking or echoing others, usually in a mocking manner).

Stream or process

Thought processes are oftentimes significantly impaired in individuals who have schizophrenia and may be evident by the presence of any of the following distortions in thought:

- **flight of ideas** (although more common in mania) (rapid and incomprehensible communication where ideas are unable to be expressed in completion before the next one commences)
- **clanging** (words are chosen for their sound, not their meaning)
- **thought control** or **broadcasting** (a belief that others can hear or control one's thoughts)
- **poverty of thought** (reduction in the quantity of thoughts)
- **thought blocking** (abrupt gaps in the flow of thoughts)
- **perseveration** (repetition of words or ideas).

Judgement

It is not uncommon for individuals experiencing schizophrenia to demonstrate poor or impaired **judgement**. The consumer who believes the police are following him may suggest violence as a way of managing an officer who stops him for a minor traffic violation. Similarly, a consumer who believes that she has an invisible force-shield protecting her may not see the danger in walking in front of traffic.

Cognition

Schizophrenia is commonly associated with issues around cognition, including difficulties with concentration (meaning you may require frequent breaks during the MSE), memory (the consumer may need reminders) and EF. EF issues are particularly important here and this information may be reported by others in the consumer's family. They may note that the consumer has difficulties with goal direction and following through with tasks (such as getting dressed in the correct order).

Insight

When acutely unwell, consumers with schizophrenia will often present with little to no insight. Understanding about their condition and causes of their experiences is often not related to a belief that they are mentally ill, and this can have serious implications for adherence to treatment and medication. A male consumer who believes that he really is pregnant with Satan's baby (and not delusional), while denying that he has schizophrenia, would be deemed insightless.

CASE **STUDY**

CARING DURING A PANDEMIC

Peter is a 27-year-old man who has been living with schizophrenia for five years. He lives at home with his disabled mother, Pamela. Peter's last psychotic episode was particularly difficult for the family because it occurred during the COVID-19 pandemic lockdown in Melbourne. Pamela noticed that Peter had become obsessed with conspiracy theories, germs and cleaning during this time and refused to leave the house. This made getting food and supplies difficult for Pamela and put a significant strain on her physical and mental health, too. Pamela ensured that all their medicines were delivered by the local pharmacy, but unbeknown to her, Peter threw out his Abilify because he believed that 'big pharma' were testing products on him. Pamela became very worried when Peter began claiming that COVID-19 was targeting men 'like him' who took unnecessary 'guinea pig medications'. Pamela noticed that Peter was spending hours on the internet, searching global news sites about the pandemic, and arguing with people on social media. Peter even tried to convince Pamela not to take her medicines for diabetes and congestive heart failure. He became so convinced these medications were poisoned that he tried to throw them out, and Pamela had to hide them from him.

During this time, Pamela began seeing a psychologist through Telehealth for her anxiety. The psychologist became concerned when Pamela hid in her closet for some Zoom appointments, in case Peter caught her talking to a 'medic'. The psychologist established that Peter was not violent or threatening towards his mother, but Pamela indicated that his lectures on 'big pharma' were tiring and she didn't want to give him 'more reasons to talk about it'. When Peter said he was going to brush his teeth with hand sanitiser, Pamela phoned his mental health case manager and Peter was brought into hospital.

This was a very difficult time for Peter and Pamela. Pamela was not permitted to visit him in hospital because of COVID-19 restrictions, and she felt incredibly guilty about this. She cried for hours after Peter phoned, begging her to let him come home. Eventually Pamela realised she was experiencing depression.

Questions

1   The COVID-19 pandemic is a good example of how people with serious mental illness can incorporate current news events into their delusional systems. Describe the different types of behaviour and thinking that indicate Peter was experiencing a relapse of his schizophrenia. Be sure to use correct terminology, as presented in Chapter 7.
2   Why do you think global issues such as a pandemic place further stress on people already vulnerable to mental illness?
3   Unsettling world events such as the COVID-19 pandemic can be particularly challenging for people who are already experiencing mental health issues, but are challenging for their carers as well. What types of services are available for carers in your area to help carers cope in these situations?

Risk assessment

In Chapter 7, we explored the importance of undertaking a comprehensive and holistic risk assessment. In this section, we explore the risk assessment in the context of schizophrenia, reviewing some of the more common areas of assessment the mental health nurse may see.

Interpersonal violence

Research suggests that about 20% of consumers in acute mental health facilities in Western society may act violently and that in terms of predicting potential violence, individuals with schizophrenia feature prominently in data (Iozzino et al., 2015). It is important to understand that a history of violence, in addition to compulsory or involuntary admission and drug and alcohol abuse, are more consistent aetiological factors in violence than diagnosis alone. Schizophrenia is not synonymous with violence. However, due to the nature of the condition and the symptomatology, caution should be exercised.

Consumers with schizophrenia may become violent due to:

■   commanding hallucinations (experiences where the consumer hears a voice/s telling them to do something – e.g. 'Go and hit that man.')
■   paranoia or suspiciousness
■   compulsory or involuntary admission coupled with poor insight into illness
■   unit dynamics (e.g. multiple admission of persons with paranoia).

SAFETY FIRST

POSITIONING DURING INTERVIEWS

Always situate yourself in a position closest to an exit when undertaking an interview with a consumer. Never place yourself in a room where you are restricted in your access to an exit, in the unlikely event of aggression directed towards you.

Deliberate self-harm/non-suicidal self-injury (DSH)

Schizophrenia has been associated with increased reporting of deliberate self-harm (DSH)/non-suicidal self-injury in inpatient settings (Larkin, Di Blasi & Arensman, 2014). **Deliberate self-harm (DSH)/non-suicidal self-injury** is an intentional act where the desire is to inflict pain or injury (such as cutting or burning skin), but not die. It is believed that around 18% of individuals presenting with a first episode of psychosis admit to DSH/non-suicidal self-injury in the stages prior to treatment. After treatment, this is reduced to around 11% (Schizophrenia Research Institute, 2014).

When undertaking a risk assessment with a consumer and exploring DSH/non-suicidal self-injury, the nurse may see:

■   commanding hallucinations (e.g. hearing a voice: 'You should cut your arm, it will make you feel better.')
■   experiences that are increasingly distressing in nature
■   previous history of self-harm
■   alcohol and other drug (A&OD) use (this is explored in Chapter 14).

Suicide

Suicide is a global health concern. **Suicide** is an intentional act where the purpose is to die. The lifetime risk of suicide in individuals with a diagnosis of schizophrenia is about 1.8%; however, this rate is thought to be as high as 5.6% in the earlier period of the condition (Schizophrenia Research Institute, 2014). The most convincing predictor of a suicide attempt is a previous history of an attempt. Having a prior history of DSH/non-suicidal self-injury and a diagnosis of schizophrenia are also risk factors, in addition to a history of depression for both suicide and DSH/non-suicidal self-injury.

Nurses who are undertaking a risk assessment with the consumer who is experiencing suicidal ideation may expect to see:

- commanding hallucinations (e.g. hearing a voice: 'You're worthless…you are better off dead…you should take all of your medication in the box right now')
- experiences that are increasingly distressing in nature
- previous history of DHS/non-suicidal self-injury
- A&OD issues
- depressive symptoms.

SAFETY FIRST ⚠

SUICIDE

The following are possible warning signs that someone with schizophrenia may be at risk of suicide:

- command hallucinations that tell them to hurt themselves
- previous suicide attempt, or past history of DSH/non-suicidal self-injury
- bereaved by suicide (friend, family)
- identifies as Aboriginal or Torres Strait Islander
- male
- recent upgrade of will
- giving away meaningful possessions
- sudden changes in mood
- pending discharge from hospital.

Altered thought process

Altered thought process is a term used to describe a series of distortions often affecting perception and may be evidenced through **disorganised speech**, and issues with thought form, stream and content.

Disturbed sleep pattern

Consumers with a mental health condition often experience issues with sleep. Sleeping issues may also be a sign of relapse in individuals who are in recovery. Negative symptoms and sedation from medication can significantly impact on sleep, making it difficult for the person to get out of bed.

During the active phase of the illness, sleep may be significantly reduced due to:

- paranoia resulting in a need to keep a vigil during normal sleeping periods
- anxiety or distress related to positive symptoms
- a need to undertake certain rituals associated with psychotic features of illness (e.g. a need to count all the cars in the street).

After treatment, issues with medication side effects can impact on sleep too. Issues such as **akathisia** and sleep apnoea due to medication-induced weight gain can be troublesome and distressing.

Self-care deficit

Due to the significant cognitive impairment that many consumers with schizophrenia experience, self-care deficits can be problematic. Issues with EF can make getting dressed difficult, and negative symptoms can exacerbate this through a loss of motivation to wash clothing, change bedding and participate in social activities where presentation is important. It is vital for the nurse to provide gentle support in addressing self-care deficits and encourage, prompt and intervene where necessary.

TREATMENT

In Chapter 4, we explored the different psychotherapeutic agents used to medically treat various mental health conditions. Now we explore antipsychotic medications and non-pharmacological treatments, including cognitive behavioural therapy. In the 1950s, with the introduction of the first antipsychotic, treatment of mental illness was revolutionised. Since then, a range of antipsychotic treatments has emerged.

First-generation (conventional/typical) antipsychotics

First-generation antipsychotics (also commonly known as conventional or typical) antipsychotics still have a place in mental health care today, although due to the increase of serious adverse side effects they are not considered first-line treatment for schizophrenia. First-generation antipsychotics are divided into two distinct classes and are categorised as phenothiazines and non-phenothiazines. Antipsychotics of the phenothiazine type are dopamine-2 (D2) receptor antagonists. This means they work by reducing the effects of dopamine in the brain. Dopamine has many functions in the brain, including assisting in memory, attention, learning, behaviour and cognition. High levels of dopamine in the brain are believed to be associated with psychosis and schizophrenia. Drugs in the typical range are known to treat the positive symptoms of schizophrenia well. They are, however, associated with poor response to treating the negative symptoms of schizophrenia and can make them worse. **Table 8.5** outlines the various phenothiazine and non-phenothiazine drugs available in Australia, including recommended dosage range and side effects.

As you will note, the side effects induced by these drugs are similar regardless of the medication administered.

TABLE 8.5
Phenothiazine and non-phenothiazine dosage and side effects

PHENOTHIAZINE DRUG NAME	DOSE RANGE	SIDE EFFECTS
Chlorpromazine (Largactil)	25–100 mg PO (max. 600–800 mg/day) 25–50 mg IMI (3–4 times/24 hr period)	• Neuroleptic malignant syndrome (NMS) • Tardive dyskinesia (TD) • Hypotension • Sedation • Convulsions • Hyperprolactinaemia • Constipation • Weight gain • Photosensitivity • Prolonged QT interval • Anticholinergic effects • Extrapyramidal side effects (EPS) (incl. akathisia, parkinsonism, tardive dyskinesia) • Agranulocytosis
Pericyazine (Neulactil)	10–75 mg/day PO	
Trifluoperazine hydrochloride (Stelazine)	2–4 mg/day PO (max. 15 mg/day)	
Fluphenazine decanoate (Modecate)	12.5–25 mg (max. 100 mg) IMI 4–6 weekly	
NON-PHENOTHIAZINE DRUG NAME	**DOSE RANGE**	**SIDE EFFECTS**
Haloperidol (Serenace)	1–5 mg PO/IMI (max. 100 mg/day)	• EPS (incl. akathisia, acute dystonic reactions, TD) • NMS • Hypotension • Anticholinergic effects • Sedation • Tremor

SOURCE: MIMS ONLINE, 2016

Second-generation (unconventional/atypical) antipsychotics

Second-generation (also commonly referred to as unconventional or atypical) antipsychotics are the first-line treatment for schizophrenia. Arriving in the 1990s, second-generation agents significantly transformed the treatment of schizophrenia and psychotic illness. These agents are known for their tolerability and efficacy, and importantly are associated with treating both negative and positive symptoms effectively. Due to their ability to target precise dopamine receptors, it is understood that this has significantly reduced the incidence of more troublesome side effects, such as EPS, which are commonly associated with typical agents. These agents come in a range of administration forms, including long-acting injections (LAI) or depots, readily dissolvable sublingual wafers, syrups and tablets, making them useful to consumers where adherence to treatment may be an issue. **Table 8.6** outlines the unconventional antipsychotics available for use in Australia to treat schizophrenia.

SAFETY FIRST

DRUGS WITH SIMILAR NAMES
Care must be taken when administering the antipsychotic zuclopenthixol. There are different methods of administration of this drug (PO, IMI and LAI). It is very important to differentiate between the IMI versions decanoate and acetate by thoroughly checking the orders on the drug chart *prior* to preparation and administration.

SAFETY FIRST

POST-INJECTION SYNDROME
Olanzapine Relprevv LAI requires post-injection monitoring for at least two hours after administration as it has been associated with incidences of 'overdose' and high concentration plasma levels. While this may be due to poor technique (e.g. not aspirating during dorsogluteal administration and injecting into a blood supply), it may be caused by small lacerations of fine blood vessels resulting in increased concentrations of medication being rapidly absorbed. The latter is not related to technique and evidence of blood vessel laceration is unlikely to be evident during aspiration.

TABLE 8.6
Unconventional antipsychotic dosage and side effects

DRUG NAME	DOSAGE AND ROUTE	SIDE EFFECTS
Aripiprazole (Abilify)	10–30 mg PO	• Headache
Asenapine (Saphris)	10–20 mg/day sublingual (max. 20 mg)	• Gastrointestinal upset
Paliperidone (Invega) Invega Sustenna	3–9 mg PO (max. 12 mg/day) 25–150 mg IMI LAI/month	• Weight changes • EPS (incl. akathisia, TD, dystonia)
Quetiapine (Seroquel)	150–750 mg PO/day	• NMS • Insomnia
Risperidone (Risperdal) Risperal Consta	4–6 mg PO/sublingual/day 25–50 mg IMI LAI/2 weeks	• Tachycardia • Dizziness • Anergia
Ziprasidone (Zeldox)	20–40 mg PO/IMI (max. 80 mg/day PO and max. 40 mg/day IMI)	• Constipation • Restlessness
Zuclopenthixol (Clopixol tablets)	10–50 mg PO/day	• Somnolence • Dry mouth
Zuclopenthixol acetate (Clopixol)	50–150 mg IMI every 2–3 days (max. 4 doses or max. 400 mg/course)	• Depression • Anxiety
Zuclopenthixol decanoate (Clopixol)	200–400 mg IMI/2–4 weeks	
Olanzapine (Zyprexa) Olanzapine (Relprevv)	10–20 mg PO/sublingual/IMI (max. 20 mg/day PO and max. 30 mg/day IMI) 210–405 mg IMI LAI/2–4 weeks	• Observe for post-injection syndrome for 2 hours after administration
Clozapine (Clopine)	Dose is titrated slowly 200–450 mg PO (max. 600–900 mg/day)	• In addition to common side effects listed above, strict blood monitoring protocol required for administration of clozapine • Myocarditis • Cardiomyopathy • Agranulocytosis

SOURCE: MIMS ONLINE, 2016

Metabolic syndrome

Metabolic syndrome (*MetSy*) is an unfortunate condition that is associated with the administration of unconventional/atypical antipsychotics, and is most commonly associated with olanzapine, clozapine and less commonly, risperidone. It is understood that metabolic syndrome caused by antipsychotic medication is exacerbated by experiences such as those included in **Table 8.7**.

To combat *MetSy*, lifestyle counselling and regular tests are important. In particular, baseline weight (and body mass index – BMI) and blood pressure readings that is taken on admission and then again at every visit (or weekly) will help to identify early excessive weight gain before it becomes more serious and difficult to manage. In addition, fasting glucose and lipids at first contact, and then every three or four months, is beneficial in tracking changes. Some clinicians consider the addition of a biguanide (such as metformin) to treat metabolic syndrome in its early stages in consumers who are taking olanzapine or clozapine as useful. Biguanides are believed to be a useful adjunct treatment for *MetSy* in olanzapine and clozapine due to the serious incidence of weight gain associated with these medications.

TABLE 8.7
Development of metabolic syndrome in schizophrenia

SYMPTOM	BEHAVIOUR	EXACERBATED BY
Thirst and hyper-salivation	• Choice of beverage (e.g. high-calorie, sugary drinks)	• Health literacy • Accessibility (easy to obtain) • Motivation to choose healthy food
Appetite stimulation	• Choice of food (highly processed, fast foods) • Availability of healthy choices	• Poverty (healthy foods generally cost more and require preparation that processed foods do not) • Knowledge, motivation and ability to prepare healthy food • Accessibility of healthy choices
Increased sedation	• Impaired motivation to exercise exacerbated by social withdrawal and/or paranoia • Impaired motivation to prepare healthy foods	• Poverty (e.g. cost of gym membership) • Health literacy
Negative symptoms	• Social withdrawal • Avolition • Anhedonia	• Opportunities to engage • Lack of social supports/skills • Temperament

Side effects

There are a number of uncomfortable, distressing and life-threatening side effects associated with the administration of antipsychotic medication and adherence rates are around 40–60% in individuals with schizophrenia (Sendt, Tracy & Bhattacharyya, 2015). Medication side effects are a common cause of non-adherence to treatment, and associated with relapse and poorer clinical outcomes. Research suggests that the individual's attitude towards medication in addition to their degree of insight play important roles in the continuation of adhering to medication regimen (Sendt, Tracy & Bhattacharyya, 2015). **Tables 8.5** and **8.6** discussed a number of side effects associated with both typical and atypical antipsychotics. This section explores the potential different types of side effects of antipsychotic medication.

Neuroleptic malignant syndrome

While neuroleptic malignant syndrome (NMS) is a rare condition, in instances where it does occur, it is fatal in 5–20% of cases (Friedman, 2015). NMS can occur in either typical or atypical antipsychotic administration, and while it can take a month to develop, the majority of affected individuals develop symptoms within hours (although it can have a more rapid onset). The clinical presentation of NMS includes:

- rigidity
- alterations in mental state (from confusion, to coma)
- hyperthermia (>38°C)
- autonomic dysfunction (tachycardia, tachypnoea, diaphoresis, labile BP).

Immediate cessation of the offending neuroleptic agent is required in the treatment and management of NMS. It is important to consider that while oral medications can be ceased immediately, LAI medication can result in prolonged symptoms of NMS and is a substantial reason why LAI should be trialled in oral format prior to commencement of IM administration. Control of hyperthermia, rigidity, airway management and fluids are used to treat NMS.

Extrapyramidal symptoms

Extrapyramidal symptoms (EPS) or side effects are a series of 'movement' symptoms affecting the central nervous system, and range in severity and intensity. Generally, EPS are more common in consumers taking typical antipsychotics. EPS comprise four different symptoms: akathisia, parkinsonism, tardive dyskinesia and acute dystonia. Akathisia is an internal state of restlessness; the individual finds it difficult to remain still, and feels a need to move. This can result in difficulties in sleeping and resting and the individual may be seen pacing around, crossing and uncrossing their legs, or rocking. Akathisia generally presents in the early stages of treatment and is treated with beta-blockers (such as propranolol), anticholinergics (such as benztropine) or benzodiazepines (such as diazepam).

Parkinsonism involves a number of movement issues typically seen in Parkinson's disease (**Figure 8.1**). Symptoms include fine tremor, shuffling gait, cogwheel rigidity, drooling, masklike facial features and rigidity. Treatment includes the administration of anticholinergic agents.

Tardive dyskinesia (TD) is a distressing and embarrassing distortion of facial features which does not always respond to treatment and is associated with long-term antipsychotic use. TD is characterised by uncontrolled tongue withering, lip smacking and fast blinking, but can also involve involuntary movements of the limbs. Treatment has sporadic success and may involve withdrawing the offending agent or reducing the dose, changing to an atypical agent or adding a benzodiazepine.

The final EPS is **acute dystonia** and this includes a series of potentially fatal muscle spasms, which can occur early in the treatment with antipsychotic agents. Spasms can occur in the neck or the back (torticollis or retrocollis) where positioning is protracted or to one side; the eyes (oculogyric crisis) where the eyes position upwards for an extended period of time; and the tongue or throat (glossopharyngeal) spasm, which may result in respiratory distress. Treatment involves the administration of intravenous or intramuscular benztropine or diphenhydramine. Dystonia is a distressing experience for the consumer and requires prompt treatment.

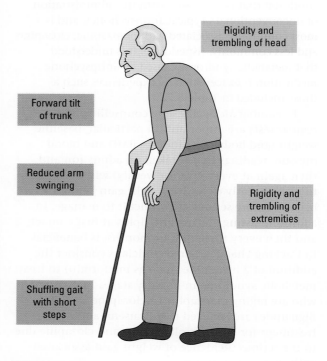

Rigidity and trembling of head

Forward tilt of trunk

Reduced arm swinging

Rigidity and trembling of extremities

Shuffling gait with short steps

FIGURE 8.1
Movement distortions common to parkinsonism

Anticholinergic side effects

Anticholinergic side effects are a common result of using antipsychotic medications and are experienced by many consumers. While they are generally more prevalent in those taking typical antipsychotics, anticholinergic side effects can occur in atypical agents too (namely clozapine). *Peripheral anticholinergic* side effects include constipation, dry mouth, urinary incontinence, blurred vision, increased heart rate, decreased sweating and sedation, while *central anticholinergic* side effects include issues with memory and cognition, and attention deficit.

Sexual dysfunction

It is understandable that people with schizophrenia may experience issues with relationships due to social withdrawal, paranoia and negative symptoms; however, medication side effects are also a significant cause of sexual dysfunction. Between 30–60% of individuals with schizophrenia who are being treated with antipsychotics experience sexual dysfunction. In men, erectile dysfunction and ejaculation delay are some of the common experiences of sexual dysfunction (Vodusek & Boller, 2015). Women may experience a reduction in lubrication, rendering intercourse difficult and painful, while both males and females can experience decreased libido with antipsychotics. Sexual dysfunction is known to play a significant role in non-adherence to antipsychotic medication.

Agranulocytosis

While agranulocytosis is a relatively rare condition occurring in around 1% of individuals, it is serious and can cause death. **Agranulocytosis** is a bone marrow suppression disorder resulting in a lowered white blood cell count and is associated with the antipsychotic clozapine; this is one of the major reasons that clozapine is only used for refractory (or treatment-resistant) schizophrenia (Stern, Fava, Wilens & Rosenbaum, 2015). Clozapine administration requires strict adherence to blood protocol monitoring and must be titrated slowly. Agranulocytosis usually occurs within the first 18 weeks of treatment (which is when blood monitoring is at its strictest) and consumers who are on clozapine must be informed to immediately report any of the following symptoms:

- sore throat
- fever
- chills
- mouth ulcers or bleeding gums
- weakness.

In the unlikely event that a consumer develops agranulocytosis, a full blood test will confirm diagnosis, and the medication believed responsible must be ceased in the short term. Depending on the severity of symptoms and blood test results, the antipsychotic agent may have to be withdrawn completely, and the individual commenced on another medication. Given that clozapine is not a first-line treatment for schizophrenia and is used for refractory cases, it is imperative that monitoring is stringent and thorough as it is likely that the consumer has tried and been unsuccessfully treated with other atypical agents in the past.

Tobacco smoking and antipsychotic medications

Individuals who identify as 'daily smokers' report levels of psychological distress in the high to very high range (AIHW, 2016) and rates of tobacco smoking in those with schizophrenia are thought to be around 60% (Greenhalgh, Bayly & Winstanley, 2015). Tobacco smoking is a known contributing factor in the lowered measurement of clozapine and olanzapine plasma concentrations in individuals being treated with antipsychotics. It is understood that this is due to an increased metabolism of medication in smokers and is impacted by as few as 7–12 cigarettes per day (Luft & Kulsaekaran, 2013). This necessitates smokers requiring higher doses of medication to achieve the same therapeutic level as non-smokers. Smokers who are on olanzapine or clozapine should be aware to report *any* reduction in their smoking pattern, or a desire to quit to their physician immediately, as a cessation of smoking can result in a dramatic increase in plasma concentration levels resulting in 'overdose'. With this overdose come increases in side effects, including potentially fatal ones as discussed earlier. Blood concentration levels have been reported at half the level of non-smokers prescribed the same dose, so while smoking reduction or cessation should always be the desire of the health care clinician, care does need to be exercised here (Luft & Kulsaekaran, 2013).

Complementary and alternative medicine

Complementary and alternative therapies (CAM) are those that provide an adjunct to traditional medicine and are considered by some to be beneficial to an individual's physical and mental well-being. Vancampfort et al. (2012) explored the use of yoga in a systematic review of research into its effectiveness as an adjunct with schizophrenia. Given that yoga has not been associated with adverse outcomes, it is considered a useful adjunct treatment, in particular given its effectiveness in promoting movement and reducing negative and positive symptoms. Acupuncture is the insertion of fine needles into the skin at various points that are thought to be meridians or lines of energy. Acupuncture was deemed an effective adjunct therapy for the treatment of schizophrenia, in particular due to its effectiveness in promotion of sleep (Bosch, van der Noort, Staudte & Lim, 2015). While CAM therapies may not always demonstrate clinical effectiveness in schizophrenia, they can have a role in adjunct therapy, providing relief from symptoms and a feeling of engagement with treatment in the consumer. Clinicians need to work collaboratively with consumers and respect and support their choices in treatment.

Non-pharmacological interventions

Music therapy has also been established as an effective adjunct to traditional methods of treatment for schizophrenia. Lu et al. (2013) noted improvement of schizophrenia symptoms in their study using group music therapy as an intervention.

Cognitive behavioural therapy (CBT) has demonstrated mixed effectiveness for use with schizophrenia. CBT is often recommended in the treatment of schizophrenia (Steel, 2013) and there is some evidence to suggest that CBT is mildly effective in the treatment of symptoms. However, there is also a breadth of evidence to suggest it has no impact whatsoever (Jauhar et al., 2014). Non-pharmacological therapies are discussed in greater depth in Chapter 4.

RECOVERY AND RELAPSE PREVENTION

A diagnosis of schizophrenia is often associated with the notion of a 'lifetime sentence' and this creates a stigma where both consumer and the community may not associate schizophrenia with potential for recovery. This is most certainly not the case. Many

individuals with schizophrenia will return to their previous (or premorbid) level of functioning. Friedrich (2014, p. 16) notes that 'there are far more people with schizophrenia who are working and going to school than who are living on the street homeless' – hence, the importance of making these individuals the face of schizophrenia rather than the stereotyped view that many people may have.

Recovery

It is important to consider the concepts around recovery-oriented practice when exploring the notion of recovery from schizophrenia; Chapter 21 explores this in greater depth. Recovery is a personal journey for each and every consumer and does not necessarily equate with symptom amelioration (which is perhaps too clinical and simplistic). Many consumers with schizophrenia live independently in the presence *or* absence of varying degrees of symptoms. Conservative estimates suggest that about 10–20% of consumers with schizophrenia will recover, but that 68% of individuals will achieve substantial improvement (APA, 2016).

Relapse

Unsurprisingly, medication non-adherence plays a major role in the relapse of schizophrenia. Non-adherence to pharmacological treatment is responsible for repeat hospitalisations, impaired quality of life, poor self-esteem and vocational and social dysfunction (Kulkarni & Reeve-Parker, 2015). In addition to these serious results of relapse, relationship strain with family and friends, costs

---

EVIDENCE-BASED PRACTICE

The lived experience of recovery in people who hear voices

Title of study
Investigating the lived experience of recovery in people who hear voices.

Authors
Adèle de Jager, Paul Rhodes, Vanessa Beavan, Douglas Holmes, Kathryn McCabe, Neil Thomas, Simon McCarthy-Jones, Debra Lampshire and Mark Hayward

Background
Personal recovery from distressing voices and the process of this journey over time is not well understood.

Design
A narrative inquiry study exploring participants' experiences of hearing voices.

Participants
11 Australian participants who have experienced schizophrenia.

Results
A need for clinicians to be sensitive and cognisant of individuals' recovery processes and their individual readiness for change.

Conclusions
Through their experiences, consumers have much to offer clinicians in understanding schizophrenia. Listening to the lived experiences of consumers is pivotal in helping clinicians to develop an understanding of individual recovery.

Implications
The path from voice hearing to recovery is not well understood. This research adds to the narrative of the lived experience of 'voice hearers' that assists clinicians in providing consumer-sensitive mental health care.

SOURCE: DE JAGER, A., RHODES, P., BEAVAN, V., HOLMES, D., MCCABE, K., THOMAS, N., MCCARTHY-JONES, S. ... HAYWARD, M. (2016). INVESTIGATING THE LIVED EXPERIENCE OF RECOVERY IN PEOPLE WHO HEAR VOICES, *QUALITATIVE HEALTH RESEARCH*, 26(10), 1409–23. RETRIEVED FROM HTTP://JOURNALS.SAGEPUB.COM/DOI/PDF/10.1177/1049732315581602.

to the health care system and the propensity for untreated or poorly treated illness to become treatment-resistant are also seen (Kulkarni & Reeve-Parker, 2015). It is believed that around 75% of consumers cease taking their prescribed medication within 18 months and frequently more than 90% will skip a dose of medication (Brown & Gray, 2015). This plays a significant role in relapse, and therefore psychoeducation, clinician–consumer rapport and consideration of alternatives to oral medication (such as LAI) are all paramount in preventing relapse.

OTHER PSYCHOTIC DISORDERS

While schizophrenia is undoubtedly the most commonly known and probably best understood of the psychotic disorders, there are others that warrant discussion. The following section explores brief psychotic disorder and puerperal psychosis.

Brief psychotic disorder

Episodes of brief psychosis were first identified by Kahlbaum in the mid-19th century and were differentiated from other mental health conditions by their acuity followed quickly by a complete recovery (Fusar-Poli et al., 2016). While Kahlbaum's notations did not receive deserving recognition at the time, we now know that he had identified what is known as brief psychotic disorder.

This chapter has extensively covered schizophrenia, and as such you should have a thorough understanding of psychosis. For many individuals who develop psychotic illness, brief psychotic disorder is their first experience of distortion of reality. As its name suggests, brief psychotic disorder is characterised by experiences of delusions, hallucinations, and speech and behavioural disorganisation. These features are also seen in schizophrenia, but negative symptoms are not characteristic of brief psychotic disorder.

DIAGNOSTIC CRITERIA

Brief psychotic disorder

A Presence of one (or more) of the following symptoms. At least one of these must be (1), (2), or (3):
  1 Delusions.
  2 Hallucinations.
  3 Disorganized speech (e.g. frequent derailment or incoherence).
  4 Grossly disorganised or catatonic behavior.
B Duration of an episode of the disturbance is at least 1 day but less than 1 month, with eventual full return to premorbid level of functioning.

C The disturbance is not better explained by major depressive or bipolar disorder with psychotic features or another psychotic disorder such as schizophrenia or catatonia, and is not attributable to the psychological effects of a substance (e.g. a drug of abuse, a medication) or another medical condition.
Specify if:
- **With marked stressor(s)** (brief reactive psychosis): If symptoms occur in response to events that, singly or together, would be markedly stressful to almost anyone in similar circumstances in the individual's culture.
- **Without marked stressor(s):** If symptoms do not occur in response to events that, singly or together, would be markedly stressful to almost anyone in similar circumstances in the individual's culture.
- **With peripartum onset:** If onset is during pregnancy or within 4 weeks postpartum.

SOURCE: REPRINTED WITH PERMISSION FROM THE *DIAGNOSTIC AND STATISTICAL MANUAL OF MENTAL DISORDERS*, FIFTH EDITION, (COPYRIGHT ©2013): AMERICAN PSYCHIATRIC ASSOCIATION. ALL RIGHTS RESERVED.

While the return to premorbid functioning is a positive feature of this condition, it is important to note that for some individuals recurrent episodes of the condition occur, resulting in significant issues with functioning during these periods of illness (Fusar-Poli et al., 2016). Despite this, it would appear that the outcomes for brief psychotic disorder are marginally better than those with schizophrenia.

Puerperal psychosis

Puerperal is a term used to define the period immediately following childbirth. **Puerperal psychosis (PP)** is a rare psychotic condition affecting about 0.1% or 1 in every 1000 women who have given birth, and is a serious mental health condition (Andrews et al., 2013; Glover, Jomeen, Urquhart & Martin, 2014). While the condition is rare, there are potentially serious ramifications including infanticide, maternal suicide and ongoing psychotic illness. In women who do not receive prompt medical treatment for PP, the potential for infanticide (murder of the infant) is up to 4% (Schub & Smith, 2016). For example, a woman with PP may experience auditory hallucinations telling her that her infant is the 'devil's spawn' and as such she may believe that if she smothers the infant, this will cleanse its soul. Commonly, women will present as overly confused or bewildered, with serious impairment to judgement and decision-making abilities. PP may mimic delirium in many women, and as such should be eliminated through means of appropriate screening of infections, for example (Berrisford, Lambert & Heron, 2015). Other clinical signs of PP include:
- insomnia
- anorexia

- agitation
- restlessness
- manic-type symptoms and arousal
- depressive symptoms (anhedonia, guilt, hopelessness)
- over-concern for an infant
- anxiety
- paranoia
- psychosis (Schub & Smith, 2016).

PP will usually occur within four weeks of childbirth and for many women psychotic symptoms will appear three days postpartum. Women who have a past history of bipolar disorder are significantly more at risk (25–50%), in addition to those who have a family history of mood disorders and have themselves experienced PP in a previous birth (Berrisford, Lambert & Heron, 2015; Glover et al., 2014). PP returns in further births in about 60% of women who have experienced it in a previous delivery (Berrisford, Lambert & Heron, 2015).

Risk factors for the development of PP include:
- low SES
- complications in pregnancy
- complications in birth

- caesarean birth
- delivering a female baby
- premature delivery
- stillbirth
- night-time delivery after a long labour that resulted in maternal sleep deprivation (Glover et al., 2014).

It is understood that PP may be caused by changes in hormone levels postpartum and appears to respond well to conventional treatments (Andrews et al., 2013). PP is often characterised by severe depressive or manic symptoms in many women, in addition to distressing psychotic symptoms. While psychotic depression is covered in more depth in Chapter 10, depressive features of PP may include negative auditory hallucinations (telling the woman to kill herself or her infant). For the vast majority of women with PP, prompt hospitalisation is necessary and, where possible and safe, this should include admission of the infant to continue bonding and promotion of infant care. Specialised mother-and-baby mental health units are an ideal inpatient setting for the treatment of PP.

NURSING CARE PLAN

PRESENTING WITH SCHIZOPHRENIA

Consumer Diagnosis: Schizophrenia (acute exacerbation)
Nursing Diagnosis: *Altered thought process* as evidenced by belief that food has been tampered with in an effort to poison him. John believes that the federal police are involved in an elaborate scheme to have him removed from his house by means of turning his neighbours against him.
Outcomes: To experience a reduction in positive symptoms as evidenced by improved thought processes.

ASSESSMENT DATA OBJECTIVE (O) SUBJECTIVE (S)	EVIDENCE-BASED RATIONALE	RATIONALE	CONSUMER RESPONSE
On assessment describes how the federal police have been watching him through both the television and microwave in his house (O)	Regular MSE to establish change from baseline	Baseline MSE enables clinicians to identify change from initial presentation and can help establish if consumer is responding to both therapeutic and psychopharmacologic interventions	John's mental state has improved from baseline and while he is still experiencing positive symptoms, he is able to challenge these perceptions at times.
	Establish rapport		
	Ensure/monitor adherence to medication regimen		
Refusing medication (O)	Attend psychoeducation groups (or 1:1) on medication once mental state improves Provide medication options, e.g. oral, wafer, liquid, IM. Attempt to negotiate with John so that he feels he has some control.	Consider obtaining plasma levels to identify adherence. Encourage adherence to oral medication; however if John does not agree, consider LAI	John has been adherent with PO medication.
Refused both lunch and dinner on the day he was admitted.	Observed by staff to refuse to eat food served on unit.	By facilitating his own food preparation this will ensure John is able to eat food and remain hydrated. It is also an important exercise in the development of trust between John and the treating team	John no longer requires food to be brought into the unit, and is comfortable eating food prepared by kitchen staff provided they serve him and no one else touches his meal.

SOURCE: ADAPTED FROM JAKOPAC & PATEL, 2009

REFLECTION ON LEARNING FROM PRACTICE

Tim's experiences of schizophrenia are not unlike many others who experience this condition. While schizophrenia is an SMI, there is hope for recovery and for returning to some degree (if not all) of previous functioning. Tim demonstrates this through his degree of insight, where he is able to acknowledge retrospectively that the experiences he endured were not based in reality. The challenging and questioning around his diagnosis is also not uncommon in schizophrenia.

Individuals such as Tim may feel guilt about their diagnosis, wondering if there was something they did to trigger it, and their loved ones may also experience concern, wondering if it was parenting style, genetics or factors that they may have contributed to in the development of the condition. Guilt and grief play a significant role in the acceptance of a diagnosis of mental illness for many consumers, and individuals like Tim need to be supported on their journey to recovery, whatever that may look like.

CHAPTER RESOURCES

SUMMARY

- Schizophrenia is multifactorial caused by biological, genetic and environmental circumstances. While schizophrenia and schizophrenia spectrum conditions are relatively uncommon, they are considered severe mental health conditions and can have significant impacts on a consumer's life and affect less than 1% of people in their lifetime.
- Individuals experiencing schizophrenia are subject to an array of confusing, frightening and challenging symptoms which often make them question their place in the world.
- Engaging someone who is psychotic can be a daunting prospect for a novice mental health nurse, and this chapter has also described aspects of the mental state examination

that may be challenging while also acknowledging the consumer's perspective.
- While there are a number of antipsychotic agents, many have serious, undesirable side effects that result in non-adherence to treatment in some consumers.
- Someone with a lived experience of schizophrenia will often experience distressing symptoms that may result in an unwillingness to engage in treatment.
- While schizophrenia is the most well-known psychotic condition, other psychotic conditions such as schizoaffective disorder and puerperal psychosis are also challenging for clinicians and need to be understood by the student nurse.

REVIEW QUESTIONS

1 What is the prodrome of schizophrenia and how is it important in the detection and treatment of schizophrenia?
2 Schizophrenia often presents in the following order:
   a Active phase, prodrome and residual phase
   b Prodrome, active phase and recovery phase
   c Prodrome, active phase and residual phase
   d Active phase, residual phase and prodrome
3 In the 'Learning from practice' vignette, differentiate between Tim's experiences of hallucinations and delusions.

4 What does the nurse need to be aware of in preventing *MetSy* in the consumer taking an atypical antipsychotic?
5 Develop five questions that you could ask a consumer to establish whether they have insight into their illness.
6 How does schizoaffective disorder differ from schizophrenia?
7 Describe two possible causes of schizophrenia.
8 What positive symptoms of schizophrenia comprise its diagnostic criteria?
9 Name some of the side effects of anticholinergic medications.

CRITICAL THINKING

1 What are some of the negative impacts of using long-acting injectable (LAI) medications?
2 Why is schizophrenia a condition of multifactorial development?

3 Earlier onset of schizophrenia is frequently associated with poor outcomes. Why is this the case?

USEFUL WEBSITES

- Health Direct – Schizophrenia: https://www.healthdirect.gov.au/schizophrenia
- One Door Mental Health: https://www.onedoor.org.au
- SANE Australia: https://www.sane.org

REFLECT ON THIS

The multidisciplinary team

Working with people who have mental health issues such as schizophrenia requires a multidisciplinary team (MDT) approach. As health care clinicians, we have unique skills that we can use to help consumers reach their individual recovery goals. There are many clinicians who make up the MDT.

1   List the skills you think the following MDT members would have, and how they can help someone with schizophrenia:
   - student nurse
   - registered nurse
   - occupational therapist
   - psychiatrist
   - general practitioner
   - dietitian
   - psychologist
   - social worker
   - medical officer/registrar.

2   As you can see, there are many clinicians who may be involved in caring for someone with a mental health condition. While this has obvious benefits, it also has the potential to become overwhelming for the consumer, particularly when different MDT members provide different advice and services. How do you think MDTs can work collaboratively with a consumer to ensure they are not overwhelmed or given conflicting advice?

REFERENCES

Akdeniz, C., Tost, H. & Meyer-Lindenberg, A. (2014). The neurobiology of social environmental risk for schizophrenia: An evolving research field. *Social Psychiatry and Psychiatric Epidemiology*, 49, 507–17. doi:10.1007/s00127-014-0858.4

American Psychiatric Association (APA). (2013). *Diagnostic and Statistical Manual of Mental Disorders (DSM-5)* (5th edn). Washington, DC: APA.

American Psychiatric Association (APA). (2016). *New Hope for People with Schizophrenia*. Retrieved from http://www.apa.org/monitor/feb00/schizophrenia.aspx.

Andrews, G., Dean, K., Genderson, M., Hunt, C., Mitchell, P., Sachdev, P. & Trollor, J. (2013) *Management of Mental Disorders* (5th edn). Sydney: School of Psychiatry, University of NSW.

Antai-Otong, D. (2008). *Psychiatric Nursing: Biological and Behavioural Concepts*. New York: Thomson Delmar Learning.

Australian Government. (2017). *Our People*. Retrieved from http://www.australia.gov.au/about-australia/our-country/our-people.

Australian Government Department of Health. (2007). What causes schizophrenia? Retrieved from http://www.health.gov.au/internet/publications/publishing.nsf/Content/mental-pubs-w-whatschiz-toc~mental-pubs-w-whatschiz-cau.

Australian Institute of Health and Welfare (AIHW). (2016). Specific population groups. Retrieved from http://www.aihw.gov.au/alcohol-and-other-drugs/ndshs-2013/ch8.

Berrisford, G., Lambert, A. & Heron, J. (2015). Understanding postpartum psychosis. *Community Practitioner*, 88(5), 22–30.

Bosch, P., van der Noort, M., Staudte, H. & Lim, S. (2015). Schizophrenia and depression: A systematic review of the effectiveness and the working mechanisms behind acupuncture. *Explore*, 11(4), 281–91. doi:10.1016/j.explore.2015.04.004

Boyer, L., Millier, A., Pertame, E., Aballea, S., Auquier, P. & Toumi, M. (2013). Quality of life is predictive of relapse in schizophrenia. *BMC Psychiatry*, 13, 15.

Brown, E. & Gray, R. (2015). Tackling medication non-adherence in severe mental illness: Where are we going wrong? *Journal of Psychiatric and Mental Health Nursing*, 22, 192–8. doi:10.1111/jpm.12186

Cunningham, C. & Peters, K. (2014). Aetiology of schizophrenia and implications for nursing practice: A literature review. *Issues in Mental Health Nursing*, 35, 732–8. doi:10.3109/01612840.2014.908441

De Hert, M., Wampers, M., Jendricko, T., Franic, T., Vidovic, D., De Vriendt, N., … van Winkel, R. (2010). Effects of cannabis use on age at onset in schizophrenia and bipolar disorder. *Schizophrenia Research*, 126, 270–6. doi:10.1016/j.schres.2010.07.003

De Jager, A., Rhodes, P., Beavan, V., Holmes, D., McCabe, K., Thomas, N., McCarthy-Jones, S. … Hayward, M. (2016). Investigating the lived experience of recovery in people who hear voices. *Qualitative Health Research*, 26(10), 1409–23. Retrieved from http://journals.sagepub.com/doi/pdf/10.1177/1049732315581602.

Fleischhacker, W.W. & Stolerman, I.P. (2014) *Encyclopaedia of Schizophrenia: Focus on Management Options*. London: Springer Healthcare.

Fresán, A., León-Ortiz, P., Robles-García, R., Azcárraga, M., Guizar, D., Reyes-Madrigal, F., Tovilla-Zárate, C.A. & de la Fuente-Sandoval, C. (2015). Personality features in ultra-high risk for psychosis: A comparative study with schizophrenia and control subjects using the Temperament and Character Inventory-Revised (TCI-R). *Journal of Psychiatric Research*, 61, 168–73. doi:10.1016/j.jpsychires.2014.12.013

Friedman, J.H. (2015). *Medication-induced Movement Disorders*. Cambridge: Cambridge University Press.

Friedrich, M.J. (2014). Researchers focus on recovery in schizophrenia. *JAMA*, 312(1), 16–18.

Fusar-Poli, P., Cappucciati, M., Christy, H., Rutigliano, G., Stahl, D.R., Borgwardt, S., … McGuire, P.K. (2016). Prognosis of brief psychotic episodes: A meta-analysis. *JAMA Psychiatry*, 73(3), 211–20. doi:10.1001/jamapsychiatry.2015.2313.

Glover, L., Jomeen, J., Urquhart, T. & Martin, C.R. (2014). Puerperal psychosis: A qualitative study of women's experiences. *Journal of Reproductive and Infant Psychology*, 32(3), 254–69.

Gottesman, I.I., Munk Laursen, T., Bertelsen, A. & Mortensen, P.B. (2010). Severe mental disorders in offspring with 2 psychiatrically ill parents. *Archives of General Psychiatry*, 67(3), 252–7.

Greenhalgh, E.M., Bayly, M. & Winstanley, M.H. (2012). 1.10 Prevalence of smoking in other high-risk sub-groups of the population. In M.M. Scollo & M.H. Winstanley (eds), *Tobacco in Australia: Facts and Issues* (4th edn). Melbourne: Cancer Council.

Horan, W.P., Blanchard, J.J. Clark, L.A. & Green, M.F. (2008). Affective traits in schizophrenia and schizotypy. *Schizophrenia Bulletin*, 34(5), 856–74. doi:10.1093/schbul/sbn083

Hur, J.W., Choi, S.H., Yun, J.Y., Chon, M.W. & Kwon, J.S. (2015). Parental socioeconomic status and prognosis in individuals with ultra-high risk for psychosis: A 2-year follow-up study. *Schizophrenia Research*, 168(1–2), 56–61. doi:10.1016/j.schres.2015.07.020

Iozzino, L., Ferrari, C., Large, M., Nielssen, O. & de Girolamo, G. (2015). Prevalence and risk factors of violence by psychiatric acute inpatients: A systematic review and meta-analysis. *PLOS ONE*, 1–18. doi:10.1371/journal.pone.0128536

Irwin, K.E., Henderson, D.C., Knight, H.P. & Pirl, W.F. (2014). Cancer care for individuals with schizophrenia. *Cancer*, 120(3), 323–34. doi:10.1002/cncr.28431

Jakopac, K.A. & Patel, S.C. (2009). *Psychiatric and Mental Health Case Studies and Care Plans*. Burlington, MA: Jones and Bartlett Learning.

Jauhar, S., McKenna, P.J., Radua, J., Fung, E., Salvador, R. & Laws, K.R. (2014). Cognitive-behavioural therapy for the symptoms of schizophrenia: Systematic review and meta-analysis with examination of potential bias. *British Journal of Psychiatry*, 204, 20–9. doi:10.1192/bjp.bp.112.116285

Jeffreys, M.R. (2015). *Teaching Cultural Competence in Nursing and Health Care: Inquiry, Action and Innovation* (3rd edn). New York: Springer Publishing Group.

Kring, A.M., Johnson, S.L., Davison, G.C. & Neale, J.M. (2012). *Abnormal Psychology* (12th edn). Hoboken, NJ: John Wiley & Sons.

Kulkarni, J. & Reeve-Parker, K. (2015). Psychiatrists' awareness of partial non-adherence to antipsychotic medication in schizophrenia: Results from the Australian ADHES survey. *Australasian Psychiatry*, 23(3), 258–64. doi:10.1177/1039856215576396

Larkin, C., Di Blasi, Z. & Arensman, E. (2014). Risk factors for repetition of self-harm: A systematic review of prospective hospital-based studies. *PLOS ONE*, 9(1), e84282. doi:10.1371/journal.pone.0084282

Lu, S.F., Kao Lo, C.H., Sung, H.C., Hsieh, T.C., Yu, S.C. & Chang, S.C. (2013). Effects of group music intervention on psychiatric symptoms and depression in patient with schizophrenia. *Complementary Therapies in Medicine*, 21, 682–8. doi:10.1016/j.ctim.2013.09.002

Luft, B. & Kulsaekaran, V. (2013). Psychotropic drugs: The effect of smoking and caffeine. *Graylands Hospital Drug Bulletin*, 20(3), 1–4.

McCarthy-Jones, S., Trauer, T., Mackinnon, A., Sims, E., Thomas, N. & Copolov, D. L. (2014). A new phenomenological survey of auditory hallucinations: Evidence for subtypes and implications for theory

and practice. *Schizophrenia Bulletin*, 40(1), 225–35. doi:10.1093/schbul/sbs156

Mental Illness Fellowship of Australia. (2008). *Aboriginal and Torres Strait Islander People*. Retrieved from http://www.sfnsw.org.au/Mental-Illness/Quality-of-Life/Indigenous#.VwGOn_I96Uk.

MIMS Online. (2018). Chlorpromazine. Retrieved from https://www.mimsonline.com.au/Search/QuickSearch.aspx?ModuleName=Product+Info&searchKeyword=Phenothiazine.

Orygen Youth Health. (2018). *Early Psychosis Prevention Intervention & Treatment Centre*. Melbourne: Orygen. Retrieved from https://oyh.org.au.

Schizophrenia Fellowship of NSW. (2008). *Schizophrenia Statistics*. Retrieved from http://www.sfnsw.org.au/Mental-Illness/Schizophrenia/Schizophrenia-Statistics#.VtOy6fl96Uk.

Schizophrenia Research Institute. (2014). *Suicide and Self Harm*. Retrieved from http://www.schizophreniaresearch.org.au/library/browse-library/course-and-outcomes/suicide-and-self-harm.

Schub, T. & Smith, N. (2016) *Postpartum Psychosis*. Los Angeles, CA: Cinahl Information Systems.

Schwartz, P.J. (2014). Can the season of birth risk factor for schizophrenia be prevented by bright light treatment for the second trimester mother around the winter solstice? *Medical Hypotheses*, 83, 809–15. doi:10.1016/j.mehy.2014.10.014

Sendt, K.V., Tracy, D.K. & Bhattacharyya, S. (2015). A systematic review of factors influencing adherence to antipsychotic medication in schizophrenia-spectrum disorders. *Psychiatry Research*, 225, 14–30.

Steel, C. (2013). *CBT for Schizophrenia*. Singapore: Wiley-Blackwell.

Stern, T.A., Fava, M., Wilens, T.E. & Rosenbaum, J.F. (2015). *Massachusetts General Hospital Psychopharmacology and Neurotherapeutics*. Elsevier Health Sciences.

Torrey, F.E. & Yolken, R.H. (2014). The urban risk and migration risk factors for schizophrenia: Are cats the answer? *Schizophrenia Research*, 159(2–3), 299–302. doi:10.1016/j.schres.2014.09.027

Vancampfort, D., Vansteelandt, K., Scheewe, T., Probst, M., Knapen, J., De Herdt, A. & De Hert, M. (2012). Yoga in schizophrenia: A systematic review of randomised controlled trials. *Acta Psychiatrica Scandinavica*, 126(1), 12–20. doi:doi.org/10.1111/j.1600-0447.2012.01865.x

Ventevogel, P., Jordans, M., Reis, R. & de Jong, J. (2013). Madness or sadness? Local concepts of mental illness in four conflict-affected African communities. *Conflict and Health*, 7, 3.

Victorian Transcultural Mental Health. (2014). *Migration, Mental Health and Accessing Mental Health Services*. Retrieved from http://www.vtmh.org.au.

Vodusek, D.B. & Boller, F. (2015). *Neurology of Sexual and Bladder Disorders: Handbook of Clinical Neurology*. Amsterdam: Elsevier.

Waters, F., Collerton, D. Ffytche, D.H., Jardi, R., Pins, D., Dudley, R., Blom, J.D., … Laroi, F. (2014). Visual hallucinations in the psychosis spectrum and comparative information from neurodegenerative disorders and eye disease. *Schizophrenia Bulletin*, 40(4), 233–45. doi:10.1093/schbul/sbu036

CHAPTER 9

BIPOLAR AND RELATED DISORDERS

Louise Alexander

LEARNING FROM PRACTICE

Being high…being manic is the most amazing thing I've ever experienced. I felt invincible and important. There wasn't anything I couldn't do. Doesn't everyone want to feel like this? I remember being so angry when I was put in hospital…told that I was 'too high' and that I was disrupting other people. Why couldn't they see what I was trying to achieve!? I was so caught up in the great feelings; I couldn't see what it was doing to my family. I don't remember caring, actually. I just remember that I had an amazing epiphany one night while baking cakes for my young children. I guess in hindsight that was my first warning. I'd had issues with depression in the past. I'd also had times where I was really happy and energised, but nothing like this. It was out of character for me to be baking and cleaning at 2 am…but I didn't think I was sick. Who would!?

I came up with this idea to feed hungry people in developing countries. My eight-year-old daughter was doing a project on famine at school and I was convinced I had a solution. I remember telling her about it, and she just looked at me like she was scared of me or something. She said it didn't make sense, but I needed to prove to her I could do this. We could do this! So I set out phoning World Vision and other charities, but they wouldn't listen.

A couple of them hung up on me, so I decided to fly to Melbourne to see them in person. I booked first class seats from Perth, and organised a week in a lavish five-star hotel in the city. It didn't matter how much I spent, this was a big breakthrough and was going to yield me millions. I just saw my lavish spending as a sort of cash advancement. I spent $25 000.00 in that week.

My husband Ed and children were beside themselves with worry. Of course, I didn't realise. I phoned them a few times (apparently at really odd hours) and tried to reassure them, but I grew tired of having to tell Ed that this would all be okay. We had a few really heated fights… I was eventually picked up by the police for causing a disturbance when I went into the offices of another charity. They took me to hospital. Gosh, I was so angry. I fought them with every ounce of energy I had. I spat, I kicked at staff. I've never been a violent person, ever. I am so ashamed. It's still hard to talk about. But now I see it was part of my illness. When I came down from my high…I spiralled into a depression – a dark, horrible depression that was enveloping and all encompassing. It was horrible. I'm so careful now with taking my medication. I know I need it. I never want to experience the highs and lows of bipolar disorder again, but I know that realistically I probably will and this scares me, but part of me misses the 'high' too…

Annie, 28, living with bipolar I disorder

Annie's description of mania provides us a small glimpse into what it may be like to be experiencing a manic

episode. Annie described feelings of resistance towards treatment. What are some of the challenges the nurse may face when working with someone like Annie, who enjoys being 'high', and how may these impact on future adherence to treatment?

INTRODUCTION

The ancient Greek physician Hippocrates was a pioneer of medicine and while his findings did not survive later critical scientific observation, there is still an eerie contextualisation in his findings from the fifth century BC with today's medical knowledge. His theories of the physiological causes of illness as opposed to religion, superstition and magic were ahead of their time. Hippocrates believed that mental illness was categorised into three distinct classifications: melancholia (depression), phrenitis (fever of the brain) and mania. Depression and mania are two components of mood, found at separate ends of the spectrum, yet equally distressing in their own right. This chapter explores some of the conditions of mood; bipolar disorder I and II, and cyclothymic disorder. Bipolar disorder (once known as manic-depression) is a serious recurrent mental health condition characterised by periods of extreme mood elevation often coupled with periods of depression interspersed over months. While bipolar disorder I and II have many similar features, bipolar I is the more serious of the two conditions. Both are associated with episodes of depression and 'normal' or euthymic moods. Bipolar I is associated with incidence of **mania** (extremely elevated or 'high' mood), while bipolar II sees **elevated mood** states, but not to the same severe state as seen in bipolar I.

Incidence

Bipolar I disorder (BDI) has a lower prevalence rate compared with the less serious **bipolar II disorder (BDII)**. In the United States, BDI affects about 0.6% of the population (APA, 2013). Karanti et al. (2015) note that the lifetime prevalence for BDI is about 0.4%, while BDII occurs more frequently at around 0.6%. Statistics in Australia tend to cluster all mood conditions together (e.g. depression, BD, dysthymia, etc.) resulting in a disproportionately high rate of 6.2% (ABS, 2009). The Australian Institute of Health and Welfare (AIHW, 2012) notes that while schizophrenia is the most common psychotic condition in Australia occurring in around 1% of populations, rates of bipolar disorders (so both I and II) are about half that, which suggests rates of bipolar disorder are similar to those in the United States.

While bipolar disorders tend to be diagnosed equally in males and females, there are notable gender differences in clinical presentations between the two, and the rates between I and II are not the same. Karanti and colleagues (2015) found that BD in women is usually seen with higher rates of depression and **hypomania**, and that women are more likely to be diagnosed with the less serious BDII.

AETIOLOGY

Much like other mental health conditions, bipolar disorders are considered to be multifactorial in cause, resulting in an interplay between genetics, environment and biological factors.

Genetic factors

Bipolar disorders have a significant degree of heritability (Yildiz, Ruiz & Nemeroff, 2015), in particular early-onset BD, which is associated with a seemingly high rate of heritability (Marangoni, Hernandez & Faedda, 2016). Twin studies have indicated a high propensity for the heritability of BD with high rates of development in both offspring, supporting the role genetics plays in its development. Individuals who develop BD often have positive histories of a first-degree relative with bipolar disorder, depression or schizophrenia; however, recent studies report many diagnoses occur without a known genetic vulnerability (Yildiz, Ruiz & Nemeroff, 2015). There is also suggestion that having a family history of BD may abnormally skew diagnosis towards this condition at the expense of other conditions that may actually be more likely (such as depression or schizophrenia). In Chapter 8 (see **Table 8.1**), we looked at the relative risk of developing schizophrenia, and bipolar disorder is included in that table.

Biological factors

Given the role of neurotransmitters in mental health and illness, it is foreseeable that these transmitters may also be linked to BD. In addition to this link, however, is one theory that suggests the role of circadian rhythms, which impact on an individual's sleep cycle (Bengesser & Reininghaus, 2013). Mania is heavily associated with insomnia and, as such, circadian rhythms have been a focus of scientific research. There is also emerging research to suggest that the female menstrual cycle may play a role in BD because of the presence of longer cycles (known as infradian rhythms) (Blows, 2016). This may also help to explain the cyclic nature and recurrence seen in BD. At the core of all this is possibly an inherent issue with signalling between multiple pertinent chemicals within the brain (Blows, 2016).

Individual factors

There are a number of individual factors that play a role in the development of BD. Ability to manage stress effectively can be an important protective factor in the prevention of mental illness. Individuals with poor or maladaptive coping mechanisms (e.g. illicit substances and alcohol use) in times of stress demonstrate higher rates of BD.

Individuals who have experienced head injury have demonstrated a higher probability of developing BD (Orlovska et al., 2014). Experiences of childhood trauma including neglect and parental death have also been associated with increased rates of BD (Marangoni, 2016). The possible link with adverse childhood experiences results in an increased propensity to demonstrate both a lifetime risk of BD and increases in 12-month prevalence of the condition (Yildiz, Ruiz & Nemeroff, 2015).

Environmental factors

BD occurs more often in high-income countries, and is seen more commonly in those with previous unsuccessful relationships (e.g. divorced or separated) and widows, as opposed to those who have not been in a relationship (APA, 2013).

A poor prenatal environment is associated with significant adverse outcomes for the resulting foetus in a wide and varying array of conditions and illnesses. There are diverse results regarding the impacts (if any) that prenatal influenza has on the development of BD in resulting children, with some studies reporting an increase while others have noted no change. Marangoni et al. (2016) noted that experiences of war prenatally were associated with higher rates of BD in the offspring if exposure occurred during the first trimester of pregnancy. Prematurity has been associated with threefold to sevenfold increases in the development of BD in offspring, in addition to experiences of birth trauma also being linked (Marangoni et al., 2016).

While schizophrenia has a clearer epidemiology of multiple factors, it would appear that currently the same environmental factors cannot be attributed to BD development, despite a possible genetic link between schizophrenia and BD development (Yildiz, Ruiz & Nemeroff, 2015). Once a child is born, the risks of environmental impact on the development of BD do not diminish. Substance misuse (e.g. cocaine, cannabis, prescription opioids, sedatives and stimulants) is significantly associated with increased risk of developing BD, and alcohol use is particularly noteworthy in this cohort.

Cultural competence and manifestations

It is important to be culturally sensitive when caring for a consumer with a diagnosis of BD, particularly if, when experiencing an episode of mania, the individual has been behaving in a manner that is frowned upon within their community. When manic, people will frequently behave in a manner that is embarrassing or distressing, and later this can result in great shame. It is also important to be aware of trends in higher rates of conditions seen in minority groups too, so that we can ensure adequate services and support are directly targeted to those groups. This section explores BD in minority groups such as migrant populations.

Migrants

Saha et al. (2015) note that Australian migrants (excluding refugees) experiencing a psychotic illness such as BD represent a smaller percentage of the demographic predicted and are more likely to have a higher education, be residing in a better socioeconomic area and be more securely employed than Australian-born individuals with psychotic illness. Migrants also tend to demonstrate lower rates of substance misuse, which is of particular importance given the negative impacts alcohol and other drugs (A&OD) have in exacerbating and triggering mental health conditions. There are a number of possible reasons why this is the case. These include the selection process of obtaining citizenship, which may eliminate individuals with mental health conditions gaining entry into Australia. Other factors may include a higher socioeconomic (SES) in their home country, and thus the ability to afford to relocate; being from a skilled worker category that is favourably viewed by the government for migrating, and thus having a higher education background; and a negative cultural perception about illicit drugs and alcohol use.

Comorbidity

A number of conditions are seen more prominently in populations diagnosed with BD. There is proportionate comorbidity for anxiety conditions, phobias, impulse-control and substance use disorders in those diagnosed with BD. In addition, there is a high correlation between attention deficit/hyperactivity disorder (ADHD) and later development of BD (APA, 2013). Major contributors of death in individuals with BD are cancer, cardiovascular disease and suicide (Yildiz, Ruiz & Nemeroff, 2015).

While the high prevalence for early mortality in those with a mental health condition is worrying in itself, what is also very troubling is the propensity for the worsening of mood disorder in the presence of physical illness (Forty et al., 2014). Metabolic syndrome (discussed in Chapter 8) is also seen frequently in those with BD.

Compared with a control group, Forty and colleagues (2014) found higher rates of the following illnesses:

- asthma (19.2% vs 10.7%)
- elevated lipids (19.2% vs 5.3%)
- hypertension (15% vs 6.2%)
- migraine headaches (23.7% vs 16.5%)
- thyroid disease (12.9% vs 2.5%).

Interesting research findings have made connections between migraine headache and BD. It is understood that they likely share aetiological similarities, resulting in this link (Forty et al., 2014); however, there does appear to be a connection between the two (Fornaro et al., 2015).

Clinical course

The average age of onset for BD is around 18 years, and while this condition can be diagnosed in children, care should always be exercised due to differential developmental variations even within chronological age (APA, 2013). Individuals who present with BD with psychotic features are more likely to do so again in successive episodes of mania (APA, 2013).

While the clinical path a condition takes will vary for every individual with the condition, there are some consistencies with clinical course, which enables practitioners to make some predictions about the sequence an individual may experience. In many cases, depression is the overarching predominant mood state affiliated with BD (Uher, Mantere, Suominen & Isometsä, 2013; Yildiz, Ruiz & Nemeroff, 2015). For many individuals, depression is also the mood episode that occurs first and therefore it is important for individuals presenting with a first episode of depression to be assessed for BD. Uher et al. (2013) also suggest that depressive episodes in BD are likely the most 'expensive' in terms of impacts on both individuals and society.

Factors associated with the onset of an episode in its early stage include stress and workplace issues, and this may result in insomnia and increasing use, or commencing use, of drugs and/or alcohol, which exacerbate the situation (Yildiz, Ruiz & Nemeroff, 2015). Substance misuse in its own right may also precede the onset of a mood episode, as may seasonal and weather changes (winter months may be associated with greater episodes of depression, while warmer months may be associated with mania). In women, almost half of those with BD will experience a depressive episode during pregnancy and into the post-delivery period (Yildiz, Ruiz & Nemeroff, 2015). This can make parenting, which is already a challenge for many new parents, extremely difficult.

Yildiz, Ruiz and Nemeroff (2015) note that generally manic episodes last around one-and-a-half to three months; hypomanic episodes last a few weeks to a few months, while an individual may endure a depressive episode for up to five months. Generally, the period between episodes of illness is stable and consistent (e.g. over time this period does not shorten *or* lengthen) and research suggests that individuals who experience depression followed by mania and then remission of episodes have worse long-term outcomes (compared with those who present with mania first) (Yildiz, Ruiz & Nemeroff, 2015).

Prognosis

As mentioned previously, BD is highly episodic in nature and therefore the likelihood of an individual experiencing further episodes of illness after the initial diagnosis are high. The episodic nature of the condition can have serious impacts on occupational and social functioning, rendering the periods of remission where the individual is not experiencing acute symptoms being influenced by their experiences of having been unwell. A large number of individuals with BD will experience chronic disordered symptoms for their entire life, significantly impacting on the psychosocial skills required within relationships and employment opportunities. Social, and in particular occupational, functioning issues can have serious impacts on SES, access to safe and affordable housing and a myriad of other important necessities.

Bipolar disorder and suicide

Many individuals diagnosed with BD also meet criteria for comorbid alcohol use disorder and in individuals experiencing both, rates of suicide attempts are higher (APA, 2013). Conservative estimates suggest between 7–20% of individuals with BD will attempt to end their life, and when compared with the broader population, the suicide risk is 30 times higher (Yildiz, Ruiz & Nemeroff, 2015).

Women with BD are more likely to have a non-violent attempt to end their life (such as an overdose) and this is consistent with broad suicide tendencies in women spanning all mental health conditions (Schaffer et al., 2015), while men represent those ending their life by suicide more often, and using more lethal and irreversible means to do so (such as hanging). All individuals with a BD diagnosis who have a substance use disorder, display more psychotic features; childhood trauma (such as abuse or neglect) and comorbid anxiety also have higher rates of death by suicide (Schaffer et al., 2015).

DIAGNOSTIC CRITERIA BIPOLAR I AND II DISORDER

In Chapter 7, we explored a range of terms that have context in the diagnostic classification of bipolar disorders. Bipolar disorders can be complex to understand because they involve three different diagnostic features that make up three different clinical presentations. **Figure 9.1** demonstrates the variations between BDI and BDII.

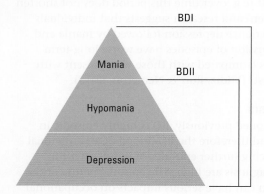

FIGURE 9.1
Variations between BDI and BDII

Table 9.2 comprises the manic episode of BDI. Mania is *only* seen in BDI. In order to be diagnosed with BDI, the consumer *must* experience at least one manic episode, which is commonly followed and/or preceded by hypomania and depression (APA, 2013). It is important to note that the consumer does not have to experience a depressive episode or hypomanic episode to be diagnosed with BDI; however, they will usually experience both through the course of this condition. This contrasts with BDII, where the consumer *must* experience both a depressive episode and hypomanic episode throughout the course of the condition, in order to be diagnosed.

Mania and hypomania

Mania is a prolonged, elevated or 'high' mood that is seen in BDI. Individuals who are experiencing mania may be grandiose, have an inflated self-esteem, have a decreased need for sleep (yet appear energetic or highly aroused) and be unable to slow down their speech, thinking and thoughts. For the vast majority of individuals who have receive a diagnosis of BD, mania usually has a rapid onset peaking in just days; however, some individuals may present with hypomania prior to the commencement of mania. Hypomania is a period of milder mania which is associated with sleeplessness and mood elevation (but not as extreme as seen in mania), and the individual does not experience psychosis or require hospitalisation. In fact, hypomania can be difficult to diagnose or detect in individuals because they may present as highly motivated or productive, require little sleep and appear happy. Most of these attributes are probably considered beneficial to an individual's work and social functioning and hence identifying them as dysfunctional may be delayed. Mania is

self-limiting and will eventually end. It is at the end of a manic or hypomanic episode that an individual often reverts to a depressive episode.

Mania and hypomania can be particularly troubling for individuals with a diagnosis of BD and the emergence of new ideas may result in serious financial consequences. For example, an individual experiencing mania may believe they are able to cure cancer by making connections between numbers that only they can see. This epiphany may have come to them while watching night-time television, when the telephone number of a telemarketer was similar to the number for a cancer charity. This may result in the individual making drastic financial decisions such as buying computers and medical equipment to set up an office, booking plane tickets for an overseas trip and quitting their job. They may do all this in a matter of hours, and not inform their family (despite usually making joint financial decisions), and therefore the results can have significant impacts on both their reputation and their relationships with loved ones. Within Western society, a need and drive to have immediate access to money, the ease of borrowing large sums of money quickly and the use of credit cards can result in serious financial destruction in very little time. Individuals may also make damaging decisions involving the use of illicit drugs and/or alcohol (with legal consequences), or become overtly sexually provocative with someone barely known to them (with health consequences), resulting in potentially dangerous sexual liaisons and potentially further damaging their reputation and existing relationships.

Now that we understand what mania and hypomania are, we look at the diagnostic criteria for both a manic episode and a hypomanic episode. **Table 9.2** outlines the DSM-5 (APA, 2013) diagnostic criteria for mania.

Table 9.3 comprises the hypomanic episode associated with both BDI and BDII. You will note that criteria 1–7 are *exactly* the same for a hypomanic episode as they are for a manic episode. The differentiation between hypomania and mania is the absence of psychotic features in the former and the duration of time mood symptoms last. Should a hypomanic episode have *any* psychotic features, the diagnosis should revert to mania (and BDI).

TABLE 9.1
Variations between BDI and BDII

CONDITION	MUST EXPERIENCE	MAY EXPERIENCE	CAN NEVER EXPERIENCE
Bipolar I disorder	Mania	Depression Hypomania Psychosis	
Bipolar II disorder	Depression Hypomania		Mania Psychosis

DIAGNOSTIC CRITERIA

Bipolar I Disorder
Manic episode

TABLE 9.2
Diagnostic criteria manic episode

For a diagnosis of bipolar I disorder, it is necessary to meet the following criteria for a manic episode. The manic episode may have been preceded by and may be followed by hypomanic or major depressive episodes.

A. A period of persistently elevated, expansive or irritable mood, and persistent increase in goal-directed activity or energy, lasting at least 1-week and present most of the day, nearly every day (duration may be decreased if hospitalization occurs).

B. During this period of mood and energy change, three (or more) of the following symptoms (four if the mood is only irritable) are present to a significant degree signifying a clear change from the individual's typical behavior:
1. Inflated self-esteem or grandiosity.
2. Decreased need for sleep (e.g. feels rested after only 3 hours of sleep).
3. More talkative than usual or pressure to keep talking.
4. Flight of ideas or subjective experience that thoughts are racing.
5. Distractibility (i.e. attention too easily drawn to unimportant or irrelevant external stimuli), as reported or observed.
6. Increased in goal-directed activity (either socially, at work or school, or sexually) or psychomotor agitation (i.e. purposelessness non-goal-directed activity).
7. Excessive involvement in activities that have a high potential for painful consequences (e.g. engaging in unrestrained buying sprees, sexual indiscretions, or foolish business investments).

C. There is sufficient severity to represent impairment to social or occupational functioning or to result in hospitalization to prevent harm to self or others, or there are psychotic features.

D. The episode is not attributable to the physiological effects of a substance (e.g., a drug of abuse, a medication, other treatment) or another medical condition.
Note: A full manic episode that emerges during antidepressant treatment (e.g., medication, electroconvulsive therapy) but persists at a fully syndromal level beyond the physiological effect of that treatment is sufficient evidence for a manic episode and, therefore, a bipolar I diagnosis.
Note: Criteria A-D constitute a manic episode. At least one lifetime manic episode is required for the diagnosis of bipolar I disorder.

DIAGNOSTIC CRITERIA

Hypomanic episode

TABLE 9.3
Diagnostic criteria hypomanic episode

A. A distinct period of abnormally and persistently elevated, expansive or irritable mood and abnormally and persistently increased activity or energy, lasting at least 4 consecutive days and present most of the day, nearly every day.

B. During the period of mood and energy change, three (or more) of the following symptoms (four if the mood is only irritable) have persisted, represent a noticeable change from usual behavior and have been present to a significant degree:
1. Inflated self-esteem or grandiosity.
2. Decreased need for sleep (e.g., feels rested after only 3 hours of sleep).
3. More talkative than usual or pressure to keep talking.
4. Flight of ideas or subjective experience that thoughts are racing.
5. Distractibility (i.e., attention too easily drawn to unimportant or irrelevant external stimuli), as reported or observed.
6. Increased in goal-directed activity (either socially, at work or school, or sexually) or psychomotor agitation (i.e. purposelessness non-goal-directed activity).
7. Excessive involvement in activities that have a high potential for painful consequences (e.g., engaging in unrestrained buying sprees, sexual indiscretions, or foolish business investments).

C. The episode is associated with an unequivocal change in functioning that is uncharacteristic of the individual when not symptomatic.

D. The disturbance in mood or changes in functioning are observable by others.

E. The episode is not severe enough to cause marked impairment in social or occupational functioning or to necessitate hospitalization. If there are psychotic features, the episode is, by definition, manic.

F. The episode is not attributable to the physiological effects of a substance (e.g., a drug of abuse, a medication, other treatment) or another medical condition.
Note: A full hypomanic episode that emerges during antidepressant treatment (e.g., medication, electroconvulsive therapy) but persists at a fully syndromal level beyond the physiological effect of that treatment is sufficient evidence for a hypomanic episode diagnosis. However, caution is indicated so that one or two symptoms (particularly increased irritability, edginess, or agitation following antidepressant use) are not taken as sufficient for diagnosis of a hypomanic episode, nor necessarily indicative of a bipolar diathesis.
Note: Criteria A -F constitute a hypomanic episode. Hypomanic episodes are common in bipolar I disorder but are not required for the diagnosis of bipolar I disorder.

The highs of mania and hypomania are often followed by the melancholy and distressing lows of depression. In fact, in BDII the individual must have at least one episode of depression. Depression is covered extensively in Chapter 10; however, here we explore the depression diagnostic criteria in relation to BDI and BDII.

DIAGNOSTIC CRITERIA

Major depressive episode

TABLE 9.4
Diagnostic criteria major depressive episode

A. Five (or more) of the following symptoms have been present during the same 2-week period and represent a change from previous functioning; at least one of the symptoms is either (1) depressed mood or (2) loss of interest or pleasure.
1. Depressed mood most of the day, nearly every day, as indicated by either subjective report (e.g., feels sad, empty, or hopeless) or observation made by others (e.g., appears tearful). (**Note:** In children and adolescents, can be irritable mood.)
2. Markedly diminished interest or pleasure in all, or almost all, activities most of the day, nearly every day (as indicated by either subjective or observation).
3. Significant weight loss when not dieting or weight gain (e.g., a change of more than 5% of body weight in a month), or decrease or increase in appetite nearly every day. (**Note:** In children, consider failure to make expected weight gain.)
4. Insomnia or hypersomnia nearly every day.
5. Psychomotor agitation or retardation nearly every day (observable by others; not merely subjective feelings of restlessness or being slowed down).
6. Fatigue or loss of energy nearly every day.
7. Feelings of worthlessness or excessive or inappropriate guilt (which may be delusional) nearly every day (not merely self-reproach or guilt about being sick).
8. Diminished ability to think or concentrate, or indecisiveness, nearly every day (either by subjective account or as observed by others).
9. Recurrent thoughts of death (not just fear of dying), recurrent suicidal ideation without a specific plan, or a suicide attempt or a specific plan for committing suicide.

B. The symptoms cause clinically significant distress or impairment in social, occupational, or other important areas of functioning.

C. The episode is not attributable to the physiological effects of a substance or another medical condition.

SOURCE: REPRINTED WITH PERMISSION FROM THE *DIAGNOSTIC AND STATISTICAL MANUAL OF MENTAL DISORDERS*, FIFTH EDITION, (COPYRIGHT ©2013). AMERICAN PSYCHIATRIC ASSOCIATION. ALL RIGHTS RESERVED.

As can be seen in these tables, bipolar disorders are complex, and involve an array of distressing and challenging symptoms that can have significant impacts on a consumer's functioning.

Cyclothymic disorder

Cyclothymic disorder is probably best thought of as a mood disorder characterised by chronic variations between mild hypomania and mild depressive states. These symptoms are insufficiently severe to warrant a confirmed diagnosis of hypomania or depression; rather, they are milder, and of reduced intensity and duration (APA, 2013). Given the nature of this condition, it is perhaps easy to understand that in some individuals a reversion into more severe illness is possible and should this occur their diagnosis also changes. Up to half of the individuals diagnosed with cyclothymic disorder will go on to develop bipolar I or II.

Cyclothymic disorder is characterised by:
- hypomanic states that do not meet criteria listed in **Table 9.3**, but have been occurring for at least two years
- depressive states that do not meet criteria listed in **Table 9.4**, but have been occurring for at least two years

- the periods in between mood states does not exceed two months
- at least half of the individual's time is spent experiencing either of these mood states (APA, 2013).

Cyclothymic disorder occurs in less than 1% of the general population and appears to affect males and females equally in those who have a relative with the condition. Like many mental health conditions, cyclothymic disorder often emerges in late adolescents or early adulthood (APA, 2013).

CLINICAL PRESENTATION AND THE MENTAL STATE EXAMINATION

Because BDs involve a series of diverse episodes, there are multiple presentations within the mental health unit. For the purpose of this chapter, we explore the clinical presentation of mania and exploration of the mental state examination (MSE). Depression is discussed in Chapter 10 and you should read that chapter if you are exploring depression and the MSE.

As with other psychotic presentations, there are myriad, diverse presentations in the context of mania and no two individuals will present with the same symptomatology. The following examples are *possible* presentations of mania a person may experience:

- incorporation of current world events into grandiose or delusional states (e.g. a belief in curing cancer; being responsible for finding life on Mars; working with high-profile actors in a major movie 'deal'; solving the global financial crisis; personally being able to resolve current world or political unrest; development of new gadget or solution to solve a problem)

- religious delusions around being 'chosen' by God, being superior to others because of this choice
- being recruited by well-known organisations for knowledge, talent or expertise (such as the FBI, federal police, NASA, etc.).

Table 9.5 explores some of the common issues that may occur with individuals who have BD, including issues the clinician may experience.

TABLE 9.5
Common issues for individuals with bipolar disorder on a mental health unit

CHALLENGE	NURSING INTERVENTION
Consumer does not sleep at night and disturbs others	This is a common and challenging issue for consumers with a diagnosis of BD and is a clinical presentation of the condition. Promoting sleep may be achieved by: • writing a sleep diary (detailing information about mood; feelings prior to sleep; use of drugs and/or alcohol prior to sleep; length of sleep; number of times woken during night; use of medication; degree of exercise) • establishing a schedule where sleep is promoted by means of dimming lighting, turning off the television or other distractions • relaxation techniques • avoiding sleeping during the day, or sleeping in • encouraging the consumer to wake at the same time every day to promote a routine • using ear plugs or eye masks to promote a quiet, dark environment • deep breathing exercises • removing caffeine from the diet at dinnertime • drinking warm milk or a calming herbal tea prior to going to bed • exercising during the day • ensuring the room temperature is conducive to sleep (not too hot or cold) • use of PRN sedative medications such as temazepam, zopiclone or melatonin. Ensuring the consumer's room is located closer to the staff station and where possible away from others can help prevent disruption to other consumers. If the consumer cannot settle, then allow them to pace or exert their energy in a manner that does not interfere with the need for sleep and rest of others (e.g. in a different area). Ensure limit setting is consistent to facilitate appropriate and safe behaviours. Directions should be clear and simple (not lengthy and complicated as concentration issues can exacerbate misunderstanding).
Consumer does not want to take medications as they will 'destroy the high' they are feeling	This is something many consumers may state when it comes time for medication (particularly in consumers who have experienced hospitalisation previously). The following options may be of assistance: • Validate their feelings and concerns (this will help establish rapport and allows the consumer to feel 'heard'). • Negotiate with the consumer where possible (this may include giving them time to make the choice to have their medication in a particular format such as liquid or tablets). • Attempt to instil insight through psychopharmacology education and illness awareness. • Explore experiences of side effects. Consumers who are prescribed medications and are aware of side effects and share these with their health care provider are more likely to remain adherent to treatment. • Substance misuse and abuse can impact on the likelihood of remaining adherent to medication and this may need to be explored. • Cognitive behavioural therapy may be beneficial in changing the consumer's beliefs and attitudes towards their need for medication. • Consider use of LAI or IMI single-dose use in the event that antipsychotic medications are being refused.
Consumer is not maintaining adequate hydration and/or nutrition	Due to the elevation of mood and need to expend energy, consumers may fail to eat and drink enough. The following options are beneficial when promoting healthy intake of diet: • high protein finger-foods that can be eaten outside of a dining area (such as sandwiches) • high-calorie shakes • ensuring the consumer has a water bottle and is routinely encouraged to drink adequate fluids (this is of particular importance to avoid lithium toxicity). Adequate hydration will also ensure that veins are more accessible for regular, routine monitoring of lithium levels • having access to foods outside of normal hospital kitchen operating hours • ensuring foods the consumer likes are available • if possible, having family bring in foods the consumer is known to enjoy • availability of snack foods that can be eaten 'on the go'

CHALLENGE	NURSING INTERVENTION
Limit setting of challenging behaviours	This is a term frequently used in the mental health setting and refers to a need to instil boundaries around behaviours, such as playing loud music at night, disrupting other consumers by being intrusive or frequently demanding needs be met immediately. To limit set, consider the following: • Ask the consumer to wait for their needs to be met and get back to them within that time frame. Remember to be realistic; individuals who are are experiencing symptoms of mania have poor perception of time and asking them to wait 20 minutes for something may result in more challenging behaviour. • Confirm that the consumer knows who their contact nurse is for the shift and ensure that they know to only seek out that person. This can ensure consistency with limit setting. • Reiterate the need to be respectful of all consumers and staff when behaviours become unmanageable and utilise de-escalation techniques as necessary.

COMMONALITIES OF THE MSE: BIPOLAR DISORDER

General appearance and behaviour

An individual experiencing symptoms of mania may present with the following anomalies in their appearance and behaviour:

- frequent changes of clothing (including trying to borrow, share or give away clothing items to other consumers)
- women may dress provocatively (heavy make-up) or in clothing that seems inappropriate for the temperature and environment (such as wearing revealing clothing for the interview and feeling the need to change clothing for this)
- extreme difficulty with sitting still for the interview, frequently trying to exit the interview room, or standing up and moving around
- dishevelled (due to failure to sleep) including hair unbrushed, men unshaven and/or **malodorous** (unpleasant smell resulting from poor hygiene).

Mood

Perhaps unsurprisingly the mood states in mania will usually fluctuate and may be described as:

- labile (labile mood is that which wavers between periods of other mood states, such as irritable, elevated and depressed)
- **irritable**
- **elevated** (mood which is overtly cheerful)
- **fatuous** (mood which is silly or foolish)
- **expansive** (individuals lack restraint in expressing their feelings or emotions and are often grandiose in their self-disclosure).

When asking the consumer to rate their mood, they may describe themselves as being 'on top of the world' or '20/10'. As we learned in Chapter 7, when exploring mood states we must also examine appetite. Individuals experiencing mania may neglect their nutritional needs and it is important to consider their degree of hydration and nutrition. They may describe having 'no time' to eat, or a need to lose weight and

focus on their appearance. Libido and sex drive may be extreme. Individuals experiencing mania may often make impulsive decisions regarding sexual encounters that they later regret. They may make provocative or suggestive comments or propositions to other consumers and/or staff on a mental health unit and, as such, may require more frequent observations. Sleep is another important area of mood assessment and is one of the most severely impacted in persons with BDs. Consumers with mania are usually energised despite not sleeping much or at all. When inquiring about sleep patterns, you may discover the consumer has 'no time for sleep' and that they are vehemently against trying to sleep.

Affect

It is likely that the affect in the consumer with BD will include those affects that are seen at the expressive end of the spectrum such as reactive, bright, broad, labile or inappropriate. The consumer may have periods where the affect is inappropriate or incongruent; for example, they may laugh when discussing something that would normally be considered upsetting (such as someone dying).

Perception

- Perceptual disturbances experienced during an episode of mania constitute psychotic symptoms and while they are relatively common, they are not seen in all persons with mania. Psychosis is a condition characterised by delusions, hallucinations and thought disorder and is predominantly seen in schizophrenia and mania. Auditory and visual hallucinations are the most common perceptual disturbances seen in mania and these disturbances are likely to be congruent with mood states and often centre on grandiose themes (Toh, Thomas & Rossell, 2015). **Grandiosity** is an inflated sense of self-esteem, self-worth, self-importance, knowledge or power. For example, a man who believes he has been chosen to be prime minister heard this after God spoke to him and told him he was 'the chosen one'; or a woman believed she was going to represent Australia at the next Olympics after receiving a message from the grave of Murray Rose. While auditory hallucinations are not the hallmark of BD, some studies have suggested they occur in over 65% of persons experiencing mania (Toh, Thomas & Rossell, 2015).

Thought

Content

For many individuals, delusions comprise a significant aspect of their experiences of mania. These delusional states typically comprise persecutory delusions, referential delusions, hypochondria and delusions of grandeur (Toh, Thomas & Rossell, 2015). Clinicians may also see **erotomanic** and religious delusions in mania. While there are various commentaries about the frequency of delusions within mania, around half of individuals will experience delusions during a manic episode and they appear to be more common than hallucinations in this cohort.

Suicide and deliberate self-harm (DHS)/non-suicidal self-injury are concerning aspects of many mental health conditions, and therefore comprise an important part of the MSE. While the majority of attempts to end their lives by suicide and acts of DSH/non-suicidal self-injury in BD occur during a depressive episode, it is still important to explore suicide in the context of command hallucinations (instructing the individual to harm themself), with the emergence of insight (where the consumer develops an understanding of their actions and experiences guilt or shame) or harm through misadventure including drug overdose and other risky behaviours. In particular, suicide rates may be higher in consumers with BD in the period after their discharge from inpatient settings (Isometsä, Sund & Pirkola, 2014). In terms of other risk areas, unplanned pregnancies are another factor of potential concern for women who have a diagnosis of BD. Marengo et al. (2015) noted that the propensity for engaging in impulsive or hypersexualised encounters associated with BD results in unplanned pregnancies for many women, possibly exposing the foetus to avoidable teratogens and resulting in treatment complications. Marengo et al. (2015) found that one-third of pregnancies in women with BD were unplanned (vs 7% in the control group), resulting in a voluntary pregnancy termination rate of over 40% in those women (vs 14% in the control group).

Form

The clinician may see disorganisation of thoughts. Are you readily able to understand what the consumer is telling you, or does their thought pattern follow no logical, discernible path? Common thought form abnormalities seen in mania include:

- loosening of associations (ideas so poorly linked they lack logical connection)
- derailment (illogical and loosely connected thoughts)
- tangentiality (irrelevant or indirect responses to questions)
- neologisms (creation of new words that have no meaning to others)
- echolalia (mimicking or echoing others, usually in a mocking manner).

Stream or process

One of the most common thought disorders in mania is flight of ideas. In flight of ideas, thinking changes rapidly and is unable to be expressed completely resulting in incomprehensible communication. This disturbance in thought can obviously make communication very difficult, and the rapid progression of thoughts can result in indecipherable speech. Because the individual's thoughts are progressing so rapidly (more rapidly than they can express), they may become easily distracted, have poor concentration (as they move onto the next thought before the first one is completed) or become irritable when others do not readily follow their patterns of thought. Other abnormalities of thought and speech include:

- clang associations or clanging (where words are chosen for their sound, not their meaning); for example, 'I'll go when I'm ready, teddy, Freddy, spaghetti, yeti'
- **pressured speech** (speech that is intense, loud, rapid and highly emphatic)
- **punning** (plays on word choices; words that sound the same but have a different meaning); for example 'Santa's helpers are known as subordinate Clauses'

Judgement

Judgement may be seriously impacted during an episode of mania, resulting in poor decision-making processes and inability to foresee the consequences of actions. This is evidenced by a propensity for risk-taking behaviours such as making impulsive financial decisions, sexual encounters, and increases in drug and alcohol use. Demonstrating a poor understanding of actions having serious consequences is a good way of measuring judgement; for example, engaging in unprotected sexual interactions with strangers demonstrates impaired judgement.

Cognition

It is not uncommon for consumers experiencing a manic episode to experience issues with their concentration and memory. In fact, they are most likely to be significantly distracted, and experience serious issues with their ability to stay focused for any length of time.

Insight

Insight is an individual's ability to decipher the causes of their behaviour and is often assessed in the context of their understanding of their illness. When psychotic, individuals are unlikely to present with good insight. One of the more complicated aspects of mania is the notion that the patient is 'too high' when in fact they may perceive themselves as simply happy or enlightened. This can result in a perception that the need for medication is about 'killing' their high when, in fact, it is about normalising and restoring their mood to a more appropriate and sustainable level. Interestingly, da Silva et al. (2016) noted in their research on BD and insight levels that individuals consistently had a poor understanding between their illness and its impact on activity and energy levels, and that increased energy levels was an illness symptom.

Risk assessment

In Chapter 7, we explored the importance of undertaking a comprehensive and holistic risk assessment. In this section, we explore the risk assessment in the context of mania, considering some of the more common areas of assessment. This list is not exhaustive, and you will need to consider other factors that are discussed in other chapters, such as medication non-adherence, self-care deficit, etc.

Disturbed sleep pattern

As we have seen, individuals with mania experience issues with a significantly reduced need for sleep, which is further impacted by an increase in goal-directed behaviours such as feeling compelled to write a book or watch the stock market on the internet. Hence, one of the important areas of risk assessment is ensuring the consumer is able to get some sleep. This may only be achieved with the use of sedatives, and individuals may require frequent limit setting (see **Table 9.5**) and redirection to make an effort to rest. Loud or disruptive behaviour when others are asleep can place them at risk of interpersonal violence, so the need for adequate sleep may also be driven by their vulnerability in such instances.

Impaired nutritional intake

Because consumers during an episode of mania are goal-driven, highly active and often have poor concentration, the concept of sitting down to three square meals a day is probably an unrealistic expectation fraught with potential disaster. **Table 9.5** identifies a number of strategies the clinician can adopt to encourage the consumer to have an adequate dietary intake. It may be necessary to place the consumer on a fluid balance chart to ensure that they are adequately hydrated and to counteract any potential issues with lithium toxicity should this be the mood stabiliser they are taking (see the 'Safety first' box).

Sexual promiscuity and vulnerability

Sexual encounters are a normal, healthy aspect of an intimate relationship and people with a mental health condition are still sexual beings who enjoy full intimate relationships. As we identified earlier, individuals who are experiencing an episode of mania may be more promiscuous and sexualised and this may result in an increased chance of negative outcomes from such behaviours. It is important to consider the following issues when exploring risk for the consumer with BD:

- women (in particular) whose presentation when experiencing a manic episode is hypersexualised may be more vulnerable to impulsive, unprotected sexual encounters that may be regretted at a later stage
- availability of prophylactics (such as condoms) in community settings
- the potential for an unknown and/or unwanted pregnancy
- ability to consent to sexual encounters with an understanding of the potential associated risks
- ratios of male and female patients, including bed locations (closer to staff station or highly visualised areas)
- staffing ratios – ensuring where possible a promiscuous consumer has a staff member of the same sex on duty
- psychoeducation, including education on sexually transmissible infections such as chlamydia and gonorrhoea (both of which are increasing in Australia).

CASE **STUDY**

SIGNS OF BIPOLAR DISORDER

Jerry is a 35-year-old man who is studying horticulture part-time at his local TAFE and working part-time for the government in a forestry role. Jerry has had bipolar disorder since his late teens, but was only officially diagnosed three years ago. Recently, Jerry has started staying up longer during the night working on his assignments, and for the past five days he has not slept at all. For the past month, Jerry has only been sporadically taking his prescribed medication.

Last week Jerry's neighbours made a complaint to the body corporate in the unit where Jerry lives after he did some gardening in his courtyard at 3 am, followed by mowing the communal areas at 4.30 am. Jerry thinks his neighbours need to 'chill' and that he was actually in the middle of a breakthrough that could result in reversing global warming. Jerry believes that his neighbours should mind their own business and stop interfering with his creativity, and he cannot understand why they are confused by his ideas. Jerry believes he is on the 'verge' of a major discovery. While he was writing his latest assignment, his research helped him unearth a discovery that will reverse global warming, resulting in him making millions of dollars. When the morning came, Jerry quit his job. Jerry's major concern now is what will happen if he accidentally reverses global warming too much and the temperature becomes too cool. While he is worried about this, he believes everything will probably be okay, because it all comes down to the word 'land' and it will 'even out', but he does want to seek clarification on this. Jerry is reassured because people live in Iceland, Greenland, Ireland and Poland and these are all cold climates. It will all balance out because there are equal numbers of countries in warmer climates that have the word 'land' in them, too, such as Swaziland, Thailand, New Zealand and the Falklands. Outcomes being 'even' is of great importance to Jerry.

Jerry's father Paul visited him a few days ago for dinner and is worried about him. Despite Paul making dinner, Jerry couldn't sit still long enough to eat it. Jerry doesn't want to talk about the possibility that he may be unwell again, because, he says, 'It's not like last time, Dad.'

Yesterday, Jerry attended the Polish embassy requesting they work with him on his project. He demanded to see the 'most senior person here' because they would be the only one who could understand his discovery. Both the Thai and Irish embassies had refused to return his calls. Jerry became upset when a representative from the Polish embassy exports department would not meet with him. Jerry was talking rapidly and loudly and staff could not follow the topic of his conversation. Jerry became irritated when staff didn't provide the information he wanted and eventually security was called. Jerry was taken to his local hospital for assessment and later admitted.

Questions

1   What signs and symptoms is Jerry demonstrating that are suggestive of a mood disorder?
2   You have been asked to formulate a risk assessment for Jerry. Based on the information in the case study, what risks would you identify?
3   Based on your understanding of bipolar disorders, do you think Jerry is exhibiting signs of mania or hypomania?

TREATMENT

There are a number of different treatments used for BD which have other clinically indicated uses in other conditions. Treatment for BD includes antipsychotics, benzodiazepines (or anxiolytics), antidepressants and, most commonly, mood stabilisers/antiepileptics (or antimanics). In Chapter 4, different medications were looked at more closely; here we explore treatments of BD in more depth. **Table 9.6** examines the different types of mood stabilisers used in treating BDs. The use of antipsychotics in BDs originated from clinical efficacy in reducing psychotic symptoms, and in the early stages of treatment they can provide sedation and emotional calming. Antipsychotics are also effective in the management of aggression, which can be seen during an episode of mania.

Benzodiazepines such as diazepam, clonazepam or lorazepam can assist in calming and can promote rest, something that individuals who are highly aroused find difficult. Sedatives such as temazepam are frequently used in an attempt to sedate a consumer with mania who is unable to relax enough to sleep from their own means, or after trying non-pharmacological methods such as those listed in **Table 9.5**. Anxiolytics such as the benzodiazepines listed here are explored in more depth in Chapter 11.

Mood stabilisers/antimanics

The effectiveness of lithium as a mood stabiliser was discovered by Australian psychiatrist Dr John Cade and has been pivotal in the treatment of BD. Aside from lithium, many of the conventional mood stabilisers are traditionally used as antiepileptic medications or anticonvulsants. Quetiapine (which is an antipsychotic) is also regarded as useful in the treatment of BD, has known efficacy as a mood stabiliser and may prevent relapse.

TABLE 9.6
Mood stabilisers: dose ranges and side effects

MEDICATION NAME	DOSE RANGE	SIDE EFFECTS AND INDICATIONS
Lithium carbonate (Lithicarb™)	Acute: 500–2000 mg PO titrated over approx. 3 days (regular blood testing required) Acute mania serum levels 0.6–1.2 mmol/L Therapeutic (maintenance) levels 0.6–0.8 mmol/L	Side effects are directly related to serum lithium levels. The following symptoms should resolve once dosage stabilises, and include: • GI upset (mild nausea, diarrhoea) • dizziness • muscle weakness. The following are more persistent side effects: • fine hand tremor • fatigue • thirst • polyuria • anorexia or weight gain (1–2 kg) • constipation • headache • ECG changes • skin conditions (e.g. acne).
Sodium valproate (anticonvulsant)	1000–2500 mg/day PO in BD dose with food Target serum levels 50–100 mg/L	Include: • nausea; • diarrhoea • vomiting • constipation • headache • sedation or fatigue • muscle twitching.
Lamotrigine (anticonvulsant)	100–400 mg/day PO in BD dose. Careful titration required as high commencing doses have been related to occurrence of life-threatening rash; see the 'Safety first' box. Serum levels are not a reliable measure of efficacy for lamotrigine.	Lamotrigine has efficacy in treating BD where depressive episodes have occurred. • Life-threatening rash • double-vision (diplopia); • dizziness; • headache; • loss of coordination (ataxia); • nausea & vomiting; • fatigue.
Carbamazepine	400–1600 mg PO Target serum levels 4–12 mg/L	Some side effects can be mitigated by commencing a low dose and titrating slowly. Side effects include: • dizziness • headache • loss of coordination (ataxia) • sedation • fatigue • double-vision (diplopia) • nausea • vomiting • fluid retention • dry mouth.

SOURCE: ANDREWS ET AL., 2013; MIMS ONLINE, 2018

REFLECT ON THIS

Australian consumers' experiences of bipolar disorder during COVID-19

Read the following article:

Van Rheenen, T.E., Meyer, D., Phillipou, A., Tan, E.J., Toh, W.L. & Rossell, S.L. (2020). Mental health status of individuals with a mood disorder during the COVID-19 pandemic in Australia: Initial results from the COLLATE project. *Journal of Affective Disorders*, 275(1), 69–77. DOI: https://doi.org/10.1016/j.jad.2020.06.037

1   What additional challenges might a pandemic pose for someone experiencing a manic episode? Your response should consider the impacts:
   ■   on executive functioning
   ■   of psychosis
   ■   of depressive episodes
   ■   of how social distancing and isolation may affect people living with mood disorders.

- community mental health nurse
- psychologist
- psychiatrist
- general practitioner.

Medications which reduce the symptoms of
depression (antidepressants) are more likely to be
adhered to by individuals with BDs, and this is
because the individual's experiences of depression
and its impacts on their life are often deemed more
distressing than those of mania or hypomania.
Generally, mania feels good. This belief resides in
the notion that an antidepressant is more necessary
and useful, because the experiences of depression
are inherently more distressing than those of mania.
Therefore, it is imperative to ensure adherence to
mood stabilisers, and where prescribed antipsychotic
medications, are adhered to also. Mood stabilisers
have clinical efficacy in treating depression in BD,
and are particularly important for individuals who
take antidepressant medications to prevent further
depressive episodes. Antidepressant medications are
discussed in great depth in Chapter 10.

SAFETY FIRST

LITHIUM TOXICITY

Lithium toxicity is a potentially fatal condition caused by
high serum lithium levels and is indicated by the following:

- tremor which is worsening
- nausea, vomiting and diarrhoea
- slurred speech
- muscle twitches
- altered consciousness.

    Care practitioners should be mindful of the following:

- When levels exceed 1.5 mmol/L, the next dose of lithium
should be withheld and the physician notified promptly.
- Serum lithium concentration levels >2 mmol/L are toxic
and dangerous.
- All consumers on lithium should be advised that
prolonged vomiting and diarrhoea may lead to lithium
toxicity. This may be a result of lithium overdose, or any
ailment such as flu, food poisoning or diarrhoeal illness
where dehydration may occur.
- Maintaining adequate hydration in hot weather is also
important. Some medications, such as diuretics, can
also impact severely on Lithium levels so consumers
should be working collaboratively with the treating

doctor and case manager to ensure that they are not
at increased risk of toxicity due to unwanted drug
interactions.

SAFETY FIRST

LAMOTRIGINE AND STEVENS-JOHNSON SYNDROME (SJS)

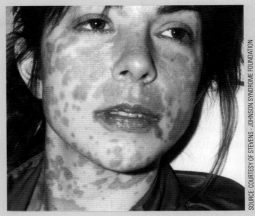

SOURCE: COURTESY OF STEVENS-JOHNSON SYNDROME FOUNDATION

FIGURE 9.2
Adult female with Stevens-Johnson syndrome (SJS)

This rash will usually present in the initial period (five
days to eight weeks) of treatment and can be serious.
Consumers taking lamotrigine should be encouraged to
report any rash, and clinicians and consumers should look
for the following:

- fever and flu-like symptoms
- initially painless (but itchy) fine red spots or any rash
on the neck, trunk or face (mouth, lips, eyes, nostrils)
or genital/anal area which may progress to rupturing
bulbous lesions
- may involve GI tract and mucous membranes
- anorexia.

Manic 'switching'

The phenomenon of **manic switching** involves
the reversion from a depressive state to a manic state
and is associated with the use of an antidepressant
medication. In essence, the antidepressant medication

raises the consumer's mood too 'high', and they proceed to mania. Recurrent treatment of depression in BD with tricyclic antidepressants (TCAs) has demonstrated a high propensity for switching to a manic state (Young & Dulcis, 2015). Bupropion (a medication used to quit smoking) has also demonstrated high rates of conversion to mania in clinical studies. The mechanism behind this occurrence is thought to result from the reuptake site blockage of noradrenaline and dopamine, increasing their levels (Young & Dulcis, 2015). Risk factors associated with manic switching in addition to the inclusion of an antidepressant include:

- being diagnosed young
- experiencing more episodes of depression and or mania
- individuals who have a history of rapid cycling in the previous 12 months
- individuals who have been treated with multiple antidepressants during their condition
- previous positive history for suicide attempt
- history of substance use (namely, amphetamines)
- treatment with the antidepressant venlafaxine (Niitsu, Fabbri & Serretti, 2015).

You will find that while exploring detailed precautions and uses of antidepressants in pharmacological databases and texts, many will note the susceptibility for some individuals to progress to mania. The addition of a mood stabiliser for individuals with BD taking antidepressants may mitigate this potential to switch to mania during the course of treatment.

RECOVERY AND RELAPSE PREVENTION

Outcomes associated with BD are often poor due to the episodic nature of the condition, and this is more so for BDI. Outcomes are also exacerbated by the degree to which individuals are supported by friends, family and the mental health team; their adherence to the treatment regimen; and use of illicit substances.

Relapse

In individuals who present with mania, over 90% will experience recurring mood episodes and more than half (60%) who experience a manic episode will follow this with a sudden depressive episode (APA, 2013). Research suggests that even for those individuals who have remained in remission for three years, the probability of relapse is high, and by seven years 82% of individuals had experienced a relapse of an episode (Yildiz, Ruiz & Nemeroff, 2015). In longitudinal studies greater than 25 years, individuals followed up had on average between five to nine episodes of bipolar illness in this

period, indicating the serious episodic nature of the condition (Yildiz, Ruiz & Nemeroff, 2015).

Individuals who experience more than four mood episodes in a 12-month period are referred to as 'rapid cycling', and this is a particularly debilitating form of BDI. Generally, individuals will return to a level of functioning between episodes that correlates with acceptable work-functioning. However, about 30% experience a severe impairment in their ability to work and this can have serious consequences on extensive aspects of an individual's life (APA, 2013). As with other mental health conditions, the more episodes of illness, the poorer the outcomes usually are.

Medication adherence also plays a significant role in outcomes of BD. MacDonald et al. (2016) note that about 41% of consumers with BD are non-adherent or inconsistently adherent with their antipsychotic medication, resulting in relapse, increased rates of hospitalisation, and suicide. In some instances, individuals will stop taking their mood-stabilising medication in order to experience the highs of mania. Invariably, this is often followed by the extreme lows of a depressive episode.

Signs of relapse (mania)

While an individual's experience of a relapse of BD will likely vary widely, there are some commonalities in these experiences. Each individual has a unique pattern of relapse, and this is known as their relapse signature. It is important for the nurse to convey the possible symptoms of relapse to the consumer and, where appropriate, carers. Being empowered with a deep understanding of BD can be helpful in preventing future mood episodes, or noticing the emergence of symptoms which warrant attention can significantly reduce the impacts of a relapse. Individuals will often experience hypomania prior to the development of manic symptoms, often culminating in grandiosity and psychotic symptoms. Some of the more common, early warning indicators of mania relapse are:

- reduction in need for sleep and/or having trouble sleeping
- colours may seem 'brighter' or 'sharper' or senses more honed (sharper hearing, smell etc.)
- more talkative than usual (and a subjective need to keep talking)
- waning concentration
- more active and social than usual
- feelings of anxiety
- emergence of new ideas or impractical plans
- becoming irritable or impatient
- elevation of mood
- emerging feelings of power, increased confidence or self-importance
- more goal-directed.

As the episode intensifies, these symptoms may be coupled with feelings of omnipotence and heightened sexual desires. Carers and friends can provide support and help in identifying a possible relapse of BD in consumers with BD. For example, consumers experiencing early relapse may make phone calls to friends or family in the middle of the night, not realising that most people are asleep at that time. Carers or friends may be in a position to identify this behaviour and direct the individual to seek appropriate help.

Mood diaries are also useful in the tracking of moods and help a consumer to identify mood states that may deviate outside of what are considered 'normal' for them personally. A mood diary is also important in helping consumers and their carers realise that everyday 'ups and downs' are a perfectly normal part of human existence and should not necessarily cause worry *unless* these experiences deviate outside set parameters.

The postnatal period in women is a time of potential relapse. Postnatal depression (PND) or mania affects about 40–50% of women who have BD, and these women are also at an increased chance to experience PND in further pregnancies (Andrews et al., 2013). The stress of pregnancy, hormonal influences and often the need to cease medications that may result in foetal developmental or congenital issues all play a role in the impacts of BD in women in the pre-, peri- and postnatal periods.

Recovery

Because the majority of individuals who experience an episode associated with a diagnosis of BD go on to experience further episodes, recovery from illness symptoms can be troublesome and difficult. Fortunately, the notion of recovery now looks at the individual's ideal around recovery, not merely symptom amelioration. **Table 9.7** outlines the possible treatment outcomes.

TABLE 9.7
Possible treatment outcomes in BD

TREATMENT OUTCOME	DEFINITION
Response	50% reduction in symptoms from baseline, initial presenting symptoms
Remission	Absence of minimal symptoms for at least one week
Recovery/sustained remission	At least 8–12 consecutive weeks of remission
Relapse/recurrence	Return to full syndrome criteria following remission of any duration
Roughening	Return of symptoms at **subsyndromal level**, perhaps representing a prodrome of an impending episode

SOURCE: YILDIZ, RUIZ & NEMEROFF, 2015

What happens after mania?

The saying 'what goes up, must come down' is relatable to many individuals experiencing a manic episode and, sadly, with insight often comes humiliation. As we saw in the lived experience of Annie in the vignette at the beginning of this chapter, she also invariably experienced a depressive episode. While the experiences of mania may be pleasurable for individuals during a manic episode, the ramifications of this pleasure are frequently not fully understood until the episode is diminishing and insight begins to return. The individual who reverts to a depressive episode following mania (which is common) may ruminate on their past failings; feeling shame, guilt and embarrassment regarding their behaviours while manic. Some of the more common experiences of mania include damage to reputation or embarrassment resulting from actions while manic. Some of these actions may include:

- damage to interpersonal relationships from their behaviour or actions
- financial implications from making impulsive and often outrageous decisions (such as buying expensive laboratory equipment to 'cure cancer', musical instruments to start a band, or expensive computer and office equipment to run their new business)
- the results of aggressive or hostile behaviour towards others (including possible legal implications)
- promiscuous sexual encounters that may be seriously damaging to existing relationships, in addition to potential for pregnancy and sexually transmitted infections
- the stigma of being identifiable as 'mentally ill'
- distress or worry about relapse
- distress about potential to pass on BD to their offspring.

Mania and legal issues

McCabe, Christopher, Pinals and Fisher (2013) note that individuals experiencing an episode of mania are five times more likely to be arrested when compared with the general population and are more frequently incarcerated. Individuals who experience episodes of mania are also more likely to have a conviction for a violent crime and it is understood that substance misuse exacerbates this issue. In addition, those individuals with criminal convictions also appear to have more frequent episodes of mania and more hospitalisations than those without (Daff & Thomas, 2014). It is important to consider that many criminal convictions within this demographic also include those convicted of non-violent offences, such as offences related to financial issues, and thus it is imperative not to make a connection between violence and bipolar disorder.

NURSING CARE PLAN

WORKING WITH TRAN

Consumer Diagnosis: Bipolar disorder I (manic episode)
Nursing Diagnosis: Impaired nutritional intake as evidenced by an inability to sit with co-consumers during meal times, reduced urinary output, and hypotension.
Nursing Diagnosis: Impaired social interactions with others related to hyperactivity and agitation as seen by intrusive behaviour towards other consumers, impaired concentration and attention span.
Outcomes: To resume regular diet and increase hydration.
Outcomes: To reduce intrusive behaviours towards other consumers and maintain safety.

ASSESSMENT DATA OBJECTIVE (O) SUBJECTIVE (S)	EVIDENCE-BASED RATIONALE	RATIONALE	CONSUMER RESPONSE
Tran has been an inpatient for 24 hours and has not been able to sit in the communal dining area for any appropriate amount of time that results in her eating a meal (O). Tran has been noted to keep interrupting conversation between other consumers, is unable to sit down with others and maintain a conversation. Several consumers have complained about her behaviour and are asking for her to be kept away from them.	Encourage high-calorie/protein finger foods that Tran can eat 'on the move'. Offer high protein shakes. This may be done in consultation with the unit's occupational therapist. Commence fluid balance chart (FBC). Continue to monitor MSE. Monitor and educate re. signs of lithium toxicity. Provide Tran with consistent limits. Ensure limits are communicated clearly and simply. Communicate limits to the whole team. Provide alternative activities for Tran that can be done in a smaller group or as a 1:1 or solitary activity Assign one nurse to be primary nurse that Tran interacts with. Engage with a dietitian to provide assistance with planning and implementation of an appropriate meal schedule for Tran. This will ensure her caloric needs are being met.	High-calorie/protein diet will provide suitable energy and sustenance without the need to have concentration levels that enable sitting down for a prepared meal. High-protein shakes will provide nourishment and fluids. Having a friend or loved one bring in favoured foods may make Tran more inclined to eat/drink. FBC will enable clinicians to prevent dehydration and ramifications of same (such as toxicity) before it becomes a more serious issue. Baseline MSE enables clinicians to identify change from initial presentation and can help establish if Tran is responding to both therapeutic and psychopharmacologic interventions. It is important that Tran is aware of the symptoms of toxicity so that she reports any adverse effects. Monitor lithium plasma levels to ensure toxicity does not occur. Providing Tran with a primary contact nurse will help to decrease distractability and increase consistency in applying any required limits. Suggesting alternative activities is more effective as Tran is easily distracted at the moment, rather than imposing punitive restrictions.	Tran has been reluctantly amenable to the diet offered by clinicians on the unit. She has continued to drink the shakes and eat the small sandwiches while she undertakes other activities. There have been no signs of toxicity and lithium levels are within the therapeutic range. While Tran has required redirection to the primary nurse allocated, this has decreased and Tran is initiating more specific requests/queries to this person. Tran continues to find it difficult to sustain her concentration for extended periods, but is more willing to engage in alternative activities as suggested by the nurse. There have been no further complaints from other consumers on the unit.

SOURCE: ADAPTED FROM JAKOPAC & PATEL, 2009

REFLECTION ON LEARNING FROM PRACTICE

Annie's experiences of mania are not unlike those of many others who experience bipolar affective disorder. One of the contributing factors for the clinician to consider in consumers such as Annie is the role that the pleasures of mania play in future adherence to treatment. We all like to feel good about ourselves; Annie is not alone in this desire, and therefore it is an important exercise in empathy to understand the motivations in non-adherence to treatment. Annie herself has said that she 'misses' the high feelings she had and this is an important concept for the clinician to consider. While bipolar disorders constitute serious disturbances of mood, there is hope for meaningful recovery.

CHAPTER RESOURCES

SUMMARY

- Bipolar disorders are a group of challenging and serious conditions that can have devastating impacts on consumers' reputation, finances, relationships and health (to name but a few areas).
- Bipolar disorders are multifactorial, comprising diverse aetiology. They occur in over 2% of the population at any given time.
- The diagnostic criteria for bipolar disorder include three different mood states.

- There are specific areas of the MSE that need careful attention when interviewing the consumer with BD.
- While there are a number of different treatments for BDs, some of these carry with them a risk of potentially life-threatening side effects.
- Consumers with BD experience a range of symptoms, but there is hope for recovery and they should actively be involved in the recovery process.

REVIEW QUESTIONS

1 How do bipolar I disorder and bipolar II disorder differ?
2 Discuss the care of the manic consumer in the inpatient mental health unit.
3 Describe the term 'grandiosity' and give one example of a delusion of grandeur.
4 Manic switching is:
   a A rapid change of mood from mania to depression induced by antidepressant medication

   b A rapid change of mood from depression to mania induced by antidepressant medication
   c A rapid change of mood from mania to depression induced by antipsychotic medication
   d A rapid change of mood from depression to mania induced by antipsychotic medication
5 What is hypomania?
6 Describe four possible causes of bipolar disorder.

CRITICAL THINKING

1 How would you care for a consumer who is hypersexualised on an acute inpatient unit?
2 Hypomania is a common symptom in bipolar disorders. How does hypomania differ from mania?

3 How would you help a consumer prevent relapse of mania?

USEFUL WEBSITES

- bipolarcaregivers.org: http://www.bipolarcaregivers.org
- Black Dog Institute: https://www.blackdoginstitute.org.au

- headspace: https://www.headspace.org.au

REFLECT ON THIS

The MDT and the consumer with bipolar disorder
A team effort is required when helping someone recover from bipolar disorder, with the consumer at the centre of this journey. There are, however, many different members in this team, each with their own skills to offer.
1 Reflect upon your understanding of mania and the challenges a person with this condition experiences. Research the following MDT members and discuss how each clinician can assist in a person's recovery journey:
   - mental health nurse
   - student nurse

- occupational therapist
- dietitian
- psychiatrist
- peer support worker.

2 As a student nurse, what are your individual goals when working with someone who has bipolar disorder? Reflect upon whether your goals are about meeting your learning needs or about helping the consumer. If your goals are more centred on yourself, how might you change them so that the consumer also benefits from your placement?

REFERENCES

American Psychiatric Association (APA). (2013). *Diagnostic and Statistical Manual of Mental Disorders (DSM-5)* (5th edn). Washington, DC: APA.

Andrews, G., Dean, K., Genderson, M., Hunt, C., Mitchell, P., Sachdev, P. & Trollor, J. (2013). *Management of Mental Disorders* (5th edn). Sydney: School of Psychiatry, University of NSW.

Australian Bureau of Statistics (ABS). (2009). *4102.0 – Australian Social Trends, March 2009.* Retrieved from http://www.abs.gov.au/AUSSTATS/abs@.nsf/Lookup/4102.0Main+Features30March%202009.

Australian Institute of Health and Welfare (AIHW). (2012). *Overview of Mental Health Services in Australia: Prevalence, Impact and Burden.* Retrieved from https://www.aihw.gov.au/getmedia/f53e4869-8bb5-44ef-b2e4-6f3981fd3359/Overview-of-mental-health.pdf.aspx.

Bengesser, S. & Reininghaus, E. (2013). *Genetics of Bipolar Disorder.* Frankfurt am Main: Peter Lang AG. Retrieved from http://www.ebrary.com.

Blows, W.T. (2016). *The Biological Basis of Mental Health* (3rd edn). London: Routledge, Taylor & Francis.

Daff, E. & Thomas, D.M. (2014). Bipolar disorder and criminal offending: A data linkage study. *Social Psychiatry Psychiatric Epidemiology*, 49, 1985–91. doi:10.1007/s00127-014-0882-4

da Silva, R.D.A., Mograbi, D.C., Bifano, J., Santana, C.M.T. & Cheniaux, E. (2016). Insight in bipolar mania: Evaluation of its heterogeneity and correlation with clinical symptoms. *Journal of Affective Disorders*, 199, 95–8. doi:10.1016/j.jad.2016.04.019

Fornaro, M., De Berardis, D., De Pasquale, C., Indelicato, L., Pollice, R., Valchera, A. ... Oedegaard, K.J. (2015). Prevalence and clinical features associated to bipolar disorder-migraine comorbidity: A systematic review. *Comprehensive Psychiatry*, 56, 1–16. doi:10.1016/j.comppsych.2014.09.020

Forty, L., Ulanova, A., Jones, L., Gordon-Smith, K., Fraser, C., Farmer, A., McGuffin, P. ... Craddock, N. (2014). Comorbid medical illness in bipolar disorder. *British Journal of Psychiatry*, 205, 465–72. doi:10.1192/bjp.bp.114.152249

Isometsä, E., Sund, R. & Pirkola, S. (2014). Post-discharge suicide of inpatients with bipolar disorder in Finland. *Bipolar Disorders*, 16(8), 867–74. doi:10.1111/bdi.12237

Jakopac, K. A. & Patel, S. C. (2009). *Psychiatric and Mental Health Case Studies and Care Plans.* Burlington, MA: Jones and Bartlett Learning.

Karanti, A., Bobeck, C., Osterman, M., Kardell, M., Tidemalm, D., Runeson, B. ... Landen, M. (2015). Gender differences in the treatment of patients with bipolar disorder: A study of 7354 patients. *Journal of Affective Disorders*, 174, 303–9. doi:10.1016/jad.2014.11.058

MacDonald, L., Chapman, S., Syrett, M., Bowskill, R. & Horne, R. (2016). Improving medication adherence in bipolar disorder: A systematic review and meta-analysis of 30 years of intervention trials. *Journal of Affective Disorders*, 194, 202–21. doi:10.1016/j.jad.2016.01.002

Marangoni, C., Hernandez, M. & Faedda, G. L. (2016). The role of environmental exposures as risk factors for bipolar disorder: A systematic review of longitudinal studies. *Journal of Affective Disorders*, 193, 165–74. doi:10.1016/j.jad.2015.12.055

Marengo, E., Martino, D.J., Igoa, A., Scápola, M., Fassi, G., Baamonde, M.U. & Strejilevich, S.A. (2015). Unplanned pregnancies and reproductive health among women with bipolar disorder. *Journal of Affective Disorders*, 178, 201–5. doi:10.1016/j.jad.2015.02.033

McCabe, P.J., Christopher, P.P., Pinals, D.A. & Fisher, W.H. (2013). Predictors of criminal justice involvement in severe mania. *Journal of Affective Disorders*, 149, 367–74. doi:10.1016/j.jad.2013.02.015

Niitsu, T., Fabbri, C. & Serretti, A. (2015). Predictors of switch from depression to mania in bipolar disorder. *Journal of Psychiatric Research*, 66(67), 45–53. doi:10.1016/j.jpsychires.2015.04.014

Orlovska, S., Pedersen, M.S., Benros, M.E., Mortensen, P.B., Agerbo, E. & Nordentolf, M. (2014). Head injury as risk factor for psychiatric disorders: A nationwide register-based follow-up study of 113,906 persons with head injury. *American Journal of Psychiatry*, 171, 463–9.

Saha, S., Morgan, V.A., Castle, D., Silove, D. & McGrath, J.J. (2015). Sociodemographic and clinical correlates of migrant status in adults with psychotic disorders: Data from the Australian Survey of High Impact Psychosis. *Epidemiology and Psychiatric Sciences*, 24, 534–41. doi:10.1017/S2045796014000535

Schaffer, A., Isometsä, E.T., Azorin, J.M., Cassidy, F., Goldstein, T., Rihmer, Z., ... Yatham, L. (2015). A review of factors associated with greater likelihood of suicide attempts and suicide deaths in bipolar disorder: Part II of a report of the International Society for Bipolar Disorders Task Force on Suicide in Bipolar Disorder. *Australian & New Zealand Journal of Psychiatry*, 1–15. doi:10.1177/0004867415594428

Toh, W.L., Thomas, N. & Rossell, S.L. (2015). Auditory verbal hallucinations in bipolar disorder (BD) and major depressive disorder (MDD): A systematic review. *Journal of Affective Disorders*, 184, 18–28. doi:10.1016/j.jad.2015.05.040.

Uher, R., Mantere, O., Suominen, K. & Isometsä, E. (2013). Typology of clinical course in bipolar disorder based on 18-month naturalistic follow-up. *Psychological Medicine*, 43, 789–99. doi:10.1017/S0033291712001523

Van Rheenen, T.E., Meyer, D., Phillipou, A., Tan, E.J., Toh, W.L. & Rossell, S.L. (2020). Mental health status of individuals with a mood disorder during the COVID-19 pandemic in Australia: Initial results from the COLLATE project. *Journal of Affective Disorders*, 275(1), 69–77. DOI: https://doi.org/10.1016/j.jad.2020.06.037

Yildiz, A., Ruiz, P. & Nemeroff, C.B. (2015). *The Bipolar Book: History, Neurobiology, and Treatment.* Oxford: Oxford University Press.

Young, J.W. & Dulcis, D. (2015). Investigating the mechanism(s) underlying switching between states in bipolar disorder. *European Journal of Pharmacology*, 759, 151–62. doi:10.1016/j.ejphar.2015.03.019

CHAPTER 10

DEPRESSIVE DISORDERS

Gylo (Julie) Hercelinskyj

LEARNING OUTCOMES

Upon completion of this chapter, you should be able to:

10.1 Identify the incidence of depressive disorders

10.2 Understand the aetiology and epidemiology of depressive disorders

10.3 Develop an understanding of the presentation associated with depressive disorders

10.4 Review the treatment options for depressive disorders including pharmacological treatment

10.5 Understand persistent depressive disorder

10.6 Understand depression in the perinatal period

10.7 Understand depression in older people

10.8 Learn about recovery and relapse prevention

10.9 Explore the ways in which mental health nurses can work with consumers and families living with the experience of a depressive disorder

LEARNING FROM PRACTICE

I met Elina when I was working as a new clinical educator in mental health. Elina had just been transferred from the acute hospital following an attempt to end her life. She arrived at the acute unit with her head and left side of her face heavily bandaged. In handover, staff had been told she was admitted following a 'serious' suicide attempt in response to 'psychotic depression'. I could see the students were struggling with this – the confused expressions on their faces suggested they had not heard of depression with psychotic symptoms before. In debriefing one student asked, 'But how can you be depressed and psychotic at the same time? Depressed is feeling really down isn't it, sometimes enough to try and take your own life, but psychotic – I just don't get it…?'

'I remember her from the general hospital,' another student blurted out. 'Do you know how she did it? 'Okay everyone,' I said. 'There is clearly a need to work through this situation. Let's begin with your question about why someone who is depressed can also be hearing voices or experiencing disturbed thinking.'

This situation was going to need careful handling. There was clearly the educational component. But the other critical thing to reflect on was professional behaviour, being judgemental and looking at the person at the centre of the event – Elina.

Conrad, mental health nurse

What are the main issues that Conrad has identified? Why would Conrad have been concerned about the direction the discussion was taking? Consider your current understanding of depression. What does it mean to say a person is experiencing an episode of psychotic depression?

INTRODUCTION

Depression (along with anxiety disorders, which are addressed in Chapter 11) is increasingly recognised as one of the most prevalent and pressing mental health issues in contemporary society. Rollo May, an American psychologist, described depression as the 'inability to construct a future' (May, n.d.). The history of depression is a long one and has been identified, discussed and written about through the ages. Originally termed melancholia, depression can be traced as far back as the Mesopotamian era where depression was viewed as a spiritual illness caused by demonic possession. This view can also be seen in the writings of the ancient Greek, Chinese and Egyptian cultures. Hippocrates (460 BCE–370 BCE) believed that personality traits and mental health conditions were related to a balance or imbalance of body fluids, which he termed humours. There were four of these humours: yellow bile, black bile, phlegm and blood. Hippocrates thought that melancholia was caused by too much black bile in the spleen and could be treated by strategies such as bloodletting, swimming, diet and exercise. In the eighteenth and nineteenth centuries, it was believed that depression was an inherited trait that reflected a weak temperament. This view resulted in people often being assigned to institutions and subjected to treatments such as water immersion, special spinning stools that were used to make a person feel dizzy (the theory being that this action would rearrange the contents of a person's brain back into the correct position), as well as special diets, enemas and vomiting.

Clearly in the twenty-first century, there is an understanding that depression is the result of multiple factors (both physiological and psychosocial) and treatment options address these multiple factors.

You will also see that **mood disorders** can be referred to as affective or emotional disorders (Andrews et al., 2013). The use of these terms refers to the ways in which mood disorders are seen to impact on a person's sense of emotional or affective regulation. As DSM-5 now uses the term depressive disorders, this chapter will use both mood disorder and depressive disorder where relevant in the discussion.

Incidence

Mood disorders such as depression have a significant impact on both the national and international burden of disease and are thought to affect approximately 300 million people worldwide (WHO, 2018).

Globally, major depressive disorder (MDD) is a recurrent mental health condition that can be a debilitating experience for people. Estimates suggest that MDD affects 5% of the global population at any given time, and that it is the second leading cause of disability (Ferrari et al., 2013). More specifically, mood disorders such as MDD and dysthymia affect 6% of people aged 16–85 years (bipolar affective disorder is also classified as a mood disorder and is addressed in Chapter 9). A higher proportion of females report mood disorders than males both in the 12 months previous to data being collected (7% compared with 5%) and during their lifetime (18% compared with 12%) (ABS, 2011). More specifically, mood disorders such as MDD and dysthymia affect approximately 6% of people aged 16–85 years (AIHW, 2018). A higher proportion of females report mood disorders than males (7% compared with 5%) in their lifetime (18% compared with 12%) (ABS, 2011).

Adolescence and young adulthood is a critical stage of transition in an individual's physical and mental development. Mental health conditions in young people can seriously disrupt their growth and development, eroding their quality of life by affecting their self-confidence, relationships, education and employment.

AETIOLOGY AND EPIDEMIOLOGY

Given the high prevalence of depression in the community, a great deal of research is available looking at the aetiology and development of MDD. Like many mental health conditions, there is no one clear cause for depression identified. Rather, the disorder is considered to be multifactorial, combining genetic, environmental and neurochemical factors.

Biological factors

The most recent investigations into biological factors influencing the development of MDD highlight the interrelationship between various neurotransmitters and their relationship to the pathophysiology of depression.

Serotonin and norepinephrine

Research has identified a relationship between mood disorders such as depression and abnormal levels of norepinephrine and serotonin. It is postulated that decreased sensitivity of β-adrenergic receptors and decreased levels of norepinephrine released following the activation of the presynaptic β_2-receptors are associated with depressive symptoms. This is further supported by the clinical effects of antidepressant drugs with noradrenergic effects. Low levels of serotonin, or the brain's poor use of this neurotransmitter, appear to be associated with depression (Bernstein, 2016). It is thought that this depletion of serotonin acts as a trigger for the onset of depression. This is supported by the enormous impact the use of selective serotonin reuptake inhibitors (SSRIs) has had in the effectiveness of treating depression (Bernstein, 2016; Kaplan, Kaplan & Ruiz, 2015).

Dopamine

Dopamine is also thought to be implicated in the onset of depression. Evidence so far suggests that dopamine activity may be decreased in a person experiencing depression. Drugs that increase dopamine levels have been shown to reduce the symptoms of depression.

Altered hormonal regulation

Additionally, studies have shown that increased hypothalamic-pituitary–adrenal-axis (HPA) activity commonly associated with stress responses in mammals can be seen in a high proportion of people receiving treatment for depression on an inpatient basis. Although not as high, this increased activity has also been identified in people receiving treatment for depression in the community (Sadock, Sadock & Ruiz, 2015).

Genetic vulnerability

Twin studies show that genetic factors account for only 50–70% of mood disorders (including both depression and bipolar affective disorder), implying that environmental/individual factors are also associated with mood disorders. This means that, while a person may have a family history of depression and this can create a genetic predisposition to the condition, environmental factors impact on whether a person actually develops depression. Family studies have shown a higher rate of depression in first-degree relatives. Additionally, first-degree relatives with depression are also more likely to experience other mental health conditions such as anxiety disorders concurrently (Sadock, Sadock & Ruiz, 2015).

Structural and functional brain imaging

Researchers using structural magnetic resonance imaging (MRI) have reported abnormalities in specific brain regions in people who experience MDD. These changes are mainly in regions of the brain related to the generation and regulation of emotions (Singh & Gotlib, 2014).

Disruptions in sleep neurophysiology

Depression has been shown to be associated with changes in sleeping patterns, specifically a loss of deep (slow-wave) sleep coupled with an increase of nocturnal arousal (Sadock, Sadock & Ruiz, 2015).

How cognition impacts on depression

Cognitive models of depression are based on the key idea that the way a person thinks will impact on their mood. In the case of depression, negative thinking that is excessive and prolonged will result in depression. Research that started in the 1970s suggested that depression results from the concept of *learned helplessness* (Seligman, 1974). Learned helplessness is described as the process where a person feels helpless and believes they lack control over events in their environment. This idea of 'giving up' is based on previous negative experiences and events. The person develops a thinking style that focuses on their inability or inadequacy on working through potential issues and it is this style of thinking, or **cognition**, that makes people particularly vulnerable to depression.

Other work on cognitive factors relating to depression include the idea of **rumination**. If a person who is depressed ruminates on the depression, they are likely to remain depressed for longer than a person who does not. It is postulated that a person who ruminates excessively will experience increased periods of depression because of this constant negative thinking. This contributes to impaired problem-solving and poor use of social supports (Bernstein, 2016).

Cultural features of major depressive disorder

Australia is a culturally diverse nation. The Australian Bureau of Statistics (ABS) estimates that in June 2015, 28.2% of Australia's population was born overseas (ABS, 2016). The ABS also predicts that by 2050, 32% of Australia's population will be overseas born (Cully & Mejoski, cited in Minas et al., 2013).

People migrate for a number of reasons and the experience of migration is profound. Adjusting to a new culture will be both an individual and group experience. The extent to which a person successfully transitions to a new culture and integrates their new and previous lives, involves an ongoing recognition and management of their emotional and physical reactions to the new environment and incorporating new perspectives into their lives, while having their own cultural beliefs understood and validated (Winkleman, 2009). Immigration can impact on people's mental health and well-being and may lead to **culture shock**, depression and feelings of suicide (Kposowa, McElvain & Breault, 2008; Meng et al., 2014). The process of resettlement brings with it many challenges, including ongoing anxiety about safety, feelings of loss and bereavement for previous lives and families remaining in the country of origin, social isolation, discrimination and racism. In 2003, Bhugra argued that rates of depression vary according to migrant status. It is estimated that 5% of refugees who resettle in developed countries such as Australia and New Zealand have been diagnosed with MDD (Fazel, Wheel & Danash, cited in May et al., 2014). The Department of Health and Human Services (2015) has noted that alongside anxiety and post-traumatic stress disorder, depression is also commonly experienced among migrants and refugees. Experiences such as torture and traumatic events are also associated with a diagnosis of depression (Steel et al., 2009). It is therefore essential that the mental health needs of migrants and refugees be identified early and that easily accessible and culturally safe mental health services are provided. The experience of depression for Indigenous Australians is discussed in Chapter 25.

CULTURAL CONSIDERATIONS

Refugees, migrants and depression

Refugees are one group of immigrants whose experiences of relocation following the trauma associated with leaving their country of birth can have a significant impact on their mental health. Factors such as the conflict occurring in their country of origin, lengthy periods in refugee camps, the involuntary detention of refugees and asylum seekers, together with limited employment opportunities after relocation, poor housing options and access to and willingness to utilise health services are just some factors that impact on mental health and well-being. For example, a large proportion of migrant women who face relocation, distant family and support networks, language barriers and potentially discriminatory or culturally insensitive care experience postnatal depression (Hennegan, Redshaw & Kruske, 2015).

People leave countries where conflict, separation and torture have forced them to flee, and seek safety and security for themselves and their families elsewhere. Their path to developed countries is often fraught with danger and exploitation. Professional and industrial health organisations, including nursing, oppose policies that segregate people into detention facilities. Effective communication and referral to appropriate health facilities that provide services staffed by clinicians with expertise in refugee health (including mental health) are among key elements of a culturally responsive and responsible health service. It is imperative that mental health nurses seize opportunities to promote positive mental health in their work with all immigrants, including refugees and asylum seekers, in order to decrease the stigma that can be associated with seeking help. Knowledge of the resources available, such as interpreting services, organisations that provide specific support and advocacy services to refugees and developing greater understanding of the issues facing refugees, are essential; as is knowing the position taken by professional organisations based on an informed understanding of the issues.

Comorbidity

Major depressive disorder has a high comorbidity with a number of physical and mental health conditions. In particular, there is a high correlation of people diagnosed with a major depressive disorder and comorbid anxiety disorder. People with a major depressive disorder can also have a comorbidity with substance use disorders (Delgadillo et al., 2013) Major depressive disorder is most frequently experienced in conjunction with generalised anxiety disorder (Van Ameringen, 2016), which is covered in Chapter 11. In Australia, 20% of the population will experience a mental health condition in any 12-month period. Of these, 11.5% have one disorder and 8.5% have two or more disorders (Black Dog Institute, 2009). Being diagnosed with both MDD and generalised anxiety disorder can often mean an increased severity of symptoms experienced, greater functional impairment and poorer response to treatment (Van Ameringen, 2016).

Major depressive disorder has also been associated with a diagnosis of physical illness, such as diabetes, cardiovascular disease, stroke and respiratory disorders. Early work by Arroyo et al. (2004) has identified depression as a major risk factor for the development of type 2 diabetes. Having a diagnosis of both depression and diabetes significantly increases the chance of developing complications (Meng et al., 2014). Depression has also been associated with metabolic syndrome (Dunbar et al., 2008). The experience of depression can act to amplify the impact of chronic medical conditions as people adjust to changes in their functional abilities, body image, and social and role identities.

There are a number of other conditions that also have depressive features. These include:

- alcohol use disorder
- anxiety disorders (generalised anxiety disorder, mixed anxiety-depressive disorder, panic disorder)
- post-traumatic stress disorder
- eating disorders (anorexia nervosa and bulimia nervosa)
- schizophrenia (Sadock, Sadock & Ruiz, 2015).

Diagnostic criteria major depressive disorder

The clinical presentation of a major depressive disorder can vary greatly, from people who experience discrete episodes of depression with many months or years between an episode to those people who rarely experience any remission with no symptoms (fortunately, this is rare).

DIAGNOSTIC CRITERIA

Major depressive disorder

A Five (or more) of the following symptoms have been present during the same 2-week period and represent a change from previous functioning; at least one of the symptoms is either (1) depressed mood or (2) loss of interest or pleasure.

 1 Depressed mood most of the day, nearly every day, as indicated by either subjective report (e.g., feels sad, empty, hopeless) or observation made by others (e.g., appears tearful). (**Note:** In children and adolescents, can be irritable mood.)

 2 Markedly diminished interest or pleasure in all, or almost all, activities most of the day, nearly every day (as indicated by either subjective account or observation).

 3 Significant weight loss when not dieting or weight gain (e.g., a change of more than 5% of body weight in a month), or decrease or increase in appetite nearly every day. (**Note:** In children, consider failure to make expected weight gain.)

 4 Insomnia or hypersomnia nearly every day.

 5 Psychomotor agitation or retardation nearly every day (observable by others, not merely subjective feelings of restlessness or being slowed down).

 6 Fatigue of loss of energy nearly every day.

 7 Feelings of worthlessness or excessive or inappropriate guilt (which may be delusional) nearly every day (not merely self-reproach or guilt about being sick).

 8 Diminished ability to think or concentrate, or indecisiveness, nearly every day (either by subjective account or as observed by others).

 9 Recurrent thoughts of death (not just fear of dying), recurrent suicidal ideation without a specific plan, or a suicide attempt or a specific plan for committing suicide.

B The symptoms cause clinically significant distress or impairment in social, occupational, or other important areas of functioning.

C The episode is not attributable to the physiological effects of a substance or another medical condition.

Note: Criteria A-C represent a major depressive episode.

Note: Responses to a significant loss (e.g., bereavement, financial ruin, losses from a natural disaster, a serious medical illness or disability) may include the feelings of intense sadness, rumination about the loss, insomnia, poor appetite, and weight loss noted in Criterion A, which may resemble a depressive episode. Although such symptoms may be understandable or considered appropriate to the loss, the presence of a major depressive episode in addition to the normal response to a significant loss should also be carefully considered. This decision inevitably requires the exercise of clinical judgment based on the individual's history and the cultural norms for the expression of distress in the context of loss.

In distinguishing grief from a major depressive episode (MDE), it is useful to consider that in grief the predominant affect is feelings of emptiness and loss, while in an MDE it is persistent depressed mood and the inability to anticipate happiness or pleasure. The dysphoria in grief is likely to decrease in intensity over days to weeks and occurs in waves, the so-called pangs of grief. These waves tend to be associated with thoughts or reminders of the deceased. The depressed mood of an MDE is more persistent and not tied to specific thoughts or preoccupations. The pain of grief may be accompanied by positive emotions and humor that are uncharacteristic of the pervasive unhappiness and misery characteristic of an MDE. The thought content associated with grief generally features a preoccupation with thoughts and memories of the deceased, rather than the self-critical or pessimistic ruminations seen in an MDE. In grief, self-esteem is generally preserved, whereas in an MDE feelings of worthlessness and self-loathing are common. If self-derogatory ideation is present in grief, it typically involves perceived failings vis-à-vis the deceased (e.g., not visiting frequently enough, not telling the deceased how much he or she was loved). If a bereaved individual thinks about death and dying, such thoughts are generally focused on the deceased and possibly about "joining" the deceased, whereas in an MDE such thoughts are focused on ending one's own life because of feeling worthless, undeserving of life, or unable to cope with the pain of depression.

D The occurrence of the major depressive episode is not better explained by schizoaffective disorder, schizophrenia, schizophreniform disorder, delusional disorder, or other specified and unspecified schizophrenia spectrum and other psychotic disorders.

E There has never been a manic episode or a hypomanic episode.

A person experiencing a major depressive disorder will experience significant changes in **mood** and affect, concentration, sleep, energy, motivation, social interaction and appetite. It is important to remember that changes in appetite, sleep and energy can also be experienced as part of other conditions. This is why the *Diagnostic and Statistical Manual of Mental Disorders* (DSM-5; APA, 2013) clearly states that one of the five symptoms must be either criterion one (1) or two (2).

CLINICAL PRESENTATION OF DEPRESSIVE DISORDER IN THE CONTEXT OF THE MENTAL STATE EXAMINATION

A person who experiences an episode of depression will typically present with a range of features that must meet the diagnostic criteria outlined above. The following 'Commonalities of the MSE' section covers the signs and symptoms typically assessed for in the MSE.

COMMONALITIES OF THE MSE: DEPRESSION

General appearance and behaviour

The person may withdraw from social activities, family and friends. A person will often experience lack of energy and inability to complete usual tasks/activities. Movements may be slowed down (psychomotor retardation) or the consumer may appear anxious and restless with agitated movements such as wringing their hands (psychomotor agitation). They will often display poor eye contact during interactions. Struggling with motivation can result in individuals being dishevelled in appearance, such as being unshaven, have unkempt hair, messy clothes and malodour.

Mood

The person may present with feelings of sadness, hopelessness or emptiness. These feelings can often be worse in the morning, reducing in intensity in the early evening. The person may have a diminished appetite. The person can describe themselves as 'feeling flat', 'depressed' or 'feeling numb'.

Sleeping patterns/habits can also be impacted, with people experiencing sleep disturbances such as difficulty falling asleep and early morning waking. Libido is also impacted by a person's mood and a person diagnosed with major depressive disorder will likely experience decreased libido. This can have a significant impact on their interpersonal communication with intimate partners.

Affect

This refers to the consumer's observable emotions – is their affect appropriate or **inappropriate** in relation to their thinking and speech? In depression, affect is usually congruent with mood. Also, the consumer will show little to no emotional expression/response; that is, the range of a person's affect can be **restricted**, blunted or flat.

Perception

A person experiencing a major depressive episode who also experiences hallucinations during this time is said to have major depression with psychotic features. Their experience of hallucinations is most likely to be in line with their thought content, and they can experience very negative hallucinations as well as command hallucinations. For example, if a person believes they have a terminal illness, they may also experience auditory hallucinations making statements such as 'You don't deserve to live'.

Thought

Content

The consumer's thoughts are usually congruent with their mood. They will often make statements such as 'I have no hope', 'I feel useless', 'I feel worthless' or 'Life is not worth living'. Statements such as these reflect the person's low self-esteem and need to be considered in relation to assessment and the risk for suicide. A consumer experiencing delusional thought content related to feelings of depression is said to have depression with psychotic features. For example, a person may believe they have a terminal illness.

Form

A person experiencing a major depressive episode will often experience what is referred to as **poverty of thought content** (thought that when verbalised gives little information, is delayed, slow to be expressed and tends to monosyllabic). This is an objective assessment detail that is observed by the mental health nurse.

Judgement

Judgement can be impaired as a consumer experiencing major depression can feel that people in their lives would be better off without them.

Cognition

A person who is depressed is most likely to be orientated to time, place and person. However, many people experiencing major depressive disorder do refer to difficulty in concentration and increased forgetfulness. For example, a person may be unable to recall what they ate at dinner the night before.

Executive functioning

Executive functioning refers to the capacity to problem solve and plan, initiate, achieve and/or complete goal-directed activities. A person who is depressed can have difficulties planning and completing daily activities such as getting out of bed, daily hygiene and work commitments.

Insight

Because depression impacts on cognition, emotion and motivation, a person may not have an accurate insight into the link between their thoughts and feelings and how other people's impressions of them do not match their own.

Risk assessment

Risk assessment for a person experiencing an episode of major depressive disorder is a key element of a comprehensive mental health assessment. Risk assessments will be completed formally as per a clinical organisation's policy as part of clinical practice guidelines and best practice. Particular elements of a risk assessment that are important to highlight include risk of harm to self (suicide) and risk of harm to others. It is essential to monitor for risk of harm to self (suicide). In the first instance, it is essential to have a good understanding of the risk factors associated with suicide, and this is addressed in some detail in Chapter 20. However, it is useful to highlight some of the following key points. Risk factors for suicide include:

- a family history of a mental health condition
- a history of previous suicide attempts
- previous family history of suicide attempts
- prior episodes of major depression
- level and persistence of suicidal thoughts
- having a plan for suicide
- having access to the means to carry out a suicidal plan
- other 'at risk' mental states (e.g. feelings of hopelessness/worthlessness/anxiety)
- feelings of guilt or shame
- experience of psychotic symptoms (e.g. command hallucinations)
- substance use (current or prior)
- a tendency to be impulsive.

It is critical that you also consider the possible protective factors that a person has in their lives. This can include supportive networks of family and/or friends, and recognising any previous times where they have accessed support networks and/or services.

Risk of harm to others must also be assessed, particularly if the person is experiencing psychotic symptoms such as command hallucinations.

Risk presentations (at risk groups) for major depressive disorder

The risk for suicidal behaviour is always a possibility whenever a person experiences a major depressive episode. Therefore, it is essential that all consumers who are depressed are assessed for degree of suicide risk. A previous history of suicide attempts or threats is a consistent risk factor for suicide behaviour. Refer to Chapter 20 for more information about this.

Aboriginal and Torres Strait Islander peoples

In 2002–03 and 2003–04, Aboriginal and Torres Strait Islander peoples were hospitalised for mental health and behavioural conditions at twice the rate of other Australians. Depression was the most frequently reported mental health–related condition reported by general practitioners for both Aboriginal and Torres Strait Islander peoples (25%) and other Australians (34%) during 2000–01 to 2004–05 (VicHealth Mental Health and Wellbeing Unit, 2007). This suggests that while mental health issues result in higher hospitalisation in Indigenous populations, such people present to their GP at lower rates. This may help explain their higher admission rates to hospital. These figures appear to have continued to increase; a review of community surveys by Jorm, Bourchier, Cvetkovski and Stewart (2012) found that Indigenous people consistently showed a higher prevalence of anxiety and depression symptoms than non-Indigenous adults. This difference was between 50% and three times. Risk factors such as unemployment, lower completion of educational qualifications, low income and adverse life events correlate with the experience of these symptoms.

TREATMENT

The best approach to treatment is early recognition and intervention. Chapter 4 explored the main psychotherapeutic agents used to treat various mental health conditions. Here, we identify the various pharmacological and non-pharmacological measures used in treating and helping people experiencing depression. These include antidepressants, psychological therapies such as cognitive behavioural therapy and electroconvulsive therapy (ECT).

Pharmacological treatment

The major group of drugs used to treat the symptoms of depression is **antidepressants**, and for many people antidepressants are the first line of treatment. However, most antidepressants take between two to four weeks to reach therapeutic levels. Please refer to Chapter 4 for further information on antidepressants.

Selective serotonin reuptake inhibitors

Before the introduction of selective serotonin reuptake inhibitors (SSRIs), antidepressants, while effective, were accompanied by a large number of side effects. They required close monitoring and were far more dangerous in the event of an overdose. Fluoxetine (Prozac®) was the first SSRI released onto the market, in 1987. **Table 10.1** identifies a range of SSRIs currently used in clinical practice.

TABLE 10.1
Selective serotonin reuptake inhibitors (SSRIs)

MEDICATION	DOSAGE	SIDE EFFECTS/CONTRAINDICATIONS
Fluoxetine (Lovan®, Prozac®)	10–60 mg	• Fatigue • Hot flushes • Headache • Tremor • Rash • Diarrhoea • Constipation • Sexual dysfunction • Nausea, vomiting • Insomnia • Hyponatraemia • Black box warning: interactions with other SSRIs, St John's wort • Should not be combined with monoamine oxidase inhibitors (MAOIs)
Escitalopram (Lexapro®)	5–20 mg	• Fatigue • Hot flushes • Headache • Tremor • Diarrhoea • Constipation • Sexual dysfunction • Black box warning: interactions with other SSRIs, St John's wort • Should not be combined with MAOIs
Citalopram (Celexa®)	10–40 mg	• Fatigue • Hot flushes • Headache • Tremor • Rash • Diarrhoea • Constipation • Sexual dysfunction • Nausea, vomiting • Insomnia • Hyponatraemia • Black box warning: interactions with other SSRIs, St John's wort • Should not be combined with MAOIs
Sertraline (Zoloft®)	25–200 mg	• Gastrointestinal (GI) upset • Headache • Sedation • Insomnia • Dry mouth • Tremor • Sexual dysfunction • Black box warning: interactions with other SSRIs, St John's Wort • Should not be combined with MAOIs

MEDICATION	DOSAGE	SIDE EFFECTS/CONTRAINDICATIONS
Fluvoxamine (Luvox®)	100–300 mg	• Fatigue • Hot flushes • Headache • Tremor • Rash • Diarrhoea • Constipation • Sexual dysfunction • Nausea, vomiting • Insomnia • Hyponatraemia • Black box warning: interactions with other SSRIs, St John's wort • Should not be combined with MAOIs
Paroxetine (Aropax®)	20–60 mg	• Black Box warning: interactions with other SSRIs, St John's wort • Should not be combined with MAOIs • Discontinuation symptoms are common • Dry mouth • Sexual dysfunction • GI upset • Drowsiness • Dizziness

SOURCE: ANDREWS ET AL., 2013; MIMS ONLINE, 2018

Tricyclic antidepressants

This group of antidepressants was the first line of treatment until the introduction of SSRIs in the late 1980s. Therefore, the interactions and side effects of these drugs are well known and documented (see **Table 10.2**).

Serotonin-noradrenaline reuptake inhibitors

Serotonin-noradrenaline reuptake inhibitors (SNRIs) were introduced in the 1990s and act by blocking the reabsorption of serotonin and norepinephrine in the brain; that is, they increase the amount of serotonin and noradrenaline available in the brain by blocking reabsorption (**Table 10.3**).

Mirtazapine (Avanza®) is not an SNRI, but its mechanism of action works to release serotonin and noradrenaline. As such, it has a similar side-effect profile and range and disadvantages.

Monoamine oxidase inhibitors

Before tricyclic antidepressants, monoamine oxidase inhibitors (MAOIs) were among the first antidepressants developed in the 1950s. They have been largely replaced by other groups of antidepressants due to their significant side-effect profile. Monoamine oxidase metabolises monoamines in the brain. The monoamines considered to have a role in depression are serotonin, norepinephrine and dopamine.

TABLE 10.2
Tricyclic antidepressants

MEDICATION	DOSAGE	SIDE EFFECTS/CONTRAINDICATIONS/PRECAUTIONS	DISADVANTAGES AND/OR BENEFITS
Amitriptyline (Endep®)	30–300 mg	• Sedation, postural hypotension, arrhythmia, tachycardia, dry mouth, constipation, urinary retention • Interact with SSRIs, increases plasma levels of alcohol, antipsychotics and MAOIs. These need to be avoided • Cardiac history	• Increased sedation • Weight gain • Disorientation/confusion in older people • Increased risk of bone fractures in people over the age of 50 (due to orthostatic hypotension) • Oldest class of antidepressants and rarely used as first treatment option
Imipramine (Tofranil®)	25–300 mg	• Excessive dosage can lead to arrhythmias, seizures	

SOURCE: ANDREWS ET AL., 2013; MIMS ONLINE, 2018

TABLE 10.3
Serotonin-noradrenaline reuptake inhibitors (SNRIs)

MEDICATION	DOSAGE	SIDE EFFECTS/ CONTRAINDICATIONS/ DISADVANTAGES
Duloxetine (Cymbalta®)	30–90/120 mg	• Dry mouth • GI upset • Constipation • Diarrhoea • Vivid dreams • Fatigue • Black box warning: interactions with MAOIs, SSRIs and St John's wort
Venlafaxine (Effexor®)	75–375 mg	• Nausea • Vomiting • Diarrhoea • Constipation • Anorexia • Fatigue • Sexual dysfunction • Headache • Black box warning: interactions with MAOIs, SSRIs and St John's wort

SOURCE: ANDREWS ET AL., 2013; MIMS ONLINE, 2018

MAOIs work by inhibiting the metabolism of this monoamine.

MAOIs are associated with a rare but potentially severe interaction with foods containing high levels of tyramine. The GI system contains a monoamine which metabolises tyramine. Because MAOIs inhibit the metabolism of monoamines, higher levels of tyramine enter the circulatory system. This leads to a hypertensive crisis. Therefore, dietary restrictions are essential for a person who is taking an MAOI. This means the restriction of food and beverages high in tyramine. This refers to aged or spoiled high-protein foods, such as all aged cheeses, aged soy products, fermented/dried meats, spoiled/improperly stored meats and liver, Marmite/Vegemite, tap beer, and fava bean pods. Some foods and beverages that were originally banned in the 1960s are now thought to be acceptable in restricted quantities/volumes (Bodkin & Goren, 2017).

CULTURAL CONSIDERATIONS

MAOIs and diet
While the dietary restrictions for a person taking a MAOI may not seem significant to some clinicians, it is essential to remember that dietary patterns can vary significantly between different cultures. Therefore, it is imperative that the mental health nurse has a good understanding of the usual dietary intake of consumers who might be considered for an MAOI antidepressant; reporting relevant information back to the health care team; and incorporating this understanding into any education required.

Issues related to the use of pharmacological treatments
While the use of antidepressants has significantly helped consumers to manage their symptoms of depression, the use of these medications is not without its issues. These issues relate to potential life-threatening side effects, which are highlighted below.

Serotonin syndrome
Serotonin syndrome is a potentially fatal complication of antidepressant therapy which results from excessive concentration of serotonin within the central nervous system, with a mortality rate of between 2–12%. There are a range of cognitive, autonomic and neuromuscular symptoms that can be experienced, which can range from mild to life-threatening. Therefore, care must be taken when a consumer is changing antidepressants, and they also must receive education on medications which are contraindicated when on antidepressants. While serotonin syndrome can occur as a result of overdosing with one single agent, it is more common when multiple serotonergic agents (even when each is at therapeutic dose) are administered concurrently. Treatment involves discontinuing the offending agent, intravenous fluids and administration of benzodiazepines along with management of **hyperthermia**. Specific signs and symptoms that are associated with serotonin syndrome are:

- at least three of the following symptoms: agitation, shivering, tremor, fever, muscle spasms, diarrhoea, **ataxia**, **diaphoresis**, **hyperreflexia**, changes in mental state (e.g. cognitive changes, hypomania)
- other symptoms include: restlessness, perceptual disturbances, nausea, vomiting, tachycardia, rapid changes in blood pressure, loss of coordination (Andrews et al., 2013).

Antidepressant discontinuation syndrome
Abruptly ceasing, discontinuing or switching antidepressant medication may cause withdrawal symptoms and is referred to as abrupt/withdrawal discontinuation syndrome. Whilst this condition is not life threatening, it can be uncomfortable. **Table 10.4** indicates the range of symptoms a person may experience.

TABLE 10.4
Discontinuation symptoms

BODY SYSTEM	SYMPTOMS
Affective	Irritability, agitation, anxiety
Gastrointestinal	Vomiting and diarrhoea, nausea, anorexia
Vasomotor	Sweating
Neurosensory	Paraesthesia (pins and needles)
Other neurological	Sleep disturbances, dizziness, vertigo, headache, lethargy

SOURCE: ADAPTED FROM LUFT, 2013

The symptoms are usually of short duration and mild. However, if a consumer abruptly stops taking their antidepressant medication, they may experience more prolonged and severe symptoms. The severity of symptoms will also be impacted by the **half-life** of the particular drug. That is, an antidepressant with a short half-life and higher dose can produce a more rapid onset of symptoms than an antidepressant with a longer half-life that is prescribed at a lower dose. Therefore, there is a need for a clearly defined and monitored tapering, titration and switching regimen to be developed (Luft, 2013).

Suicidality and antidepressant use

A black box warning represents the strongest level of warning included in the packaging of a medication. In 2004, the US Food and Drug Administration issued a black box warning on antidepressants and the associated risk with an increase in suicidal thoughts, feelings and behaviour in young people: suicidality. An example of such a warning is shown in **Figure 10.1**.

SOURCE: U.S. FOOD AND DRUG ADMINISTRATION

Suicidality and Antidepressant Drugs

Antidepressants increased the risk compared to placebo of suicidal thinking and behavior (suicidality) in children, adolescents, and young adults in short-term studies of major depressive disorder (MDD) and other psychiatric disorders. Anyone considering the use of [Insert established name] or any other antidepressant in a child, adolescent, or young adult must balance this risk with the clinical need. Short-term studies did not show an increase in the risk of suicidality with antidepressants compared to placebo in adults beyond age 24; there was a reduction in risk with antidepressants compared to placebo in adults aged 65 and older. Depression and certain other psychiatric disorders are themselves associated with increases in the risk of suicide. Patients of all ages who are started on antidepressant therapy should be monitored appropriately and observed closely for clinical worsening, suicidality, or unusual changes in behavior. Families and caregivers should be advised of the need for close observation and communication with the prescriber. [Insert Drug Name] is not approved for use in pediatric patients. [The previous sentence would be replaced with the sentence, below, for the following drugs: Prozac: Prozac is approved for use in pediatric patients with MDD and obsessive compulsive disorder (OCD). Zoloft: Zoloft is not approved for use in pediatric patients except for patients with obsessive compulsive disorder (OCD). Fluvoxamine: Fluvoxamine is not approved for use in pediatric patients except for patients with obsessive compulsive disorder (OCD).] (See Warnings: Clinical Worsening and Suicide Risk, Precautions: Information for Patients, and Precautions: Pediatric Use)

FIGURE 10.1
A black box warning (US Food and Drug Administration)

In Australia, this is referred to as a boxed warning, and is administered by the Therapeutic Goods Administration (TGA) and included in the product information sent to prescribers. There has been controversy over the decision to release the black box warning in the United States, with authors such as Friedman (2014) arguing that the data shows a decrease in the diagnosis and treatment in younger people, but also in adults, who were not the intended population for this warning. However, he does state that the decrease in diagnosis and prescribing only correlates with the introduction of the warning, and does not demonstrate a causal link. Friedman concludes that that the FDA should consider removing the warning or at a minimum consult with the medical profession regarding its efficacy

and suitability. Gordon and Melville (2013, p. 622), reporting on recent work, concluded that adolescents have a small but increased risk of experiencing suicidal thoughts and behaviours 'at least in the short term'. While there may be controversy and continued debate, it is essential to recognise the importance for assessment, monitoring, appropriate individualised treatment and support for a person experiencing depression by the entire multidisciplinary team, including mental health nurses (Gordon & Melville, 2013).

Non-pharmacological approaches to treatment

While many people will be familiar with the use of antidepressants to treat depression, not every consumer will find the use of antidepressants effective or see this as the only way to manage their symptoms. As part of holistic, recovery-oriented practice, people are increasingly using a combination of both medications and non-pharmacological approaches to managing symptoms of depression.

Cognitive behavioural therapy

Cognitive behavioural therapy (CBT) has been shown to be an effective treatment option when used alone or in combination with medication. The aim of CBT is to assist consumers to develop practical and workable self-help strategies they can use when they are experiencing an episode of depression as well as help with any future episodes (Hughes, Heron & Younge, 2014). This process can help consumers to experience success, build self-esteem and begin the process of challenging negative thought patterns. Guidi, Tomba and Fava (2016) conducted a meta-analysis of the literature on the effectiveness of CBT as part of a sequential approach to reducing the risk of relapse in major depressive disorder. Their results indicated that CBT, used alone or in combination with continued use of antidepressants following successful response to medication in the acute phase, showed an overall decrease in risk of relapse of approximately 20%. CBT is discussed in detail in Chapter 4.

Behavioural strategies

Strategies such as exercise, opportunities for social interaction, scheduling activities, structured problem-solving and goal planning are key examples of behavioural strategies that can be implemented when working with a consumer experiencing major depression (Andrews et al., 2013). The aim in using behavioural strategies is to assist the consumer to maintain a regular routine. A person experiencing depression will often isolate themselves from others and have little energy to undertake the activities in which they previously engaged. Collaborating on behavioural strategies with a consumer can facilitate an increase in self-esteem as they begin to realise they have control over aspects of their daily life again. It is in experiencing these small, but significant, successes that habits become established (or re-established).

Cognitive strategies

Cognitive strategies focus on helping consumers to review and revise the way in which their thinking patterns consistently focus on negative assumptions and outcomes, such as self-blame, low self-esteem and feelings of worthlessness. Thinking patterns then are over-generalised; that is, if a person does poorly in one aspect of their life or one activity, there is a tendency to generalise this behaviour to all aspects of their life (including interactions with others). The aim of a cognitive approach is to assist consumers to reappraise their patterns of thinking and involves identifying these underlying beliefs and assumptions that their thinking is based on. Refer to Chapter 4 for further details.

Interpersonal therapy

Interpersonal therapy refers to a therapeutic approach in which a person addressees specific interpersonal issues that may have resulted due to a major life transition such as bereavement leading to a complicated grief reaction, divorce, workplace bullying, or postnatal depression associated with a difficult transition to the parenting role (Andrews et al., 2013).

Mindfulness-based cognitive therapy

Mindfulness is a process whereby a person pays attention to their experience and the thoughts and feelings that are occurring at the time; that is, in the present moment. Mindfulness-based cognitive therapy is based on the practice of meditation-based mindfulness integrated with cognitive therapy strategies. Current research suggests that it can be effective in reducing the risk of relapse for people who have experienced recurrent episodes of depression (McDonald, 2016).

Reminiscence therapy

In reminiscence therapy, a person is involved in a conversation regarding past events and experiences. The aim of this therapeutic strategy is to review, evaluate and validate their lives (Kampfe, 2015).

EVIDENCE-BASED PRACTICE

Consumers and their preferred treatment

Title of study

Are treatment preferences relevant in response to serotonergic antidepressants and cognitive behavioral therapy in depressed primary patients?

Authors

R. Mergl, V. Henkel, A.K. Allgaier, D. Kramer, M. Hautzinge, R. Kohnen, R. … U. Hergerl

Background

The authors identified that there is little information regarding consumers' preferred treatment options and expectations when experiencing depression. The aim of the study was to investigate the efficacy of an antidepressant (sertraline) and cognitive behavioural group therapy (CBT-G) in treating patients diagnosed with mild-to-moderate depression who were treated in a primary care setting.

Design

A randomised control trial was employed to allocate participants to a group where either treatment with Sertraline alone, or in a group where participants undertook a course of CBT-G, or a third group where participants could choose their preferred treatment option.

Participants

A total of 145 participants diagnosed by their primary care provider with mild-to-moderate depression took part in this study over a four-year period (2000–04).

Results

Consumers with a diagnosis of depression who received their preferred treatment, whether Sertraline or CBT-G, responded significantly better than those who did not receive their preferred therapy.

Conclusions

Identified that consumers receiving their preferred treatment (whether pharmacotherapy or psychotherapy) respond significantly better than those who do not receive their preferred therapy.

Implications

It is essential as a nurse to support and advocate when necessary for consumers' preferred treatment option whether that is medication or talking therapies or a combination of both.

SOURCE: MERGL, R., HENKEL, V., ALLGAIER, A.K., KRAMER, D., HAUTZINGE, M., KOHNEN, R., … HERGERL, U. (2011). ARE TREATMENT PREFERENCES RELEVANT IN RESPONSE TO SEROTONERGIC ANTIDEPRESSANTS AND COGNITIVE BEHAVIORAL THERAPY IN DEPRESSED PRIMARY PATIENTS? *PSYCHOTHERAPY AND PSYCHOSOMATICS*, 80, 39–47. DOI:10.1159/000318772

Physical treatments

The main physical treatment options for managing depression are **electroconvulsive therapy (ECT)** and **transcranial magnetic stimulation (TMS)**. These treatment options can be used in conjunction with antidepressants and non-pharmacological approaches to manage symptoms of depression. There are specific indications for the use of both treatment options.

Electroconvulsive therapy (ECT)

Perhaps the most misunderstood and emotive treatment option used in contemporary mental health service delivery is ECT. Films such as *One Flew Over the Cuckoo's Nest* (1975), *Frances* (1982), *Girl Interrupted* (1999) and *A Beautiful Mind* (2001) evoke an image of ECT that both creates and reflects the attitudes of the public. Research in 2002 regarding medical students' knowledge about ECT demonstrated a poor understanding that reflected negative attitudes, which were reinforced by media portrayals of the procedure (Walter, McDonald, Rey & Joseph, 2002).

These representations are grounded in the history of ECT, which began in the 1930s in Italy, where it was recognised that inducing seizures could relieve symptoms of a mental health condition (Sadowsky, 2017). However, in addition to the physical risk associated with its use, historically ECT has also been used as a form of social control of consumers.

Yet consumers and mental health clinicians such as nurses know that contemporary use of ECT practice is a safe and effective treatment for major depression.

In Australia, there is legislation governing the use, duration and consent of ECT and there are very few side effects. All staff involved in using ECT are registered health professionals who are required to have undergone specific education and training in this procedure.

ECT is a fully supervised medical procedure performed under general anaesthesia and muscle relaxation. ECT is thought to work by stimulating the dopaminergic pathways of the brain with electricity – a modified seizure is produced by the selective passage of an electrical current through the brain. The electrical current is passed by placing electrodes on specific parts of a person's scalp. ECT is administered by either **bilateral** or **unilateral** placement of the electrodes on the individual's scalp, as illustrated in **Figure 10.2**. **Table 10.5** lists some important features of ECT.

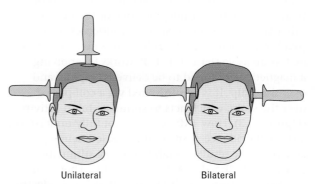

Unilateral   Bilateral

FIGURE 10.2
Electrode placement for unilateral and bilateral ECT

TABLE 10.5
Significant features of ECT

Indications	Major depressive disorder. ECT is effective when: • psychotic or somatic symptoms are present • the consumer has responded well to ECT in the past • the person had little success from other treatment options such as talking therapies (e.g. CBT) and/or medications or a combination of both • the consumer is acutely suicidal and immediate treatment is required • the consumer is unable to tolerate and/or medications are contraindicated. ECT can also be used for other serious mental health conditions, such as schizophrenia, mania and catatonia.
Course of treatment	Most commonly given on an inpatient basis. A person is likely to have 2–3 sessions/week for a total of 6–12 sessions. Maintenance ECT frequencies vary, but may include, for example, one treatment monthly, or once every six months. A review of the consumer's clinical response to ECT must be formally conducted at least weekly by the authorised psychiatrist. Ongoing daily assessment by nursing staff is essential to complement this.
Pre-procedure	A complete physical assessment must be completed. Medications are reviewed and any medication that may raise or lower the seizure threshold or is known to cause increased post ECT confusion should be ceased or the dosage reduced. The individual will need to fast for a period prior to receiving ECT to prevent the risk of aspiration of gastric contents.
Procedure	The consumer is administered a general anaesthetic and muscle relaxant by a specialist anaesthetist who will monitor their airway and breathing throughout the procedure. An induced seizure of between 70–150 volts via electrodes is administered by the authorised psychiatrist who is trained to administer ECT. Motor activity is assessed visually for evidence of a seizure. All consumers will have an EEG tracing completed during the procedure to record the duration of seizure activity in the brain. Seizure activity (motor and brain wave activity) lasts ~30–60 seconds.

Post-procedure	Post-anaesthetic care is provided. Following approval by the anaesthetist, a consumer will be transferred to a recovery bay where they will be monitored continuously by nursing staff. Nurses are responsible for ensuring the consumer maintains a patent airway and monitors the pulse and blood pressure until stable. Oxygen can be given via a face mask and can be discontinued when the consumer can engage in conversation. Regular observations of pulse, blood pressure and oxygen saturation levels (even if the consumer is not wearing an oxygen mask) need to be taken and documented. There should be a continuous nursing presence and observation until reorientation is achieved.
Side effects	Include: • transient short-term memory loss • headache • confusion • nausea • muscle aches.
Legislation	All states and territories in Australia have specific legislation in their Mental Health Acts in relation to ECT. This includes issues related to consent, and maximum number of treatments and length of time over which ECT may be administered.

SOURCE: ADAPTED FROM DEPARTMENT OF HEALTH, 2013

Transcranial magnetic stimulation (TMS)

Transcranial magnetic stimulation (TMS) is an option for consumers who do not tolerate other forms of treatment, such as antidepressants, or to augment other treatment options such as antidepressants and psychotherapeutic interventions. It is considered to be less invasive than ECT. TMS works by applying a magnetic field timed to be delivered rapidly and over the scalp. It is administered via a coil placed over the scalp, which acts to stimulate brain activity (**Figure 10.3**). How TMS works is not fully understood, although evidence posits that increased neural activity is the result of high frequency stimulation (Diefenbach, Bragdon & Goethe, 2013). There is a low risk of seizure activity with TMS as it uses electric currents. Additional side effects, while uncommon, include headaches, facial twitching related to the TMS pulses and temporary hearing problems.

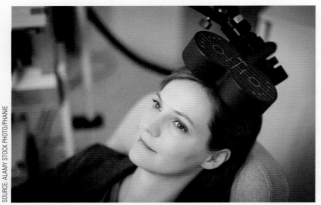

SOURCE: ALAMY STOCK PHOTO/PHANIE

FIGURE 10.3
Transcranial magnetic therapy

TMS treatment protocols vary, but Galletly and colleagues (2015) suggest that a typical course of treatment might involve 18–30 treatments (each lasting about 30 minutes) over 4–6 weeks. Fitzgerald (2012) provided a useful comparison of the characteristics of TMS and ECT (**Table 10.6**).

TABLE 10.6
Characteristics of repetitive transcranial magnetic stimulation and electroconvulsive therapy

	REPETITIVE TRANSCRANIAL MAGNETIC STIMULATION	ELECTROCONVULSIVE THERAPY
Action	Non-convulsive	Convulsive
Indications	Treatment-resistant depression Failure to tolerate other treatments for depression Possible first-line treatment based on patient choice	Severe depression Treatment-resistant depression Catatonia Emergency treatment of depression requiring urgent clinical response
Efficacy	Moderately well established Response rates <50%	Well established Response rates >50%
Safety	Low risk of seizure induction No cognitive adverse effects No general anaesthetic	Risks associated with general anaesthesia Memory impairment, possible other cognitive adverse effects

SOURCE: FITZGERALD, 2012 © NPS MEDICINEWISE. AUSTRALIAN PRESCRIBER.

PERSISTENT DEPRESSIVE DISORDER (DYSTHYMIA)

Whereas the experience of major depressive disorder is often described as being an overwhelming despair and hopelessness, persistent depressive disorder (known previously as **dysthymia**) accounts for **depressed mood** for a period of two years, where the person experiences a depressed mood for more days than they do not (APA, 2013). This contrasts with major depressive disorder, where a depressed mood or loss of interest or pleasure in nearly all activities for a period of at least two consecutive weeks is the key feature along with recovery typically beginning within three months of the onset of symptoms. A person experiencing persistent depressive disorder can describe their mood as gloomy or down in the dumps. The DSM-5 (2013) criteria for diagnosis list a range of criteria in addition to the primary one of depressed mood for most of the day on more days than not for at least two years (Criterion A). Criterion B lists a range of features, of which a person must experience a minimum of two:

- poor appetite or overeating
- insomnia or hypersomnia
- low energy or fatigue
- low self-esteem
- poor concentration or difficulties making decisions
- feelings of hopelessness.

For a diagnosis to be confirmed, a person cannot be symptom free (as described in Criteria A and B) for more than two months (APA, 2013). The 12-month prevalence of dysthymia was 1.3% of the Australian population in 2007 (ABS, 2008). A person diagnosed with persistent depressive disorder is at a higher risk of experiencing other mental health conditions such as substance or anxiety disorders.

DEPRESSION IN THE PERINATAL PERIOD

Pregnancy is a time of both great joy and challenges. For the childbearing woman, **perinatal depression** (and perinatal anxiety) is identified by Austin and Priest (2005) as the most common mental health condition among psychiatric disorders in industrialised nations. Austin and Priest note prevalence rates of 13% in the first few postpartum weeks and up to 20% in the first year.

The term perinatal depression is used to highlight that a woman can experience depression across the childbearing continuum. The DSM-5 outlines the key criteria for a diagnosis of a mental health condition; namely, symptoms, duration of symptoms and severity of symptoms (APA, 2013). To be diagnosed with depression, a woman must meet the diagnostic criteria for major depressive disorder, identified earlier in this chapter. The DSM-5 (2013) uses a time specifier to classify depression in the postnatal period. To be diagnosed with major depressive disorder following childbirth, a woman must meet the criteria for major depressive disorder in the four weeks following the birth of a child. This is referred to as depression with peripartum onset (APA, 2013). However, **postnatal depression** in its broadest sense is depression that has its onset within the first 12 months following the birth of a child (Andrews et al., 2013; beyondblue, 2018; Centre for Perinatal Excellence, 2019).

Antenatal depressive symptoms are as common as postnatal symptoms (Austin, 2004; Leigh & Milgrom et al., 2008); depression identified postnatally begins antenatally in up to 40% of women (Austin, 2004). Additionally, anxiety disorders may be as common as depression in the perinatal period (Austin & Priest, 2005; Fairbrother et al., 2015; Wenzel, Haugen, Jackson & Brendle, 2005). Between 20% and 40% of women with a past episode of depression in the postnatal period will relapse after the birth of a subsequent child (Austin & Priest, 2005; Milgrom et al., 1995).

The experience of depression can range from postnatal (baby) blues through to postnatal depression and puerperal psychosis. However, remember that a woman can also experience depression in the antenatal period as well as after the postnatal period. **Table 10.7** illustrates the key differences between these experiences.

TABLE 10.7
Differences between baby blues and perinatal depression

	BABY BLUES	PERINATAL DEPRESSION
Usual onset	48–96 hours postpartum; often coincides with full lactation	Antenatal: woman must meet the criteria for diagnosis as outlined in the DSM-5 DSM-5 specifier for depression with peripartum onset stipulates that symptoms must present with the first 4 weeks postnatally A broader definition of postnatal depression considers the onset from the first month to 3–6 months in the postnatal period and in some literature even up to one year following birth
Duration	Transient, <72 hours May persist up to ~10 days	Generally, lasts weeks to months Usually remits around 4–6 months 15–25% continue for 12 months Factors that influence duration/severity: delay in diagnosis, severity of symptoms and response to treatment
Aetiology/ contributing factors	Unknown, likely hormonal and/or electrolyte changes – decrease in oestrogen and progesterone	Past history Personal or family history of mental health problems Current AOD use Lack of available support or socially isolated Current or past history of abuse Negative or stressful life events – including birth trauma Multiple births Baby issues – feeding, sleeping Sole parent Young mother

	BABY BLUES	PERINATAL DEPRESSION
Incidence	50–80%	~10.15%
Signs and symptoms	Tearfulness Tiredness Irritability/labile mood Heightened sensitivity Physical aches and soreness	Persistent (greater than 2 weeks) experience of low mood, sleep disturbance (insomnia or excessive sleeping), anger/irritability, changes to cognition (poor memory/decision making), feelings of helplessness or hopelessness, thought about harming self or baby
Management strategies	Supportive strategies – **sleep hygiene**, emotional support/understanding, promoting physical comfort (food, fluids, being pain free)	Medication: antidepressant SSRI Psychotherapy: counselling, support group The woman may need hospitalisation if symptoms severe or risk of harm Exercise, nutrition, other complementary therapies Enhanced maternal child health nurse/midwife Postpartum depression rarely resolves without intervention

SOURCE: ADAPTED FROM APA, 2013; BEYONDBLUE, 2018; DIXON, 2010

Postpartum (puerperal) psychosis

Postpartum psychosis affects approximately 0.1% of the population and has its onset usually within the first two weeks following birth, although symptoms can manifest as soon as 48–72 hours following delivery (Higgins, 2011). There are several risk factors associated with the development and onset of postpartum psychosis and these include a personal and/or family history of bipolar disorder, postpartum psychosis or major depressive disorder, first-time mothers, discontinuation of mood stabilisers and obstetrical complications (Monzon di Scalea & Pearlstein, 2014; Sadock, Sadock & Ruiz, 2013).

Postpartum psychosis is considered a mental health emergency. A number of clear signs and symptoms are present, and **Table 10.8** outlines these using the mental state format.

TABLE 10.8
Clinical features of postpartum psychosis

DOMAIN	CLINICAL FEATURES
Behaviour	Restlessness
Speech	Talkative, rambling
Mood and affect	Irritability, labile mood
Sleep	Insomnia
Thought	Delusions, disorganised thinking
Perception	Hallucinations (command type)
Cognition	Confusion, difficulty concentrating

SOURCE: ADAPTED FROM HIGGINS, 2011; MONZON DI SCALEA & PEARLSTEIN, 2014

Delusions are said to be mood congruent and often involve thoughts of the baby being killed or hurt in some way, ideas of reference and delusions of control. Though rare, there is an estimated 4% risk of infanticide and 5% risk of suicide, and therefore risk assessment, early identification management and support are essential (Sadock, Sadock & Ruiz, 2013).

The management for postpartum psychosis has traditionally been medically oriented (Glover, Jomeen, Urquhart & Martin, 2014). Management will involve hospital admission as it is a mental health emergency. Ideally, the admission would be for both mother and baby, although this depends on the availability of specialist perinatal mental health services. This is important, as one of the potential consequences of postpartum psychosis is disrupted bonding and attachment between mother and infant, which is exacerbated if the woman is admitted separately. Pharmacological treatment may be used but it is considered on a case-by-case basis, which will consider factors such as any previous history of postpartum psychosis and treatment received together with the woman's response to this. Breastfeeding is also a factor that must be reviewed, as it is not recommended with a number of psychotropic medications (e.g. lithium) (Di Florio, Smith & Jones, 2013).

Nursing collaboration with women experiencing postpartum psychosis provides education, information on the condition, its management, and support for the mother, partner and other involved family members. Crucial aspects of nursing management are helping to dispel ideas regarding postpartum psychosis being something the woman can resist, and encouraging family support networks and understanding (Glover et al., 2014).

DEPRESSION AND OLDER PEOPLE

A person can experience depression at any point in their lives. This is as true for young people, adolescents and adults as it is for an older person. However, it is not true that depression is something all older people will experience; that is, depression is not a normal part of ageing. Depression is estimated to affect between 10% to 15% of older people (ABS, 2009) and is thought to impact older adults living in supported accommodation (e.g. residential care facilities) at a higher rate of approximately 35% of people (ABS, 2009).

In contrast with younger people, however, an older person experiencing depression may not refer to emotional symptoms as frequently. Instead, they may experience and present with symptoms that are more physical in nature, such as difficulty in sleeping (hypersomnia, insomnia), problems with their appetite, memory problems, agitation or referring to their 'nerves' rather than using language that is more emotionally based. An older person may not associate these symptoms with depression as they and others may believe they are experiencing changes related to the ageing process. However, the criteria for diagnosing depression in an older person remain the same as those listed earlier in this chapter.

There are some specific risk factors that may increase an older person's risk of experiencing depression. Factors such increasing physical health problems, chronic illness/pain, immobility, changes in independent living arrangements and the experience of loss through death of a spouse, friends and increased social isolation can impact on an older person's experience of depression.

Assessment of the older person who may be experiencing depression is essential. Symptoms such as anhedonia, sleeping difficulties, difficulty in concentrating, a decrease in energy and motivation can all be experienced and need to be assessed for. Risk assessment for suicidal thoughts is also an essential component when assessing the older person who is at risk of experiencing depression.

Treatment of depression includes pharmacological treatments, physical treatment such as ECT, problem-solving strategies and lifestyle strategies that aim to increase opportunities for social inclusion, support and physical activity, diet and sleep hygiene.

NURSING CARE PLAN

WORKING WITH ED

Ed Dorcas is a 45-year-old man who is married to Sarah and has two sons – Joel who is 10 years old and Noah who is 13 years old. Ed works as an accountant in a large firm and lives in an inner-city suburb of a major city. Ed has been vying to become a partner in the firm for the past nine months, but recently another accountant was hired. Ed began feeling down about seven months ago when one of the partners left the firm, and the stress of trying to gain the position commenced. He began increasing his alcohol intake approximately six months ago and stood down as football coach to the under 10 football team he had been involved with for the past four years. Ed was found by Sarah on the floor of the garage with an injured arm after a failed suicide attempt. The rope broke during his attempt to hang himself, and he received minor abrasions to his neck and a sprained wrist. The following nursing care plan outlines the relevant features of Ed's mental health assessment (including the mental state examination), care priorities and rationale.

MENTAL STATE EXAMINATION	ASSESSMENT DATA COLLECTED
Appearance	Dishevelled, unshaven male, poorly dressed
Behaviour	No eye contact; psychomotor retardation
Mood	Depressed; tearful; rates mood 2/10, feels 'utterly hopeless' and distressed by current circumstances – namely, that his suicide attempt did not result in his imminent death: 'I can't even get that right'. Presents with anhedonia, anergia and avolition
Appetite	Poor; feels eating is a chore, no motivation to cook or eat. Has lost about 5 kg
Sleep	Interrupted. Finds it difficult to get out of bed, but does not feel rested when he has slept Some napping during the day; no sleep routine and denies use of sedatives current or previous
Libido	Last sexually active with wife three months ago, but was impotent during attempt. States he has absolutely no desire to have sex: 'Can't be bothered'
Speech	Latency of responses; monosyllabic in conversation
Perception	Denies perceptual disturbance
Thought	Content: • Rumination regarding failed suicide attempt • Guilt at being a 'shitty father' • Still wants to die • Feels like a bad parent • Nil obsessions Guilt delusions. Wife claims he accused her of having an affair but it is possible he did this to try and force her to leave him.

MENTAL STATE EXAMINATION	ASSESSMENT DATA COLLECTED
Judgement	Understands consequences of suicide attempt but feels there is no other way out
Insight	Good understanding of presence of depression but doesn't believe he is worth saving Agreeable to taking medications but admits to feeling 'beyond help'
Memory	Good
Orientation	NAD (nothing abnormal detected)
Intelligence	Not formally assessed but appears above average
Risk assessment	Suicide – high: • Thoughts – yes • Plan – partial • Method – yes • Lethality – yes • Self-harm – denies • Homicide – denies

From the above mental health assessment, Ed is likely to show a number of behaviours. These include sleep disturbances, poor nutritional intake, loss of interest and pleasure in usual activities including intimate relationships with Sarah, decreased attendance to activities of daily living such as hygiene and grooming, reduced levels of energy and decreased activity, reduced interaction with other people, thoughts that are unpleasant, negative and persistent, resulting in low self-esteem.

The role the mental health nurse plays in working with Ed demonstrates the special contribution they make to the multidisciplinary team. Based on the symptoms described above, the nurse would be considering a range of care priorities. Importantly, the care priorities and strategies implemented should involve Ed to the extent that he feels up to being involved and be based on collaboration with him and others as he agrees or requests to be involved. Many of the strategies implemented now may well become important strategies that Ed can use on an ongoing basis as his personal recovery journey continues.

SYMPTOM	CARE PRIORITY	STRATEGIES AND RATIONALE
Low mood Social withdrawal	Establish rapport with Ed and begin the process of his personal recovery journey	Use of therapeutic interpersonal skills is essential. Attending, paraphrasing, reflection of feelings together with empathy, genuineness and a non-judgemental presence help demonstrate therapeutic presence.
Persistent negative thoughts Suicide risk	Maintain safety	Risk assessment to ascertain Ed's level of risk for suicide is essential to maintain safety and provide the ongoing opportunity for Ed to speak about his current thoughts related to suicide in a safe and non-judgemental space.
Poor hygiene and grooming Disrupted sleep patterns	Support maintenance of activities of daily living Implement collaborative strategies to regain a more regular sleeping pattern	Develop a plan for a regular time to rise and go to bed. Attend to personal hygiene at the same time. Offer assistance to a level that enables Ed to increasingly assume control over his own personal care. Avoid sleeping during the day. Avoid caffeine drinks at night. Do not lie awake at night for an extended period. Establishing routines such as these while in hospital will help Ed with his transition back home.
	Provide education and support to Ed, Sarah and their sons	Educate Ed on any medications he is prescribed. Include Sarah in this activity with Ed's consent. Review Ed's experience of his symptoms and assist him to place these symptoms in the context of understanding his experience of depression. This will promote self-efficacy in that Ed will learn to recognise his triggers and when to seek increased support.
Discharge planning	Review the supports that Ed has/may wish to access in the community Liaise with the potential case manager as required Construct a recovery and relapse prevention plan with Ed as he feels able to contribute to the process	Thinking about and planning for discharge early increases the supports Ed has available, provides a structured framework for Ed and his family to follow in seeking assistance as they require it, and builds confidence in Ed's capacity to manage his health and well-being into the future.

RECOVERY AND RELAPSE PREVENTION

A person's experience of major depressive disorder will be as varied and unique as people themselves are. People can experience an episode of major depressive disorder at any age; however, about 25% of people who develop a depressive disorder will do so before the age of 20 years, and 50% before the age of 30 years (Kessler et al., 2005).

Depressive symptoms begin to decrease usually within three months of the onset of symptoms in approximately 40% of people diagnosed with a major depressive disorder and up to 80% of people diagnosed with major depressive disorder within one year (APA, 2013). While this is good news for those individuals, there are a proportion of people who will experience delayed and/or less successful outcomes. Factors that are associated with slower and/or lower recovery rates include people who experience depression with psychotic features, pronounced anxiety, personality disorder and severe symptoms.

The risk of recurrence decreases the longer the period between episodes of major depressive disorder. However, the risk of a recurrence of depression is increased if a person has experienced severe symptoms in the previous episode, or has had multiple episodes of depression. Additionally, young people and those individuals who have ongoing mild symptoms of depression even when in remission are at a higher risk of experiencing depression in the future (APA, 2013).

Relapse prevention is an important component of a consumer's recovery journey. Having the knowledge and understanding about how to promote ongoing well-being and to access supports if and as required promotes confidence and a sense of control a person has as they move into the future. Aspects to consider in a relapse prevention plan include:

- *Self-monitoring of mood:* Various tools such as a mood worksheet enable a consumer to rate their mood at different times and in relation to different circumstances.
- *Symptom monitoring:* This is a useful strategy whereby a consumer learns to identify specific symptoms (or warning signs) that may be indicative of a change in their mood and the triggers precipitating these changes; for example, increasing difficulty in concentrating or an increase in negative thinking. Learning what events or circumstances can trigger these symptoms is important in how a consumer then addresses them.
- *Developing strategies that promote health and well-being:* For example, effective sleep hygiene practices, ways to manage stress and developing work/life balance.
- *Having an action plan:* This lists specific actions to be taken such as who to contact, what early interventions may be necessary; for example important contact numbers of health clinicians.

THE FAMILY'S EXPERIENCE OF DEPRESSION

Families play an important role in providing support and information to consumers who have a diagnosis of major depression. It is crucial that nurses recognise the impact that this care-giving role can have on individual family members as well as the family unit, as whole families can experience increased stress that impacts on their own physical and emotional health and well-being, causes disruption to employment, social contacts, and roles and expectations of various family members. This can be experienced as a sense of having to live life around the needs of the consumer, and having to learn to manage a new and sometimes unexpected range of emotions towards the consumer. Families in the early stages of living with a consumer who has been diagnosed with major depression are often on an enormous learning curve themselves in relation to what depression is and gaining insight into it. Some family members describe their lives as 'walking on egg shells' or just trying to 'stay out of the way'.

Support and education are vital for families – not only because these increase their understanding of the reality of what is happening to their loved one, but so that they can support them more effectively in the short to long term. Mental health nurses play a pivotal role through providing education and support to families, that includes education regarding what depression is, the ways in which they may be able to support their family member and, importantly, how to look after themselves. Online resources available through organisations such as SANE Australia, beyondblue, the Black Dog Institute and government resources such as Health Direct are available online and provide information and links to supports that are easily accessible and clearly presented. Sometimes families will also benefit from more specialised support with specialised clinicians such as psychologists. General practitioners also provide a valuable level of support to families.

EVIDENCE-BASED PRACTICE

Families of people living with depression

Title of study

Relatives of patients with depression: experiences of everyday life

Authors

Hege Skundberg-Kletthagen, Sigrid Wangensteen, Marie Louise Hall-Lord and Brigitta Hedelin

Background

Depression is a mental health condition experienced by people across the globe. Families who live with a loved one experiencing symptoms of depression are impacted emotionally, socially, occupationally and physiologically in the context of their caring role. The aim of this project was to describe the experiences of everyday life as a relative of a person diagnosed with depression.

Design

Using a phenomenographic approach, the authors interviewed 24 relatives to illuminate participants' experience and understanding of their everyday experiences.

Results

The major findings from this project identified and described how relatives negotiated the range of feelings experienced, their changing roles in the relationship, the adjustment to daily living, focusing on their own health and managing the situation characterised by a range of contradictions and tension between feeling a duty of care and also experiencing a sense of frustration and negative thoughts

at the way in which caring for a relative impacted on their lives.

Conclusions

Knowledge regarding depression was an important factor in helping relatives understand their role and addressing their own feelings such as shame and hope. This understanding is crucial in that it impacts on how relatives understand and respond to the symptoms of depression, and also importantly how they respond to their relative.

Implications

As part of the multidisciplinary team, mental health nurses have an important role to play in early identification of support needs and education for relatives and developing appropriate interventions to support family members.

QUESTIONS

1 The authors of this article spoke of the need for mental health nurses to be involved in early identification of support needs, education and interventions to appropriately support family members. However, the multidisciplinary team comprises a range of people, including the consumer and their family. How can mental health nurses provide this support through collaboration?

2 Why is it essential to involve the consumer and family in such decision-making?

3 How confident do you feel at this point in taking on such a role?

SOURCE: SKUNDBERG-KLETTHAGEN, H., WANGENSTEEN, S., HALL-LORD, M. & HEDELIN, B. (2014). RELATIVES OF PATIENTS WITH DEPRESSION: EXPERIENCES OF EVERYDAY LIFE. *SCANDINAVIAN JOURNAL OF CARING SCIENCES*, 28(3), 564–71. DOI:10.1111/SCS.12082

REFLECTION ON LEARNING FROM PRACTICE

The emotional turmoil experienced by a person living with a diagnosis of major depressive disorder is unique to them. While two people may have the same diagnosis, to presume that their experience will follow a typical pattern is short sighted and lacks an understanding of the complexity of the condition and the individual circumstances that impact on a person's experience of it.

The comments made by the students reflected their lack of understanding of the complexity of depression and the unique human response to people's experience of it. The event also reminds us that while the circumstances surrounding Elina's experience were extreme, statements such as those made by the students reflected not only a

lack of understanding of depression but objectified Elina's experience. This was potentially unprofessional practice and not reflective of person-centred and recovery-oriented care.

The mental health nurse must position themselves as a collaborator with the consumer. The mental health nurse must be a champion of hope. They must facilitate and help the consumer to build hope and in order to do this, they must have hope themselves.

One mental health nurse stated, 'Consumers have asked me, Why do you stay here? Why do you put up with that?' I say, 'It's because I know that that person is going to get well. You know, I know I'm going to see that person get back to their lives' (Hercelinskyj, 2010).

CHAPTER RESOURCES

SUMMARY

- Major depression is a highly prevalent disorder that impacts on people's lives globally. Major depression is experienced by men and women with a higher proportion of females reporting mood disorders than males.
- There are a variety of theories surrounding the aetiology of major depressive disorder.
- The clinical presentation and assessment of a person experiencing major depressive disorder is multifaceted and must be holistic in order to identify appropriate care priorities with the consumer, and implement relevant strategies. Assessment of suicide risk is an essential element of the mental health nurse's professional responsibilities.
- There are a range of pharmacological, non-pharmacological and physical treatment options available. Treatment is tailored to the specific needs of the consumer and can involve a combination of treatment options.
- Persistent depressive disorder was previously referred to as dysthymia. The key feature of persistent depressive disorder is where a consumer experiences a depressed mood for a period of two years and their depressed mood is experienced more days than not. A person experiencing persistent depressive disorder can describe their mood as 'gloomy' or 'down in the dumps'.

- Major depression can be experienced at any time during the perinatal period. The term perinatal depression is used to highlight that a woman can experience depression across the childbearing continuum. The experience of depression can occur in the antenatal period as well as the postnatal period. In the postnatal period, depression can range from postnatal (baby) blues through to postnatal depression and puerperal psychosis.
- A person can experience depression at any point in their lives. However, depression is not a normal part of ageing. Older people can also experience depression differently to younger people and psychosocial factors can impact on an older person's experience of depression.
- Mental health nurses must work collaboratively with consumers to develop an individualised recovery relapse plan that accounts for the consumer's lived experience of a major depressive episode and is congruent with the recovery journey.
- Major depression is a complex multifaceted condition that impacts on consumers and their families. While there are a range of symptoms associated with depression, each person's experience of this condition is uniquely individual. The mental health nurse has a pivotal role in supporting and working with consumers and families living with the experience of a depressive disorder.

REVIEW QUESTIONS

1 When assessing the consumer with dysthymia, the nurse should expect to find which of the following?
   a Chronic and mild depression
   b Episodic cycles of low and high moods
   c Chronic anxiety superimposed with severe depression
   d Sleep disturbances associated with daytime sleepiness

2 A consumer who has started on an antidepressant medication complains of a dry mouth. The nurse's most appropriate response is to:
   a Call the doctor immediately
   b Offer sugarless gum or sips of water
   c Assess blood pressure
   d Interpret the behaviour as attention seeking

3 During a mental health assessment, the nurse asks the consumer how they are feeling. What domain of the mental state examination is the nurse assessing?
   a Perception
   b Affect
   c Though form
   d Mood

4 Anhedonia is a lack of:
   a Pleasure and enjoyment
   b Speech
   c Thoughts as evidenced by reduced conversation
   d Energy and motivation

5 In addition to depressed mood and sleep disturbance, what are other common symptoms of a major depressive episode?
   a Depersonalisation, self-harm and suicidal ideation
   b Poor concentration, delusions of guilt and anhedonia
   c Apathy, labile mood, incongruent affect
   d Anergia, anhedonia and social withdrawal

6 Mary is a 24-year-old woman who is experiencing a major depressive episode. She has recently commenced on antidepressant medication. What drug classification does Sertraline belong to, and what are the common side effects associated with this drug?

CRITICAL THINKING

1 Has someone you know experienced depression? What signs and symptoms did they experience? What strategies did they find helpful? What were the most challenging moments of their experience?

2 Mental health nurses work closely with consumers who have a lived experience of depression and their families. What are the challenges in their role? How can mental health nurses care for themselves as part of their professional role?

3 What is the difference between grief and depression?

4 What factors increase a person's vulnerability to depression?

5 There is increasing recognition of the experience of depression during the perinatal period. Yet women can be reluctant to accept they are depressed and/or seek help. Why do you think this is the case?

6 Public sporting and media personalities such as Serena Williams, Jessica Rowe, Owen Wilson and Leisel Jones have spoken about their lived experience of depression. What impact do you believe their stories may have on people's understanding of depression and to what extent do you believe this helps to de-stigmatise depression?

USEFUL WEBSITES

- beyondblue: https://www.beyondblue.org.au
- Health direct: https://www.healthdirect.gov.au
- PANDA: https://www.panda.org.au

REFLECT ON THIS

Reflecting on natural disasters
The 2009 Black Saturday and 2019–20 summer bushfires in Victoria had catastrophic consequences for people's mental health across a range of domains, including emotionally and psychologically. To better understand the mental health ramifications of natural disasters such as bushfires, read the following information from beyondblue: https://www.beyondblue.org.au/the-facts/bushfires-and-mental-health

In 2020, the COVID-19 pandemic commenced in the midst of bushfires in some parts of Australia. Consider the potential impact on people's psychological and emotional wellbeing from the pandemic occurring at the same time as the bushfire emergency. The following document from the Black Dog Institute provides information related to the

psychological ramifications of the COVID-19 pandemic: https://www.blackdoginstitute.org.au/wp-content/uploads/2020/04/20200319_covid19-evidence-and-reccomendations.pdf

After reading the article from the Black Dog Institute, reflect on the following questions:

1 What populations are at increased risk in this pandemic situation?

2 What strategies does the document outline for dealing with the mental health ramifications?

3 Based on your understanding of the issues and the information provided, how could you use the suggested strategies in your clinical practice?

REFERENCES

American Psychiatric Association (APA). (2013). *Diagnostic and Statistical Manual of Mental Disorders (DSM-5)* (5th edn). Washington, DC: APA.

Andrews, G., Dean, K., Genderson, M., Hunt, C., Mitchell, P., Sachdev, P. & Trollor, J. (2013). *Management of Mental Disorders* (5th edn). Sydney: School of Psychiatry, University of NSW.

Arroyo, C., Hu, F.B., Ryan, L.M., Kawachi, I., Colditz, G.A., Speizer, F.E. & Manson, J. (2004). Depressive symptoms and risk of type 2 diabetes in women. *Journal of Diabetes Care*, 27(1), 129–33. doi:10.2337/diacare.27.1.129%

Austin, M.-P. & Priest, S.R. (2005). Clinical issues in perinatal mental health: New developments in the detection and treatment of perinatal mood and anxiety disorders. *Acta Psychiatrica Scandinavica*, 112(2), 97–104. doi:doi:10.1111/j.1600-0447.2005.00549.x

Australian Bureau of Statistics (ABS). (2008). *National Survey of Mental Health and Wellbeing: Summary of Results,*

2007. ABS: Canberra. Retrieved from http://www.abs.gov.au/ausstats/abs@.nsf/Latestproducts/4326.0Main%20Features32007?opendocument&tabname=Summary&prodno=4326.0&issue=2007&num=&view=.

Australian Bureau of Statistics (ABS). (2009). *National Survey of Mental Health and Wellbeing: Summary of Results*. 4326.0. ABS: Canberra.

Australian Bureau of Statistics (ABS). (2011). *Gender Indicators, Australia, Jul 2011. 4125.0*. Canberra: ABS. Retrieved from http://www.abs.gov.au/ausstats/abs@.nsf/Lookup/by%20Subject/4125.0~Jul%202011~Main%20Features~Mental%20health~3150.

Australian Bureau of Statistics (ABS). (2016). *Migration, Australia, 2014–15*. ABS: Canberra. Retrieved from http://www.abs.gov.au/ausstats/abs@.nsf/mf/3412.0.

Australian Institute of Health and Welfare (AIHW). (2018). *Mental Health Services in Australia*. Canberra: AIHW. Retrieved from https://www.aihw.gov.au/reports/mental-health-services/

mental-health-services-in-australia/report-contents/summary-of-mental-health-services-in-australia/prevalence-and-policies.

Bernstein, D. (2016). *Psychology: Foundations and Frontiers*. Clifton Park, NY: Cengage Learning.

beyondblue. (2018). *Maternal Mental Health and Wellbeing. Perinatal Depression*. Retrieved from https://healthyfamilies.beyondblue. org.au/pregnancy-and-new-parents/maternal-mental-health-and-wellbeing/depression.

Bhugra, D. (2003). Migration and depression. *Acta Psychiatrica Scandinavica*, 108(s418), 67–72. doi:doi:10.1034/j.1600-0447.108. s418.14.x

Black Dog Institute. (2009). *Facts and Figures about Mental Health and Mood Disorders*. Retrieved from http://www.blackdoginstitute.org. au/docs/Factsandfiguresaboutmentalhealthandmooddisorders.pdf.

Black Dog Institute. (2020). The mental health ramifications of COVID-19: The Australian context. Retrieved from https://www. blackdoginstitute.org.au/wp-content/uploads/2020/04/20200319_ covid19-evidence-and-reccomendations.pdf

Bodkin, J.A. & Goren, J.J. (2017). Not obsolete: Continuing roles for TCAs and MAOIs. *Psychiatric Times*. Retrieved from http://www. psychiatrictimes.com/articles/not-obsolete-continuing-roles-tcas-and-maois.

Centre of Perinatal Excellence. (2019). Postnatal depression. Retrieved from http://cope.org.au/first-year/postnatal-mental-health-conditions/postnatal-depression.

Delgadillo, J., Godfrey, C., Gilbody, S. & Payne, S. (2013). Depression, anxiety and comorbid substance use: Association patterns in outpatient addictions treatment. *Mental Health and Substance Use*, 6(1), 59–75.

Department of Health. (2013). *Nursing Practice: Working with People Prescribed and Undergoing Electroconvulsive Therapy. Department of Health Guideline*. Melbourne: Mental Health, Drugs and Regions Division, Department of Health, Victorian Government.

Department of Health and Human Services. (2015). *Refugee and Asylum Seeker Health*. Retrieved from http://www.health.vic.gov.au/ diversity/refugee.htm.

Di Florio, A., Smith, S. & Jones, I. (2013). Postpartum psychosis. *The Obstetrician & Gynaecologist*, 15, 145–50. doi:10.1111/tog.12041

Diefenbach, G.J., Bragdon, L. & Goethe, J.W. (2013). Treating anxious depression using repetitive transcranial magnetic stimulation. *Journal of Affective Disorders*, 151(1), 365–8. doi:http://dx.doi. org/10.1016/j.jad.2013.05.094

Dixon, L. (2010). Supporting women becoming mothers. In S. Pairman, S.K. Tracy, C. Thorogood & J. Pincombe (eds), *Midwifery: Preparation for Practice* (2nd edn, pp. 574–91). Sydney: Churchill Livingstone/Elsevier.

Dunbar, J.A., Reddy, P., Davis-Lameloise, N., Philpot, B., Laatikainen, T., Kilkkinen, A., Bunker, S.J., Best, J.D., Vartiainen, E., Kai Lo, S., … Janus, E.D. (2008). Depression: An important comorbidity with metabolic syndrome in a general population. *Diabetes Care*, 31(12), 2368–73.

Fairbrother, N., Young, A.H., Janssen, P., Antony, M.M. & Tucker, E.J.B.P. (2015). Depression and anxiety during the perinatal period. *BMC Psychiatry*, 15(1), 206. doi:10.1186/s12888-015-0526-6

Ferrari, A.J., Somerville, A.J., Baxter, A.J., Norman, R., Patten, S.B., Vos, T. & Whiteford, H.A. (2013). Global variation in the prevalence and incidence of major depressive disorder: A systematic review of the epidemiological literature. *Psychological Medicine*, 43(3), 471–81. doi:10.1017/S0033291712001511

Fitzgerald, P.B. (2012). Transcranial magnetic stimulation-based methods in the treatment of depression. *Australian Prescriber*, 35, 59–61, Table 1. Retrieved from https://www.nps.org.au/australian-prescriber/articles/transcranial-magnetic-stimulation-based-methods-in-the-treatment-of-depression.

Friedman, R.A. (2014). Antidepressants' black-box warning – 10 years later. *New England Journal of Medicine*, 371(18), 1666–8. doi:10.1056/ NEJMp1408480

Frisch, N. & Frisch, L.E. (2011). *Psychiatric Mental Health Nursing* (4th edn). Clifton Park, NY: Delmar Cengage Learning.

Galletly, C.A., Loo, C.K., Malhi, G.S., Mitchell, P.B. & Fitzgerald, P. (2015). Why repetitive transcranial magnetic stimulation should be available for treatment resistant depression. *Australian & New Zealand Journal of Psychiatry*, 49(2), pp. 182–3.

Glover, L., Jomeen, J., Urquhart, T. & Martin, C.R. (2014). Puerperal psychosis – a qualitative study of women's experiences. *Journal of Reproductive and Infant Psychology*, 32(3), 254–69. doi:10.1080/0264 6838.2014.883597

Gordon, M. & Melville, G. (2013). Selective serotonin re-uptake inhibitors: A review of the side effects in adolescents. *Australian Family Physician*, 42(9), 620–3. Retrieved from http://search.informit. com.au/documentSummary;dn=537153851446265;res=IELHEA.

Guidi, J., Tomba, E. & Fava, G.A. (2016). The sequential integration of pharmacotherapy and psychotherapy in the treatment of major depressive disorder: A meta-analysis of the sequential model and a critical review of the literature. *American Journal of Psychiatry*, 173(2), 128–37. doi:10.1176/appi.ajp.2015.15040476

Hennegan, J., Redshaw, M. & Kruske, S. (2015). Another country, another language and a new baby: A quantitative study of the postnatal experiences of migrant women in Australia. *Women and Birth*, 28(4), e124–e133. doi:10.1016/j.wombi.2015.07.001

Hercelinskyj, G. (2010). Perceptions of professional identity in mental health nursing and the implications for recruitment and retention. Unpublished Doctoral thesis (Doctor of Philosophy), Charles Darwin University, Darwin.

Higgins, A. (2011). Postpartum psychosis. In C.R. Martin (ed.), *Perinatal Mental Health: A Clinical Guide* (pp. 165–72). Keswick, Cumbria: M&K Publishing.

Hughes, C., Heron, S. & Younge, J. (2014). *CBT for Mild to Moderate Depression and Anxiety: A Guide to Low-intensity Interventions*. Maidenhead, Berkshire: McGraw Hill Education.

Jorm, A.F., Bourchier, S.J., Cvetkovski, S. & Stewart, G. (2012). Mental health of Indigenous Australians: A review of findings from community surveys. *Medical Journal of Australia*, 196(2), 118–21. doi:10.5694/mja11.10041

Kampfe, C.M. (2015). *Counseling Older People: Opportunities and Challenges*. Hoboken, NJ: Wiley.

Kaplan, B.J., Kaplan, V.A. & Ruiz, P. (2015). *Kaplan & Sadock's Synopsis of Psychiatry. Behavioral Sciences/Clinical Psychiatry* (11th edn). Philadelphia, PA: Wolters Kluwer.

Kessler, R.C., Berglund, P., Demler, O., Jin, R., Merikangas, K.R. & Walters, E.E. (2005). Lifetime prevalence and age-of-onset distributions of DSM-IV disorders in the National Comorbidity Survey Replication. *Archives of General Psychiatry*, 62(6), 593–602.

Kposowa, A.J., McElvain, J.P. & Breault, K.D. (2008). Immigration and suicide: The role of marital status, duration of residence, and social integration. *Archives of Suicide Research*, 12(1), 82–92. doi:10.1080/13811110701801044

Leigh, B. & Milgrom, J. (2008). Risk factors for antenatal depression, postnatal depression and parenting stress. *BMC Psychiatry*, 16, 8–24. doi:10.1186/1471-244X-8-24

Luft, B. (2013). Antidepressant switching strategies. *Graylands Hospital Drug Bulletin*, 20(1).

May, R. (n.d.). BrainyQuote.com. Retrieved from BrainyQuote.com, https://www.brainyquote.com/quotes/quotes/r/rollomay158690.html.

May, S., Rapee, R.M., Coello, M., Momartin, S. & Aroche, J. (2014). Mental health literacy among refugee communities: Differences between the Australian lay public and the Iraqi and Sudanese refugee communities. *Social Psychiatry and Psychiatric Epidemiology*, 49(5), 757–69. doi:10.1007/s00127-013-0793-9

McDonald, S. (2016). Mindfulness is not a waste of time – it can help treat depression. *The Conversation*, 27 May. Retrieved from http://theconversation.com/mindfulness-is-not-a-waste-of-time-it-can-help-treat-depression-59100.

Meng, Z., Molyneaux, L., McGill, M., Shen, X. & Yue, D.K. (2014). Impact of sociodemographic and diabetes-related factors on the presence and severity of depression in immigrant Chinese Australian people with diabetes. *Clinical Diabetes*, 32(4), 163–9. doi:10.2337/diaclin.32.4.163

Mergl, R., Henkel, V., Allgaier, A.K., Kramer, D., Hautzinge, M., Kohnen, R., ... Hergerl, U. (2011). Are treatment preferences relevant in response to serotonergic antidepressants and cognitive behavioral therapy in depressed primary patients? *Psychotherapy and Psychosomatics*, 80, 39–47. doi:10.1159/000318772

MIMS Online. (2018). *Monthly Index of Medical Specialities Online*. St Leonards, NSW: MIMS Australia. Retrieved from http://www.mims.com.au.

Minas, H., Kakuma, R., San Too, L., Vayani, H., Orapeleng, S., Prasad-Ildes, R., ... Oehm, D. (2013). *Mental Health Research and Evaluation in Multicultural Australia: Developing a Culture of Inclusion*. Brisbane: Mental Health in Multicultural Australia. Retrieved from http://www.mhima.org.au/pdfs/2093%20MHiMA%20CALD%20REPORT_06-2.pdf.

Monzon, C., Lanza di Scalea & Pearlstein, T. (2014). Postpartum psychosis: Updates and clinical issues. *Psychiatric Times (Special Reports)*. Retrieved from http://www.psychiatrictimes.com/login?referrer=http%3A//www.psychiatrictimes.com%2Fspecial-reports.

Sadock, B.J., Sadock, V.A. & Ruiz, P. (2015). *Kaplan & Sadock's Synopsis of Psychiatry* (11th edn). Philadelphia, PA: Wolters Kluwer.

Sandowsky, J. (2017). Electroconvulsive therapy: A history of controversy, but also of help. *The Conversation*. Retrieved from http://theconversation.com/electroconvulsive-therapy-a-history-of-controversy-but-also-of-help-70938.

Seligman, M.E.P. (1974). Depression and learned helplessness. In R.J. Friedman & M.M. Katz (eds). *The Psychology of Depression:*
Contemporary Theory and Research (pp. 83–113). Washington, DC: Winston.

Singh, M. & Gotlib, I.H. (2014). The neuroscience of depression: Implications for assessment and intervention. *Behaviour Research and Therapy*, 62, 60–73. doi:http://dx.doi.org/10.1016/j.brat.2014.08.008

Skundberg-Kletthagen, H., Wangensteen, S., Hall-Lord, M. & Hedelin, B. (2014). Relatives of patients with depression: Experiences of everyday life. *Scandinavian Journal of Caring Sciences*, 28(3), 564–71. doi:10.1111/scs.12082

Steel, Z., Chey, T., Silove, D., Marnane, C., Bryant, R.A. & van Ommeren, M. (2009). Association of torture and other potentially traumatic events with mental health outcomes among populations exposed to mass conflict and displacement: A systematic review and meta-analysis. *JAMA*, 302(5), 537–49. doi:10.1001/jama.2009.1132

Van Ameringen, M. (2016). Comorbid anxiety and depression in adults: Epidemiology, clinical manifestations and diagnosis. Retrieved from http://www.uptodate.com/contents/comorbid-anxiety-and-depression-in-adults-epidemiology-clinical-manifestations-and-diagnosis#H32457364.

VicHealth Mental Health and Wellbeing Unit. (2007). *Burden of Disease Due to Mental Illness and Mental Health Problems 2007. Research Summary 1*. Retrieved from https://www.vichealth.vic.gov.au/media-and-resources/publications/burden-of-disease-due-to-mental-illness-and-mental-health-problems.

Walter, G., McDonald, A., Rey, J.M. & Rosen, A. (2002). Medical student knowledge and attitudes regarding ECT prior to and after viewing ECT scenes from movies. *Journal of ECT*, 18(1), 43–6.

Wenzel, A., Haugen, E.N., Jackson, L.C. & Brendle, J.R. (2005). Anxiety symptoms and disorders at eight weeks postpartum. *Journal of Anxiety Disorders*, 19(3), 295–311. doi:https://doi.org/10.1016/j.janxdis.2004.04.001

Winkelman M. (2009). *Culture and Health. Applying Medical Anthropology*. San Francisco, CA: John Wiley & Sons.

World Health Organization (WHO). (2018). *Depression. Fact Sheet*. Retrieved from https://www.who.int/news-room/fact-sheets/detail/depression.

CHAPTER 11

ANXIETY DISORDERS

Louise Alexander and Gylo (Julie) Hercelinskyj

LEARNING OUTCOMES

Upon completion of this chapter, you should be able to:

11.1 Gain an understanding of the different anxiety disorders

11.2 Develop an understanding of the aetiology of anxiety disorders, including external causes of disorders

11.3 Understand the key diagnostic criteria for a range of anxiety disorders

11.4 Develop a comprehensive understanding of the treatments associated with anxiety disorders, including the non-pharmacological treatment options associated with anxiety disorders

11.5 Understand nursing interventions for someone experiencing anxiety

LEARNING FROM PRACTICE

I was young…about three or four and we were visiting people on a farm. There were many people there, it was loud and I went along with the other children watching from the sidelines. Suddenly I heard that we were going to get the chicken from outside. They killed the chicken and without warning the carcass was floundering around, blood spurting out and it was all (carcass and blood) heading in my direction. I remember running inside terrified, crying straight into my father's arms and everyone laughed at the little girl crying and screaming. I am nearly 60 now and I have never forgotten that moment. I am terrified of birds. I cannot prepare chicken or duck or any bird. Going to Wilsons Promontory was a nightmare, so is the bird sanctuary in Queensland. I have never watched *Birds* by Alfred Hitchcock, I have hidden in terror from budgerigars… but that's another story.

Juniper, 59, a consumer living with a specific phobia

As evidenced by this vignette, phobias can be very distressing and often involve what may be considered harmless objects or animals by other people. They are, however, extremely distressing and often debilitating to the individual who is afraid of them, and can result in avoidance or isolative behaviours. Everyone has experienced anxiety at some stage in their life. Consider something in your life that has made you feel anxious. What did you do to combat those feelings, and were your techniques successful?

INTRODUCTION

Everyone has experienced **anxiety** at some point in their life. This may have been in the form of apprehension about an upcoming exam or sitting a test for a driver's licence. Anxiety is a normal human response, and for many people it is useful in motivating them to act on something. For example, some people may need to feel the anxiety of potentially failing an exam to be motivated to study for it. Anxiety can come in many forms, including fear, physical reactions such as tightness in the chest, and avoidance behaviours such as failing to go outside. When anxiety becomes overwhelming and impedes someone from living their life, or occurs in the absence of an obvious trigger, this may be indicative of an **anxiety disorder**. One of the main factors associated with anxiety disorders is that the response (anxiety or fear) is deemed disproportionate to the stimulus (e.g. the exam). This chapter explores the different kinds of anxiety disorders:

- generalised anxiety disorder
- specific phobia
- social anxiety disorder
- panic disorder
- agoraphobia.

Table 11.1 outlines the fears commonly experienced by people with anxiety disorders. By understanding these fears, the nurse can assist the individual in working through their anxiety.

TABLE 11.1
Anxiety: feelings, causes and responses

COMMON FEELINGS	CAUSES	RESPONSE
'I feel like I am going mad.'	People often have preconceived ideas about mental illness and these, combined with the symptoms associated with anxiety disorders, can result in significant destabilisation of their perceptions of their own mental health.	Reassurance here is important. Anxiety is extremely common, and responds well to treatment. While the feeling of anxiety is frightening, these feelings are real and not imaginary or the result of a psychotic experience.
'I think I am having a heart attack.'	Panic attacks mimic a heart attack and it is therefore not surprising that this is someone's first line of thought in the presence of physical symptoms such as chest pain or shortness of breath. People with anxiety also tend to be more worrisome in general, and may be more prone to fear of illness, thus exacerbating anxiety symptoms.	After eliminating cardiovascular involvement, reassurance that an individual cannot be physically harmed by anxiety is very important. When the individual is assured that they are not experiencing a heart attack, many will be able to calm down from this knowledge alone. A reminder that they have experienced these symptoms previously without any harm may also be beneficial.
'I'm going to embarrass myself in front of everyone.'	Imagine that you feel like you may faint or be unable to speak in front of people, or that you will try to flee in a perceived stressful situation around others. These are some of the fears experienced by a person with anxiety. The fight or flight response is a primal response aimed at keeping us safe but for people with anxiety, it can cause embarrassment. Unfortunately, worry or concern about this only makes the anxiety worse.	Again, reassurance is key here. Taking the person to a private, quiet area where others cannot observe them is important for the preservation of dignity and can assist in making the individual feel less embarrassed.

WHAT IS ANXIETY?

We use the term 'anxiety' frequently, but what does it actually mean? Anxiety is intense worry, apprehension or unease regarding a particular situation or outcome. There are different components to the experience of anxiety, including physical, psychological and behavioural aspects, as shown in **Table 11.2**. For most people, anxiety occurs in response to a stimulus or trigger; however, for those with an anxiety disorder, anxiety symptoms occur even in the absence of a trigger and can be very distressing. Anxiety is the most common mental health condition in Australia, affecting 14% of the population (ABS, 2008).

TABLE 11.2
Domains of anxiety

PHYSICAL DOMAIN	PSYCHOLOGICAL DOMAIN	BEHAVIOURAL DOMAIN
Palpitations and tachycardia	Feeling of impending doom	Isolation
Dry mouth	Irritable or low tolerance for stress	Avoidance behaviours
Chest pain	Rumination	Aggression towards others
Sweating	Hypervigilance	Increasing consumption of alcohol/illicit drugs
Shortness of breath	Impaired concentration	
GI upset (including nausea and/or diarrhoea)	Feeling 'on edge'	
Headaches	Extreme or irrational fear	
Hot flashes		
Muscle tension		
Insomnia or difficulty 'turning off'		
Trembling, jittering		

What is the difference between anxiety and an anxiety disorder?

You can probably relate to many of the symptoms listed in **Table 11.2**, and it would be more worrisome if you had never experienced anxiety! There are, however, some telltale warnings about everyday, normal anxiety versus disordered worry. These include the duration of anxiety. If the anxiety lasts for a considerable period after the stressful situation has resolved, then this may be suggestive of something more pathological. In addition, disordered anxiety is usually more severe (or becomes progressively intense) and involves behavioural responses (such as avoidance) in an attempt to control situations that are more anxiety provoking. The response is also out of proportion to the potential risk (if any) associated with the stimulus.

It is important to consider the causes and commonalities particular to individuals with anxiety disorders. The next section looks at the aetiology and epidemiology of anxiety disorders as a cluster of conditions rather than individually.

AETIOLOGY

The causes of anxiety disorders are both myriad and multifaceted. While one of the major contributing factors associated with the development of anxiety disorders is genetics; environmental factors are also likely to be a factor rather than genetics alone (Maniglio, 2012). Experiences of childhood trauma and adversity are highly associated with the development of anxiety disorders; in particular, events such as sexual abuse, physical abuse and neglect (Hovens et al., 2012). Rates of anxiety are also higher in children where a parent is also anxious. In terms of parenting characteristics often seen in anxious children, the following have been noted:

- controlling parenting
- over-protectiveness
- over-involved parenting
- critical parenting style that is low in warmth (Rapee, 2014).

Temperament is also a contributing factor associated with the development of many mental health conditions, including anxiety. Childhood temperamental factors associated with anxiety include:

- distress when separated from the primary care provider
- shyness
- withdrawal from social situations including interacting with peers
- fear of new situations
- reluctance to interact with foreign objects or new people (Rapee, 2014).

It is also important to note the impact of external factors when exploring the aetiology of anxiety. In particular, poor resilience (see Chapter 21) and a lack of protective factors are associated with the development and exacerbation of many mental health conditions. Some of the different kinds of *external* issues that may result in anxiety are:

- serious physical illness
- stress associated with work or school
- relationship issues (e.g. divorce)
- response to trauma (e.g. grief from the sudden loss of a spouse)
- use of illicit drugs (e.g. speed, cocaine, 'crack')
- overuse of caffeine
- financial worries
- abuse (verbal, physical, sexual, emotional, bullying)
- sudden life changes (e.g. pregnancy).

Incidence and epidemiology

Anxiety disorders are more prevalent in females and have an average age of onset of 11 years of age (Rapee, 2014). Approximately three-quarters of anxiety disorders emerge by the age of 21 years, making anxiety a particularly prevalent and detrimental condition of childhood and youth.

Comorbidity

Anxiety disorders have a higher comorbidity with depressive disorders and substance-use disorders. In the case of substance-use disorders, it is important to consider whether the use of the substance is in *response* to anxiety (e.g. 'I drink alcohol because it helps me leave the house when I'm anxious') or the *cause* of it (e.g. 'My anxiety started when I started snorting cocaine'). For those with alcohol dependency, what may have begun as 'social lubrication' may have quickly developed into a dependency on alcohol.

Certain mental health conditions are also associated with experiences of anxiety. For example, individuals with autism spectrum disorder (ASD) often present with higher levels of anxiety, and anxiety is one of the clinical features of the condition. Individuals with ASD may also experience other anxiety-type conditions such as compulsions, phobias and social awkwardness that may complicate the process of diagnosis and treatment (Kerns et al., 2015). Often anxiety disorders are seen in the presence of other conditions, and for some conditions such as panic disorder, agoraphobia and generalised anxiety disorder, this comorbidity is highly likely (APA, 2013).

REFLECT ON THIS

Anxiety and COVID-19

A global pandemic is a testing time and even the most resilient person with exceptional mental health would probably admit to struggling with the uncertainty, isolation and unpredictability of this time. The way a person responds to adversity is affected by a number of things, such as their support systems, financial situation, resilience and health. In times of crisis, such as a pandemic, those who may be more susceptible to stress include:

- people with poor physical or mental health or underlying conditions
- carers
- frontline workers
- people whose employment and income have been impacted upon
- those who are socially isolated
- minority populations
- homeless people
- people who use substances (Centers for Disease Control & Prevention, 2021).

Francourt et al. (2020) found that anxiety and depression rates were higher in their UK sample in the early stages of lockdown restrictions, but these rates improved rapidly as people adapted to the new situation. They note the importance of supporting people before and in the early stages of a lockdown to prevent anxiety and depression increasing (Francourt, Steptoe & Bu, 2020).

1   Consider the role of primary healthcare in responding to anxiety symptoms during a period of lockdown. What services/resources are available to support general practitioners in responding to people with increased anxiety in your local area?

2   Consider resources in your local area, in addition to web-based supports. What suggestions can we make to individuals to improve their stress responses and coping mechanisms?

DIAGNOSTIC CRITERIA

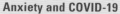

As a cluster of conditions, anxiety disorders include social anxiety disorder, panic disorder, social phobias, agoraphobia and generalised anxiety disorder. Each of their respective diagnostic criteria are listed in their descriptions below.

Social anxiety disorder (social phobia)

Social anxiety disorder (SAD) is a condition associated with considerable anxiety when in social situations. While the idea of giving a speech or presentation to an audience is something that many people will identify as causing some anxiety, for people with SAD, this fear and anxiety is debilitating and interferes with their life considerably. Many people experiencing SAD will simply be unable to do it. For those experiencing SAD, this anxiety occurs in most social situations and the idea of being judged or scrutinised by others is very distressing. The fear of being observed by others may also result in the person being unable to eat in public, and often acute awareness of their anxiety symptoms (such as blushing, sweating or difficulty speaking) results in isolative or avoidance behaviours. The following situations are frequently feared by those with SAD:

- public speaking
- consuming food or drinks in view of others
- social gatherings such as parties
- taking public transport
- waiting in a queue
- speaking to strangers
- using a public toilet (Andrews et al., 2013).

The individual with SAD may experience a panic attack in public, or at the thought of having to make a presentation, for example, and the anticipatory anxiety results in avoiding such situations altogether (APA, 2013). For diagnostic criteria, see **Table 11.3**.

DIAGNOSTIC CRITERIA

Social anxiety disorder (social phobia)

TABLE 11.3
Diagnostic criteria social anxiety disorder (social phobia)

A.	Marked fear or anxiety about one or more social situations in which the individual is exposed to possible scrutiny by others. Examples include social interactions (e.g., having a conversation, meeting unfamiliar people), being observed (e.g., eating or drinking), and performing in front of others (e.g., giving a speech). **Note:** In children, the anxiety must occur in peer settings and not just during interactions with adults.
B.	The individual fears that he or she will act in a way or show anxiety symptoms that will be negatively evaluated (i.e., will be humiliating or embarrassing; will lead to rejection or offend others).
C.	The social situations almost always provoke fear or anxiety. **Note:** In children, the fear or anxiety may be expressed by crying, tantrums, freezing, clinging, shrinking, or failing to speak in social situations.
D.	The social situations are avoided or endured with intense fear or anxiety.
E.	The fear or anxiety is out of proportion to the actual threat posed by the social situation and to the sociocultural context.
F.	The fear, anxiety, or avoidance is persistent, typically lasting for 6 months or more.
G.	The fear, anxiety, or avoidance causes clinically significant distress or impairment in social, occupational, or other important areas of functioning.
H.	The fear, anxiety, or avoidance is not attributable to the physiological effects of a substance (e.g., a drug of abuse, a medication) or another medical condition.
I.	The fear, anxiety, or avoidance is not better explained by the symptoms of another mental disorder, such as panic disorder, body dysmorphic disorder, or autism spectrum disorder.
J.	If another medical condition (e.g., Parkinson's disease, obesity, disfigurement from burns or injury) is present, the fear, anxiety, or avoidance is clearly unrelated or is excessive.

Specify if:
* **Performance only:** If the fear is restricted to speaking or performing in public.

The lifetime prevalence of SAD in Australia is around 11%, making it a common mental health condition (ABS, 2008). For the majority of individuals diagnosed with SAD, the condition onsets between 8–15 years of age (APA, 2013). Perhaps unsurprisingly, SAD comorbidity is often in the realm of other anxiety disorders, substance use disorders and depression (APA, 2013).

Panic disorder

Panic disorder is a physically symptomatic condition characterised by recurring and unexpected **panic attacks** (see **Table 11.4** for details). The individual experiences a distressing array of symptoms occurring in the absence of a trigger, often resulting in panic attacks that become expected or anticipated in similar situations. For many people who experience panic attacks, they will occur when they are resting, relaxing or when they awake from sleep (APA,

2013). Often the individual will think they are having a heart attack, and as such may phone for an ambulance or attend an emergency department.

As with other anxiety conditions, the fear and distress caused by the condition often results in avoidance behaviours, such as avoiding physical exertion. Panic attacks are typically seen (comorbidity) in individuals who also have anxiety disorder, depression or substance use disorders (APA, 2013). For the vast majority of those with panic disorder, agoraphobia and anxiety disorder are common precursors to its development (APA, 2013). In Australia and New Zealand, about 1–2% of the population experience panic disorder, often commencing in early adulthood (Department of Health, 2005). The symptoms (1 to 13 in **Table 11.4**) associated with panic disorder can occur in any anxiety disorder and occur in around 11% of adults (APA, 2013).

DIAGNOSTIC CRITERIA

Panic disorder

TABLE 11.4
Diagnostic criteria panic disorder

A. Recurrent unexpected panic attacks. A panic attack is an abrupt surge of intense fear or intense discomfort that reaches a peak within minutes, and during which time four (or more) of the following symptoms occur: **Note:** The abrupt surge can occur from a calm state or an anxious state. 1. Palpitations, pounding heart, or accelerated heart rate. 2. Sweating. 3. Trembling or shaking. 4. Sensations of shortness of breath or smothering. 5. Feelings of choking. 6. Chest pain or discomfort. 7. Nausea or abdominal distress. 8. Feeling dizzy, unsteady, light-headed, or faint. 9. Chills or heat sensations. 10. Paraesthesias (numbness or tingling sensations). 11. Derealization (feelings of unreality) or depersonalization (being detached from one-self). 12. Fear of losing control or "going crazy." 13. Fear of dying.
B. At least one of the attacks has been followed by 1 month (or more) of one or both of the following: 1. Persistent concern or worry about additional panic attacks or their consequences (e.g. losing control, having a heart attack, "going crazy"). 2. A significant maladaptive change in behavior related to the attacks (e.g., behaviors designed to avoid having panic attacks, such as avoidance of exercise or unfamiliar situations).
C. The disturbance is not attributable to the physiological effects of a substance (e.g. a drug of abuse, a medication) or another medical condition (e.g. hyperthyroidism, cardiopulmonary disorders).
D. The disturbance is not better explained by another mental disorder (e.g. the panic attacks do not occur only in response to feared social situations, as in social anxiety disorder, in response to circumscribed phobic objects or situations, as in specific phobia; in response to obsessions, as in obsessive-compulsive disorder; in response to reminders of traumatic events, as in posttraumatic stress disorder; or in response to separation from attachment figures, as in separation anxiety disorder).

Specific phobia

Phobias are actually quite common. Many people would be able to relate to being afraid of spiders or snakes, for example. What varies with a specific phobia is the degree to which the stimulus causes distress, and the individual's proclivity to avoid situations where the stimulus may be; for example, avoiding visiting family because they will have to take an elevator to reach their apartment. The very idea of taking the elevator is anxiety provoking and results in intense fear. **Table 11.5** outlines the diagnostic criteria for specific phobias. Specific phobias are clustered to identify the stimulus that is fear provoking; for example, it may be flying (situational phobia), mice (animal phobia), thunderstorms (natural environment phobia) or having blood drawn (blood-injection-injury phobia). While the stimulus is very different between these types of phobias, what remains the same is the *response*; the feelings of intense fear and anxiety in relation to the stimulus, and a need (often irrational) to immediately exit what is perceived to be a dangerous situation.

It is not uncommon for individuals to experience a phobic response to more than one stimulus (APA, 2013). Most people experiencing a specific phobia are aware that their fear is irrational, but they are unable to control the anxiety and fear associated with the stimulus. Prevalence rates for specific phobia are between 7–9%, affecting females more frequently (2:1) (APA, 2013).

For some people with a specific phobia, the condition develops in response to a traumatic event, such as a fear of spiders after being bitten by one, but for many individuals the condition is largely unexplained. Comorbidity for specific phobias includes other anxiety-based disorders, and dependent personality disorder (APA, 2013).

Agoraphobia

Imagine that you are crippled with fear and anxiety at the thought of leaving your home or being in a crowd. This is the reality of someone living with **agoraphobia**. Agoraphobia is an intense fear or anxiety state in response to being in open or enclosed spaces (see **Table 11.6** for diagnostic criteria). People with agoraphobia may experience a panic attack at the thought of, or when immersed in, the situation of their fear. For many people with agoraphobia, catastrophising a situation is common. They may feel that they have no ability to escape or exit an enclosed space, or that something horrible will happen to them (APA, 2013). Avoidance behaviours are a common response to potentially distressing situations,

DIAGNOSTIC CRITERIA

Specific phobia

TABLE 11.5
Diagnostic criteria specific phobia

A.	Marked fear or anxiety about a specific object or situation (e.g. flying, heights, animals, receiving an injection, seeing blood). **Note:** In children, the fear or anxiety may be expressed by crying, tantrums, freezing, or clinging.
B.	The phobic object or situation almost always provokes immediate fear or anxiety.
C.	The phobic object or situation is actively avoided or endured with intense fear or anxiety.
D.	The fear or anxiety is out of proportion to the actual danger posed by the specific object or situation and to the sociocultural context.
E.	The fear, anxiety, or avoidance is persistent, typically lasting for 6 months or more.
F.	The fear, anxiety, or avoidance causes clinically significant distress or impairment in social, occupational, or other important areas of functioning.
G.	The disturbance is not better explained by the symptoms of another mental disorder, including fear, anxiety, and avoidance of situations associated with panic-like symptoms or other incapacitating symptoms (as in agoraphobia); objects or situations related to obsessions (as in obsessive-compulsive disorder); reminders of traumatic events (as in posttraumatic stress disorder); separation from home or attachment figures (as in separation anxiety disorder); or social situations (as in social anxiety disorder).

Specify if:
- **Animal** (e.g., spiders, insects, dogs).
- **Natural environment** (e.g., heights, storms, water).
- **Blood-injection-injury** (e.g., needles, invasive medical procedures).
- **Situational** (e.g., airplanes, elevators, enclosed places).
- **Other** (e.g., situations that may lead to choking or vomiting; in children, e.g., loud sounds or costumed characters).

DIAGNOSTIC CRITERIA

Agoraphobia

TABLE 11.6
Diagnostic criteria agoraphobia

A.	Marked fear or anxiety about two (or more) of the following five situations: 1. Using public transportation (e.g. automobiles, buses, trains, ships, planes). 2. Being in open spaces (e.g. parking lots, marketplaces, bridges). 3. Being in enclosed places (e.g. shops, theaters, cinemas). 4. Standing in line or being in a crowd. 5. Being outside of the home alone.
B.	The individual fears or avoids these situations because of thoughts that escape might be difficult or help might not be available in the event of developing panic-like symptoms or other incapacitating or embarrassing symptoms (e.g. fear of falling in the elderly; fear of incontinence).
C.	The agoraphobic situations always provoke fear or anxiety.
D.	The agoraphobic situations are actively avoided, require the presence of a companion, or are endured with intense fear or anxiety.
E.	The fear or anxiety is out of proportion to the actual danger posed by the agoraphobic situations and to the sociocultural context.
F.	The fear, anxiety or avoidance is persistent, typically lasting for 6 months or more.
G.	The fear, anxiety, or avoidance causes clinically significant distress or impairment in social, occupational or other important areas of functioning.
H.	If another medical condition (e.g. inflammatory bowel disease, Parkinson's disease) is present, the fear, anxiety, or avoidance is clearly excessive.
I.	The fear, anxiety, or avoidance is not better explained by the symptoms of another mental disorder – for example, the symptoms are not confined to specific phobia, situational type; do not involve only social situations (as in social anxiety disorder); and are not related exclusively to obsessions (as in obsessive-compulsive disorder), perceived defects or flaws in physical appearance (as in body dysmorphic disorder), reminders of traumatic events (as in posttraumatic stress disorder), or fear of separation (as in separation anxiety disorder).

and this is also common for agoraphobia. The individual may *never* leave their home in response to anticipated panic or fear at this very prospect.

Agoraphobia is much more common in females and occurs in almost 2% of the population. For most, the condition is chronic in nature (APA, 2013).

Generalised anxiety disorder (GAD)

Generalised anxiety disorder (GAD) is a condition characterised by disproportionate worry and anxiety, and is often associated with restlessness and poor concentration (APA, 2013). This worry impacts an individual's life significantly and is diagnosable by the criteria listed in **Table 11.7**.

DIAGNOSTIC CRITERIA

Generalised anxiety disorder

TABLE 11.7
Diagnostic criteria generalised anxiety disorder

A.	Excessive anxiety and worry (apprehensive expectation), occurring more days than not for at least 6 months, about a number of events or activities (such as work or school performance).
B.	The individual finds it difficult to control the worry.
C.	The anxiety and worry are associated with three (or more) of the following six symptoms (with at least some symptoms having been present for more days than not for the past 6 months): **Note:** Only one item is required in children. 1. Restlessness or feeling keyed up or on edge. 2. Being easily fatigued. 3. Difficulty concentrating or mind going blank. 4. Irritability. 5. Muscle tension. 6. Sleep disturbance (difficulty falling or staying asleep, or restless, unsatisfying sleep).
D.	The anxiety, worry, or physical symptoms cause clinically significant distress or impairment in social, occupational, or other important areas of functioning.
E.	The anxiety is not attributable to the physiological effects of a substance (e.g. a drug of abuse, a medication) or another medical condition (e.g. hyperthyroidism).
F.	The disturbance is not better explained by another mental disorder (e.g. anxiety or worry about having panic attacks in panic disorder, negative evaluation in social anxiety disorder (social phobia), contamination or other obsessions in obsessive-compulsive disorder, separation from attachment figures in separation anxiety disorder, reminders of traumatic events in posttraumatic stress disorder, gaining weight in anorexia nervosa, physical complaints in somatic symptom disorder, perceived appearance flaws in body dysmorphic disorder, having a serious illness in illness anxiety disorder, or the content of delusional beliefs in schizophrenia or delusional disorder).

SOURCE: REPRINTED WITH PERMISSION FROM THE *DIAGNOSTIC AND STATISTICAL MANUAL OF MENTAL DISORDERS*, FIFTH EDITION, (COPYRIGHT ©2013). AMERICAN PSYCHIATRIC ASSOCIATION. ALL RIGHTS RESERVED.

COMMONALITIES OF THE MSE: GENERALISED ANXIETY DISORDER

General appearance and behaviour

Psychomotor agitation (restlessness/agitation) may be present. The consumer may appear to be sweating and shaky, with muscle tension. They may find it difficult to sit still, and may complain of nausea or other gastrointestinal upset. They may demonstrate behaviours or physical symptoms related to hyperarousal such as increased respiratory rate (or if severe, hyperventilation). A consumer with anxiety may be amenable to being interviewed, but may be fearful or distressed during the interview.

Speech

The consumer's speech rate may be increased.

Mood

The person may have disturbed sleep patterns (insomnia, difficulty getting to or staying asleep), including rumination. Fatigue may be excessive. Appetite disturbances (poor appetite) may be present and may also be impacted by GI upsets such as nausea and vomiting and diarrhoea. Mood may present as low or depressed (consider the relationship between depression and anxiety), and the person may demonstrate irritability.

Thought content

The consumer may constantly worry about numerous issues and events. This worry is out of proportion to the actual circumstances. Themes relate to anxiety and worry regarding the specific event or situation. This may be something others may consider 'minor' or of little consequence. Catastrophising may occur. A consumer may describe their sense of being unable to exert any control over a situation or events. Consumers engage in negative self-talk regarding their inability to control events and situations and the consequences of this.

Cognition

The consumer may experience difficulties in concentration and be easily distracted. They may also experience memory impairment (e.g. they cannot remember daily commitments/responsibilities, etc).

Insight

While a consumer will usually understand that their fear/anxiety is unwarranted, they are unable to manage their anxiety effectively and continue to feel overwhelmed (adapted from APA, 2013; Johnson, 2018).

CASE **STUDY**

MAJOR LIFE EVENTS AND EXPERIENCE OF ANXIETY

Andrew is a recently widowed 66-year-old man with three adult children. Andrew's wife of 40 years died two years ago and he has been living alone since then with good family supports. Recently, his employer of 22 years went through a restructure, and Andrew's job has become much more technical and challenging. Andrew now has to present reports to a number of senior managers on a semi-regular basis. Andrew wants to retire in a few years, but is not enjoying the sudden changes to his role and is starting to experience extreme reactions to public speaking. There are many younger workers in his department, with more tertiary qualifications, and sometimes he feels like a rabbit being surrounded by prey. They all seem to want his job and are so confident that he feels they probably would do a better job. Andrew admits that when the company went through the restructure, he was still grieving the loss of his wife and did not concentrate in the seminars on the expectations of his new role, and feels both unprepared and confused. Lately, in the week prior to presenting to his managers, Andrew finds it difficult to sleep and spends hours looking over his report, but he cannot concentrate on it enough to make any changes. On the day of his presentation, Andrew won't eat breakfast as he feels he may be sick, he has sweaty palms and a racing heart. He is so nervous and self-conscious during his presentation that he forgets important information, and has trouble answering simple questions. He is convinced he looks like a fool! At home he is distracted, and has been avoiding social situations with his children (which is very out of character). Last week Andrew's manager requested a meeting to discuss his performance. Andrew is convinced he is about to be performance-managed out of the company.

Questions

1 How would you differentiate between anxiety and an anxiety disorder?
2 Andrew's experiences are not uncommon for someone who is both newly widowed and approaching retirement in a restructured working environment. He is exhibiting a number of physiological, psychological and behavioural changes. List your findings for each change in Andrew's presentation.

About 3% of adults have GAD, and for many there are physical symptoms associated with the condition, such as gastrointestinal upset or sweating (APA, 2013). In addition, GAD is more commonly seen in females, and may be exacerbated by lifetime periods of stress (e.g. job changes, family issues, physical illness, etc.). For most people who experience GAD, the condition is preceded by a typically anxious experience of life, and for many with this disorder the course is chronic.

TREATMENT OF ANXIETY DISORDERS

Like all mental health conditions, recommendations for treatment of anxiety disorders are a combination of both pharmacological and psychotherapeutic interventions, such as cognitive behavioural therapy.

Pharmacological treatment

Fortunately, pharmacological treatment is readily available and effective for those experiencing anxiety disorders. Clinically indicated long-term treatment of anxiety disorders is antidepressants and beta-blockers, and on a short-term basis, anxiolytics such as diazepam are used.

If individuals experience *occasional* panic attacks, diazepam, clonazepam and lorazepam are effective medications in eliminating the symptoms of a panic attack. Safe long-term pharmacological treatment for anxiety and prevention of panic attacks are antidepressants, including sertraline, fluoxetine and paroxetine. It is important to consider that the side effects of benzodiazepine (see **Table 11.8**) will usually render

SAFETY FIRST

HYPERVENTILATION AND ANXIETY

Hyperventilation is common during panic attacks and usually makes anxiety worse. Aside from distress and apprehension, hyperventilation usually causes the individual to feel:

- dizzy
- palpitations
- breathless
- tingling in hands or feet
- lightheaded or like they are going to faint.

During a panic attack the following strategies may be useful to implement:

- have the person sit down. Rapid respirations associated with hyperventilation are caused by elevated oxygen levels (and too little carbon dioxide), causing constriction of blood vessels to the brain and resulting in the individual losing consciousness. If they do not sit down, they may fall and injure themselves
- have them take slow, normal breaths from their belly, or breathe slowly through their nose
- take normal breaths and hold them before exhaling; for example, take a breath in, hold for five seconds, and take five seconds to release this breath
- utilise practised panic attack strategies such as mindfulness or relaxation techniques.

Panic attacks can mimic a cardiac arrest and this means it is important to consider that this may be a more serious health care issue. In the event that you are unsure, always consult a doctor.

TABLE 11.8
Medications for anxiety disorders

MEDICATION	ANXIETY CONDITION
SELECTIVE SEROTONIN REUPTAKE INHIBITORS (SSRIs)	
Fluoxetine	SAD, GAD, panic disorder
Fluvoxamine	SAD, GAD, panic disorder
Sertraline	SAD, GAD, panic disorder
Paroxetine	SAD, GAD, panic disorder
Escitalopram	SAD, GAD, panic disorder
Citalopram	GAD, panic disorder
SEROTONIN-NOREPINEPHRINE REUPTAKE INHIBITORS (SNRIs)	
Venlafaxine	SAD, GAD, panic disorder
Duloxetine	SAD, GAD, panic disorder
BETA-BLOCKERS	
Propranolol	SAD
Atenolol	SAD
ANTIANXIETY	
Buspirone hydrochloride	GAD, panic disorder

SOURCE: ANDREWS ET AL., 2013; MIMS ONLINE, 2018

driving and operating machinery dangerous. As such, individuals who take benzodiazepine for an acute episode of panic in a place other than their home may need to consider how the medication will affect them for the time period following. Beta-blockers are also increasingly prescribed for anxiety and include propranolol and atenolol. **Table 11.8** discusses the use of antidepressants in anxiety disorders. For more detailed information on individual medications, refer to Chapter 10.

Anxiolytics

Anxiolytics from the benzodiazepine family are potent anxiolytics, well understood and can be useful in the treatment of acute anxiety symptoms, such as in the event of a panic attack. However, as mentioned in the 'Safety first' box, benzodiazepines are well known for their addictive properties and as such are only used on a short-term (no longer than 2–3 weeks) basis, or as treatment for sporadic, acute anxiety attacks. It is also the nurses responsibility to be aware of, and recognise, signs of overdose.

Table 11.9 outlines the different types of antianxiety medications, including dose ranges and side effects.

Beta-blockers

Beta-blockers are now more commonly prescribed for individuals who experience panic symptoms, as they can address many of the debilitating physical symptoms such as palpitations. When administering a beta-blocker, it is important to consider that while elevated heart rate may resolve with the medication, hypotension may also occur. As such, the consumer needs to be informed of the signs of hypotension, such as:

- dizziness
- light-headedness
- fainting
- unsteadiness
- blurred vision
- nausea.

In the event that hypotension occurs, individuals should be warned of the potential for fainting and dizziness, and referred to their primary health care worker for medication review.

SAFETY FIRST

USE OF ANXIOLYTICS

While anxiolytics such as diazepam are effective in controlling the distressing symptoms of panic, they are clinically indicated for short-term use only. Diazepam, in particular, is clinically useful in managing panic attacks because it is rapid-acting and, due to its longer half-life, is the least addictive of what is essentially a *very* addictive group of medications. Benzodiazepines are notoriously addictive and this is one of the major reasons they are infrequently (or reluctantly) prescribed.

Care should always be used when administering PRN benzodiazepines that mental health consumers avoid dependence on medications that are both difficult to obtain from a doctor and easy to become dependent on. Nurses should actively seek non-pharmacological ways to assist consumers in managing their anxiety and distress to enhance effective coping in the absence of clinical staff and reduce reliance on medication. Consider the impacts on a consumer who not only has to manage their mental health condition, but additionally a reliance to a medication that can easily turn into a substance use disorder.

TABLE 11.9
Antianxiety medications

MEDICATION NAME	DOSE RANGE	SIDE EFFECTS AND INDICATION
Alprazolam	0.5–1.5 mg daily in divided doses (max. 4 mg daily)	Short-term use for anxiety, and panic disorder. Side effects: • drowsiness • light-headedness • dizziness.
Clonazepam	1 mg/day Maintenance 4–8 mg/day Max. 20 mg daily	Short-term use for anxiety. Side effects: • drowsiness • somnolence • ataxia • behavioural problems • hypersalivation • fatigue • muscle weakness • vertigo.
Diazepam	5–40 mg is the usual adult dose in divided doses. Dosage needs to be adjusted for consumers who have hepatic or renal disease and lower doses are required for older people.	Short-term use for acute anxiety. Side effects are dose related and include: • drowsiness • fatigue • muscle weakness • ataxia.
Lorazepam	2–3 mg in divided doses (with a range between 1–10 mg)	Short-term relief of anxiety. Side effects: • amnesia • dizziness • sedation • unsteadiness • weakness.
Oxazepam	Mild–moderate anxiety 7.5–15 mg (TDS-QID) Severe anxiety 15-30 mg (TDS-QID)	Short-term use for anxiety. Side effects: • drowsiness.
Clobazam	10–30 mg/day	Short-term use (<4 weeks) for acute anxiety and sleep disturbance associated with anxiety. Side effects: • sedation • tiredness • drowsiness.

SOURCE: MIMS ONLINE, 2018

Why is anxiety treated with antidepressants?

There are reasons why antidepressants are not only indicated in the treatment of anxiety, but they are highly successful too. This can be a little confusing, and cause people to think that anxiety and depression are the same, or a similar, condition. While anxiety and depression are separate conditions, both impact on the same neurotransmitters in the brain, and as such can be treated with similar medications. Antidepressants affect the neurotransmitter serotonin, which plays an important role in regulating anxiety. Antidepressants are useful in alleviating anxiety and reducing repetitive thinking (as seen in OCD) in addition to successfully treating depression.

SSRI antidepressants have proven effective in alleviating symptoms of anxiety *regardless* of its origin or diagnostic label. For example, SSRIs work well for people with post-traumatic stress disorder (PTSD), OCD, anxiety disorders, self-harm and eating disorders. The similarity or pattern here is the alleviation of anxiety, which is of multiple diagnostic causes. What they all have in common is the experience of anxiety; what is dissimilar, is its manifestation.

Non-pharmacological interventions

While many people will find medications useful in managing the symptoms of their anxiety either short-or long-term, the individual also needs to think about how they can begin to retrain how they respond to situations and events that cause feelings of anxiety or panic. The decision to use either a combination of pharmacological and non-pharmacological treatments or a single approach is developed by the consumer together with their treating team. **Table 11.10** outlines some common non-pharmacological approaches used in managing anxiety.

TABLE 11.10
Non-pharmacological approaches used in managing anxiety

THERAPY	DESCRIPTION	NOTES
Graded exposure	Graded exposure aims to help a person break the pattern of avoidance to feared objects or situations. The goal of a graded approach is to help the consumer develop a fear hierarchy in which they rank the feared object/situation in terms of the level of anxiety they experience in confronting it.	Graded exposure sits under the umbrella of exposure therapy. There are several types of exposure therapy. The term 'graded exposure' refers to the pacing of the therapy.
Systematic desensitisation (SD)	A therapeutic approach based on the principles of classical conditioning. Exposure to a feared object/situation is combined with relaxation exercises to help a person feel more in control and able to manage their feelings. The feared object/situation is ranked in terms of the level of anxiety experienced from least to most feared. The person learns to associate the feared objects, activities or situations with relaxation. The person reconditions the way they respond to the situation. Classical conditioning is explained in Chapter 2.	SD sits under the umbrella of exposure therapy but includes specific behaviour management techniques. Developed by Wolpe (1958) in the mid-20th century, SD is based on the idea that it is impossible to be simultaneously afraid and relaxed. Implementing relation/breathing techniques and feeling calm in low-anxiety producing situations then enables a person to progress to more intense situations. SD is increasingly used through the process of virtual reality or virtual desensitisation. This provides the possibility of using realistic situations which can be monitored in the safety of the therapeutic environment as opposed to a person having to encounter feared objects/situations in the external world, potentially unsupported (Bernstein, 2016).
E-therapies	Effective for mild to moderate anxiety. Based on cognitive behavioural principles, a person is taught to identify and change thought patterns that are impeding their ability to overcome their anxiety. E-therapy is self-paced and can incorporate support from an external counsellor.	E-therapies are said to be cost-effective, have the potential to reach vulnerable and disenfranchised groups and are accessible to people living in rural and remote areas (Wodarski & Frimpong, 2014).
Cognitive behavioural therapy	CBT is covered in Chapter 4. It is used in the treatment of anxiety disorders to help a person recognise unhelpful patterns that are contributing to their anxiety, in order for them to be able to make changes to replace these thoughts with thoughts that reduce anxiety and improve their coping skills.	As part of the treatment process, CBT will utilise a number of behavioural techniques, such as progressive muscle relaxation, breathing techniques and graded exposure. Cognitive strategies such as challenging 'faulty' thinking (e.g. overgeneralisation or catastrophising) and cognitive restructuring are used.
Acceptance and commitment therapy (ACT)	ACT is covered in Chapter 4. It is a therapeutic approach for learning skills to help a person accept what is outside their personal control (such as never experiencing feelings of anxiety) and committing to action that enriches their lives. In the context of anxiety disorders, this means that a person works on understanding their anxiety/fear/panic and how they can relate to it, rather than learning techniques to avoid the feelings of anxiety.	All people experience anxiety; it is part of the range of human responses that can be experienced. Using mindfulness-based techniques, a person can learn to work with these feelings as opposed to trying to ignore or escape them.
Relaxation methods	These methods include, for example, progressive muscle relaxation, whereby a person is taught to progressively tense different muscles and then release that tension before moving on to the next muscle group (Park, 2013). Chen et al. (2009) found that progressive muscle relaxation was effective in managing anxiety for consumers who had a diagnosis of schizophrenia.	A more recent systematic review of the benefits of progressive muscle relaxation for individuals receiving chemotherapy (Pelekasis, Matsouka & Koumarianou, 2017) concluded that while it may improve symptoms of anxiety for this population group, more rigorous studies need to be conducted in order to provide higher quality evidence.

SOURCE: ADAPTED FROM BERNSTEIN, 2016; BEYONDBLUE, 2016; PARK, 2013; PELEKASIS, MATSOUKA & KOUMARIANOU, 2017; WODARSKI & FRIMPONG, 2014

HOW DO MENTAL HEALTH NURSES ASSIST A PERSON EXPERIENCING ANXIETY?

Nursing approaches to assisting a person experiencing anxiety focus on supportive interventions, therapeutic communication and education. Earlier in this chapter, we introduced specific strategies to assist a person who is experiencing a panic attack.

Supportive interventions are based on principles of promoting a sense of emotional and physical safety. Sitting with a consumer, decreasing the amount of stimulation they are encountering in the immediate area, remaining calm and using clear concise language are all ways in which the mental health nurse can assist a person who is experiencing anxiety. The use of PRN (when necessary) medications may be indicated

if the person is experiencing high levels of anxiety, but it is a short-term alternative. In addition, it is very important to promote the use of deep breathing and relaxation techniques that a person can use to prevent/manage/reduce the impact of anxiety. This knowledge empowers a person to be in control at a time when anxiety can strip a person of their feeling of control. When the person is less anxious, provide opportunities for exploring possible catalysts that increase feelings of anxiety and strategies that the person has used previously that have been successful. Working from a strengths-based perspective is a powerful reinforcer for the individual, as it shows them they do have skills and strengths they can draw on. Reinforcing and supporting a person in these ways are part of what is the *core business* of mental health nursing. The following nursing care plan draws together a number of these ideas.

NURSING CARE PLAN

MANAGING PANIC ATTACKS

Consumer Diagnosis: Panic Attacks
Nursing Diagnosis: Extreme fear/panic whereby Maeve experiences feelings of intense dread and anxiety, tightness in the chest, palpitations, sweating and difficulty breathing.
Outcomes: Develop strategies to manage any future episodes of panic.

Maeve is a 42-year-old woman who recently presented to the emergency department. Maeve was driving to work along a busy arterial road when she suddenly felt faint and

experienced tightness in her chest and difficulty breathing. She managed to turn into a side street, where she continued to experience these symptoms for several minutes before they subsided. Eventually, the symptoms settled down, which enabled Maeve to contact her partner. She attended the emergency department, where a range of tests were performed with all results being within normal parameters. Since this first visit, Maeve has experienced several more of these episodes. As nothing physiological was identified, Maeve has been asked to visit her local GP, who has referred her for assessment to the practice nurse.

ASSESSMENT DATA OBJECTIVE (O) SUBJECTIVE (S)	EVIDENCE-BASED RATIONALE	RATIONALE	CONSUMER RESPONSE
Maeve describes how she feels a sudden, severe and uncontrollable anxiety (S). She does not understand what is happening to her and why the ED staff won't take her concerns seriously (S). States, 'I feel like I am having a heart attack or am going to suffocate.' (S)	Provide psychoeducation that encompasses information and education about anxiety. Be non-judgemental and empathic.	Education provides Maeve with information to help her understand the possible context of the symptoms she is experiencing. Maeve has already encountered possible negative attitudes from health care staff. Panic attacks are a terrifying experience for a person and this must be acknowledged.	Maeve begins to understand the connections between events, her thinking and response. She increasingly implements strategies to manage any future episode of panic. She feels supported and maintains an ongoing relationship with her GP, practice nurse and other health care professionals.

SECTION 2

ASSESSMENT DATA OBJECTIVE (O) SUBJECTIVE (S)	EVIDENCE-BASED RATIONALE	RATIONALE	CONSUMER RESPONSE
Maeve is worried about driving and being alone in case she has further episodes of this intense anxiety. She has subsequently gone on sick leave and is increasingly restricting her activities socially (S). Electrocardiogram (ECG): NAD (O) Blood test results: NAD (O)	Implement strategies that Maeve can learn to implement to manage any episode of panic. Refer to appropriate health care professional after discussion with Maeve and GP. Maeve with her GP will also discuss the usefulness of any pharmacological treatment.	Interventions such as CBT can help Maeve understand the process she is going through and the way in which her faulty thinking is impacting on her emotions and physiological response behaviour. Homework can assist Maeve to identify possible triggers that precede an episode of panic. Using active strategies such as deep breathing, positive coping statements, distraction techniques, etc. can help Maeve develop different ways to manage symptoms of panic in the early stages. ACT can help Maeve develop an awareness of her bodily sensations and help her to learn to understand the difference between bodily symptoms as a phenomenon that all people can experience and thinking which interprets them as something to be fought against.	

SOURCE: ADAPTED FROM JAKOPAC & PATEL, 2009

REFLECTION ON LEARNING FROM PRACTICE

Juniper's experience of anxiety reflects a number of ideas presented in this chapter. Juniper has avoided activities and situations which bring her into contact with her feared object and these restrictions have often isolated her from activities that others would see as either normal daily activities (cooking) or pleasure activities (camping).

She has traditionally used humour as a way to try and deflect the odd looks she gets from people when they find out about her fears. She uses relaxation and deep breathing whenever she is at the market with her husband and jokes that she married a man who enjoys cooking so that she wouldn't have to deal with that side of things. These coping strategies have worked for her in the context of her life. She knows that for others, their experience of anxiety is far more debilitating.

CHAPTER RESOURCES

SUMMARY

- Anxiety is intense worry, apprehension or unease regarding a particular situation or outcome. Anxiety is a response that all people experience, and can actually be a motivating experience.
- Anxiety becomes 'disordered' when the duration and severity of the experience are extreme and the response is out of proportion to the perceived risk. Behaviours engaged in by the person to control the situation are also extreme.

- Diagnostic criteria for anxiety disorders are varied and can have significant impacts on individuals.
- Treatment for anxiety disorders involves pharmacological treatment as well as behavioural strategies.
- The mental health nurse can implement a range of strategies to assist a person experiencing anxiety.

REVIEW QUESTIONS

1   A specific phobia is characterised by the following feature:
    a   Marked fear or anxiety about a specific object or situation
    b   Feelings of intense hatred towards the specific object
    c   Excessive anxiety and worry
    d   Intense anxiety related to public speaking

2   Warren avoids using public transport and being in enclosed spaces. Each time he finds himself in these situations, he experiences extreme anxiety and has a panic attack. He has increasingly isolated himself at home, stating, 'There's no need to go out. I can do everything from my computer.' Warren is likely to be experiencing:
    a   Social anxiety disorder
    b   Generalised anxiety disorder
    c   Agoraphobia
    d   Specific phobia

3   Evan is 60, a registered nurse who works in a disaster response team attached to a major hospital in remote Australia. Following a recent natural disaster, Evan was involved in a mass casualty event resulting in a high death toll, including the loss of several members of the medical team of which he was part. Following a mandatory debriefing and counselling process, Evan returned to work in the operating theatre at his local hospital. Several weeks after his return to work, while he was preparing to assist in a surgical case, Evan started to feel his heart race; he felt dizzy, he could not focus on what he was doing and his chest was tight. He was to taken to the emergency department, where he described that he felt he was having a heart attack.
    a   What condition is Evan experiencing?
    b   What specific actions could the mental health nurse implement at this time?

4   Imagine you are asked to give an education session to other students on generalised anxiety disorder. How would you explain the key features of this condition to them?

5   What education should the mental health nurse provide to a consumer who has been prescribed benzodiazepine for the treatment of their anxiety disorder?

6   Why are antidepressants used in the treatment of anxiety disorders?

CRITICAL THINKING

1   Anxiety and depression are often mistaken as being the same condition, or believed to go hand-in-hand. Why is this?

2   Describe the physiological, psychological and behavioural symptoms of anxiety.

3   Sarah has a phobia to needles and you need to draw blood for an urgent test. Discuss how you would approach this.

USEFUL WEBSITES

- Anxiety and Depression Association of America (ADAA): https://adaa.org
- beyondblue: https://www.beyondblue.org.au

- Way Ahead – Mental Health Association of Australia: http://wayahead.org.au

REFLECT ON THIS

National response to crisis situations

Australia frequently experiences devastating bushfires. As noted in earlier chapters, the summer of 2019–20 saw massive areas of the country destroyed by bushfires that, in some instances, burned for months. These types of crisis events can have a devastating impact on people's mental health. Navigating normal responses to trauma, such as fear and stress, while being aware that these responses can transition into more serious responses such as PTSD, is important. Our mental health is also affected by our financial situation, employment and housing.

Using your computer's search engine, research the national response by mental health services for people impacted by bushfires. How are people affected by bushfires supported during and after such crises?

REFERENCES

American Psychiatric Association (APA). (2013). *Diagnostic and Statistical Manual of Mental Disorders (DSM-5)* (5th edn). Washington, DC: APA.

Andrews, G., Dean, K., Genderson, M., Hunt, C., Mitchell, P., Sachdev, P. & Trollor, J. (2013). *Management of Mental Disorders* (5th edn). Sydney: School of Psychiatry, University of NSW.

Australian Bureau of Statistics (ABS). (2008). *National Survey of Mental Health and Wellbeing: Summary of Results, 2007.* Cat. no. 4326.0. Canberra: ABS.

Bernstein, D. (2016). *Psychology: Foundations and Frontiers.* Toronto: Cengage Learning.

beyondblue. (2016). *Psychological Treatments for Anxiety.* Retrieved from https://www.beyondblue.org.au/the-facts/anxiety/treatments-for-anxiety/psychological-treatments-for-anxiety.

Centers for Disease Control & Prevention. (2021). Coping with stress. Retrieved from https://www.cdc.gov/coronavirus/2019-ncov/daily-life-coping/managing-stress-anxiety.html.

Chen, W.-C., Chu, H., Lu, R.-B., Chou, Y.-H., Chen, C.-H., Chang, Y.-C., … Chou, K.-R. (2009). Efficacy of progressive muscle relaxation training in reducing anxiety in patients with acute schizophrenia. *Journal of Clinical Nursing*, 18(15), 2187–96. doi:10.1111/j.1365-2702.2008.02773

Department of Health. (2005). *What Is Panic Disorder and Agoraphobia?* Australian Government, Department of Health. Retrieved from http://www.health.gov.au/internet/publications/publishing.nsf/Content/mental-pubs-p-panic-toc~mental-pubs-p-panic-wha.

Francourt, D., Steptoe, A. & Bu, F. (2020). Trajectories of anxiety and depressive symptoms during enforced isolation due to COVID-19 in England: A longitudinal observational study. *The Lancet.* https://doi.org/10.1016/S2215-0366(20)30482-X

Hovens, J.G.F.M., Giltay, E.J., Wiesma, J.E., Spinhoven, P., Pennix, B.W.J.H. & Zitman, F.G. (2012). Impacts of childhood life events and trauma on the course of depressive and anxiety disorders. *Acta Psychiatrica Scandinavica*, 126(3), 198–207.

Jakopac, K. A. & Patel, S. C. (2009). *Psychiatric and Mental Health Case Studies and Care Plans.* Burlington, MA: Jones and Bartlett Learning.

Johnson, S. (2018). *Therapist's Guide to Clinical Intervention: The 1-2-3s of Treatment Planning* (2nd edn). London: Academic Press.

Kerns, C.M., Kendall, P.C., Zickgraf, H., Franklin, M.E., Miller, J. & Herrington, J. (2015). Not to be overshadowed or overlooked: Functional impairments associated with comorbid anxiety disorders in youth with ASD. *Behaviour Therapy*, 46, 29–39.

Maniglio, R. (2012). Child sexual abuse in the etiology of anxiety disorders: A systematic review of reviews. *Trauma, Violence & Abuse*, 14(2), 96–112.

MIMS Online. (2018). Retrieved from https://www.mimsonline.com.au/Login/Login.aspx?ReturnUrl=%2f.

Park, C. (2013). Mind-body CAM interventions: Current status and considerations for integration into clinical health psychology. *Journal of Clinical Psychology*, 69(1), 45–63. doi:10.1002/jclp.21910

Pelekasis, P., Matsouka, I. & Koumarianou, A. (2017). *Progressive Muscle Relaxation as a Supportive Intervention for Cancer Patients Undergoing Chemotherapy: A Systematic Review* (vol. 15), pp. 465–73. Cambridge: Cambridge University Press.

Rapee, R.M. (2014). Preschool environment and temperament as predictors of social and non-social anxiety disorders in middle adolescence. *Journal of the American Academy of Child and Adolescent Psychiatry*, 53(3), 320–8.

Wodarski, J.S. & Frimpong, J. (2014). Application of e-therapy programs to social work practice. In J.S. Wodarski & S.V. Curtis (eds), *E-therapy for Substance Use and Co-morbidity.* Cham: Springer International.

Wolpe, J. (1958). *Psychotherapy by Reciprocal Inhibition.* Palo Alto, CA: Stanford University Press.

PERSONALITY DISORDERS

Louise Alexander

LEARNING OUTCOMES

Upon completion of this chapter, you should be able to:

12.1 Define personality disorders and understand general personality disorder as a baseline for all 10 behaviours and conditions discussed in this chapter

12.2 Understand the characteristics of cluster *A*, *B* and *C* personality disorders

12.3 Develop a comprehensive understanding of antisocial personality disorder aetiology, epidemiology, treatment and management

12.5 Develop a comprehensive understanding of borderline personality disorder aetiology, epidemiology, treatment and management

LEARNING FROM PRACTICE

There are times when I wonder how anyone in my family can put up with me. Life has been difficult ever since I can remember and I guess I didn't know how to cope with it. At the time, cutting seemed like a way of managing my overwhelming feelings of pain…not physical pain, but emotional pain. It started as a one-off thing…probably like when people take drugs. Cutting is my drug I guess. Other girls at school were doing it too, it didn't seem so unusual. It wasn't until I finished school and then realised it was the way I dealt with everything that I knew I actually needed the help my family had been trying to make me get for years. My relationship with my mum and sisters was so chaotic. I would get so angry at them for the stupidest of things, and then wonder why they wouldn't forgive me when I said I was sorry.

I moved out when I was 19 and things really haven't gotten better. I am 24 now and have a part-time job but the struggle not to cut, to see my blood seep, to feel the relief is there all the time. I don't actually want to die, but people don't get that…think I'm crying out for help or being a drama queen.

They don't understand. I don't really understand myself, so how can I expect other people to? I've been in hospital a few times, usually after a break-up with my boyfriend where I lose all control. Sometimes being in hospital helps, and talking with my psychologist helps, and we've developed strategies for me to use instead of cutting. Sometimes these help, but not always. I hope one day, I won't need to rely on therapy to get through a bad day.

Tara, 24-year-old consumer who has a diagnosis of borderline personality disorder

Tara's experiences of borderline personality disorder are common for consumers with this condition. As we can see Tara's behaviour has impacted on not only her, but on the lives of those around her. What do you think may be some of the family impacts associated with borderline personality disorder? In your response consider what typical family responses may be to Tara's behaviours.

INTRODUCTION

Conditions of personality are complex and frequently involve disturbances in behavioural, cognitive and emotional regulation. These patterns are generally enduring, often commencing early in life, and may be associated to comorbidity with other mental health conditions, resulting in significant distress for the consumer and those around them. This chapter explores the notion of 'personality', while providing an overview of the different personality disorders, their clinical manifestations and treatment options. Not all personality disorders feature prominently in mental health acute care settings; in fact, some consumers will have a personality disorder as a secondary comorbidity, resulting in reduced emphasis on management and care in the clinical environment. Of all the personality disorders seen in acute care settings, however, borderline personality disorder (BPD) is often perceived to be the most challenging for mental health clinicians and thus is more extensively explored in this chapter. Much like BPD, antisocial personality disorder (ASPD) can create a number of challenges for clinicians working in mental health, and as such this condition is also thoroughly explored.

DEFINING PERSONALITY AND UNDERSTANDING GENERAL PERSONALITY DISORDER

People use the term 'personality' frequently, but what exactly is our personality? There have been many proffered explanations; however, generally, personality is a:

> dynamic integration of the totality of a person's subjective experience and behaviour patterns, including both (1) conscious, concrete, and habitual behaviours, experiences of self and the surrounding world, conscious, explicit psychic thinking, and habitual desires and fears and (2) unconscious behaviour patterns, experiences and views, and intentional states. (Kernberg, 2016, p. 145)

As can be seen in Kernberg's description, the concept of personality is multifaceted and is impacted by both internal and external factors, and particularly how the individual responds to these factors. When exploring personality, it is important to note that *cognition* (our ability to understand, and acquire knowledge of our environment), *perception* (our interpretation of the environment) and *affect* (our responses or reactions) are all significant in this experience.

Personality traits

Psychologists have identified the common **personality traits** among humankind, and these are colloquially known as the 'big five'. The 'big five' personality inventory is considered one of the most rigorous methods of exploring personality; that is, most individuals will fall within one of these five traits. While the list is not exhaustive, it is common for individuals to identify certain aspects of personality that fall within one of the five traits listed below. For some people, aspects of one trait may be stronger, but they may demonstrate characteristics across different traits. Indeed, it is not uncommon to have a diagnosis of more than one personality disorder that comprises characteristics from different traits. As we delve deeper into understanding personality disorders in this chapter, you will begin to see that many of the characteristics of personality disorders are also characteristic of one of these five traits. Individuals will usually identify with characteristics of one or more of the traits, but not necessarily demonstrate all, or even many, of the characteristics described. The 'big five' traits are:

- neuroticism
- extraversion
- openness
- agreeableness
- conscientiousness.

Table 12.1 outlines the characteristics of the 'big five'; perhaps you see elements of your own personality within these – most people will!

TABLE 12.1
The 'big five' personality traits

NEUROTICISM	EXTRAVERSION	OPENNESS	AGREEABLENESS	CONSCIENTIOUSNESS
• Prone to anger and anxiety • Nervous • 'Moody' • Temperamental • Prone to worry • May be impulsive	• Talkative • Assertive • May be perceived as domineering and attention-seeking	• Curious • Imaginative • Creative • Emotive • May also be distractible and unpredictable	• Acquiescent • Kind • Trusting • Warm • Compassionate • May be perceived as naïve or subservient	• Organised • Thorough • Reliable • Dependable • Self-disciplined • Dutiful • May be stubborn or obsessive • Can be inflexible

Now that we have looked at the five common personality traits, we consider which trait may be more associated with challenging behaviours. Perhaps you identified that those individuals prone to neuroticism present with the most challenges from a mental health perspective. While most of these five traits have positive aspects to them, there are opportunities to view these as potential negative traits too, given the right (or wrong) situation. For example, being amenable and kind (as seen in the agreeableness trait) may result in an individual who is easily taken advantage of. Generally, when an individual presents with a personality that is rigid and maladaptive, resulting in significant disruption to their life, one may consider the diagnosis of a personality disorder. It is important to note that these traits are not 'abnormal', and are common to many individuals, yourself included. However, when an individual presents with *many* characteristics from these traits, it may be indicative of a personality disorder. You will see some of the characteristics of the personality traits reflected in diagnostic criteria for many of the personality disorders discussed below.

General personality disorder

Personality disorders are inherently conditions associated with impairment in *cognition*, *affectivity*, *impulse control* and *interpersonal functioning*. These patterns are enduring (continuous or long-lasting) and result in significant impairment in the individual's ability to function successfully in a social, occupational and interpersonal manner. They also impact on others; namely, those personally involved with the individual such as family, intimate partner, work colleagues and friends. General personality disorder (GPD) is a condition that forms the basis of *all* personality disorders discussed in this chapter.

GPD is a relatively new addition to psychiatry and is still debatable. We can consider GPD as the overarching or umbrella for personality disorders, while the different clusters comprise more specific signs and symptoms. While GPD is not a specific diagnosis, it is a helpful and important consideration when exploring all personality disorders. As you gain an understanding of the other personality disorders, you will see that characteristics of GPD are carried over into them too. This is because GPD comprises the basic characteristics of a disordered personality at an elemental level. Therefore, the personality disorders listed in **Table 12.3**, **Table 12.4** and **Table 12.9** are factors seen in *addition* to those listed in **Table 12.2**, which outlines the *Diagnostic and Statistical Manual of Mental Disorders* (DSM-5; APA, 2013) criteria for GPD.

DIAGNOSTIC CRITERIA

General personality disorder

TABLE 12.2
Diagnostic criteria general personality disorder

A. An enduring pattern of inner experience and behavior that deviates markedly from the expectations of the individual's culture. This pattern is manifested in two (or more) of the following areas:
  1. Cognition (i.e., ways of perceiving and interpreting self, other people, and events).
  2. Affectivity (i.e., the range, intensity, lability, and appropriateness of emotional response).
  3. Interpersonal functioning.
  4. Impulse control.

B. The enduring pattern is inflexible and pervasive across a broad range of personal and social situations.
C. The enduring pattern leads to clinically significant distress or impairment in social, occupational, or other important areas of functioning.
D. The pattern is stable and of long duration, and its onset can be traced back at least to adolescence or early adulthood.
E. The enduring pattern is not better explained as a manifestation or consequence of another mental disorder.
F. The enduring pattern is not attributable to the physiological effects of a substance (e.g., a drug of abuse, a medication) or another medical condition (e.g., head trauma)

SOURCE: REPRINTED WITH PERMISSION FROM THE *DIAGNOSTIC AND STATISTICAL MANUAL OF MENTAL DISORDERS*, FIFTH EDITION, (COPYRIGHT ©2013). AMERICAN PSYCHIATRIC ASSOCIATION. ALL RIGHTS RESERVED.

INTRODUCING CLUSTER *A*, *B* AND *C* PERSONALITY DISORDERS

There are 10 distinct different personality disorders and these are separated into what are known collectively as 'clusters'. Personality clusters exist as a means to categorise their descriptive similarities, and different clusters are categorised because conditions in these sections have similar-type features. For example, Cluster *A* personality disorders have a series of similar behaviours and characteristics that are typically seen in that group of conditions. This section describes the different personality disorders within the clustered groups. The three distinct clusters are simply known as clusters *A*, *B* and *C*.

Cluster *A* personality disorders

Cluster *A* personality disorders include those that refer to behaviours that are defined as odd, eccentric or paranoid. Consumers with a cluster A personality are prone to withdrawal and may exhibit isolative or secretive tendencies. Cluster *A* personality disorders share some of the characteristics of schizophrenia; however, there is a distinct lack of distortion of reality. **Table 12.3** outlines in detail the diagnostic criteria of cluster *A* personality disorders. Which personality traits from **Table 12.1** can you see reflected in these personality disorders?

DIAGNOSTIC CRITERIA

Cluster A personality disorders

TABLE 12.3
Diagnostic criteria cluster *A* personality disorders

Paranoid personality disorder

A. A pervasive distrust and suspiciousness of others such that their motives are interpreted as malevolent, beginning by early adulthood and present in a variety of contexts, as indicated by four (or more) of the following:
1. Suspects, without sufficient basis, that others are exploiting, harming, or deceiving him or her.
2. Is preoccupied with unjustified doubts about the loyalty or trustworthiness of friends or associates.
3. Is reluctant to confide in others because of unwarranted fear that the information will be used maliciously against him or her.
4. Reads hidden demeaning or threatening meanings into benign remarks or events.
5. Persistently bears grudges (i.e., is unforgiving of insults, injuries, or slights).
6. Perceives attacks on his or her character or reputation that are not apparent to others and is quick to react angrily or to counterattack.
7. Has recurrent suspicions, without justification, regarding fidelity of spouse or sexual partner.

B. Does not occur exclusively during the course of schizophrenia, a bipolar disorder or depressive disorder with psychotic features, or another psychotic disorder and is not attributable to the physiological effects of another medical condition.

Schizoid personality disorder

A. A pervasive pattern of detachment from social relationships and a restricted range of expression of emotions in interpersonal settings, beginning by early adulthood and present in a variety of contexts, as indicated by four (or more) of the following:
1. Neither desires nor enjoys close relationships, including being part of a family.
2. Almost always chooses solitary activities.
3. Has little, if any, interest in having sexual experiences with another person.
4. Takes pleasure in few, if any, activities.
5. Lacks close friends or confidants other than first-degree relatives.
6. Appears indifferent to the praise or criticism of others.
7. Shows emotional coldness, detachment, or flattened affectivity.

B. Does not occur exclusively during the course of schizophrenia, a bipolar disorder or depressive disorder with psychotic features, another psychotic disorder, or autism spectrum disorder and is not attributable to the physiological effects of another medical condition.

Schizotypal personality disorder

A. A pervasive pattern of social and interpersonal deficits marked by acute discomfort with, and reduced capacity for, close relationships as well as by cognitive or perceptual distortions and eccentricities of behavior, beginning by early adulthood and present in a variety of contexts, as indicated by five (or more) of the following:
1. Ideas of reference (excluding delusions of reference).
2. Odd beliefs or magical thinking that influences behavior and is inconsistent with subcultural norms (e.g., superstitiousness, belief in clairvoyance, telepathy, or "sixth sense"; in children and adolescents, bizarre fantasies or preoccupations).
3. Unusual perceptual experiences, including bodily illusions.
4. Odd thinking and speech (e.g., vague, circumstantial, metaphorical, overelaborate, or stereotyped).
5. Suspiciousness or paranoid ideation.
6. Inappropriate or constricted affect.
7. Behavior or appearance that is odd, eccentric, or peculiar.
8. Lack of close friends or confidants other than first-degree relatives.
9. Excessive social anxiety that does not diminish with familiarity and tends to be associated with paranoid fears rather than negative judgments about self.

B. Does not occur exclusively during the course of schizophrenia, a bipolar disorder or depressive disorder with psychotic features, another psychotic disorder, or autism spectrum disorder.

As you can see, there are many similar characteristics of cluster *A* personality disorders, including:
- the way the individual relates to others, and the way they perceive others to relate to them
- reduced need for personal and/or intimate relationships
- a preference to be alone, whether it be due to trust, fear or a simple desire to avoid others
- concerns about the motivations of others.

After reading the characteristics of the cluster *A* personality disorders listed in **Table 12.3**, you can see that the picture of odd, eccentric and paranoid behaviours are good general descriptions of what these cluster *A* disorders are like. Now we will look at the specific behaviours associated with each condition in cluster *A*.

Characteristics of paranoid personality disorder

Paranoid personality disorder (PPD; see **Table 12.3**) is thought to occur in about 2–4 in every 100 people and is more often diagnosed in males (APA, 2013). There may be a dual diagnosis (a co-occurring substance use disorder and mental health condition) with this condition and its development is often noted in childhood and adolescence. Individuals experiencing PPD are often rather challenging to get along with, particularly given they are prone to assuming the actions of others (be they positive *or* negative) to be vindictive or malicious and are generally untrusting of others. This behaviour results in further isolation and distance between themselves and others. Generally, individuals with PPD may be reticent to share their feelings because they are wary of others, anticipating that their motives are potentially harmful, thus making interpersonal relationships and trust difficult. Consider the challenges of making friends or establishing an intimate relationship when you are inherently doubtful that the other person is not trying to hurt you or take advantage of you. On the other hand, imagine trying to establish a relationship with someone who does not share their feelings or thoughts with you because they simply do not trust you. It is not surprising that people with PPD find relationships difficult. Indeed, for most people relationships that are healthy and trusting still require effort, and having PPD significantly compounds the potential difficulty for healthy relationships with others.

Characteristics of schizoid personality disorder

Schizoid personality disorder (**SZPD**; see **Table 12.3**) occurs in approximately 3 in every 100 people and is only slightly more common to males (APA, 2013). Features of this condition predominantly involve a desire to avoid close personal relationships and a preference to be alone, because engaging with others is generally an anxiety-provoking experience. Consumers may experience difficulty with social interactions, present as aloof and generally find the experience of social interaction unpleasant. Due to affective restrictions, individuals with SZPD may present with a blunted or flat affect and this is in line with their restricted range of emotions. Because individuals with SZPD are unaffected by the emotions or attitudes of those around them, they are frequently unresponsive to criticism or praise.

Characteristics of schizotypal personality disorder

Schizotypal personality disorder (**STPD**; see **Table 12.3**) is the most closely related to schizophrenia (see Chapter 8) of the entire cluster *A* disorders and is, in fact, believed by many to be a schizophrenia-spectrum condition. Notably, STPD consists of disturbed thinking and behaviour; however, it is not severe enough to warrant a diagnosis of schizophrenia. Nonetheless, some people with STPD will later go on to develop schizophrenia, and this is increased in individuals with a genetic link to someone with schizophrenia. Rates of STPD

are varied depending on geographic location, with results varying from below 1% to over 4%, and the condition is marginally more common in males (APA, 2013). While the prevalence may be slightly varied, in terms of the development of the condition, it usually emerges in adolescence, as evidenced by a reduced ability to maintain peer relationships, poor academic achievement, being unsociable and a propensity for the odd, eccentric traits common to cluster *A* types resulting in bullying (APA, 2013). While psychotic features are not common to the condition, in periods of extreme stress or anxiety, brief psychotic symptoms not warranted in escalating a diagnosis may occur.

As with SZPD, disturbance of affect is often observed. Affect that is generally restricted is more common; however, incongruent or inappropriate affectivity may also be evident. Disturbance of speech is common to STPD. In particular, presence of tangential speech may be apparent. Cognitive impacts are more severe and individuals are often significantly impacted by paranoia, illusions, magical thinking or ideas of reference.

Magical thinking is a concept probably best defined by the statement 'thinking equates to doing'. Individuals demonstrating magical thinking believe what is termed 'a plausible link of causation', meaning events are influenced by other events despite a lack of causal link. This implies that there are causal relationships between events and actions or thoughts that in fact do not exist. Magical thinking is believing, for example, 'Because I could only get a seat on the right side of the bus today, it is going to be a bad day'. Magical thinking, which is also seen in obsessive-compulsive disorder (OCD; see Chapter 17), is often linked to superstitions or lucky sayings, rituals or numbers.

Cluster *B* personality disorders

Cluster *B* personality disorders can be challenging for consumers, family members/carers and clinicians alike. Typically, cluster *B* personality disorders are composed of those behaviours that are seen to be emotional and dramatic, often with strong manipulative behaviours present. Prone to dramatic flair, individuals with a cluster *B* personality disorder can be highly stigmatised within the mental health system, and these conditions are often characteristically considered unstable. The DSM-5 (APA, 2013) criteria for cluster *B* personality disorders are listed in **Table 12.4**. In this section, we introduce these personality disorders. Following the introduction of cluster *C* personality disorders, we go into much greater depth for both antisocial personality disorder (APD) and borderline personality disorder (BPD) later in the chapter.

DIAGNOSTIC CRITERIA

Cluster B personality disorders

TABLE 12.4
Diagnostic criteria cluster B personality disorders

Antisocial personality disorder

A. A pervasive pattern of disregard for and violation of the rights of others, occurring since age 15 years, as indicated by three (or more) of the following:
  1. Failure to conform to social norms with respect to lawful behaviors, as indicated by repeatedly performing acts that are grounds for arrest.
  2. Deceitfulness, as indicated by repeated lying, use of aliases, or conning others for personal profit or pleasure.
  3. Impulsivity or failure to plan ahead.
  4. Irritability and aggressiveness, as indicated by repeated physical fights or assaults.
  5. Reckless disregard for safety of self or others.
  6. Consistent irresponsibility, as indicated by repeated failure to sustain consistent work behavior or honor financial obligations.
  7. Lack of remorse, as indicated by being indifferent to or rationalizing having hurt, mistreated, or stolen from another.

B. The individual is at least age 18 years.

C. There is evidence of conduct disorder with onset before age 15 years.

D. The occurrence of antisocial behavior is not exclusively during the course of schizophrenia or bipolar disorder.

Borderline personality disorder

A pervasive pattern of instability of interpersonal relationships, self-image, and affects, and marked impulsivity, beginning by early adulthood and present in a variety of contexts, as indicated by five (or more) of the following:
1. Frantic efforts to avoid real or imagined abandonment. (**Note:** Do not include suicidal or self-mutilating behavior covered in Criterion 5.)
2. A pattern of unstable and intense interpersonal relationships characterized by alternating between extremes of idealization and devaluation.
3. Identity disturbance: markedly and persistently unstable self-image or sense of self.
4. Impulsivity in at least two areas that are potentially self-damaging (e.g., spending, sex, substance abuse, reckless driving, binge eating).
   (**Note:** Do not include suicidal or self-mutilating behavior covered in Criterion 5.)
5. Recurrent suicidal behavior, gestures, or threats, or self-mutilating behavior.
6. Affective instability due to a marked reactivity of mood (e.g., intense episodic dysphoria, irritability, or anxiety usually lasting a few hours and only rarely more than a few days).
7. Chronic feelings of emptiness.
8. Inappropriate, intense anger or difficulty controlling anger (e.g., frequent displays of temper, constant anger, recurrent physical fights).
9. Transient, stress-related paranoid ideation or severe dissociative symptoms.

Histrionic personality disorder

A pervasive pattern of excessive emotionality and attention seeking, beginning by early adulthood and present in a variety of contexts, as indicated by five (or more) of the following:
1. Is uncomfortable in situations in which he or she is not the center of attention.
2. Interaction with others is often characterized by inappropriate sexually seductive or provocative behavior.
3. Displays rapidly shifting and shallow expression of emotions.
4. Consistently uses physical appearance to draw attention to self.
5. Has a style of speech that is excessively impressionistic and lacking in detail.
6. Shows self-dramatization, theatricality, and exaggerated expression of emotion.
7. Is suggestible (i.e., easily influenced by others or circumstances).
8. Considers relationships to be more intimate than they actually are.

Narcissistic personality disorder

A pervasive pattern of grandiosity (in fantasy or behavior), need for admiration, and lack of empathy, beginning by early adulthood and present in a variety of contexts, as indicated by five (or more) of the following:
1. Has a grandiose sense of self-importance (e.g., exaggerates achievements and talents, expects to be recognized as superior without commensurate achievements).
2. Is preoccupied with fantasies of unlimited success, power, brilliance, beauty, or ideal love.
3. Believes that he or she is "special" and unique and can only be understood by, or should associate with, other special or high-status people (or institutions).
4. Requires excessive admiration.
5. Has a sense of entitlement (i.e., unreasonable expectations of especially favorable treatment or automatic compliance with his or her expectations).
6. Is interpersonally exploitative (i.e., takes advantage of others to achieve his or her own ends).
7. Lacks empathy: is unwilling to recognize or identify with the feelings and needs of others.
8. Is often envious of others or believes that others are envious of him or her.
9. Shows arrogant, haughty behaviors or attitudes.

Characteristics of antisocial personality disorder

Antisocial personality disorder (APD; see **Table 12.4**) is a condition characterised by failure to conform to social norms and violation of the rights of others. As a significant personality disorder, this chapter contains a comprehensive detailing of characteristics, prevalence, aetiology, epidemiology, treatment and management of APD following this overview of cluster *A*, *B* and *C* personality disorders (see page 212).

Characteristics of histrionic personality disorder

Histrionic personality disorder (HPD; see **Table 12.4**) is a condition characterised by attention-seeking behaviours and, consequently, a need to be the centre of attention. HPD affects around 1.84% of the population, and the condition is diagnosed more often in females (APA, 2013). Those with HPD will often develop relationships with others quickly, and overemphasise the intimacy of these relationships and fluctuate in their emotional intensity. It is common for those with HPD to use sexual promiscuity or their appearance to attempt to seduce or impress others. Friends or acquaintances may view the consumer as shallow, because while they are often dramatic in their expression (e.g. such as becoming distressed over something minor, or hugging or embracing in an inappropriate display of affection), these feelings or emotions are shallow and fleeting. Interpersonal and intimate relationships are often fleeting because HPD individuals may find it hard to keep another's genuine interest and, as such, will be drawn to those who react to their suggestiveness and fulfil their need to be the centre of attention. Long-term intimate relationships are difficult to sustain.

While the potential suicide risk for HPD is not well known, their tendency for dramatic and attention-seeking behaviours means suicide gestures (such as threats or proclamations) and self-harming (non-suicidal self-injury) behaviours, in an effort to be noticed or receive better care, *are* known (APA, 2013). Individuals with HPD demonstrate higher rates of suicide attempts (often using poorly enacted non-lethal means) versus actual deaths resulting from suicide. Can you see some correlation between the extraversion traits listed in **Table 12.1** and HPD?

Characteristics of narcissistic personality disorder

Narcissistic personality disorder (**NPD**; see **Table 12.4**) is aptly named after the Greek myth of Narcissus. Narcissus rejected the romantic advances of another, and instead became enamoured with his own reflection, falling in love with the sight of his own face reflected from a pool of water (see **Figure 12.1**). Like its namesake, those with NPD inherently believe that they require the admiration of others, are grandiose and will only seek out the acquaintance of those they perceive to be worthy of their company. One of the characteristics of this condition is the lack of *actual* accomplishment, yet the overt belief that others should be impressed and they must only engage with other 'like-minded' elitists. NPD is also characterised by a lack of empathy and overvalued sense of accomplishment and entitlement (Paris, 2015).

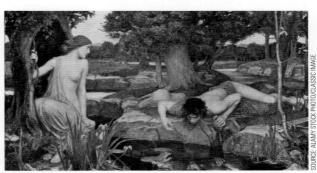

FIGURE 12.1
In Greek mythology, Narcissus fell in love with his own reflection, and Echo who despite trying could not attract his attention

NPD has had a contentious relationship with psychiatry, and there is a distinct lack of research and literature on this condition, and it is not recognised in the International Classification of Diseases (ICD-10). Unsurprisingly, individuals with NPD will often experience significant issues in both their vocational and intimate relationships, and demonstrate higher rates of both unemployment and divorce (Paris, 2013). Prevalence rates of NPD are difficult to determine, with results as diverse as 0–6.2% (APA, 2013), although more recently rates of 0.7–1.2% seem more realistic (Paris, 2015). NPD is more common in men (APA, 2013). Because narcissistic traits are frequently seen in healthy adolescents, care must be taken when suspecting the condition in younger people.

Of the few dedicated NPD researchers, Ogrodniczuk (2013) has been imperative in contributing to the small pool of literature on this condition and notes that it is often comorbid conditions that result in individuals with a diagnosis of NPD engaging mental health services for help. NPD has a high correlation with substance misuse, anxiety and mood disorders, and suicide attempts may also be one of the behaviours that result in contact with mental health services. Ogrodniczuk (2013) notes individuals with NPD demonstrate higher rates of death from suicide, especially those who are employed in the military, which appears to be a vocation attracting individuals with NPD (in one study at rates of around 20%) when compared with civilian populations.

Characteristics of borderline personality disorder

Borderline personality disorder (BPD; see **Table 12.4**) is a condition characterised by emotional dysregulation and chaotic interpersonal relationships. As a significant personality disorder, this chapter contains a comprehensive detailing of characteristics, prevalence, aetiology, epidemiology, treatment and management of BPD following this overview of cluster *A*, *B* and *C* personality disorders (see page 212).

Cluster *C* personality disorders

There are three **cluster *C* personality disorders** making up the final set of conditions within the family of personality disorders. Typically, these personality disorders are known as the anxious or fearful type of conditions, and are characterised by high degrees of stress. **Table 12.5** outlines the DSM-5 (APA, 2013) criteria for cluster *C* disorders.

DIAGNOSTIC CRITERIA

Cluster C personality disorders

TABLE 12.5
Diagnostic criteria cluster *C* personality disorders

Avoidant personality disorder

A pervasive pattern of social inhibition, feelings of inadequacy, and hypersensitivity to negative evaluation, beginning by early adulthood and present in a variety of contexts, as indicated by four (or more) of the following:

1. Avoids occupational activities that involve significant interpersonal contact because of fears of criticism, disapproval, or rejection.
2. Is unwilling to get involved with people unless certain of being liked.
3. Shows restraint within intimate relationships because of the fear of being shamed or ridiculed.
4. Is preoccupied with being criticized or rejected in social situations.
5. Is inhibited in new interpersonal situations because of feelings of inadequacy.
6. Views self as socially inept, personally unappealing, or inferior to others.
7. Is unusually reluctant to take personal risks or to engage in any new activities because they may prove embarrassing.

Dependent personality disorder

A pervasive and excessive need to be taken care of that leads to submissive and clinging behavior and fears of separation, beginning by early adulthood and present in a variety of contexts, as indicated by five (or more) of the following:

1. Has difficulty making everyday decisions without an excessive amount of advice and reassurance from others.
2. Needs others to assume responsibility for most major areas of his or her life.
3. Has difficulty expressing disagreement with others because of fear of loss of support or approval. (**Note:** Do not include realistic fears of retribution.)
4. Has difficulty initiating projects or doing things on his or her own (because of a lack of self-confidence in judgment or abilities rather than a lack of motivation or energy).
5. Goes to excessive lengths to obtain nurturance and support from others, to the point of volunteering to do things that are unpleasant.
6. Feels uncomfortable or helpless when alone because of exaggerated fears of being unable to care for himself or herself.
7. Urgently seeks another relationship as a source of care and support when a close relationship ends.
8. Is unrealistically preoccupied with fears of being left to take care of himself or herself.

Obsessive-Compulsive personality disorder

A pervasive pattern of preoccupation with orderliness, perfectionism, and mental and interpersonal control, at the expense of flexibility, openness, and efficiency, beginning by early adulthood and present in a variety of contexts, as indicated by four (or more) of the following:

1. Is preoccupied with details, rules, lists, order, organization, or schedules to the extent that the major point of the activity is lost.
2. Shows perfectionism that interferes with task completion (e.g., is unable to complete a project because his or her own overly strict standards are not met).
3. Is excessively devoted to work and productivity to the exclusion of leisure activities and friendships (not accounted for by obvious economic necessity).
4. Is overconscientious, scrupulous, and inflexible about matters of morality, ethics, or values (not accounted for by cultural or religious identification).
5. Is unable to discard worn-out or worthless objects even when they have no sentimental value.
6. Is reluctant to delegate tasks or to work with others unless they submit to exactly his or her way of doing things.
7. Adopts a miserly spending style toward both self and others; money is viewed as something to be hoarded for future catastrophes.
8. Shows rigidity and stubbornness.

Avoidant personality disorder

The overwhelming features of **avoidant personality disorder (AVPD)** are an overt presence of distress or discomfort experienced in social, occupational or interpersonal situations, coupled with a low self-esteem (see **Table 12.5** for a full list of diagnostic criteria). These feelings are exacerbated by an overall feeling of inadequacy while in the presence of others, and extreme sensitivity to criticism (even minor). Individuals with AVPD will avoid developing new friendships or taking on new work roles, unless they feel guaranteed to be liked and accepted by others. This fear of being criticised or rejected by others is manifested in avoidance of situations where this may occur, and they are noted to have a low threshold for tolerating these responses in others (APA, 2013). This can result in perceived overreactions to what were meant as minor comments. To others, those with AVPD may appear withdrawn and shy and their interactions are often seriously inhibited due to fear of embarrassing themselves. AVPD has been likened to social phobia as there are a number of similarities between the two.

As with other personality disorders, traumatic or negative childhood experiences are a common aetiological factor. AVPD is associated with high rates of emotional neglect in childhood, in addition to physical abuse and environments where love and affection are not demonstrated by parents (Eikenaes, Egeland, Hummelen & Wilberg, 2015). AVPD is comorbid with other anxiety-based conditions such as social anxiety disorder and agoraphobia (fear of public places). Occurring in about 2.4% of the general population in equal proportions of males and females, AVPD behaviours are frequently observed in childhood, commencing as shyness and manifesting in avoidant behaviours such as evading strangers and unfamiliar situations (APA, 2013). While critical periods of the condition are often around adolescence, which is a pivotal time for increasing avoidant behaviours, the condition is often seen to diminish as individuals age.

Dependent personality disorder

Dependent personality disorder (DPD) is a condition characterised by submissiveness and the need to be taken care of by another person, resulting in 'clinginess' and separation anxiety (see **Table 12.5** for a full list of diagnostic criteria). This person relies on another to make important decisions (such as major financial ones) and very minor decisions (such as how to do their hair, what to eat or what shampoo to buy). Individuals with DPD experience extreme difficulty in making daily decisions and require elaborate amounts of guidance and support from others to reach a decision. Due to this passiveness, they may also find it very difficult to challenge another person (and in fact do not become appropriately upset in situations where they *have* been wronged), or stand up for themselves out of worry of losing their support (APA, 2013). Because of inherent poor self-esteem, they often lack conviction in their abilities and struggle to undertake activities independently, or initiate them at all. This can have a major impact on their ability to undertake their work at an acceptable level. Because of their low self-confidence and need to be supported, they will often undertake tasks which are unpleasant and may stay in dysfunctional or violent relationships (enduring sexual, physical or emotional abuse). When a relationship they are dependent on ends, they will frantically seek to replace this person immediately.

DPD is understood to affect about 0.6% of the population and appears to be more common in females (APA, 2013). DPD is linked to parenting styles that are authoritarian and over-protective, resulting in adolescents who find it difficult to make choices such as who they befriend, what classes they study and what they want to do with their life.

CULTURAL CONSIDERATIONS

Cultural differences in dependent personality disorder
It is important to remember that different cultures may manifest conditions in different ways, or that some behaviours are more culturally acceptable and as such may not be truly 'disordered'. Conditions such as DPD should only be diagnosed when exhibited behaviours manifest in a manner that exceeds cultural norms. This is particularly an important consideration in cultures where it is acceptable to defer to a male partner or elder, and where passive behaviours are expected (APA, 2013).

Obsessive-compulsive personality disorder

Not to be confused with obsessive-compulsive disorder, **obsessive-compulsive personality disorder (OCPD)** is a condition associated with perfectionism, controlling behaviours and a need for uniformity resulting in serious interpersonal and occupational dysfunction (see **Table 12.5** for a full list of diagnostic criteria). These traits occur at the expense of flexibility, and individuals with OCPD can be rigid and unwilling to compromise (APA, 2013). Finding structure and order necessary, individuals with OCPD find spontaneity and relaxation difficult, and prefer it when tasks and their time are highly organised and structured (Cain, Ansell, Simpson & Pinto, 2015).

In the workplace, this can cause significant issues. Due to the need to control situations and details, those with OCPD may find it incredibly difficult to delegate tasks (and when they do, micromanage the situation), resulting in others feeling inadequate and frustrated. Because of a misperception that others will not do a good enough job, individuals with OCPD may end up taking on 'all the work', but because they spend so much of their time writing lists, planning (rather than actioning) and redoing their work because they are unsatisfied with its quality, much of their work ends up not being done at all. This results in poor work performance, but also significantly impacts workplace relationships. Strict adherence to 'rules', a tendency to 'hoard' inconsequential items and inflexibility are other characteristics of the condition. One way of imagining how long an individual with OCPD may go unnoticed is to consider how long they can maintain important areas of their lives without their condition creating serious impacts for *others*. If OCPD has potentially significant issues with employment, perhaps it is best to consider how long an individual could keep working while demonstrating the behaviours outlined in **Table 12.5** before it becomes an issue for those around them. They are, therefore, often bound only by how long others are able to endure their actions. Given that we all have our own unique traits, it is also possible that someone with OCPD may work alongside someone who lacks in confidence, is timid and prefers direction, and is therefore more willing to be supervised in a controlling manner by someone else. In other words, someone who is happy to be micromanaged would likely not have an issue with this type of colleague and may even prefer it.

The margins of prevalence for OCPD are large, at between 2.1–7.9% outside clinical populations (APA, 2013), while being slightly higher and more consistent within clinical populations (Cain et al., 2015) and twice as common in males. Given the potential positive outcomes with this condition (e.g. work colleagues cede to their controlling behaviours), the condition may be more common than is reported. It is important to note that prevalence rates can be inherently difficult to predict for conditions that do not readily result in hospitalisation and treatment (such as some of the personality disorders in this chapter). Can you see some correlation between the conscientiousness traits noted in **Table 12.1** and OCPD?

CLINICAL OBSERVATIONS

The difference between OCD and OCPD

The inclusion of what are two different conditions with very similar names can be very confusing (and frustrating!) for students, consumers and clinicians alike. Probably the easiest way to differentiate between OCD and OCPD is:

- Obsessive-compulsive disorder (OCD) is characterised by intrusive thoughts (obsessions), which *create* anxiety – for example, 'germs are everywhere… everything I touch is dirty' – and repetitive behaviours (compulsions) which, when undertaken, alleviate anxiety – 'when I wash my hands, the germs go, and I am clean.' So these intrusive thoughts are alleviated somewhat by undertaking this ritualistic behaviour. OCD is inherently an anxiety disorder.
- Obsessive-compulsive *personality* disorder (OCPD), on the other hand, is a pattern of *behaviours* that result in distress and interference with daily functioning. The individual with OCPD is 'obsessed' with order, a need for perfectionism and control to the detriment of flexibility, openness and productivity. As such, OCPD is inherently a personality disorder.

OCD is often usually easier to detect than OCPD, as it is often so highly debilitating and those experiencing OCD are more likely to seek help.

ANTISOCIAL PERSONALITY DISORDER (APD)

Antisocial personality disorder (APD) became more prevalent after the Second World War, suggesting that the rapid changes to social structures at that time yielded individuals with a prevalence for more impulsive and disruptive behaviours (Paris, 2015). The terms *sociopath* and *psychopath* are sometimes used interchangeably with APD, although they themselves are not classified mental health conditions.

The difference between APD and psychopathy is fraught, complicated and not yet fully understood. **Psychopathy** is defined as a series or set of characteristics and behaviours affiliated with the exploitation of other people for personal gain (Ficks, Dong & Waldman, 2014). It is proposed that this is one of the main differences between psychopathy and APD, as the consumer with APD may not be as fixated on exploiting others as a psychopath. In addition, it has been suggested that a psychopath will exhibit an unyielding absence of empathic responses to others or situations, and will always present with what is known as a superficial affect, which results in the person seeming constantly callous and aloof

(Ogloff, Campbell & Shepherd, 2016). In contrast, the consumer with a diagnosis of APD may make an effort to express empathy and a range of emotions that they do not genuinely feel. It has been suggested that psychopathy and APD are effectively the same condition, and that psychopathy is a more severe form of APD, but more research is required into the specifics to draw a definitive conclusion.

Individuals with APD are often highly impulsive, without regard for the actions that their behaviour may cause other people, and this lack of empathy or concern makes it easy for them to victimise others. For example, most people would not imagine 'conning' an older couple out of their pension – mostly because it is amoral and unlawful, but also because we have regard for the negative consequences our actions could have on others. We are concerned and empathic. The older couple may lose their home if we steal money from them. They may not be able to afford food, utility bills and medicines. The individual with APD does not care about this. They care about what they will be able to do with the money, how they can avoid getting caught, and perhaps who their next target is. The APD individual pays no mind to the ramifications for this couple, and their only concern is the potential consequences to *themself.*

Characteristics of antisocial personality disorder (APD)

Antisocial personality disorder (see **Table 12.4**) is characterised by evidence of conduct-distorted behaviours in the individual *prior* to the age of 15, and can only be diagnosed in individuals older than 18 years who have evident conduct disorder (CD) behaviours. CD is a complex disruptive or impulse-control disorder characterised by a pattern of disturbing behaviours that include (but are not limited to) aggression directed towards people or animals, property destruction, deceitfulness or theft, and rule violations (APA, 2013). As CD is not a personality disorder, it will not be further explored in this chapter; however, it is important to become familiar with CD to properly understand the scope of APD as the two are intimately linked. There is a more thorough description of CD in Chapter 19.

Traditionally, individuals with a diagnosis of APD have issues with impulse control and delaying gratification and these behaviours are frequently associated with illegal consequences such as speeding, taking illegal substances and physical altercations with little or no provocation. Individuals with APD often present as confident, arrogant and egotistical and they will often have serious issues maintaining relationships with others due to their behaviours, lack of empathy and general mistreatment of others.

Incidence and epidemiology

Rates of APD in the community are hard to assess and vary considerably from country to country, with rates as low as 0.2% and as high as 3% reported (APA, 2013). The lifetime prevalence is thought to be 1% in females and 3% in males (Andrews et al., 2013). What is consistent despite location is that APD is significantly more prevalent in males. Men diagnosed with APD are more likely to engage in activities that draw the attention of police and/or criminal charges compared with women with the same diagnosis (Sher et al., 2015). It is also probably not surprising to imagine that APD has a high incidence in prison and forensic settings – in some studies as high as 80% of inmates – as they frequently violate laws and the rights of others (APA, 2013; Black, 2015). Males tend to demonstrate the more aggressive features of the condition than females, although there is suggestion that a lack of overt aggression in women results in a reduced inclination for diagnosis in this cohort which may not be epidemiologically correct. This implies that society may expect to see less aggressive tendencies demonstrated by females and, as such, diagnosticians may avoid a diagnosis if there is a lack of violence despite other prominent clinical features being evident. It appears that APD is a predominantly Westernised condition, with infrequent occurrence in developing countries or developed countries where there is maintenance of strong cultural ties or customs (Paris, 2015).

Aetiology

Because APD requires CD behaviours in youth, it is important to explore the aetiology of CD. As with other mental health conditions, the causes and patterns of APD are complex and involve an interplay of multiple different factors that are discussed in more detail below.

Genetic factors

Family history of CD or APD is often positive, in addition to increased rates of substance misuse and incarcerations. Ficks, Dong and Waldman (2014) note that genetic studies suggest genes play a significant role in development of APD and CD. Personality traits that are seen in APD, such as impulsiveness, reduced empathy and involvement in criminal behaviours, are believed to be highly heritable (Paris, 2015). It is understood that aggressive traits are also highly heritable, and aggressive behaviour has strong links to criminal behaviour. It is important to note, however, that both genes and environment (in particular, child abuse) play a significant role in the development of APD (APA, 2013).

Biological and individual factors

Young people with CD will often have lower intelligence quotient (IQ) rates than the average (APA, 2013) and it is believed that subtle brain structural variations in white matter in the frontal lobes may also play a role in violence and APD (Paris, 2015). It is possible that these structural brain abnormalities impact the individual's ability to process the feelings or emotions of both themselves and others. Paris (2015) proposes that for some individuals with APD it is quite simply the notion of a 'bad seed' and that the callous, unemotional traits seen in this condition permit some individuals to 'survive' or even thrive in battle conditions (such as during war), while others are unable to cope with the atrocities of such experiences.

Other individual factors include poor affective regulation, which is aggravated by issues with the expression and understanding of emotions (effectively emotional regulation) in both themselves and others. There is also often an inclination to respond quickly and with anger to minor situations and a more pronounced ability to detect anger in other people – which they then, in turn, respond to with anger themselves (Fox et al., 2015).

As with all other mental health conditions, temperament and individual variances also play a role in the development of APD. Generally, persons with a diagnosis of APD typically display personality traits such as narcissism (which, simplistically, is a strong belief in one's self-importance above all others) and a high degree of manipulative behavioural traits, in addition to impulsivity and poor control over self-gratification (Buck, 2015).

Jackson and Beaver (2015) note that diet and nutrition may play a role in the development of characteristic traits associated with APD. Poor nutrition can have a negative effect on memory, learning, cognition and executive functioning, and poor diet in childhood may result in increased externalising and aggressive behaviours later in life. Poor diet may also be seen in children who are neglected which is, in and of itself, a risk factor for APD.

Environmental factors

One of the strongest indicators of APD is a family environment that is fraught with dysfunction (Paris, 2015). Individuals with APD frequently come from families where there is a history of neglect, violence, rejection, abuse, substance misuse and inadequate supervision (APA, 2013). Of significant importance is a lack of the parental discipline (or inconsistent discipline) that is necessary to regulate impulsive behaviours consistent with this diagnosis. Parental relationships are often strained, and there may be a lack of expressed warmth and poor or insecure attachment (Buck, 2015).

Childhood abuse and neglect are strongly associated with significant risks to mental health and well-being and, in particular, the development of callous or unemotional personality traits that are highly associated with APD (Carlson, Oshri & Kwon, 2015). Fox et al. (2015) note that 90% of juvenile offenders have a past history of childhood trauma, and that 30% met criteria for post-traumatic stress disorder. In addition, childhood trauma or abuse increases the potential for violence in young offenders by over 200% (Fox et al., 2015).

Domestic violence is also linked to higher rates of childhood involvement in juvenile justice up to five years after it is experienced, and high scores of scales that measure adverse childhood experiences are common to those youth with criminal involvement (Fox et al., 2015). The more childhood damage the youth is exposed to or experiences, the more likely they will engage in serious, chronic offences later in life. It has been suggested that this inclination towards violence, as a result of childhood trauma, may result in damage to chromosomes, hormone imbalances and issues with biological chemicals responsible for the regulation of stress mechanics (Fox et al., 2015).

Individuals exposed to childhood abuse and neglect appear to demonstrate an inclination as adolescents to participate in risk-taking behaviours such as sexual promiscuity, substance misuse and violence. This increase may be a result of poor coping mechanisms in stressful situations (such as using illicit drugs to manage distress related to sexual abuse), genetics and the role of growing up in such an abusive environment.

Individuals with APD demonstrate higher rates of unemployment, homelessness and violence (Le Corff & Toupin, 2014). Issues with employment retention are often aggravated by impulsiveness, a tendency to be arrogant and a poor ability to develop and maintain relationships with colleagues. Issues associated with an inability to manage responsibilities (such as workload, financial obligations and parenting) can also result in significant issues. APD is more prevalent in individuals originating from low socioeconomic regions, and is generally more common to urban locations (APA, 2013).

APD and the law

Given the inclination to demonstrate reduced capacity for empathy and a tendency to take advantage of others and be impulsive, it is perhaps unsurprising that individuals with APD often find themselves in the criminal justice system. Incarcerations for theft, violence and assault are not uncommon, and the prevalence of more sadistic sexual crimes and homicides is also consistent with the traits of APD. Lack of remorse, coupled with an affinity not to learn from previous mistakes or punishment, makes recidivism in APD likely (Andrews et al., 2013).

Males who demonstrate angry behaviours, and whose mothers suffered from postnatal depression with antisocial traits, are more likely to be engaged in unlawful activities later in life (DeLisi & Vaughn, 2015). There are strong links between aggression, genetics and involvement in crime. González-Tapia and Obsuth (2015, p. 60) point out that 'within any given community approximately 10% of families may be responsible for more than 50% of criminal offences'. This highlights the role genetics likely plays in APD traits and criminal behaviour. Fox and colleagues (2015) support this notion, stating that 50% of serious crimes committed in the United States by juveniles are committed by the same 10% of juvenile offenders. Individuals with APD have higher rates of death through violent means, such as homicide, accidents or suicide, and this increased risk is likely the result of their inclination to react to situations impulsively.

Comorbidity

APD has significant comorbidity with a variety of other mental health issues, but most commonly with substance misuse such as alcohol, and disorders such as depression or anxiety affecting about 25% of individuals with APD (Andrews et al., 2013; APA, 2013; Black, 2015). Substance use disorders occur more commonly in APD than in *any* other mental illness (Ogloff, Campbell & Shepherd, 2015). Andrews et al. (2013) observe that comorbidity of mental illness in APD is around 90%, while Sher et al. (2015) note that in some studies, men with BPD are probably over-diagnosed with APD due to the antisocial elements of BPD and, as such, a possible higher comorbidity may be overrepresented in this cohort. Women with a diagnosis of APD were more likely to be diagnosed with comorbid borderline or histrionic personality disorders, and men and women have high comorbidity with alcohol use disorder. Rates of cannabis and cocaine use disorders were also significant (Sher et al., 2015).

Clinical course

Typically, these early childhood disruptive behaviours emerge before the age of eight years, and the vast majority (around 80%) will have symptoms by age 11 (Black, 2015). This is particularly evident in boys, who usually demonstrate earlier onset of disruptive or impulsive behaviours, while girls may not present with symptoms until puberty (APA, 2013). There have been a number of studies exploring the rate of young individuals who proceed from CD to develop

APD. Research suggests that the greater the conduct-distorted behaviours evident in youth, the more likely the individual will proceed to APD, with predicted escalation ranges being 35–50% (Le Corff & Toupin, 2014) or 40–70% (Andrews et al., 2013). In particular, behaviours within CD that are identified as *overt* (such as violence and assault) are more likely to result in progression to APD, versus those that are seen as *covert* (such as lying and breaking rules), which demonstrate a reduced susceptibility to escalate (Le Corff & Toupin, 2014). Women tend to have a more complicated or chaotic presentation of APD, whereas males appear to be more consistent in their behavioural issues, which are more chronic (Andrews et al., 2013).

As with most other mental health conditions, APD is pervasive and may be chronic in its nature, but as the individual ages, can become less evident in those engaging in criminal activities (APA, 2013). By the 40th year, most individuals with APD are not as impulsive and exploitative. The fact that those diagnosed with APD have a higher premature mortality rate is also an important factor to consider when exploring such data.

Treatment

Medication is not indicated in the treatment of APD. Personality disorders can be notoriously difficult to treat and individuals with APD rarely voluntarily seek help for their condition outside of enforced court-appointed programs, or drug and alcohol rehabilitation. In fact, Thylstrup and Hesse (2016) note that those with a diagnosis of APD are more likely to be omitted from treatment entirely and they propose that due to the susceptibility for alcohol and other drug (A&OD) issues with this population, that facilities for APD should be entwined with such services. A high proportion of consumers with APD will withdraw from programs aimed at helping them and this makes treatment challenging at best. Thylstrup and Hesse (2016) propose that psychoeducation may be an effective method of treatment where the consumer is educated about the condition, resulting in a more educated decision-making process.

Traditional models of treatment whereby the individual is expected to adopt the feelings and experiences of their victim are particularly ineffective, because the individual with APD lacks empathy and targeting their empathic understanding of another's experiences is not worthwhile or effective. At best, programs that focus on helping the APD individual achieve what they want without hurting others (or getting caught) are more worthwhile.

Typically, cognitive behaviour therapies are the current treatment options for APD with the main objective being refraining from future offending behaviours. Aside from A&OD treatment, anger management, domestic violence groups and behavioural modification, in addition to social skills training, may be beneficial (Andrews et al., 2013). It is very important to understand the consumer's motivations for seeking treatment as this may significantly impact on its success.

Given the wealth of information around childhood trauma and higher incidence for APD, one of the most important measures in reducing rates of APD is *prevention*. Ensuring that children are safe can seriously reduce the incidence of conditions such as APD, which have long-lasting personal and community ramifications.

Management

It is important to be mindful of behavioural tendencies such as manipulation and aggression in the clinical environment. Much of the management of APD revolves around preventing future offending through use of cognitive and behaviour therapies (see Chapter 4). The manipulative nature of individuals with APD requires an experienced mental health team, effective at setting limits and enforcing boundaries around acceptable behaviours (Andrews et al., 2013).

One treatment that has been successful in managing offending behaviours is *reasoning and rehabilitation* (R&R). R&R focuses on social skills training, cognitive abilities and the development of ideals necessary for positive social engagement (Andrews et al., 2013). Other areas of importance include development of self-control, and the ability to reduce impulsive behaviours and actions, and delay gratification.

BORDERLINE PERSONALITY DISORDER

The name 'borderline personality disorder' is somewhat misleading, as it suggests an individual who sits on the 'borderline' of another diagnosis. Although this is the origin of its moniker – coined to suggest a 'borderline' somewhere between neurosis and psychosis – in reality, **borderline personality disorder (BPD)** fits somewhere in the realm of emotional dysregulation and chaotic interpersonal relationships. Individuals diagnosed with BPD often experience abrupt mood fluctuations and impulsivity, but are highly prone to help-seeking (unlike people diagnosed with many other personality disorders).

In terms of significance within the clinical setting, BPD is the most common personality disorder that is encountered and is generally considered the most severe of all the personality disorders. Individuals with BPD tend to see others as either good or bad,

and experience difficulty acknowledging that good people may do bad things, and vice versa. This creates serious issues with interpersonal relationships and functioning. This section explores this condition in more detail.

Characteristics of BPD

Borderline personality disorder (see **Table 12.6**) is characterised by a long-enduring pattern of dysfunction in relationships, emotional regulation, self-esteem, impulsiveness, mood instability and suicide and self-harming/non-suicidal self-injuring behaviours. While the mood instability can appear to mimic major depressive disorder (and MDD *is* a common comorbidity to BPD), this variability does not tend to be enduring, but may last only hours or days, and return to normal. Individuals with BPD are highly influenced by their environment and, as such, their moods may often reflect the chaos around them, with rapidly shifting periods of intense dysphoria, hypomania and extreme anger not uncommonly experienced in succession. For many individuals with BPD, suicidality and self-harm/non-suicidal self-injury are strong features of their condition, and are in fact common maladaptive coping mechanisms in response to times of stress. Relationships (particularly romantic ones) with others are usually chaotic and intense, resulting in frequent quarrels and an insecurity or dependence exacerbated by an intense fear of abandonment (which may or may not be real). **Table 12.6** includes diagnostic criterion 2: 'a pattern of unstable and intense interpersonal relationships characterised by alternating between extremes of idealisation and devaluation' (APA, 2013, p. 663). This refers to the notion of 'good' and 'bad' within people and the inability of the individual with a diagnosis of BPD to see 'grey' areas, including in themselves. For example, a woman diagnosed with BPD may state initially that she has a wonderful relationship with her psychologist, and feels very comfortable sharing intimate details of her life. However, when her psychologist is unable to keep her next appointment, this changes to loathing, verbal abuse and reluctance to continue appointments. One week later, she reverts back to liking her therapist again. As with most personality disorders, there is a need for firm limit setting. In DSM-5 (2013) criterion 1, we see a 'frantic efforts to avoid real or imagined abandonment' p. 663), and this may be evidenced by extreme reactions to normal passages of time (such as appointments coming to an end or a clinician's shift ending) wherein the individual feels they are being abandoned and that they therefore must be inherently bad. This fulfils their belief that they are worthless and fits criterion 3 (identify disturbance) well.

DIAGNOSTIC CRITERIA

Borderline personality disorder

TABLE 12.6
Diagnostic criteria borderline personality disorder

A pervasive pattern of instability of interpersonal relationships, self-image, and affects, and marked impulsivity, beginning by early adulthood and present in a variety of contexts, as indicated by five (or more) of the following:

1. Frantic efforts to avoid real or imagined abandonment (**Note:** Do not include suicidal or self-mutilating behaviour covered in Criterion 5).
2. A pattern of unstable and intense interpersonal relationships characterised by alternating between extremes of idealisation and devaluation.
3. Identity disturbance: markedly and persistently unstable self-image or sense of self.
4. Impulsivity in at least two areas that are potentially self-damaging (e.g., spending, sex, substance abuse, reckless driving, binge eating).
   (**Note:** do not include suicidal or self-mutilating behaviour covered in Criterion 5).
5. Recurrent suicidal behaviour, gestures or threats, or self-mutilating behaviour.
6. Affective instability due to a marked reactivity of mood (e.g., intense episodic dysphoria, irritability or anxiety usually lasting a few hours and only rarely more than a few days).
7. Chronic feelings of emptiness.
8. Inappropriate, intense anger or difficulty controlling anger (e.g., frequent displays of temper, constant anger, recurrent physical fights).
9. Transient, stress-related paranoid ideation or severe dissociative symptoms.

Transitory auditory hallucinations in times of extreme stress occur in about half of those people who have a diagnosis of BPD, but they are not associated with delusions (or psychosis) and often occur in the context of negative (e.g. 'You are worthless') or commanding (e.g. 'You should kill yourself') experiences. While in the past antipsychotics have been a common treatment of BPD (and had some efficacy in managing aggression as well as perceptual disturbance), medication is generally only used to treat symptoms as they occur.

COMMONALITIES OF THE MSE: BORDERLINE PERSONALITY DISORDER

A person presenting with BPD will typically present with a range of features that are the diagnostic criteria listed in **Table 12.6** as expressed through behaviours. It should be noted, however, that BPD can be difficult to identify. BPD assessment requires effective, non-judgmental communication and observation of behaviours that are reported or observed. This section explores aspects of the MSE that have particular characteristics that may be relevant to BPD. You will note, this is not a complete MSE.

General appearance and behaviour

The individual may be cooperative with the interview and any issues related to appearance are likely related to their mood at the time (e.g. if they are unkempt or dishevelled, this may be because their mood is depressed). They may present with poor eye contact. The consumer may present with old self-harm scars on their arms, wrists or legs (see **Figure 12.2**) and there may be evidence of more recent lacerations (such as bandages, bleeding, etc.). The individual may pick at their wounds during the interview, depending on how distressed they are.

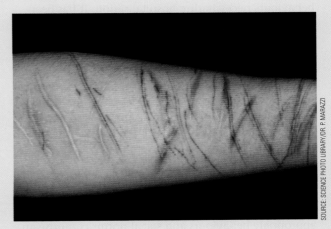

SOURCE: SCIENCE PHOTO LIBRARY/DR. P. MARAZZI

FIGURE 12.2
A person presenting with self-harm marks from cutting

Mood

For many consumers with BPD, fluctuations in mood are very common. Mood states such as agitation, anxiety, irritability, tearfulness and distress are not uncommon. These moods may also fluctuate (labile) rapidly, and can be very intense. Individuals with BPD may partake in risky sexual behaviours, making them vulnerable to exploitation. Individuals with BPD may also demonstrate unhealthy eating patterns such as binge eating, resulting in issues with self-esteem and self-image.

Affect
Due to the frequency of mood changes in BPD, there may also be notable changes in affect, resulting in instability of affect.

Thought content
For many consumers with BPD, their thoughts will focus on self-harm/non-suicidal self-injury and/or suicide and their inability to control impulses about acting out these thoughts. Thought content may also involve negative self-perceptions or image, poor relationships with others, and a perception that others will leave them or abandon them.

Insight
Individuals with BPD may have good insight into their condition, but demonstrate little control over their behaviour or actions. In the event that medication is prescribed, many consumers will adhere to their regimen until they believe that medication is no longer helping.

Incidence and epidemiology
Borderline personality disorder occurs at rates of about 1% (Paris, 2015), is seen in around 20% of mental health unit inpatients (APA, 2013) and, as such, is of significant clinical concern. This rate is reportedly as high as 50% in Australian adolescent inpatient mental health units (Kaess, Brunner & Chanen, 2014). BPD is significantly more common in females in inpatient settings (making up around 75%); however, rates of BPD in community settings are reported as equal among males and females (Ishibashi, 2014; Paris, 2015). This suggests that females are more likely to seek help for their condition, and that they are more prone to self-harming/non-suicidal self-injuring behaviours necessitating hospitalisation. It has been suggested that men may be more likely to receive a diagnosis of antisocial personality disorder, even when the symptoms suggest BPD, and this distribution may be reflective of diagnostic bias (Ishibashi, 2014; Kaess, Brunner & Chanen, 2014). Males are more likely to die from suicide, and to have a co-occurring substance misuse diagnosis, and so may be admitted to the A&OD rehabilitation arena, not the inpatient mental health setting (Paris, 2015).

Aetiology
Conditions that affect an individual's personality and their ability to interact within the constructs of appropriate behaviours and social norms comprise an aetiology with origins of multiple different bases. This section explores the aetiology of BPD.

Genetic factors
BPD appears to be more common in those with a familial history of substance misuse, affective disorders and APD, and is around five times more likely in individuals with a first-degree relative with BPD (APA, 2013). Paris (2015) notes that around 50% of BPD diagnoses are inherited. Temperamental traits such as introversion, impulsiveness and negative emotionality are more likely to be features of an individual diagnosed with BPD, in addition to susceptibility to stress (Kaess, Brunner & Chanen, 2014).

Biological and individual factors
Some studies have indicated brain imaging changes and other biological factors being responsible for affective instability, impulsiveness and stress vulnerability in individuals with a diagnosis of BPD (Paris, 2015). Risk factors for developing BPD from a biological perspective include having a first-degree relative with the condition and this, in addition to adverse childhood experiences such as neglect or abuse, results in a higher chance of developing the condition (Amad et al., 2014). Amad and colleagues (2014) note that in twin studies the prevalence of developing BPD was estimated at between 35–69%. Other hypotheses include issues with serotonin transportation genes and dysfunctions of dopamine. In particular, it would appear that aetiological hypotheses of BPD development are heavily influenced by genetics, but that psychosocial factors only further increase this risk (Amad et al., 2014).

Environmental factors
Sadly, as with other PDs a history of childhood trauma such as abuse and neglect are commonly seen in those with people who have a diagnosis of BPD (Kaess, Brunner & Chanen, 2014). Traditionally, it was believed that a diagnosis of BPD was usually highly correlated with a history of sexual abuse; however, more recently it has been understood that many childhood adversities may be co-occurring with sexual abuse and as such this factor is more complicated to separate. Nonetheless, sexual abuse is still considered by many to be a prominent aetiological feature of the condition. Paris (2015) notes that childhood abuse

or adversity is *not* an indicator in about one-third of those diagnosed, which suggests there is more at play. It is possible that temperamental vulnerabilities are involved in the individual's ability to deal with adversity (such as childhood trauma), and as such plays a vital role in the development of not only BPD, but all mental illnesses. Sharp and Tackett (2014) note in a meta-analysis of sexual abuse in BPD that between 40–71% of those diagnosed with BPD were sexually abused, as compared to the control group, where abuse was identified in 19–46% of individuals. They also note that in one study comparing BPD individuals to those with a different mental illness, the rates varied, being 53% versus 17%.

Low SES is correlated to BPD, as it is with many other adverse health conditions. Those with a diagnosis of BPD are also more likely to come from families where separation, divorce or parental death have occurred (Sharp & Tackett, 2014). Parental influences are also inherent in this diagnosis. Parental emotional instability or emotional withdrawal are possible catalysts for BPD in some young people and actual physical separation for long periods of time were also common (Sharp & Tackett, 2014). Adverse adolescent relationships with peers and bullying are factors associated with higher rates of BPD, and family dysfunction and neglect are also indicated (Paris, 2015).

Comorbidity

Much like other conditions where impulsiveness plays a role, BPD is highly correlated to comorbid substance use disorders, in particular alcohol use disorder. In addition, there are comorbidities to mood disorders such as depression, bipolar affective disorder and anxiety disorders (Carpenter, Wood & Trull, 2016). Tomko et al. (2014) also note a correlation between antisocial personality disorder and BPD. Additionally, the comorbidity rates are consistently high for BPD with the lifetime prevalence of mood disorders and anxiety disorders in the range of 85%, and substance-use disorders around 79% (Bateman et al., 2016).

Individuals with BPD also have higher rates of comorbid physical illness. In particular, higher rates of diabetes, cardiovascular disease and sexually transmitted infections are noted within this population (NHMRC, 2013).

Clinical course

Symptoms of BPD often emerge in adolescence and the unstable pattern of dysfunction often continues into adulthood, with severe mood and impulse-control unpredictability progressing into adulthood (APA, 2013). BPD is at its most volatile in the early-adult period, when there is also the greatest danger of suicide; however, the dysfunctional elements of the condition tend to diminish the older the individual gets, until the 40th year, when most individuals have a more stabilised pattern of behaviour. Kaess, Brunner and Chanen (2014) note that 10 years post-diagnosis, 85% of individuals with BPD no longer meet enough diagnostic criteria to be diagnosed with the condition. After 16 years, this increases even further, to 99%.

Suicide and self-harm/non-suicidal self-injury

The patterns of suicidality and self-harm/non-suicidal self-injury in BPD are enduring and chronic and are often a long-lasting feature of the illness. **Table 12.7** outlines some of the possible signs of impending suicide or self-harm/non-suicidal self-injury in someone with a diagnosis of BPD. While every suicide attempt should be taken seriously, suicide actions in BPD are often an expression of distress and an attempt to communicate this to others or a way of dealing with a crisis. However, as attempts progress, the ante is often 'upped' and this can have catastrophic results. Around 10% of individuals with BPD will eventually die from suicide, and this number is made up of individuals with traits that are more suggestive of impulsiveness and agitation (Paris, 2015). It is important to differentiate between self-harm/non-suicidal self-injury and suicide, as the two are not interchangeable (see Chapter 20). One of the most clinically effective ways of detecting suicide is through a thorough risk assessment (see Chapter 7). Current research indicates that suicide and self-harm/non-suicidal self-injury is more successfully managed with therapeutic interventions such as 'talk therapy' over medication-based treatments alone (NHMRC, 2013).

TABLE 12.7
Possible indicators impending of self-harm/non-suicidal self-injury/ suicide in individuals with BPD

POSSIBLE INDICATORS
• Recent or impending discharge from hospital (including following a breach of management plan/contract)
• Variations to normal patterns of self-harm/non-suicidal self-injury
• Decompensating mental state
• Increases in substance misuse
• Recent adverse life changes such as relationship issues, financial or employment issues or legal problems
• Lethality of previous suicide attempts

SOURCE: BASED ON NHMRC, 2013

CASE **STUDY**

TEAGAN'S STORY

Teagan is a 21-year-old woman and living with her partner, Amita. Teagan and Amita have been together for 15 months; their relationship is volatile and they have separated a number of times. Last night, Teagan broke up with Amita again in a fiery exchange of insults and anger. Teagan believed that Amita was about to leave her and fearing this relationship breakdown, she thought she would 'get in first'. Amita admits things have been tumultuous between them for months now, and that neither is happy, but wanted to work things out by seeing a relationship counsellor. Amita is also concerned about Teagan's use of cannabis. Amita claims that Teagan's responses to small indiscretions are extreme and that she is quick to make judgements about people or situations with little information. Recently, Teagan decided that a friend of Amita's wasn't allowed to come to their house because she had made some 'throwaway' comments about their dog. Amita says Teagan does this often, liking people quickly for frivolous reasons, and disliking others for similar reasons.

Teagan has been cutting herself since she was 13 years old. She finds it difficult to articulate why she does it, only that she gets relief from cutting. On a few occasions she has contemplated suicide, and many more times she has threatened it. Amita finds this aspect of their relationship very difficult to deal with and frequently feels as though Teagan's threats to self-harm or suicide are a way of manipulating her.

Questions

1   Now that we have explored the different diagnostic criteria and symptoms of BPD, can you identify any specific symptoms Teagan exhibits in the case study?
2   How do you think members of the multidisciplinary team (MDT) could assist Teagan? What would their roles be in working with her?
3   Which MDT member/s would you most like to see 'in action' as they work with Teagan?
4   What do you hope to learn from observing and participating with the MDT?

Treatment

Like most mental health conditions, early intervention is key to treating BPD. However, this needs to be mitigated with the tendency within modern medicine to label and 'diagnose' individuals. This is of particular importance given that many of the symptoms of BPD (like most other mental health conditions) emerge in critical adolescent periods, and BPD can be a highly stigmatised condition within psychiatry. There are a number of reasons why BPD is stigmatised in health care; some of these reasons include clinicians' poor understanding about the motivation for self-harming/non-suicidal self-injuring behaviours; a perception that the individual is manipulative; poor or varied responses to treatment; and cycling crises and readmissions. The National Health and Medical Research Council (NHMRC, 2013), in its *Clinical Practice Guidelines for*

the Management of Borderline Personality Disorder, has developed a comprehensive and evidence-based set of Australian standards for the contemporary management of BPD that provides a complete document for clinicians, consumers, carers and students.

Non-pharmacological treatment

While many individuals with a diagnosis of BPD are committed to engaging in treatment of their condition, dropout rates still vary from 10–50% and treatment requires committed clinicians to ensure the consumer remains engaged (Merced, 2015). Non-pharmacological treatments where appropriate are always more preferable than medication. Where medications *cannot* be avoided, then a combination of both 'talk' and traditional medication-based therapies is recommended. The most common non-pharmacological therapies are described in **Table 12.8**.

TABLE 12.8
Contemporary 'talk therapies' for BPD

THERAPY	DEFINITION	BENEFITS
Dialectical behavioural therapy (DBT)	DBT was specifically developed to treat suicidal and self-harming behaviours inherent in BPD, using principles of cognitive and behavioural therapy. DBT helps the individual manage emotions common to interpersonal relationships such as romantic feelings, anger and reactive tendencies during times of stress. DBT focuses on the individual's strengths and challenges assumptions they may have about themselves and others.	DBT has efficacy in: • reducing self-injurious behaviours • improving self-esteem and self-image • reducing 'interfering' behaviours associated with reducing life quality and those that impact on success of therapy • reducing trauma-associated symptoms of distress.
Cognitive behavioural therapy (CBT)	CBT is designed to help individuals identify faulty thinking and promote thought restructuring to more positive patterns. CBT can be helpful in managing mood states and assist the individual in developing practical strategies to challenge unhelpful thought processes.	CBT has efficacy in: • managing anger/impulsiveness • substance misuse • low self-esteem and poor self-image • behavioural challenges.

THERAPY	DEFINITION	BENEFITS
Schema-focused therapy (SFT)	Useful in managing chronic conditions, SFT can be beneficial in addressing maladaptive coping strategies (such as self-harm or risk-taking behaviours). SFT is a combined therapy that seeks to challenge 'schemas', which are patterns of thinking that people develop when they are young and can result in maladaptive behaviours characteristic of many mental health conditions.	SFT has efficacy in: • addressing enduring patterns of maladaptive coping strategies and internal negative thought processes (such as 'I'm unworthy') which are common to BPD.
Mentalised-based treatments	Another therapy designed specifically for BPD as a result of disorganised attachment, mentalisation therapy assists individuals to differentiate their own personal feeling and thoughts from those around them.	MBT has efficacy in: • helping the individual see the experiences and views of others • improving self-regulation of emotional states and interpersonal relationships with others.
Acceptance and commitment therapy (ACT)	ACT uses mindfulness (an awareness practice that enables the individual to engage in their life 'in the moment'). This permits them to take full advantage of their potential and to have meaningful and rewarding relationships with others.	ACT has efficacy in: • helping the individual live in the 'here and now' and to accept their life by minimising the negative impacts painful experiences can have.
Transference-focused therapy (TFT)	TFT is another model designed specifically for BPD to address the disrupted interpersonal relationships experienced as a result of distorted perceptions of self and others.	TFT has efficacy in: • addressing repetitive self-injurious behaviour • developing control over behaviours • managing emotional fluctuations • improving interpersonal relationships • goal achievement.
Systems training for emotional predictability and problem solving (STEPPS)	Modified DBT, STEPPS is a group-based therapy combining skills training and CBT; it is not an individual therapy. STEPPS is an intensive therapy requiring a dedication to undertaking the 'homework', and is of lengthy duration (20 weeks). STEPPS provides participants with psychoeducation regarding BPD, emotional management/regulatory training and behavioural management training.	STEPPS has efficacy in: • improving the individual's understanding of BPD, and how to effectively manage their behaviours and emotions.

Given the potential for difficulties with interpersonal relationships with BPD, it is of vital importance the clinician is cognisant of issues such as boundaries, ensuring that the parameters of the therapeutic relationship are understood and adhered to for the protection of both the clinician and the consumer. Individuals with a diagnosis BPD often require firm limit-setting, and treatment that is structured. Setting meeting time limits is important for many consumers, and those with BPD may benefit from this structure perhaps more than others. This means that interactions should run to schedule and that the consumer is aware of when they will end. This can help mitigate inherent abandonment issues in BPD.

There are a number of contemporary non-pharmacological treatment options indicated and this list is not exhaustive. Chapter 4 explores therapeutic psychotherapies in greater detail.

Pharmacological treatments

Currently there is no medication specifically indicated for the treatment of BPD in Australia. Due to the complexity and challenges associated with treating BPD, over the years most of the major psychotropic medications have been used (albeit largely unsuccessfully) to treat the condition (Crawford, MacLaren & Reilly, 2014). Antidepressants are useful in the treatment of individuals who have affective instability and for those with impulsive behaviours (Bellino, Bozzatello & Bogetto, 2015); however, there is also significant research to suggest that they are not useful and, in the case of tricyclics, may do more harm than good (Andrews et al., 2013). **Table 12.9** outlines the use of psychotropic medications for BPD in Australia, including the rationales behind usage.

Crawford, MacLaren and Reilly (2014) note that despite research to the contrary, the majority of patients with BPD are treated with antidepressants, with little or no obvious improvement to their mental health. Medication use in BPD should always be an adjunct to therapy-based interventions, as discussed in **Table 12.8**, and care should always be taken with prescribed amounts of medication due to the risk associated with suicide attempts.

Management

The current contemporary management of BPD suggests that, unless unavoidable, inpatient treatment is *not* the best place for individuals with this condition. Where suicide intent is high, imminent or lethal, a short-stay inpatient admission *may* be beneficial; however, there is a degree of contention about its efficacy and there are many who believe an admission is more harmful than beneficial (both to the consumer with BPD and the clinical inpatient environment, which may include other

TABLE 12.9

Pharmacological management of BPD and rationales

MEDICATION	USE
Antipsychotics	In limited trials, aripiprazole demonstrated efficacy in managing agitation, anger, hostility, depression, anxiety and interpersonal functioning. In clinical trials, olanzapine demonstrated efficacy in managing BPD symptoms, hostility, irritability and improving general functioning.
Antidepressants	Many clinicians prescribe treatment of BPD with antidepressants under the assumption that they can be effective in managing the repetitious self-harming behaviours associated with the condition. Clinical trials on limited ADs, however, have not supported this belief. Clinical trials have suggested fluvoxamine has efficacy in treating BPD symptoms overall, while the MAOI phenelzine has been indicated in improving hostility.
Mood stabilisers	To control the fluctuations or mood instability common to BPD. Mood stabilisers are gaining more momentum as an effective treatment of BPD among some prescribers. Sodium valproate has demonstrated efficacy in treating irritability, depression and interpersonal functioning in BPD in clinical trials, while lamotrigine has been indicated as useful in treating anger. Of all the mood stabilisers, topiramate has been shown to be the most effective in clinical trials, assisting in addressing hostility, anxiety and interpersonal functioning.
Anxiolytics*	For short-term management of crisis states such as severe anxiety and distress.

SOURCE: BASED ON NHMRC, 2013

*Anxiolytics are currently contraindicated for a variety of reasons, including their tendency to be abused, but also due to behavioural disruption (Andrews et al., 2013). You may, however, still see them being prescribed for consumers with BPD.

consumers who are highly suggestive towards the active self-harming behaviours of others) (Avery & Bradshaw, 2015). The NHMRC (2013) notes that psychological interventions such as CBT are effective in reducing rates of hospitalisation in individuals with BPD. It also notes that hospitalisation should be for crisis management, of a short duration, and that lengthy stays should be avoided as community-based treatment programs are most effective.

In addition, hospitalisation may actually reinforce self-harming/non-suicidal self-injuring behaviours and validate the notion of 'being ill' in an era where self-responsibility and promoting autonomy for health and treatments are encouraged. The decision to admit a consumer with a diagnosis of BPD is often based on risk aversion and a tendency to 'play it safe' in the event the consumer makes a lethal suicide attempt after being refused an inpatient admission. Every service will have a different way of managing consumers with BPD, but it is important to be aware of the multitude of complexities regarding the decision to admit in addition to the impacts on services that need to mitigate risk with priority of admissions and bed capacity.

Transference and countertransference

Transference and countertransference are two phenomena not uncommon to BPD or the realm of psychology. Transference occurs when the consumer unconsciously transfers feelings or emotions that were experienced previously (usually during childhood) to their current relationship with their nurse or doctor. For example, the nurse reminds the consumer of their aunt Sarah (whom they had a poor relationship with) and so they transfer these negative feelings and emotions to their interactions. This transference can be positive or negative and impacts on the therapeutic relationship and therapy progression for the consumer. Countertransference occurs when the clinician transfers their feelings of previous experiences onto another consumer. Often the countertransference is associated with negative experiences with a condition, the type of behaviours exhibited or a client with the same type of behaviours or symptoms.

Because individuals with BPD are prone to viewing others as all 'good' or all 'bad', the mental health team needs to be mindful of the potential for this behaviour to cause division within the team. For example, particular staff may be exposed to the more undesirable behaviours (e.g. aggression, verbal abuse, self-harming/non-suicidal self-injury) and become more disheartened by all interactions with that consumer. On the other hand, other clinicians may encounter the more amiable aspects of the individual (e.g. idealisation) and may have an increased threshold for tolerating interactions. This can result in division among staff and needs to be closely monitored. Previously, behaviours that seek to divide a team were referred to as 'staff splitting', and you may hear this term used clinically. It is thus imperative that firm boundaries are set and that all clinical staff adhere to the same set of boundaries. Individuals with BPD may be more likely to note discrepancies within a team and use this to their advantage and so consistency among the treating team is imperative. One way of ensuring this consistency is to develop a management plan.

Management plans (see **Table 12.10**) have been used in mental health services for many years, particularly for the treatment of BPD. Individually personalised management plans for crisis management should be discussed with the consumer and their carer where appropriate. Management plans ensure that consumers, carers and clinical staff are aware of expectations, agree on treatment objectives and can remain safe in times of crisis (NHMRC, 2013).

TABLE 12.10

Requirement of management plan for BPD consumers

MANAGEMENT PLAN INCLUSIONS FOR BPD
• Diagnosis
• Short-term goals
• Long-term goals
• Circumstances which may cause or exacerbate risk
• Personalised effective coping strategies in times of distress
• Self-management strategies
• Emergency contact details (such as case manager, psychologist, family/support person, local hospital emergency department)
• Roles and responsibilities of primary care providers and contact details
• Roles of carers/partner/friends and their contact details
• Review dates
• Names of individuals who have a copy of the management plan

SOURCE: BASED ON NHMRC, 2013

NURSING CARE PLAN

WORKING WITH BETH

Consumer Diagnosis: Beth Adamson, 27 (diagnosed with borderline personality disorder)

Nursing Diagnosis: Increase in self-harming/non-suicidal self-injuring behaviours since relationship breakdown with partner.

Outcomes: To manage impulses to self-harm.

Beth is a 27-year-old woman who was recently diagnosed with borderline personality disorder. Beth was admitted to the mental health unit after an increase in self-harming behaviours. Beth moved out of her family home when she was 17 years old to live with a friend's family. Beth states her father sexually abused her on a regular basis and acknowledges that, as a result, she has issues with her self-esteem and interpersonal relationships. Beth has a tumultuous relationship with her current boyfriend Simon, and the pair recently broke up. Beth threatened to self-harm if Simon left her. Beth has been prone to outbursts of anger, including physical aggression, and concedes that this was one of the reasons she and Simon have broken up. She states that she has broken furniture, punched holes in the walls and thrown things at Simon. Beth also states that she apologises after such events, when she calms down, and admits that controlling her impulsive behaviours has been an issue for her in the past. Beth states that this time Simon is refusing to accept her apology, and has moved out of their share-house.

ASSESSMENT DATA OBJECTIVE (O) SUBJECTIVE (S)	EVIDENCE-BASED RATIONALE	RATIONALE	CONSUMER RESPONSE
On assessment Beth has numerous superficial lacerations to upper thighs and arms (O). States that she feels 'relief' when she cuts and is distressed by the breakdown of her relationship (S). Observed by staff to isolate herself in her room, teary and upset when approached (O).	Establish rapport. Regular risk assessment. Follow Beth's management plan (developed by Beth and her community case manager). Close visual observations (15/60). Room search and removal of harmful objects. Encourage and/or facilitate positive coping, self-soothing strategies in times of distress.	Conducting regular risk assessments promotes interaction with Beth and establishes her level of risk to herself. Establishing a 'benchmark' can assist in noticing changes to level of risk. Development of rapport is important in facilitating a relationship where Beth feels comfortable disclosing urges to self-harm so that staff can support other agreed-on alternative coping strategies. It is important to be consistent with Beth and ensure that her community-developed management plan can be followed where possible. 15/60 visual observations mean staff will need to observe/interact with Beth and ensure that she is safe. Removal of objects that are used to self-harm ensures safety. Adopting positive self-soothing strategies is important in managing BPD. Beth should be encouraged to adopt practices such as using ice on areas she wants to cut to enable her to feel pain without the risk of permanent scarring. Other strategies include journal writing, exercising which helps release physical tension and feelings of distress or relaxation techniques.	Beth has approached staff on three separate occasions when she felt strong urges to self-harm. With assistance and encouragement Beth was able to talk about her distress and used ice on her thigh to cause non-permanent pain, rather than pick at her leg with a pen (which she wanted to do).

SOURCE: ADAPTED FROM JAKOPAC & PATEL, 2009

REFLECT ON THIS

Experiences of trauma and BPD

Paula is a 35-year-old woman who has been living with a diagnosis of borderline personality disorder for 14 years. Until recently, Paula had been able to manage her condition, frequently seeing her psychologist and developing strategies to manage her emotional reactions. This all changed, however, when her father, Antonio, died last month. Paula had been sexually abused by her father and was estranged from him and other family members for many years. Paula reconnected with some family upon hearing of her father's death and found it incredibly difficult to hear what a 'wonderful person' Antonio was, as cited numerous times at his funeral and wake.

Questions

1   Discuss the role stress can play in the exacerbation of a mental state. How might Antonio's recent death have contributed to Paula's declining mental state? Your answer should include context of protective and risk factors.

2   Many people with BPD have experienced adverse childhood experiences (ACE), such as abuse and neglect. Discuss the role of these ACEs in the development of BPD.

REFLECTION ON LEARNING FROM PRACTICE

Tara has articulately explained her experiences living with BPD. After reading this chapter, can you identify certain clinical features or experiences she describes that align with her diagnosis? Consider the isolation associated with such a diagnosis and the impacts that behavioural issues may have on employment, family and relationships with others.

These behavioural issues may result in further experiences of isolation, discrimination and subsequent diagnoses of other conditions such as depression and anxiety. BPD is a complex condition that requires complex psychological approaches and clinicians that are compassionate, yet firm in limit setting.

CHAPTER RESOURCES

SUMMARY

- Personality disorders are a complex array of particular behavioural traits that clinically can be very difficult to manage. Typically, personality disorders encompass a range of emotional, behavioural and interpersonal issues with functioning.
- There are three clusters encompassing suspicion (cluster *A*), dramatic engagement with others (cluster *B*) and fearful interactions (cluster *C*).
- Antisocial personality disorder has a complex aetiology, and is more likely to occur in males. Treatment for antisocial personality disorder is difficult to achieve and pharmacological agents are not recommended.
- Borderline personality disorder is more common in individuals with a first-line relative with the condition, and is more frequently seen in females. There are no specific pharmacological treatments indicated for the management of borderline personality disorder and as such medical treatment tends to focus on symptoms.

REVIEW QUESTIONS

1   Antisocial personality disorder is characterised by:
   a   Emotional interpersonal relationships with others
   b   A need to be the centre of attention
   c   A need to be admired by others
   d   Disregard for the rights of others

2   Individuals with borderline personality disorder will benefit from:
   a   Intensive psychotherapy and hospitalisation
   b   A combination of pharmacological and psychotherapeutic therapies
   c   Therapies such as DBT or mindfulness
   d   Medications such as antidepressants and mood stabilisers

3   Discuss the characteristics of cluster *A*, *B* and *C* personality disorders:
   • Cluster *A*: Odd, eccentric and paranoid
   • Cluster *B*: dramatic and emotional
   • Cluster *C*: anxious and fearful
4   Typical characteristics of borderline personality disorder are:
   a   A need for perfectionism
   b   Unstable or intense interpersonal relationships
   c   Grandiose self-image
   d   Disregard for others

5   Raj is a 35-year old man on the mental health unit. Raj frequently engages in deceitful, manipulative and impulsive behaviours. Which personality disorder is Raj likely to have?
   a   Paranoid
   b   Schizotypal
   c   Borderline
   d   Antisocial

CRITICAL THINKING

1   Borderline personality disorder is associated with 'a pattern of unstable and intense interpersonal relationships characterised by alternating between extremes of idealisation and devaluation' (APA, 2013, p. 663). What do you think this means?

2   Consider your own personality. Which personality traits do you think you have of the characteristics listed in **Table 12.1**, and why? Give examples to support your answers.
3   Females are more likely to receive a diagnosis of BPD, and males APD. Discuss one of the possible reasons for this.

USEFUL WEBSITES

- Australian BPD Foundation: https://bpdfoundation.org.au
- BPD Resources: http://www.bpdresources.net
- Emotions Matter: https://emotionsmatterbpd.org

REFLECT ON THIS

BPD and the MDT: utilising specialty expertise
While nurses comprise a large portion of the mental health workforce, they are not the only members of this team. Members of the multidisciplinary team (MDT) have many skills and attributes to share with students on placement and they respond positively when students are enthusiastic, engaged and prepared. Think of one question about borderline personality disorder that you would like to ask

the following MDT members that relates to their clinical speciality or expertise:
- consumer
- mental health nurse
- social worker
- occupational therapist
- psychologist
- medical officer
- psychiatrist.

REFERENCES

Amad, A., Ramoz, N., Thomas, P., Jardri, R. & Gorwood, P. (2014). Genetics of borderline personality disorder: Systematic review and proposal of an integrative model. *Neuroscience and Biobehavioral Reviews*, 40, 6–19.

American Psychiatric Association. (2013). *Diagnostic and Statistical Manual of Mental Disorders (DSM-5)* (5th edn). Washington, DC: APA.

Andrews, G., Dean, K., Genderson, M., Hunt, C., Mitchell, P., Sachdev, P. & Trollor, J. (2013). *Management of Mental Disorders* (5th edn). Sydney: School of Psychiatry, University of NSW.

Avery, M. & Bradshaw, T. (2015). Improving care for people with borderline personality disorder. *Mental Health Practice*, 18(6), 33–7.

Bateman, A., O'Connell, J., Lorenzini, N., Gardner, T. & Fonagy, P. (2016). A randomized controlled trial of mentalization-based treatment versus structured clinical management for patients with comorbid borderline personality disorder and antisocial personality disorder. *BMC Psychiatry*, 16(304), 1–14.

Bellino, S., Bozzatello, P. & Bogetto, F. (2015). Combined treatment of borderline personality disorder with interpersonal psychotherapy and pharmacotherapy: Predictors of response. *Psychiatry Research*, 226, 284–8.

Black, D.W. (2015). The natural history of antisocial personality disorder. *Canadian Journal of Psychiatry*, 60(7), 309–14.

Buck, K.A. (2015). Understanding adolescent psychopathic traits from early risk and protective factors: Relations among inhibitory control, maternal sensitivity, and attachment representation. *Journal of Adolescence*, 44, 97–105.

Cain, N.M., Ansell, E.B., Simpson, H.B. & Pinto, A. (2015). Interpersonal functioning in obsessive-compulsive personality disorder. *Journal of Personality Assessment*, 97(1), 90–9.

Carlson, M., Oshri, A. & Kwon, J. (2015). Child maltreatment and risk behaviours: The roles of callous/unemotional traits and conscientiousness. *Child Abuse & Neglect*, 50, 234–43.

Carpenter, R.W., Wood, P.K. & Trull, T.J. (2016). Comorbidity of borderline personality disorder and lifetime substance use disorders in a nationally representative sample. *Journal of Personality Disorders*, 30(3), 336–50.

Crawford, M.J., MacLaren, T. & Reilly, J.G. (2014). Are mood stabilisers helpful in treatment of borderline personality disorder? *BMJ*, 349, 1–3.

DeLisi, M. & Vaughn, M.G. (2015). Ingredients for criminality require genes, temperament, and psychopathic personality. *Journal of Criminal Justice*, 43, 290–4.

Eikenaes, I., Egeland, J., Hummelen, B. & Wilberg, T. (2015). Avoidant personality disorder versus social phobia: The significance of childhood neglect. *PLOS ONE*, 1–14. doi:10.1371/journal.pone.0122846

Ficks, C.A., Dong., L. & Waldman, I.D. (2014). Sex differences in the etiology of psychopathic traits in youth. *Journal of Abnormal Psychology*, 123(2), 406–11.

Fox, B.H., Perez, N., Cass, E., Baglivio, M.T. & Epps, N. (2015). Trauma changes everything: Examining the relationship between adverse childhood experiences and serious, violent and chronic juvenile offenders. *Child Abuse & Neglect*, 46, 163–73.

González-Tapia, M.I. & Obsuth, I. (2015). 'Bad genes' and criminal responsibility. *International Journal of Law & Psychiatry*, 39, 60–71.

Ishibashi, N.L. (2014). *Arguing With the DSM-5: Reflections from the Perspectives of Social Work*. Chicago, IL: Lulu Press.

Jackson, D.B. & Beaver, K.M. (2015). The influence of nutritional factors on verbal deficits and psychopathic personality traits: Evidence of the moderating role of the MAOA genotype. *International Journal of Environmental Research and Public Health*, 12, 15 739–55. doi:10.3390/ijerph121215017

Jakopac, K.A. & Patel, S.C. (2009). *Psychiatric and Mental Health Case Studies and Care Plans*. Burlington, MA: Jones and Bartlett Publishers.

Kaess, M., Brunner, R. & Chanen, A. (2014). Borderline personality disorder in adolescence. *Pediatrics*, 134(4), 782–93.

Kernberg, O.F. (2016). What is personality? *Journal of Personality Disorders*, 30(2), 145–56.

Le Corff, Y. & Toupin, J. (2014). Overt versus covert conduct disorder symptoms and the prospective prediction of antisocial personality disorder. *Journal of Personality Disorders*, 28(6), 864–72.

Merced, M. (2015). The beginning psychotherapist and borderline personality disorder: Basic treatment principles and clinical foci. *American Journal of Psychotherapy*, 69(3), 241–68.

National Health and Medical Research Council (NHMRC). (2013). *Clinical Practice Guidelines for the Management of Borderline Personality Disorder*. Melbourne: NHMRC. Released under CC BY 3.0 AU. Link to license: https://creativecommons.org/licenses/by/3.0/au/.

Ogloff, J.R.P., Campbell, R.E. & Shepherd, S.M. (2016). Disentangling psychopathy from antisocial personality disorder: An Australian analysis. *Journal of Forensic Psychology Practice*, 16(3), 198–215. doi:10.1080/15228932.2016.1177281

Ogloff, J.R.P., Talevski, D., Lemphers, A., Wood, M. & Simmons, M. (2015). Co-occurring mental illness, substance use disorders, and antisocial personality disorders among clients of forensic mental health services. *Psychiatric Rehabilitation Journal*, 38(1), 16–23.

Ogrodniczuk, J.S. (2013). *Understanding and Treating Pathological Narcissism*. Washington, DC: American Psychological Association.

Paris, J. (2015). *A Concise Guide to Personality Disorders*. Washington, DC: American Psychiatric Association.

Sharp, C. & Tackett, J.L. (2014). *Handbook of Borderline Personality Disorder in Children and Adolescents*. New York: Springer Science & Business.

Sher, L., Siever, L.J., Goodman, M., McNamara, M., Hazlett, E.A., Koenigsberg, H.W. & New, A.S. (2015). Gender differences in the clinical characteristics and psychiatric comorbidity in patients with antisocial personality disorder. *Psychiatry Research*, 229, 685–9.

Thylstrup, B. & Hesse, M. (2016). Impulsive lifestyle counseling to prevent dropout from treatment for substance use disorders in people with antisocial personality disorder: A randomized study. *Addictive Behaviors*, 57, 48–54.

Tomko, R.L., Trull, T.J., Wood, P.K. & Sher, K.J. (2014). Characteristics of borderline personality disorder in a community sample: Comorbidity, treatment utilization, and general functioning. *Journal of Personality Disorders*, 28(5), 734–50.

CHAPTER **13**

EATING DISORDERS

Louise Alexander

LEARNING OUTCOMES

Upon completion of this chapter, you should be able to:

13.1 Understand clinical manifestations of anorexia nervosa, including aetiology, diagnostic criteria, treatment, relapse and recovery

13.2 Understand clinical manifestations of bulimia nervosa, including aetiology, diagnostic criteria, treatment, relapse and recovery

13.3 Understand the diagnostic criteria, aetiology and epidemiology, and treatment options for binge-eating disorder

13.4 Understand the differences in presentation of eating disorders in male clients

LEARNING FROM PRACTICE

Fat! Disgusting! Ugly! Shameful! Ordinary! You are unworthy of love! Unworthy of life! YOU ARE SICKENING!!

These are just some of the berating labels that have been reverberating in my head, like a broken record, for more than two decades. This all-too-familiar domineering female voice has echoed in my ears, from my earliest memories as a child. At a time in your life where you are free. Free to be a child and play. Free to explore and colour outside of the lines, and although I did do this, it was always controlled. Something or someone governing me to stay between the lines, often accompanied by a sickening feeling deep in my belly, brought on by this voice that would tell me that this was bad. That I was bad! I was continuously reminded of my stupidity every time I answered a question in school incorrectly. There was never any room for error. An error is a flaw and flaws are unacceptable, the voice would remind me. This soon translated to my face and my body. Little did I know at the age of eight that life as I knew it would never be the same. It would consume me, my life, my every waking thought. Even my sleep was taken over by this beast within. I would lay there night after night, starving, exhausted, yet unable to sleep. I would simply lie there and do my ritualised safety check. I would first lay on my back and feel the bony protrusion of my hip bones, then

my ribs, followed by my sternum. Only to finish the ritual by laying on my side with my knees bent and pressed together, ensuring that at no point along my inner thighs that they met. Confirming that I was safe.

Nothing in this life has frightened me more than the thought and fear of being fat and losing control. Like all things it starts small, harmlessly cutting out one thing and then another… Until all I felt safe consuming was water. No voice of reason stood a chance against this force within me. A force that had one mission, one sole purpose, and that was to be thin and beautiful. It was all that mattered, and sadly it was worth dying for.

Belle, a 25-year-old woman with a lived experience of anorexia nervosa

Belle has provided an emotive account of her experiences of living with anorexia nervosa. Consider the social norms of our society. How might these norms contribute to the development of anorexia nervosa? Belle notes that her negative feelings about her body were evident at age 8. While this may seem early, this is consistent with current research and findings. What influences do you think could contribute to the development of anorexia nervosa in an eight-year-old child?

INTRODUCTION

Feeding and eating disorders (ED) encompass a number of disordered behaviours associated with issues around the intake of food and fluid. While eating disorders came to prominence in the second half of the 20th century, historically it is thought that descriptions of self-inflicted starvation date back to the 12th and 13th centuries. Eating disorders are highly stigmatised. While stigma is attached to most mental health conditions to varying degrees, eating disorders are often labelled as behavioural, believed to be a condition of 'choice' and not deemed serious despite significant morbidity and mortality rates (Bannatyne & Abel, 2015). In adolescence, eating disorders are believed to affect about 15% of females and 3% of males, making them all too familiar in the child and adolescent mental health context (Allen, Byrne & Crosby, 2015). Because eating disorders are so dangerous, it is important to ensure that health care professionals screen for them appropriately.

Table 13.1 outlines the SCOFF Questionnaire (Morgan, Reid & Lacey, 1999), which was devised as a quick tool to recognise potential disordered eating behaviours. This tool provides a baseline of information that any health care clinician can obtain and will identify individuals who are deemed potentially 'at risk'; as such, it enables the health care practitioner (especially those clinicians working outside of mental health) to make an informed decision to refer for more specialised care.

TABLE 13.1
The SCOFF Questionnaire

THE SCOFF QUESTIONNAIRE
• Do you make yourself SICK because you feel uncomfortably full?
• Do you worry you have lost CONTROL over how much you eat?
• Have you recently lost more than ONE stone (6 kg) in a three-month period?
• Do you believe yourself to be FAT when others say you are too thin?
• Would you say that FOOD dominates your life?
One or two 'YES' answers suggest concerning eating behaviours possibly suggestive of an eating disorder warranting further investigation.

SOURCE: MORGAN, REID & LACEY, 1999; NSW MINISTRY OF HEALTH, 2014

The most commonly known eating disorders are anorexia nervosa and bulimia nervosa; however, this chapter will also cover the lesser known binge-eating disorder.

ANOREXIA NERVOSA

The word 'anorexia' has its roots in the Latin term meaning 'without appetite', while 'nervosa' implies a stress or nervous cause of this reluctance to eat.

Anorexia nervosa was first described by William Gull in the late seventeenth century where he observed four young girls who presented with self-induced weight loss (Sharan & Sundar, 2015). **Anorexia nervosa (AN)** is a condition where the individual fails to maintain acceptable weight in relation to their age and gender, and is often associated with distorted body image and an intense fear of gaining weight despite being seriously underweight. In the general nursing setting, you may have heard or even used the term 'anorexia' to describe a patient's lack of appetite. It is the addition of the word 'nervosa' that indicates a pathological origin of anorexia in the mental health context. AN is notoriously fatal, and is in fact the most deadly of *all* mental health conditions, requiring a balance of medical and mental health input to ensure the consumer is both medically and psychologically stable.

Clinical manifestations

The most common clinical symptom of AN is deliberate weight loss resulting in low weight. **Figure 13.1** outlines the ranges of severity of AN in relation to **body mass index (BMI)** and it is this measure that enables medical staff to assess the consumer. BMI is calculated using the following simple equation:

$$BMI = \frac{weight\ (kg)}{[height\ (m)]^2}$$

Many individuals with AN will use a range of methods to facilitate weight loss, and prevent weight gain. These include:

- vigorous exercising
- restricting food and fluid intake
- misuse of laxatives, other aperients or diuretics
- self-induced vomiting or purging.

Consumers with AN *are* hungry. Unfortunately, these feelings of hunger often help to reinforce the consumer's belief that they are 'fat' because they are *always* hungry, not because they are, in fact, starving themselves to death. It is perhaps unsurprising that AN is a condition frequently associated with control: the control of what is eaten, control of weight, and control of body shape through exercise.

Individuals with AN will also use a range of methods to hide their eating behaviours, exercising

BMI ranges
Mild: BMI ≥ 17 kg/m²
Moderate: BMI 16–16.99 kg/m²
Severe: BMI 15–16.99 kg/m²
Extreme: BMI < 15 kg/m²

SOURCE: APA, 2013

FIGURE 13.1
BMI ranges and severity

patterns and general physical state (see **Table 13.2**). Some of these common methods of hiding AN include:

- wearing 'baggy' oversized clothing to hide weight loss
- cooking for other people, particularly family and friends, yet eating little or none of this prepared food themselves
- lying about the food and/or quantities they have eaten (such as cutting food up into small pieces to make it appear as though some has been eaten, dirtying plates and cutlery, etc.)
- claiming to be allergic or intolerant to certain foods (to avoid eating them without raising suspicion)
- eating alone, or being absent during family/communal meal times
- refusal to eat previously enjoyed foods
- major changes to diet, such as suddenly becoming vegetarian or vegan.

Vigorous, compulsive or problematic exercise is a frequent presentation of AN and has been referred to by many as 'hyperactive' exercising (Rizk et al., 2015). There are a number of hypotheses as to why compulsive exercise is undertaken by those with a diagnosis of AN. Obviously, weight loss is the major factor; however, it is not as simple as this. Alleviation of stress through vigorous exercise and management of depressive symptoms are also likely influences in the overuse of exercise common to those with AN (Rizk et al., 2015). Individuals with a diagnosis of AN will often continue this extreme pattern of exercise regimen regardless of poor weather (including extreme heat or cold) and injury (Harrington, Jimerson, Haxton & Jimerson, 2015). As the condition worsens, individuals with AN may experience stress fractures and other injuries associated with exercising excessively.

As the individual becomes more emaciated and starved, they will begin to demonstrate more obvious signs of AN. **Table 13.3** identifies the physical signs of AN. They may experience palpitations, bradycardia and postural hypotension (Harrington et al., 2015). Ongoing misuse of aperients can result in haemorrhoids and in some cases even rectal prolapse, and seizures caused from low blood sugar may also occur (Harrington et al., 2015).

Prevalence

Fortunately, AN is fairly rare. In the United States, one in every 200 females has the condition and the vast majority who have AN (95%) are aged between 12–25 years (Harrington et al., 2015) and these prevalence rates are consistent with *Diagnostic and Statistical Manual of Mental Disorders* (DSM-5; APA, 2013) rates of about 0.4%. While AN is historically a condition associated with females (90%), more males (Harrington et al., 2015) are increasingly being diagnosed at ratios of 10:1 (APA, 2013). Recently, there has been increased concern regarding the emerging growth of AN in very young populations (Mustelin

TABLE 13.2
Behaviours often associated with AN

ASSOCIATED BEHAVIOURS
• Preoccupation with body image and size, checking themselves in the mirror often
• Weighing/counting foods
• Missing meals, or refusing to eat and making excuses about eating
• Overly sensitive about comments regarding their appearance
• Frequently weighing themselves
• Excessively chewing food
• Becoming upset, anxious or fearful around meal times
• Claiming to need to exercise to 'burn off' calories
• Exercising despite inclement weather or injury
• Demonstrating ritualistic behaviours around food (such as placing food on their plate in a particular way, cutting food into tiny pieces, eating food in a certain order, painstakingly pulling foods apart before eating, only eating at certain times)
• Complaining about their weight
• Seeking assistance with weight loss (e.g. from the general practitioner)
• Avoiding eating in public places or social settings
• Substituting food with liquid
• Excessive interest in foods, recipes, cookbooks, diets, weight loss strategies/websites, etc.
• Associating foods with being either 'good' or 'bad'
• Self-worth and self-esteem that is highly influenced by their weight
• Only eating a restricted diet containing certain foods (usually those with low calories/fat)
• Misuse of stimulants to suppress appetite
• Adopting narrow eating patterns, or becoming vegan or vegetarian
• Calorie counting or knowing verbatim the exact amount of calories (or fat, carbohydrates, etc.) in foods

TABLE 13.3
Physical signs of anorexia nervosa

PHYSICAL SIGNS
• Weight below expected level
• Amenorrhoea
• Loss of libido (males)
• Weakness, lethargy, fatigue
• Dry skin
• Sleep disturbance
• Dehydration
• Brittle nails
• Constipation and haemorrhoids
• Intolerance to cold temperatures and hypothermia
• Hypotension
• Bradycardia
• Lanugo (fine fluffy hair covering body)
• Thin, damaged hair that may fall out
• Erosion of teeth enamel
• Dorsal hand scars from knocking teeth during purging (known as Russell's sign)
• Hoarse voice from purging
• Some may have an impaired gag reflex from purging
• Delayed wound healing and lowered immunity
• Fainting or dizziness
• Blood analysis abnormalities (in liver enzymes, potassium, calcium, sodium, phosphorus, magnesium, folate, blood glucose, urea and electrolytes (U&E), etc.).

SOURCE: APA, 2013; PALMER, 2014.

et al., 2015). By the age of 20 years, around 13% of young people will be diagnosed with an ED and 15–47% of young people will demonstrate distorted thinking patterns and behaviours around eating (Culbert, Racine & Klump, 2015).

Aetiology and epidemiology

Like all other mental health conditions, the development of AN is attributable to a number of different possible causes. Unlike most other mental health conditions, AN is impacted by factors such as media and negative experiences in childhood around body image; for example, teasing. This section will explore the causes and characteristics of individuals affected by AN.

Genetic factors

Individuals who develop AN (or any other ED) often have a family history of a mental health condition, in particular, eating disorders, depression and substance misuse and dependency issues (Zeppegno & Gramaglia, 2014). A number of studies have suggested 'moderate-to-high heritability' (Culbert, Racine & Klump, 2015, p. 1143) of AN and it is thought that the remaining individuals who go on to develop AN (or another ED) do so due to other, non-biological reasons (e.g. environment, bullying, etc.). Studies on twins have suggested the heritability of AN to be in the order of 56–76%, which strongly supports the role genetics plays (Peterson et al., 2015).

Biological factors

There is some evidence to suggest that the genes responsible for regulating serotonin may be affected in women with EDs (Culbert, Racine & Klump, 2015). Issues identified regarding dopamine receptor genes have also been seen in individuals who develop AN and have a past history of abuse. There has also been consideration in the role puberty plays in girls who develop AN, given the hormonal surge that occurs during this time, and the possibility that body changes influence self-image, and this is an area that requires further investigation.

Individual factors

Some individuals with AN will have a history of parental abuse and neglect, in particular parents who are highly critical (Culbert, Racine & Klump, 2015). Particular temperamental traits are commonly seen in certain types of mental health conditions and AN is no different. It is also important to remember that personality traits are understood to be highly heritable and while these are considered individual factors, there is often a genetic link too (Culbert, Racine & Klump, 2015). In essence, individuals with AN have an inherent dread of becoming overweight. Individuals with AN have issues with self-esteem, self-image and a notoriously negative and distorted attitude towards their body. Many people with AN are sensitive to the emotional states of those around them, but lack insight into their own emotional states, and have difficulty understanding and expressing their feelings and emotions. Traits commonly seen in those with AN include a need for control, perfectionism and a highly critical evaluation of perceived failures (Zeppegno & Gramaglia, 2014). Perfectionism is a personality trait seen in EDs and there is overlap with co-occurring obsessive-compulsive personality disorder (see Chapter 12) in this population. Also seen are neurotic (indicated by purging symptoms and striving to be thin) and impulsive personality traits in individuals who have AN (Culbert, Racine & Klump, 2015). Impulsive traits, however, are generally only seen in individuals with binge-eating and **purging behaviours** (Culbert, Racine & Klump, 2015). Consumers with AN will often set extremely high standards for themselves and are highly self-critical when they cannot meet these often unrealistic goals. This need for control is manifested in the control of what the individual eats and how much exercise they can do – it is the epitome of control; that is, controlling what goes in one's mouth. For some individuals diagnosed with AN, the condition is triggered by a traumatic event such as the death of a parent.

Environmental and social factors

There are a variety of possible causes of the fear of being overweight, but for many, AN has resulted from bullying. A desire (either through bullying, peers, media or family/culture) to fit the ideal body type often results in this restricted pattern of eating and dieting. For some, this pressure comes from sporting clubs where size is deemed important (such as gymnastics or ballet). In fact, individuals with AN participate in sport and exercise at rates higher than with any other mental health condition (Rizk et al., 2015). Copeland et al. (2015) identified bullying by peers in childhood as significant factors in the development of eating disordered behaviours seen in AN and bulimia nervosa (BN). Bullying has been attributed to a series of adverse mental health issues including suicide and psychotic symptoms. When bullying targets an individual's appearance, it can result in the experience of negative self-body image, and impact on confidence and self-esteem (Copeland et al., 2015). This poor self-image can result in restrictive dieting in an attempt to modify body shape or appearance into what is seen to be more socially acceptable; that is, being thin.

Stressful family situations and parental relationship issues may be affiliated with AN to some degree. While previously parental style was thought to be a *cause* of AN, this has largely been proven unfounded; connections of parenting styles to AN seem tenuous, and at best seem to be more prominent when observed collectively with other issues (Harrington et al., 2015). These 'other' issues include family dysfunction and tension and family stress, which can result in anxiety reactions and traits common to eating disorders in offspring. Other family contributing factors include households where expectations are high. When expectations are increasingly hard to achieve, the child may revert to controlling what they *do* have control over; that is, what they eat and how they look (Harrington et al., 2015).

Unsurprisingly, societal expectations of how people (particularly women) should look are contributing factors when considering the impacts of eating disorders (Harrington et al., 2015). It appears that many individuals with AN place significant importance on image and appearance, and associate many common adverse stereotypes with being overweight such as being less deserving, unintelligent and unattractive (Zeppegno & Gramaglia, 2014) – see **Figure 13.2**. This perception fuels the desire to continue to lose weight.

Undoubtedly, the media also play a role in eating-disordered behaviours. Individuals who present as 'at risk' for the development of AN and are exposed to media personalities who are underweight (such as

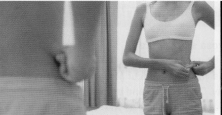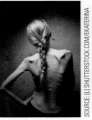

SOURCE: ILI SHUTTERSTOCK.COM/EKATERINA VIDYASOVA; (R) ALAMY STOCK PHOTO/CTK

FIGURE 13.2
These women are at different stages of anorexia

models or actresses) are believed to have a higher risk of developing the condition (Yom-Tov & Boyd, 2014). Individuals considered 'at risk' are those with disordered eating behaviours, dissatisfaction with their body and those who perceive 'thin' as the most ideal body shape (White et al., 2016). Photographs of thin celebrities from mass media often reflect the aspirations of ideal weight and body shape for young women and these images help to reinforce idealisation of thinness and a desire to emulate that appearance. This media exposure to thin celebrities may result in increased eating disordered behaviours (White et al., 2016). Young girls who are exposed to print images in magazines appear to demonstrate higher rates of eating disordered characteristics, but the role genetics plays in this development is also important to consider. Females are particularly partial to society's idealisation of being thin, and exposure to television and media that exemplifies this belief exacerbates this notion in women and young girls who may already be vulnerable to questioning their appearance (Culbert, Racine & Klump, 2015) – see **Figure 13.3**).

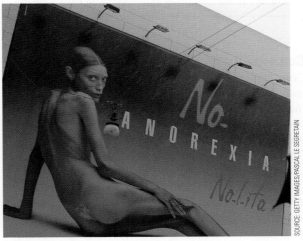

SOURCE: GETTY IMAGES/PASCAL LE SEGRETAIN

FIGURE 13.3
Before her death at age 28, French model Isabelle Caro contributed to advertisements warning against the dangers of anorexia nervosa

CULTURAL CONSIDERATIONS

Anorexia nervosa and culture

While AN is not a condition only seen in developed countries, it does appear to occur at higher rates in Western society. Cases of AN and bulimia nervosa are considered rare in many countries with prevalence rates in, for example, Korea, as low as 0.005% (Sharan & Sundar, 2015). Dissatisfaction with body shape and size is considered a growing area of concern in developing countries with Western influences and likely contributes to the development of eating disorders. Interestingly, studies exploring body attitudes in non-Western countries demonstrate similar dysfunctional eating behaviours as in Western countries; however, the aspiration or motivations for thinness in the non-Western cohort was not deemed as tenacious (Sharan & Sundar, 2015). It is hypothesised that the motivators for disordered eating behaviours in non-Western society are probably driven by factors other than body dissatisfaction. Supporting the hypothesis that media indoctrination of 'thinness' in Western society is a significant contributor to the development of EDs and ED behaviours is the fact that in communities where Western cultures have only been recently introduced, EDs have increased (Culbert, Racine & Klump, 2015). In particular, this notion was observed in studies conducted in Fiji where Western television programs depicting thin actors are believed to have led to an increase in disordered eating behaviours and dieting in individuals who were earlier indifferent to such issues (Culbert, Racine & Klump, 2015; Sharan & Sundar, 2015). It has also been suggested that for some individuals who migrate to Western societies, disordered eating may be a response to the difficulties associated with such a move.

Comorbidity

Comorbidities in other conditions where control is an issue are not uncommon in this cohort. In particular, mood disorders such as depression (see Chapter 10), obsessive-compulsive disorder (see Chapter 17), obsessive-compulsive personality disorder (see Chapter 12), post-traumatic stress disorder (see Chapter 18) and deliberate self-harming behaviours (see Chapter 20) are seen (Zeppegno & Gramaglia, 2014). Rates of depression in the past or as a comorbid feature of AN are seen in more than half of individuals diagnosed with an eating disorder (Harrington et al., 2015). There is also evidence to support the suggestion that comorbid mental health issues in individuals with AN significantly impair recovery and can impact on relapse. About 40% of individuals with AN will experience a co-occurring mood disorder, and about 30% will also have obsessive-compulsive disorder (Andrews et al., 2013).

Clinical course

For the vast majority of individuals with AN, dieting is the catalyst for the condition and this usually commences in adolescence, often around puberty. The use of dieting may be a logical solution to attaining a more healthy weight in the beginning, but while the majority of people who diet stop after achieving their desired weight, individuals with AN continue trying to lose more weight at alarming rates (Zeppegno & Gramaglia, 2014). While it is rare for AN to develop in young children, there has been a concerning increasing trend in very young people being treated for AN and other EDs. Late development of AN is also rare, particularly after the 30th year (APA, 2013).

Prognosis

AN is the most deadly of all mental health conditions with a mortality rate that increases the longer the individual lives with the condition (5% per decade) (Berends et al., 2016). A mortality rate as high as 20% has been noted in a 20-year follow-up (Andrews et al., 2013). Even among individuals who are in remission of AN, relapse is still common and the condition can manifest throughout the lifetime, alternating between remission and recurrence, and resulting in a number of long-term health issues (see **Table 13.4**).

TABLE 13.4
Health issues associated with anorexia nervosa

ASSOCIATED HEALTH ISSUES
• Osteoporosis and bone density loss
• Infertility
• Cardiac arrhythmias
• Infections
• Anaemia
• Muscle wasting/loss
• Suppression of bone marrow
• Hypotension and resulting cardiac problems

According to Keski-Rahkonen and colleagues (2014), one in every five individuals with AN will experience the condition in a chronic capacity, further increasing the potential for death to result from the illness. In addition, there are other factors associated with worsening the prognosis of AN. Individuals with AN who had symptoms of a mental health condition prior to the development of AN demonstrate a poorer prognosis. Those who also have obsessive-compulsive disorder (see Chapter 17), BN and purgative behaviours and who experience rapid weight loss are also inclined to have a poor outcome (Keski-Rahkonen et al., 2014). In one study, outcomes are also poorer for AN sufferers who were living alone and unemployed, experienced depressive symptoms prior to the development of AN and were in an unhappy relationship (Keski-Rahkonen et al., 2014).

AN, suicide and self-harm/non-suicidal self-injury

The DSM-5 (APA, 2013) reports that rates of suicide are higher in individuals with AN at 12 per 100 000 deaths annually. AN is a condition with one of the highest reported rates of suicide and is responsible for about 20% of deaths related to AN (Thornton et al., 2016). Suicidal behaviours in individuals with AN have been explored; however, the results are highly variable, with reported lifetime prevalence between 3–29% (Thornton et al., 2016). It is suggested that prolonged suffering through food deprivation fulfils the interpersonal theory of suicide (for more see Chapter 20) notion that pain tolerance is necessary (in addition to fearlessness) to go through with an attempt to end one's life (Thornton et al., 2016). Reporting of self-harming/non-suicidal self-injury in AN varies widely at rates of between 14–68% (Cucchi et al., 2016).

Diagnostic criteria

The diagnosis of AN is based on the presentation of a number of diverse criteria and behaviours, with particular attention given to the individual's BMI. **Table 13.5** outlines the diagnostic criteria for AN.

DIAGNOSTIC CRITERIA

Anorexia nervosa

TABLE 13.5
Diagnostic criteria anorexia nervosa

A.	Restriction of energy intake relative to requirements, leading to a significantly low body weight in the context of age, sex, development trajectory, and physical health. *Significantly low weight* is defined as a weight that is less than minimally normal or, for children and adolescents, less than that minimally expected.
B.	Intense fear of gaining weight or of becoming fat or persistent behavior that interferes with weight gain, even though at a significantly low weight.
C.	Disturbance in the way in which one's body weight or shape is experienced, undue influence of body weight or shape on self-evaluation, or persistent lack of recognition of the seriousness of the current low body weight.

Specify whether:
Restricting type: During the last three months, the individual has not engaged in recurrent episodes of binge eating or purging behavior (i.e., self-induced vomiting or the misuse of laxatives, diuretics, or enemas). This subtype describes presentations in which weight loss is accomplished primarily through dieting, fasting, and/or excessive exercise.
Binge-eating/purging type: During the last three months, the individual has engaged in recurrent episodes of binge eating or purging behavior (i.e. self-induced vomiting or the misuse of laxatives, diuretics, or enemas)
Specify current severity:
The minimum level of severity is based, for adults, on current body mass index (BMI) (see below) or, for children and adolescents, on BMI percentile. The ranges below are derived from World Health Organization categories for thinness in adults; for children and adolescents, corresponding BMI percentiles should be used. The level of severity may be increased to reflect clinical symptoms, the degree of functional disability, and the need for supervision.
Mild: BMI ≥ 17 kg/m^2
Moderate: BMI 16–16.99 kg/m^2
Severe: BMI 15–16.99 kg/m^2
Extreme: BMI <15 kg/m^2

CASE **STUDY**

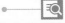

ERIN'S STORY

Erin is a 19-year-old university student in her second year at university. Erin is bright and has always been a high achiever at school, and her parents have been keen to prompt her to follow her dreams and encourage her pursuits. Erin loves cooking for her family, particularly her older brother Josh. In order to achieve the best possible Year 12 score, Erin's parents decided to move her to a private school for girls that had a good reputation for university acceptance. Erin's mother took on extra work to pay for the school fees. While Erin was sad to leave her old school and friends, she agreed that this was the best choice for her academically.

Things did not go as well as planned, however, and Erin was subjected to distressing bullying from the beginning of Year 12 until she finished the school year. Erin has always been conscious of her health and weight, but was targeted because she had 'fat legs' and the bullies sent her text messages of 'fat people' and memes with derogatory messages about her. Because her parents had made sacrifices for her to attend this school, Erin didn't want to tell them that she was being bullied, so she kept it to herself. This bullying had a devastating impact on Erin's self-esteem and she began dieting. People would comment on how great she looked, so she continued dieting. She felt she had some control over what she ate, and this made her feel better.

When her local gym had a special rate for new members, Erin joined. When she wasn't at the gym, she was studying. Because she was working out so much, and restricting her diet, Erin became seriously constipated. So, she went to her local pharmacy and began buying laxatives. Erin noticed that they helped with her constipation, but they also reduced her weight (Erin would weigh herself daily), so she began taking them all the time. It got to the point where her local pharmacy would not sell them to her any more, so she began buying them from multiple pharmacies and online. Despite the turmoil at school, Erin did well academically and achieved exceptionally high marks in her final exams. She got her first preference for courses, and enrolled in a Bachelor of Dietetics at a well-regarded university. Recently, however, wearing baggy clothing and restricting her food intake has been causing suspicions. Her mother has told her she is too thin, and her brother and father have expressed concern about her – but Erin doesn't see it this way. When Erin looks in the mirror she sees the fat girl who was bullied in Year 12. Erin has collapsed at her gym a number of times, and staff have expressed concern about her weight. Erin worried that as with the pharmacy, she will need to find another gym. At 1.62 cm tall and weighing 41 kg, Erin's BMI is 15.6.

Questions

1 What are some of the physical risks associated with Erin's behaviours?

2 Erin is exhibiting many different behaviours consistent with ED. Describe what these are.

3 Who are some of the key members of the multidisciplinary team that Erin would benefit from working with? Think also about her family: who could they seek support from?

Treatment

Eating disorders can be difficult to treat. This is because dealing with the enduring patterns of low self-image and low self-esteem is a pivotal factor in combating the condition, *regardless* of weight attainment. Not only do clinicians need to focus on the need to increase weight, but they must also help them change their feelings towards food, in addition to addressing low self-esteem and poor body image. Any one of these areas alone may be challenging. Treatment involves exploration of self, and developing appropriate strategies to recognise and express feelings and emotions, rather than suppressing these and use dieting and exercising in managing the distress associated with being unable to do this.

No single therapy is indicated in the treatment of AN. In the initial stages of treatment, medical stabilisation is imperative and electrolyte imbalances and arrhythmias often require urgent care. Roux and colleagues (2016) note that many individuals with AN (up to 40%) leave hospital before they have recovered and as such their recovery is negatively impacted. They also note that withdrawal from treatment was exacerbated in individuals who:

■ were >18 years old

■ had a disagreement with clinicians on target BMI (individuals with insight into their illness and a desire to recover do better)

■ were insightless into patterns of restricting dieting and the impact this has on their illness (Roux et al., 2016).

Individuals commencing treatment for AN will experience many challenges. In particular, being required to address behaviours towards eating and food, and challenging these patterns, can be difficult for someone who has very distinct attitudes towards particular foods (Fogarty & Ramjan, 2016). Recurrent failures at addressing behaviours and attitudes towards food can also hinder treatment and recovery in AN. **Table 13.6** explores the goals of BN and AN management.

TABLE 13.6

Eating disorder (AN and BN) management goals

GOALS OF EATING DISORDER MANAGEMENT
● Returning to and sustaining healthy body weight for their individual shape and size
● Cessation of dysfunctional eating and behaviours such as binging, purging, over-exercising and use of laxatives/diuretics
● Through use of psychological interventions such as CBT, addressing negative cognitive thinking patterns related to weight, body shape and food intake, and addressing issues related to self-image and self-esteem
● Treatment of comorbid physical and mental health conditions
● Relapse prevention

SOURCE: ADAPTED FROM SHARAN & SUNDAR, 2015

Pharmacological management

After medical stabilisation, medication *may* be considered. There is, however, little evidence to suggest that medication-based treatments in isolation are effective. Small doses of antipsychotic medication such as olanzapine may be beneficial in aiding weight gain (increase in appetite with olanzapine is very likely and serious weight gain in individuals with schizophrenia who are treated with olanzapine is common). Given the tendency for comorbid depression to occur in individuals with AN, antidepressants may also be useful. The antidepressant fluoxetine has been successful in the prevention of relapse in individuals with AN who have recovered (Sharan & Sundar, 2015). While the use of medication is limited in efficacy in treating AN, it must always be administered in conjunction with a psychological intervention that seeks to address, for example, cognitive patterns in thinking about food, body image, family dynamics and attitudes towards food (Galsworthy-Francis & Allan, 2014).

Non-pharmacological management

While bulimia nervosa has a specific, evidence-based 'talk therapy' (CBT) there is no precise treatment indicated for AN (Galsworthy-Francis & Allan, 2014). Nonetheless, treatments such as CBT can be beneficial in empowering consumers to challenge the dysfunctional thinking patterns and emotional reactions associated with the condition. Distorted perceptions about food and body image can also benefit from CBT (Galsworthy-Francis & Allan, 2014). While Galsworthy-Francis and Allan (2014) identify that CBT is the most commonly used treatment for AN (indicated for use by 88–92% of eating-disorder clinicians), there is a lack of empirical evidence to support its effectiveness.

Family-based therapy (FBT; or Maudsley Family Therapy) is used to treat adolescents with AN, and evidence to establish its effectiveness in treatment is evident (Chen et al., 2016). FBT is a series of structured sessions incorporating the parents, initially controlling weight recovery for their child (so essentially controlling eating), and then handing the gradual restoration of eating control back to the child as they begin to improve. Over time, the child is also supported to become independent in their relationship with their parents (Chen et al., 2016). FBT helps the consumer to address their perception of their body shape and image, patterns of disordered eating, and re-engage with friends socially (Harrington et al., 2015). In one study, FBT was implicit in recovery of weight in between 50–60% of patients, and was pivotal in the maintenance of weight up to four years later (Chen et al., 2016). The benefits of FBT include faster weight recovery, reduction in hospitalisation and its value in terms of costs.

Motivational interviewing (MI) is another technique that may be helpful in the treatment of AN. MI incorporates empathy in an effort to facilitate the drive to change behaviours in individuals with AN (Vella-Zarb et al., 2015). MI is explored in more depth in Chapter 4).

Refeeding and refeeding syndrome

First described in prisoners of the Holocaust in the Second World War, **refeeding syndrome** is a serious physiological response to starvation. As the war drew to a close in 1945, allied forces had the duty of liberating severely malnourished captives from Eastern European concentration campus, and did as almost anyone in their circumstances would: they gave the survivors whatever food they had, such as chocolate. Many of these survivors died. This phenomenon is known as refeeding syndrome and can result in cardiac failure, among other things. When refeeding is rapid and aggressive, refeeding syndrome can occur. Essentially, refeeding syndrome results in a potentially lethal shift of fluids and electrolyte imbalance, including decreased blood levels of magnesium, potassium and sodium (Crook, 2014; Palmer, Matthews & Owens, 2016).

The National Institute for Health and Care Excellence guidelines (NICE, 2006) identify refeeding risk based on the severity of a number of factors outlined in **Table 13.7**.

TABLE 13.7
NICE guidelines for refeeding risk

EXTREME RISK	VERY HIGH RISK	HIGH RISK	SOME RISK
Any of the following: • BMI <14 kg/m^2 – Negligible intake for >15 days.	Any of the following: • BMI <16 kg/m^2 • In past 3–6 months involuntary weight loss >15% • Negligible intake for >10 days • ↓ potassium, ↓ phosphate or ↓ magnesium serum levels	Two or more of the following: • BMI <18.5 kg/m^2 • In past 3–6 months involuntary weight loss >10% • Negligible intake for >5 days • History of AN, alcohol dependence or malnutrition	• Negligible intake for >5 days

SOURCE: ADAPTED FROM NICE, 2017

Refeeding syndrome is not only associated with AN, as it can occur in patients who are medically ill, malnourished or alcohol dependent. While the major features of refeeding syndrome are disturbances of electrolytes, some of the clinical signs of refeeding syndrome are:

- softening of bones (osteomalacia)
- anaemia
- muscle pain
- arrhythmias
- coma
- respiratory failure
- congestive heart failure
- delirium and confusion
- hyperglycaemia
- increased risk of infections and renal and liver impairment/failure
- pins and needles (paraesthesia)
- constipation
- muscle pain
- thrombocytopaenia (bleeding and reduced clotting)
- nausea and vomiting (adapted from Crook, 2014).

Due to potential risks associated with refeeding, consumers with AN will need to resume fluids and nutrition under the specialised care of dietetics and this may include oral, enteral (via nasogastric tube) or parenteral (intravenous) feeding.

Relapse prevention

While the individual with a diagnosis of AN may return to a healthy or stable weight while hospitalised, relapse rates are high in individuals whose self-image issues have not also been addressed, suggesting that treatment needs to involve exploration of self-image in order to be successful (Zeppegno & Gramaglia, 2014). Rates of relapse among individuals with AN at the 18-month post-treatment rate are around 35–41%, making relapse of the condition fairly common (Berends et al., 2016). If relapse does occur, it is most likely to do so between 4–17 months into recovery and, in one study, by five years post-treatment over 50% of individuals with AN had relapsed. Galsworthy-Francis and Allan (2014) note that less than 50% of people with AN will fully recover from the condition, while 20–30% will be affected by continuing symptoms, 10–20% will be seriously incapacitated by the condition and a further 5–10% will die.

Recovery

Recovery from AN is more likely when there is a positive improvement in self-esteem and body image in addition to successful emotional expressions and the development of healthy coping mechanisms (Zeppegno & Gramaglia, 2014). About 50% of

individuals with AN will recover fully, while 30% will recover moderately and the remaining 20% will be seriously and chronically incapacitated by the condition (Harrington et al., 2015).

Clinical management

Given the list of potential physical implications and behavioural and cognitive issues associated with AN, it is perhaps unsurprising that the management of the condition can be challenging. AN has been recognised as the most complicated and difficult mental health condition to treat (Martinez & Craighead, 2015). When a consumer is hospitalised, it is important to consider the immense distress this causes. Individuals with AN have significant fear around gaining weight and eating food, and hospitalisation means they are confronted with both of these fears at the same time (NSW Ministry of Health, 2014). This fear is also exacerbated by the forcefulness of treatment and the impacts this has on an individual's decision-making and autonomy. Due to intense fear of gaining weight, consumers with AN will go to extraordinary lengths to prevent weight gain and to increase weight loss.

Common challenges of nursing the consumer with AN

There are a number of challenges when nursing a consumer who has a diagnosis of AN, and many of these challenges are around behaviours that may be both difficult to identify (because they are hidden) or challenging because they stem from behaviours the consumer has been doing for a long time. Behaviours such as food tampering or hiding (in the room, under the bed, down the sink, in the rubbish bin, etc.) and vomiting (in sinks, toilets, rubbish bags, drink bottles, tissues, etc.) can be common practices for someone with an ED. It is also common for consumers with AN to be able to vomit without making any sound whatsoever.

When on bed rest, exercising such as going to the toilet and doing exercises, or pacing to burn calories may be observed. Misuse of laxatives is not uncommon in EDs and obtaining laxatives from an outside source (such as an unsuspecting parent or friend) may occur. It is important, therefore, that all visitors are aware that medicines (which may seem harmless) are not able to be brought into the hospital. Staff who are new or do not usually work on an ED unit must also be aware that the AN consumer may attempt to manipulate individuals they believe to be unfamiliar with feeding policy and processes.

While an inpatient in a hospital setting, weighing is a frequent and often distressing time for a consumer. In order to appear to have put on weight, consumers with an ED may resort to drinking large quantities of water prior to a weigh or placing heavy objects in their clothing (such as rocks). Consequently, weighing should be done in a hospital gown and underwear only.

For consumers who are receiving nasogastric tube (NGT) feeding there are also a number of issues that may occur. Tampering, kinking and removing of NGTs are commonly seen in individuals with AN. Aside from the obvious reasons (not wanting to gain weight from food), NGT insertion requires an X-ray to confirm the placement, and removal of tubing will likely result in delays to feeding and longer periods without nutrition. When this pattern of behaviour is frequent, it can result in serious issues with dietary intake. Other behaviours include turning the NG pump off at the wall outlet or attempting to interfere with its operation.

The consumer's belongings will need to be searched, according to hospital policy, to look for items such as aperients, diet pills, sugar-free gum or sweets (which have a laxative effect) and medications such as diuretics. Mealtimes can be a particularly anxiety-provoking and unsettled time for consumers with AN as they are usually highly supervised and communal (unless bed-restricted), with staff eating too. Consumers who are unable or unwilling to eat their meal will usually have it replaced with a nutritional supplement often in the form of an NGT feed. Use of the bathroom after eating is restricted (e.g. toileting always occurs *prior* to meals and not within one hour after) or highly supervised, and consumers who are particularly distressed by feeding (such as NGT feeds) may be given PRN anxiolytics or sedatives to ensure feeding can continue safely.

Clinical management needs to include the enforcement of treatment plans in a supportive and compassionate manner. Mental health clinicians who work in ED units need to balance this enforcement in addition to engaging with the consumer's concerned family, and developing and maintaining therapeutic rapport. There is no doubt that this poses a challenging environment for all concerned.

COMMONALITIES OF THE MSE: ANOREXIA NERVOSA

A mental state examination (MSE) is a pivotal part of the role of the mental health nurse and the MSE is an important part of diagnosing AN. It is important, however, to ensure that the consumer is physically capable and stable enough for a thorough MSE. Consider the impacts or challenges of undertaking an MSE with someone who is intoxicated with alcohol, or who has a low Glasgow Coma Scale (GCS) rating. In such instances, it would be best to wait until they are more coherent. The same may be considered when interviewing someone with AN who is significantly malnourished. Their ability to engage in the MSE may be significantly impaired by their declining physical state and starvation.

General appearance and behaviour
Unlike other conditions, this section is one where you may see overt physical signs of illness evident. Individuals with AN will be extremely thin (but may be trying to cover this up with baggy clothing), and have little or no body fat. In females, breast tissue may be absent or reduced. Individuals may also be covered in fine hair (lanugo) on their face and neck, have brittle nails and dry hair. Cyanosis of finger tips may be evident, and extremities may have a 'dusky' colour to them. They may look gaunt, have delayed or slowed growth (depending on when AN began) and describe being cold. If the consumer purges, they may have issues with their teeth, and scars (Russell's sign) on their knuckles from putting their fingers down their throat (see **Figure 13.4**). It may be difficult for the individual to remain still, because exercising is a way of burning calories and periods of hyperactivity are not uncommon.

Mood
Mood disturbance is common in individuals with AN. In particular, the consumer may describe feeling anxious or guilty and having a depressed or low mood. Their mood may present as labile with fluctuations between distress, agitation and euthymia. Appetite will be severely restricted and talking about food may result in increases in anxiety and distress. The individual will consume a significantly restricted diet that may consist of water or black tea or coffee, a small amount of porridge, and some vegetables or fruit. Skipping meals frequently and fasting is common and they may consume only 200–300 calories per day, maintained consistently for months. There may be periods of binge eating (or a belief that they have eaten too much). Libido may be reduced. Individuals with AN often have very low self-esteem and body image, so they may struggle with a belief that they are sexually attractive. Nutritional deficit may result in constant feelings of fatigue.

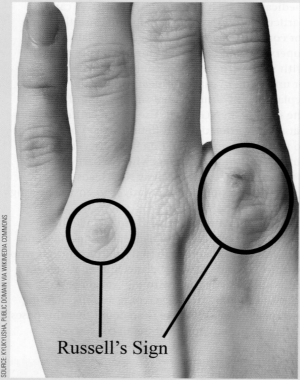

SOURCE: KYUKYUSHA, PUBLIC DOMAIN VIA WIKIMEDIA COMMONS

Russell's Sign

FIGURE 13.4
Russell's sign or scars are commonly seen in individuals who purge. The process of purging results in the knuckles and hand having contact with incisor teeth in an attempt to induce the gag reflex, and the more frequently this is done, the more likely it will result in calluses

Affect
Affect is likely congruent to mood. Individuals who experience AN may also have symptoms of depression or anxiety and as such a restriction of affect may be seen.

Thought content
Individuals with AN are generally consumed by thoughts that they are fat and that they must exercise, purge or restrict their dietary intake. They may also demonstrate an exorbitant knowledge of the calories or fat content of foods that exceeds most people's understanding. They may be experiencing suicidal thoughts or thoughts to self-harm, and it is important to explore substance use history, particularly including over-the-counter medicines such as laxatives and prescription weight-loss medications.

Cognition
Cognitive impairment is a common feature of AN and likely caused by malnutrition and its impacts on brain functioning or depressed mood. The individual may have issues with their memory, concentration and alertness. They may be easily distracted and struggle to remain focused.

Insight
Given that generally the individual with AN believes they are overweight, poor insight is common. This can make increases in caloric intake and restrictions to exercising difficult concepts for the consumer.

BULIMIA NERVOSA

The word 'bulimia' emerged before the fifteenth century from the Latin and Greek variants of terms that describe insatiable or ravenous hunger. While the term 'bulimia' has origins in history, the condition itself is very new to modern medicine. **Bulimia nervosa (BN)** was not noted until 1979, where it was seen as a variant of AN (Sharan & Sundar, 2015). BN is an eating disorder associated with a pattern of cognitive and behavioural issues related to body weight and food. This section explores BN in greater depth.

Clinical manifestations
The main features of BN are the consumption of large quantities of food (more than what the average person would consume) in a relatively short period of time. The individual has no control over their binge-eating behaviours, or at the very least, *feels* that they lack control. While many individuals who engage in binge-eating behaviours will choose foods that are unhealthy or deemed 'junk' foods, this is not a requirement of the condition; rather it is the *volume* of food consumed in a limited time frame (APA, 2013). Most individuals with BN are within a normal weight range (Andrews et al., 2013). For the vast majority of those with people who

have a diagnosis of BN, binge eating is something that brings them great shame, and so it is usually done in private. Some other emotional and behavioural clinical manifestations of BN are:

- continuing to eat despite being painfully full
- continuing to eat despite feeling physically sick
- eating when not hungry
- feelings of self-loathing and disgust at eating behaviours
- lack of control around amount of food consumed
- eating rapidly
- eating on 'auto pilot'
- ongoing eating without specific mealtimes
- eating when alone or hiding eating behaviours
- frequent dieting (with or without weight loss)
- weight fluctuations
- hiding packaging/wrappers of eaten food
- feelings of dysphoria, guilt or embarrassment after a binge-eating episode
- eating to relieve stress or in response to stressful situations
- hiding or hoarding food to be eaten later
- poor body image and low self-esteem
- Russell's signs
- purging after eating.

The signs and symptoms outlined above occur at least weekly, and for many they will occur many times per week. Individuals with BN may go to the toilet numerous times to accommodate binging and purging behaviours (Harrington et al., 2015). Purging behaviours range from 56–86% (vomiting), 26–56% (aperient abuse) and 49% diuretic abuse in individuals with eating disorders (Forney, Buchman-Schmitt, Keel & Frank, 2016). Much like a person with AN, individuals with BN may also exercise excessively despite injuries and illness.

Dental decay and erosion are common conditions seen in BN. Individuals who purge even only weekly face a fourfold increase in dental erosion, and those who frequently purge may experience rates up to 18 times higher than those who do not (Whiteway, 2015). This is possibly exacerbated by the impacts stomach acids have on dental enamel in the absence of teeth-brushing before and after purging. Complications associated with purging behaviours are outlined in **Table 13.8**.

Incidence and epidemiology

Bulimia nervosa usually emerges in late childhood, with a peak period in adolescence (APA, 2013). With a 12-month prevalence in the realm of 1–1.5%, BN is significantly more common in females (10:1). Between 5–10% of adolescents report engaging in uncontrolled binge eating and they represent the highest proportion of individuals to experience such behaviours (Goldschmidt et al., 2016). At five- and six-year follow-up, around half of those individuals are still engaging in binge-eating behaviours.

Aetiology

Given that eating-disordered behaviours have similar characteristics and somewhat similar manifestations, it is perhaps not unsurprising that they also have similar causes. The dual-pathway model of bulimia nervosa (Stice, Shaw & Nemeroff, 1998) is seen by some as fundamental in the development of BN (Allen, Byrne & Crosby, 2015). This model suggests that sociocultural pressures (from family, friends or media) to adhere to the slim body type results in a cascade of cognitions and behaviours, as listed in **Figure 13.5**.

The following section explores the various causes of BN in addition to prevalence rates.

Genetic factors

It is understood that genetic factors play a significant role in the development of BN, and genetics possibly plays a role in the development of BN and AN in as many as 50% of cases (Sharan & Sundar, 2015). In twin studies, the rate of heritability of BN is understood to be between 28–83%, demonstrating that the condition is likely heritable, but significantly varied (Peterson et al., 2015). There is also suggestion that serotonin levels and other biological factors may be responsible. It is likely that genetic vulnerability at the very least plays a role in the development or emergence of risk factors, such as certain personality traits, that are highly prevalent in eating-disordered individuals.

Biological factors

Brain derived neurotrophic factor (BDNF) is a gene that may be associated with the development of BN. BDNF appears to be connected with eating behaviours and in clinical trials many individuals with BN and AN have lower plasma levels of BDNF while those who are obese have higher levels (Phillips, Keane & Wolfe, 2014).

Individual factors

There are a number of commonalities seen in individuals who have BN, and many of these are

TABLE 13.8
Complications associated with purging

BEHAVIOUR	COMPLICATIONS
Vomiting	• Dental erosion (seen in around 63% of people who have a diagnosis of BN) • Parotid gland swelling resulting in pain and in severe cases salivary gland surgery • Tonsillitis • Oesophagitis or reflux (heartburn) • Possible elevated rates of oesophageal cancers • Rectal prolapse • Sclera bleeds (called subconjunctival haemorrhage where the white part of the eye has a red appearance due to bleeding from the pressure caused by vomiting) • Cardiac complications such as arrhythmias
Use of aperients	• 'Cathartic colon' (associated with severe, long-term abuse of laxatives rendering it unable to operate correctly) • Decreased creatinine removal in kidneys • Possible colorectal cancer (inconclusive)
Use of diuretics	• Electrolyte distortion particularly of potassium, sodium and chloride • Tubulointerstitial nephritis (inflammation of kidney tubules) • Kidney stones • Renal failure

SOURCE: ADAPTED FROM FORNEY ET AL., 2016

SECTION 2

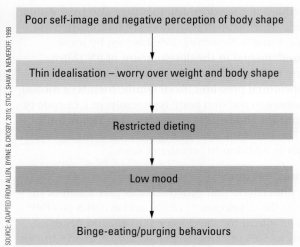

FIGURE 13.5
Dual-pathway model of bulimia nervosa

believed to emerge through experiences in childhood. In particular, traumatic or negative childhood experiences are seen in individuals with BN, in addition to poor self-esteem, parental history of a mental health condition and negative experiences of their weight. While the development of AN is not aetiologically associated with sexual abuse, past abuse in BN appears to be a risk factor (Harrington et al., 2015). One theory in support of sexual assault as an aetiological factor in BN is that the individual views their body negatively, feels embarrassment and humiliation, and is unhappy with their body image after the assault (Madowitz, Matheson & Liang, 2015). Another theory explores the psychological impacts of assault, resulting in the need for control, maladaptive coping mechanisms (such as binging and purging) and emotional regulation. In around 75% of females who develop BN, serious adverse experiences or problems occurred during the onset of the condition (Goncalves, Machado, Martins & Machado, 2014). While recently males are increasingly represented in those diagnosed with BN (and EDs in general), there is a need for further literature exploring the factors associated with the development of BN in males.

Those with BN may also present with a past history of childhood obesity and dieting, as well as a parent who is obese (Allen, Byrne & Crosby, 2015). Negative experiences in childhood, particularly where parents are openly critical about their child's weight, are associated with the development of eating disorders in adolescence before the age of 14. While these experiences can occur in an obvious manner, whereby the parent explicitly identifies the child as needing weight-control and as such makes comments or controls their diet, it can also be more subtle; for example, in the form of encouraging dieting behaviours or complimenting the slimness of others (Allen, Byrne & Crosby, 2015). While the

dual-pathway model of bulimia nervosa (Stice, Shaw & Nemeroff, 1998) identifies a possible cascade in the development of BN, what it is lacking is a time frame. Most researchers suggest that the time frame from sociocultural exposure to diagnosis of BN is around two years (Allen, Byrne & Crosby, 2015).

Certain personality variables have been indicated in the development of BN and also in other eating disorders. Traits associated with negative body image and negative emotionality are identified as possible precipitators of future BN behaviours (Cooper, 2015). Other individual factors include early-onset menstruation and parental alcohol misuse.

Teasing, bullying and peer pressure are also factors associated with eating-disorder behaviours and EDs. Interestingly, it has been noted that negative weight comments or advice from individuals in positions of power such as health care practitioners, sports coaches or teachers are also influential in the development of BN (Sharan & Sundar, 2015). Individuals with BN also report higher levels of physical abuse and fear (Goncalves et al., 2014).

One of the major individual features of BN is that it is significantly more common in females (at a ratio of 10:1) (APA, 2013). There are a few hypothesised reasons as to why this may be the case. It would appear that females may be more influenced by sociocultural factors, such as the impacts of media, and cultural considerations about size and how this relates to perceived 'worthiness' (Cooper, 2015). In addition, females tend to demonstrate lower levels of self-esteem and self-image compared with males, and females may be more inclined to assimilate value and approval with how they look. The impact of puberty on females is often a difficult time for many girls and this is also a factor (Cooper, 2015).

Particular vocations and sports have been associated with higher rates of BN development. Much like AN, rates of BN in those participating in ballet appear to be higher (Cooper, 2015). It is thought that the focus on weight and diet, in addition to peer influences, in ballet may be responsible for these higher rates. Gymnasts, elite athletes, ice-skaters and those participating in sports that are weight-dependent (such as boxing, judo, karate, etc.) may also be more inclined to demonstrate BN behaviours (Cooper, 2015).

Environmental and social factors

As with AN, social idealisation of body image and shape, which is often heavily influenced by media and the entertainment industry, is an aetiological factor in the development of BN (Harrington et al., 2015). While there is not an abundance of epidemiological research on BN in terms of environmental and social development, as with AN it does appear to be a 'Western' condition. It has even been suggested that the development of BN requires many modern conveniences that are frequently only available in Western nations; for example, availability of inexpensive palatable food, modern sanitation whereby purging can occur in private, and the desire to be thin (Keel, 2012).

Cultural competence and manifestations
While the development of eating disorders is significantly influenced by individuals who fear gaining weight and in those who diet, these behaviours may differ culturally. Latzer, Merrick and Stein (2011) suggest that while these factors are important, so too are factors where individuals feel disconnected from their culture, and in those who find the transition between cultures to be difficult. It is suggested that EDs are influenced by *internal* factors (psychological) and factors that are considered *external* (social and interpersonal). Of concern are external influences that depict contemporary representations of existing cultural values or norms (e.g. slim models and advertisements in cultures that are modernising and modelling Western culture) (Latzer, Merrick & Stein, 2011). This places greater emphasis on appearance and weight where perhaps this was not the case previously. It is suggested that these types of changes may be influential in EDs.

Comorbidity
There is some evidence to suggest that BN and the affective impacts of the condition and resulting poor self-esteem and mood can result in depressive symptoms that are perhaps more severe than seen in other eating disorders (Allen, Byrne & Crosby, 2015). BN has also been associated with increased impairments in psychological functioning. Comorbidity in BN is characterised by high rates of mood disorders (68%) and conditions impacting impulse control, such as alcohol misuse (32%) and substance misuse (39%) (Andrews et al., 2013).

In terms of physical illness and disease, BN has been found in higher rates in individuals with insulin dependent diabetes mellitus (IDDM), probably due to the need to be focused on food and eating behaviours as a means of managing the illness (Cooper, 2015). Studies have suggested rates of BN in IDDM as high as 35%, although a conservative figure between 7.9–15% is probably more likely (yet still high). It is understood that any medical condition or illness that places an emphasis on eating patterns and behaviours (such as coeliac's disease) may be associated with a higher rate of BN development.

Clinical course
BN is a condition that commonly commences in adolescence and it is rare for it to begin after the 40th year or prior to puberty (APA, 2013). BN usually develops in individuals during the course of, or subsequent to, a period of dieting and may be exacerbated (or even onset) during episodes of stress.

In the early stages of the condition, adolescents may be diagnosed with binge-eating disorder or purging disorder first; however, as the condition progresses, their eating behaviours become more disordered and they may be diagnosed with BN (Allen, Byrne & Crosby, 2015). Like many conditions, there may be periods of remission from binging behaviours, and in individuals who are symptom-free for over one year the long-term outcomes are better (APA, 2013). Around 10–15% of individuals diagnosed with BN will revert to AN, and there is a tendency for these individuals to oscillate between the two conditions (APA, 2013).

Prognosis
While the health conditions associated with BN are not as severe as seen in AN, there remain a number of serious health factors associated with this condition. Most afflictions associated with BN concern the gastrointestinal system. Medical conditions associated with BN are:
- imbalances in electrolytes (sodium, potassium, chloride), which may result in cardiac arrhythmia
- gastric ulcers
- pancreatitis
- gastric rupture from binging
- oesophageal inflammation or rupture from binging
- symptoms similar to irritable bowel due to misuse of laxatives
- staining and erosion of teeth due to gastric acids from purging (adapted from Andrews et al., 2013).

Bulimia nervosa, suicide and self-harm/non-suicidal self-injury
Bulimia nervosa is associated with a 2% increase in death per decade lived with the condition (APA, 2013). This includes deaths associated with illness from the condition and suicide. While rates of death do not appear as high as in AN, this still constitutes a serious risk. In those with BN, around 25–55% of individuals are thought to engage in self-harming behaviours (Cucchi et al., 2016).

Diagnostic criteria
The diagnosis of BN is somewhat more convoluted than AN, requiring the presence of a number of behaviours and attitudes towards self. **Table 13.9** outlines the diagnostic criteria of BN.

Treatment
Serious physical complications are not as commonly seen in BN as they are in AN and treatment is often more conservative. Having said this however, there *can* be serious implications to BN. Gastric (from binging) and oesophageal (from purging) ruptures and electrolyte imbalances are potential complications of the condition (see **Table 13.10**). Psychoeducation is an important factor in the treatment of all mental health conditions and BN is not exempt from this necessity.

DIAGNOSTIC CRITERIA

Bulimia nervosa

TABLE 13.9
Diagnostic criteria bulimia nervosa

A. Recurrent episodes of binge eating. An episode of binge eating is characterized by both of the following:
    1. Eating, in a discrete period of time (e.g., within any 2-hour period), an amount of food that is definitely larger than what most individuals would eat in a similar period of time under similar circumstances.
    2. A sense of lack of control over eating during the episode (e.g., a feeling that one cannot stop eating or control what or how much one is eating).

B. Recurrent inappropriate compensatory behaviors in order to prevent weight gain, such as self-induced vomiting; misuse of laxatives, diuretics, or other medications; fasting; or excessive exercise.
C. The binge eating and inappropriate compensatory behaviors both occur, on average, at least once a week for 3 months.
D. Self-evaluation is unduly influenced by body shape and weight.
E. The disturbance does not occur exclusively during episodes of anorexia nervosa.   *Specify* if: • **In partial remission:** After full criteria for bulimia nervosa were previously met, some, but not all, of the criteria have been met for a sustained period of time.   • **In full remission:** After full criteria for bulimia nervosa were previously met, none of the criteria have been met for a sustained period of time.   *Specify current severity:*   The minimum level of severity is based on the frequency of inappropriate compensatory behaviors (see below). The level of severity may be increased to reflect other symptoms and the degree of functional disability.   • **Mild:** An average of 1–3 episodes of inappropriate compensatory behaviors per week.   • **Moderate:** An average of 4–7 episodes of inappropriate compensatory behaviors per week.   • **Severe:** An average of 8–13 episodes of inappropriate compensatory behaviors per week.   • **Extreme:** An average of 14 or more episodes of inappropriate compensatory behaviors per week.

Psychoeducation enables the individual to understand their condition, develop insight into what are the triggers and how best to manage them. Education around the way food is metabolised is of particular importance for individuals with purging behaviours. For example, an individual will still absorb 50% of calories even immediately after purging as absorption occurs as soon as food enters the mouth (Andrews et al., 2013). A mere 10% of calories are eliminated with the use of laxatives. Because the vast majority of individuals diagnosed with BN are adolescents or young people, many are still living in the family home and thus treatment often involves a family approach.

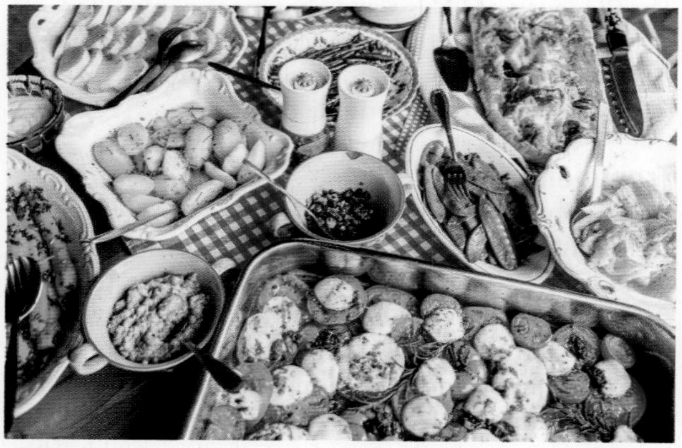

FIGURE 13.6
Meal times can be difficult for an individual with an eating disorder

This section explores the pharmacological and non-pharmacological management of BN.

Pharmacological management

There is no specific pharmacological treatment for the management of BN; however, some studies have indicated effectiveness of antidepressants, such as selective serotonin reuptake inhibitors (SSRIs) in reducing binging and purging frequencies (Harrington et al., 2015). Individuals who have not responded to traditional psychological interventions and who have demonstrated dysthymia may also benefit from an antidepressant. The SSRI antidepressant fluoxetine may be beneficial in the treatment of BN in high doses (60 mg) (Sharan & Sundar, 2015).

Non-pharmacological management

While it may seem simplistic that a food diary may be beneficial in the treatment of BN (or in AN, too), this is not the case. Completing a food diary is an important part of the treatment of EDs and provides the writer an opportunity to write about not only the food consumed, but the quantities, triggers, feelings and behaviours associated with such eating. A food diary (see **Figure 13.7**) encourages the individual to write:

- when they eat
- motivating factors or triggers for eating
- what foods they eat, and the quantity consumed
- where the food was consumed (for example in their bedroom, in the bathroom)

- if they purged or consumed laxatives after eating
- if they exercised after.

Other interventions used to treat BN include cognitive, behavioural and interpersonal therapies, which have demonstrated success in treating the condition (Harrington et al., 2015). Group therapies are common interventions with eating disorders, and mindfulness has also been successfully implemented.

Recovery and relapse prevention

Rates of relapse for BN have been reported in the realm of 25–63% and pose a significant risk for individuals diagnosed with the condition (Olmsted et al., 2015). Harrington and colleagues (2015) note that around 20% of individuals with BN will relapse and that these individuals pose significant challenges for clinicians and contribute to the mortality rates of eating disorders. There are a number of common factors associated with individuals whose condition relapses in the period following remission. Some of these factors include:

- more frequent periods of purge behaviours during treatment period (e.g. relapse behaviours)

- being younger
- concerns about body weight and shape
- persistent disordered eating behaviours and attitudes
- life events that have potential to create stress
- post-treatment reduced psychosocial coping (Olmsted et al., 2015).

Unsurprisingly, some of these relapse-potential signs and behaviours are similar to those seen in individuals with AN who also relapse. The most troubling symptoms in BN, and those that are more commonly associated with increased potential to relapse, are the consumer's remaining disordered eating behaviours. Rates of remission in adults with BN are lower than in those with binge-eating disorder (Allen, Byrne & Crosby, 2015).

Recovery of BN is more promising than that of AN. Longitudinal research into recovery patterns of BN are limited, but it is well understood that early detection results in the most positive outcomes in the management of all eating disorders. Andrews et al. (2013) note that around 70% of those with BN

When/where..?	What..?	Purging..?	Triggers..?	Exercise..?
13/12/2020 When I got home from school, I went into my bedroom and raided my stash…even though no one was home I went into the bathroom and locked the door.	Large packet of chips. One block of chocolate. Left-over pasta in fridge. Bottle of diet lemonade.	Yes and I took laxatives too	I had an argument with mum before school and it set the tone for the whole day. This is so hard…I'm so very out of control but no one understands…	No.
17/12/2020 Home, bathroom during my 'shower'.	Chocolate. Bag of jelly beans. Half-loaf of bread.	Just vomiting	Christmas is coming up and there is so much food in the house. I am so fat and hideous. All my friends will be at the beach this summer but I'm just gross. I have no control over my eating, I'm so ashamed.	Rode the exercise bike for 2 hours.
26/12/2020 My grandparents' ensuite. They think I am lying down.	Christmas pudding with custard. A left-over plate of pork and crackling. A box of chocolates. 1.25 L diet cola.	Laxatives and vomiting	I had been doing so well. I'm so disappointed with myself. This is such a hard time of year for me. I'm such a loser. I got some clothes from my aunt for Christmas and none of them fit me…	No, I feel too sick…

FIGURE 13.7
Example of a food diary entry

will demonstrate short-term recovery; however, it is understood that around half of these individuals will continue to demonstrate ED behaviours. Harrington and colleagues (2015) observed that total remission from BN is achievable in almost 80% of individuals with the condition. Perhaps predictably, individuals who are more severely afflicted with BN will demonstrate poorer rates of recovery, and those with poor impulse control who exhibit behaviours such as substance misuse, self-harm, binge eating and promiscuous sexual behaviours exhibit poor long-term outcomes (Andrews et al., 2013).

BINGE-EATING DISORDER

First identified in 1959, **binge-eating disorder (BED)** did not make its way into the DSM until as late as 1994, and this neglect has been compounded by a lack of research into the condition (Keel, 2012). BED is characterised by the ingestion of large quantities of food where the individual seemingly has little or no control over their eating behaviour. Individuals with BED are often embarrassed or ashamed of their binge-eating behaviour and will often eat in secrecy, hiding food wrappers and eating in solitary places where they cannot be 'caught'. Binge-eating episodes may be triggered by stressful situations, negative feelings about body shape/size/weight or even boredom (APA, 2013).

BED affects about 0.8% of males and 1.6% of females; the disparity between males and females is far more contained in BED than for other EDs (APA, 2013). For many individuals with BED, being overweight or obese as a child is a characteristic of the condition, and many will have a history of dieting behaviours. Remission of the condition occurs at rates higher than for BN and AN, and so BED is seen as more responsive to treatment and intervention. There is very little research into BED, but that which has occurred has shown there is often a past history of the condition in the family and the comorbidities of the condition are similar to BN and AN (APA, 2013).

Diagnostic criteria

The criteria listed in **Table 13.10** must occur for at least three months, on a weekly (at least) basis).

DIAGNOSTIC CRITERIA

Binge-eating disorder

TABLE 13.10
Diagnostic criteria binge-eating disorder

A. Recurrent episodes of binge eating. An episode of binge eating is characterised by both of the following:
   1. Eating, in a discrete period of time (e.g., within any 2-hour period), an amount of food that is definitely larger than what most people would eat in a similar period of time under similar circumstances.
   2. A sense of lack of control over eating during the episode (e.g., a feeling that one cannot stop eating or control what or how much one is eating).

B. The binge-eating episodes are associated with three (or more) of the following:
   1. Eating much more rapidly than normal.
   2. Eating until feeling uncomfortably full.
   3. Eating large amounts of food when not feeling physically hungry.
   4. Eating alone because of feeling embarrassed by how much one is eating.
   5. Feeling disgusted with oneself, depressed, or very guilty afterward.

C. Marked distress regarding binge eating is present.
D. The binge eating occurs, on average, at least once a week for 3 months.
E. The binge eating is not associated with the recurrent use of inappropriate compensatory behavior as in bulimia nervosa and does not occur exclusively during the course of bulimia nervosa or anorexia nervosa. *Specify if:* • **In partial remission:** After full criteria for binge-eating disorder were previously met, binge eating occurs at an average frequency of less than one episode per week for a sustained period of time. • **In full remission:** After full criteria for binge-eating disorder were previously met, none of the criteria have been met for a sustained period of time. *Specify* current severity: The minimum level of severity is based on the frequency of episodes of binge eating (see below). The level of severity may be increased to reflect other symptoms and the degree of functional disability. • **Mild:** 1–3 binge-eating episodes per week. • **Moderate:** 4–7 binge-eating episodes per week. • **Severe:** 8–13 binge-eating episodes per week. • **Extreme:** 14 or more binge-eating episodes per week.

How is binge-eating disorder different to bulimia nervosa?

You may be somewhat confused by the differentiation of binge-eating disorder and bulimia nervosa. The two conditions have similar characteristics; however, there *are* differences between the two. Differences include:

- In BED there is typically no dieting or restrictive eating pattern in an attempt to modify body shape or weight.
- There is a lack of compensatory behaviours such as exercising and purging in BED.
- There are better responses to treatment in BED compared with other EDs (APA, 2013).

While it is clear that there are commonalities among eating disorders, and in particular ED behaviours, it is important to consider what differentiates these patterns of behaviour when considering diagnosis.

Aetiology and epidemiology

Onset of BED is in the early-to-mid-20s, which is later than other EDs (Keel, 2012). The most commonly understood risk factors for the development of BED are being female and having parents who view them as overweight between ages 7–11. This cascades into the development of body shape concerns, and worry over their eating and weight by age 14 (Allen et al., 2014).

Allen, Byrne and Crosby's (2015) mediated model of binge eating outlines a trajectory of disordered eating and cognitions that include age as a factor. This model follows the pattern outlined in **Figure 13.8**.

Age is an important factor to consider in the development of EDs because children and adolescents are particularly vulnerable to EDs. Because BED is not as well researched and understood as the other EDs, many of the aetiological and treatment factors are similar to those of BN and AN.

Recovery

In the very limited information available on the remission of BED, one longitudinal (five-year follow-up) study demonstrated that 82% of sufferers were recovered or improved and around 4% continued to display diagnostic criteria indicative of a diagnosis of BED (Keel, 2012). This data is similar to other studies on recovery of BED.

MALES AND EATING DISORDERS

Given the significant propensity for females to develop EDs, it is natural that the majority of interventions and literature relate to females. Females account for up to 95% of all EDs. However, males are increasingly being diagnosed with EDs. One of the possible reasons for this is the change in more recent times from athletic, muscular male model images, to thin, androgynous models appearing in the media. In addition, society is more tolerant of men with mental health conditions, and increases in diagnosis may also be attributed to seeking help. This section briefly explores this phenomenon in more detail. While BN is more common in males than AN, it is believed that the numbers of both are underrepresented due to a reluctance to seek help and the inadequacies of clinicians' understanding of EDs in males (Cohn & Lemberg, 2014).

Generally, males with EDs have often been overweight or obese prior to the development of an ED, and this varies from females where there is more a *perception* of being overweight rather than actual obesity (Cohn & Lemberg, 2014). It is understood that males are more likely to undertake exercise to avoid physical complications of obesity (which they observed in their fathers) compared with females, who appear to exercise to be thin. Males are also more likely to be influenced by participation in sports that require training or weight loss, or where physique is judged (Cohn & Lemberg, 2014). Other aetiological factors associated with male EDs include:

- a history of sexual abuse/trauma (which is often underreported)
- issues with sexual orientation (EDs are more common in gay and bisexual males)
- depression
- embarrassment about their body
- substance dependency and misuse (and a propensity to be diagnosed with a substance use disorder only, despite the individual taking, for example, stimulants to reduce weight)
- influences of the media (Cohn & Lemberg, 2014).

Treatment of EDs in males can be difficult and requires a clinician who is experienced with addressing the subtle differences between the presentations of EDs.

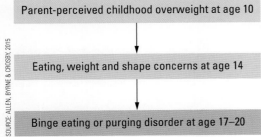

SOURCE: ALLEN, BYRNE & CROSBY, 2015

FIGURE 13.8
Allen, Byrne and Crosby's mediated model of binge eating

REFLECT ON THIS

Role of the dietitian in treating eating disorders

Engaging in psychological treatment for an eating disorder is not ideal when a person's body and brain are starving. That is why it is important to ensure the consumer is medically stable prior to commencing psychological interventions. One of the key members of the multidisciplinary team is the dietitian. Dietitians are skilled at challenging the social diet culture that exists in Western society. Dietitians are also important in supporting flexible eating behaviours, and weight. This is all underpinned by expertise in how the body uses and processes foods. A dietitian therefore is imperative for guiding other members of the MDT in formulating dietary plans that will enable the consumer to safely return to an acceptable body weight, which can support psychological intervention.

1   Consider the role of the mental health nurse in monitoring and responding to issues associated with refeeding syndrome. How might the mental health nurse and dietitian work together to safely ensure the consumer increases their body weight?

2   As we have seen, males are also increasingly affected by EDs. Reflect on some of the nuances or differences that may occur when working with male consumers with EDs.

REFLECTION ON LEARNING FROM PRACTICE

Anorexia nervosa is a serious mental health condition that has the highest mortality rate of any mental health condition. As Belle indicated in her lived experience, AN is a condition that is more complex than simply 'not eating', and consists of highly controlled feelings and behaviours that have significant implications for both physical and psychological well-being. Given that AN is frequently diagnosed in very young children, this condition has wider implications for parents, siblings, schools and society as a whole. What role do you see schools playing in the recognition of AN, and in all eating disordered behaviours? What challenges do you think parents and schools face with balancing healthy eating behaviours and exercise, without focusing on body image 'perfection' and social stereotypes?

CHAPTER RESOURCES

SUMMARY

- Anorexia nervosa (AN) is a rare condition most commonly seen in young females which results in increased morbidity and mortality. AN is associated with extreme fear of weight gain, very low BMI, restrictive dieting and eating, and may include purging, misuse of aperients/diuretics and extreme exercising. It is associated with a range of significant health conditions related to starvation and in severe cases can be fatal.

- Bulimia nervosa (BN) is a condition associated with a lack of control over eating behaviours, consumption of large quantities of food (which is usually hidden from others), and behaviours such as purging, over-exercise, restriction of intake and misuse of aperients and diuretics in order to prevent weight gain or to encourage weight loss.

- Binge eating disorder (BED) is characterised by the ingestion of large quantities of food where the individual seemingly has little or no control over their eating behaviour and often tries to hide the behaviour from others. Remission of BED occurs at rates higher than that of BN and AN, and as such it is seen as being more responsive to treatment and intervention.

- While females account for up to 95% of all EDs males are increasingly being diagnosed with EDs. BN is more common in males than AN, but the numbers of both are believed to be underrepresented due to a reluctance to seek help and inadequacies of clinicians' understanding of EDs in males.

REVIEW QUESTIONS

1 Refeeding syndrome is a serious condition seen in eating disorders (most commonly anorexia nervosa) and is caused by an electrolyte imbalance characterised by:
   a Decreased blood levels of magnesium, potassium and sodium
   b Decreased blood levels of calcium and bicarbonate ions
   c Increased blood levels of magnesium, potassium and sodium
   d Increased blood levels of calcium and bicarbonate ions
2 Signs of bulimia nervosa disorder include:
   a Eating great amounts of food in a short time and high BMI
   b Purging and low BMI
   c Secretive eating and purging
   d Intense fear of weight gain and secretive eating
3 How does the media negatively impact on eating disorders? Describe three interventions the media could adopt to reduce stereotypes and perceptions of women.
4 Which eating disorder results from a distorted body image?
   a Bulimia nervosa
   b Binge-eating disorder
   c Anorexia nervosa
   d All of the above
5 Individuals with binge-eating disorder have:
   a Excessive control over eating
   b No control over eating
   c Excessive control over exercising
   d No control over exercising
6 Describe one of the differences between the development of eating disorders in males and females.

CRITICAL THINKING

1 While anorexia nervosa and bulimia nervosa are both eating disorders, how do their symptoms differ?
2 What issues may recovery from AN be affected by?
3 Males are increasingly being diagnosed with eating disorders; however, it is understood that this number is likely underrepresented. What are some of the possible reasons for this?

USEFUL WEBSITES

- Butterfly Foundation for Eating Disorders: https://thebutterflyfoundation.org.au/support-for-australians-experiencing-eating-disorders
- headspace: https://headspace.org.au/health-professionals/understanding-eating-disorders-for-health-professionals
- National Eating Disorders Association: https://www.nationaleatingdisorders.org

REFLECT ON THIS

EDs and mirror exposure therapy
Working with consumers who have an eating disorder can be challenging. It is hard to imagine how the person sees themselves as 'fat' when what we see is an emaciated and starving person. People with eating disorders also often have issues with correct perception of body signals such as hunger, thirst and feeling full. The person with an eating disorder will often focus their attention on their appearance instead. This is why it is very important to understand the 'psychology' behind eating disorders, in addition to understanding our own perceptions of people with eating disorders.

Using the Google Scholar function, research the term 'mirror exposure therapy' and choose an article to read. What are the benefits of this form of therapy?

REFERENCES

Allen, K.L., Byrne, S.M. & Crosby, R.D. (2015). Distinguishing between risk factors for bulimia nervosa, binge eating disorder, and purging disorder. *Journal of Youth and Adolescence*, 44, 1580–91. doi:10.1007/s10964-014-0186-8

Allen, K.L., Byrne, S.M., Oddy, W.H., Schmidt, U. & Crosby, R.D. (2014). Risk factors for binge eating and purging eating disorders: Differences based on age of onset. *International Journal of Eating Disorders*, 47(7), 802–12.

American Psychiatric Association (APA). (2013). *Diagnostic and Statistical Manual of Mental Disorders (DSM-5)* (5th edn). Washington, DC: APA.

Andrews, G., Dean, K., Genderson, M., Hunt, C., Mitchell, P., Sachdev, P. & Trollor, J. (2013). *Management of Mental Disorders* (5th edn). Sydney: School of Psychiatry, University of NSW.

Bannatyne, A.J. & Abel, L.M. (2015). Can we fight stigma with science? The effect of aetiological framing on attitudes towards anorexia and the impact on volitional stigma. *Australian Journal of Psychology*, 67, 38–46. doi:10.1111/ajpy.12062

Berends, T., van Meijel, B., Nugteren, W., Deen, M., Danner, U., Hoek, H.W. & van Elburg, A.A. (2016). Rate, timing and predictors of relapse in patients with anorexia nervosa following a relapse prevention program: A cohort study. *BMC Psychiatry*, 16(316), 1–7. doi:10.1186/s12888-016-1019-y

Chen, E.Y., Weissman, J.A., Zeffiro, T.A., Yiu, A., Eneva, K.T., Arlt, J.M. & Swantek, M.J. (2016). Family-based therapy for young adults with anorexia nervosa restores weight. *International Journal of Eating Disorders*, 49(7), 701–7.

Cohn, L. & Lemberg, R. (2014). *Current Findings on Males with Eating Disorders*. Philadelphia, PA: Routledge.

Cooper, M. (2015). *The Psychology of Bulimia Nervosa: A Cognitive Perspective*. Oxford: Oxford University Press. doi:10.1093/med:psych/9780192632654.001.0001.

Copeland, W.E., Bulik, C.M., Zucker, N., Wolke, D., Lereya, S.T. & Costello, E.J. (2015). Does childhood bullying predict eating disorder symptoms? A prospective, longitudinal analysis. *International Journal of Eating Disorders*, 48(8), 1141–9.

Crook, M.A. (2014). Refeeding syndrome: Problems with definition and management. *Nutrition*, 30, 1448–55.

Cucchi, A., Ryan, D., Konstantakopoulos, G., Stroumpa, S. Kacar, S., Renshaw, S., … Kravariti, E. (2016). Lifetime prevalence of non-suicidal self-injury in patients with eating disorders: A systematic review and meta analysis. *Psychological Medicine*, 46, 1345–58. doi:10.1017/S0033291716000027

Culbert, K.M., Racine, S.E. & Klump, K.L. (2015). Research review: What we have learned about the causes of eating disorders: Synthesis of sociocultural, psychological, and biological research. *Journal of Child Psychology and Psychiatry*, 56(11), 1141–64. doi:10.1111/jcpp.12441

Fogarty, S. & Ramjan, L.M. (2016). Factors impacting treatment and recovery in anorexia nervosa: Qualitative findings from an online questionnaire. *Journal of Eating Disorders*, 4(18), 1–9. doi:10.1186/s40337-016-0107-1.

Forney, K.J., Buchman-Schmitt, J.M., Keel, P.K. & Frank, G.K.W. (2016). The medical complications associated with purging. *International Journal of Eating Disorders*, 49(3), 249–59.

Galsworthy-Francis, L. & Allan, S. (2014). Cognitive behavioural therapy for anorexia nervosa: A systematic review. *Clinical Psychology Review*, 34, 54–72. Retrieved from https://www.ncbi.nlm.nih.gov/pubmed/24394285.

Goldschmidt, A.B., Wall, M.M., Zhang, J., Loth, K.A. & Neumark-Sztainer, D. (2016). Overeating and binge eating in emerging adulthood: 10-year stability and risk factors. *Developmental Psychology*, 52(3), 475–83. doi:doi.org/10.1037/dev0000086

Goncalves, S.F., Machado, B.C., Martins, C. & Machado, P.P.P. (2014). Eating and weight/shape criticism as a specific life-event related to bulimia nervosa: A case control study. *Journal of Psychology*, 148(1), 61–72.

Harrington, B.C., Jimerson, M., Haxton, C. & Jimerson, D.C. (2015). Initial evaluation, diagnosis, and treatment of anorexia nervosa and bulimia nervosa. *American Family Physician*, 91(1), 46–53.

Keel, P.K. (2012). *The Oxford Handbook of Eating Disorders*. Oxford: Oxford University Press.

Keski-Rahkonen, A., Raevouri, A., Bulik, C.M., Hoek, H.W., Rissanen, A. & Kaprio, J. (2014). Factors associated with recovery from anorexia nervosa: A population-based study. *International Journal of Eating Disorders*, 47(2), 117–23.

Latzer, Y., Merrick, J. & Stein, D. (2011). *Understanding Eating Disorders: Integrating Culture, Psychology and Biology*. New York: Nova Science.

Madowitz, J., Matheson, B.E. & Liang, J. (2015). The relationship between eating disorders and sexual trauma. *Eating & Weight Disorders*, 20, 281–93. doi:10.1007/s40519-015-0195-y

Martinez, M.A. & Craighead, L.W. (2015). Toward person(ality)-centered treatment: How consideration of personality and individual differences in anorexia nervosa may improve treatment outcome. *Clinical Psychology: Science and Practice*, 22(3), 296–314.

Morgan, J.F., Reid, F. & Lacey, J.H. (1999). The SCOFF questionnaire: Assessment of a new screening tool for eating disorders. *BMJ*, 319(4), 1467–8.

Mustelin, L., Raevuori, A., Bulik, C.M., Rissanen, A., Hoek, H.W., Kaprio, J. & Keski-Rahkonen, A. (2015). Long-term outcomes in anorexia nervosa in the community. *International Journal of Eating Disorders*, 48, 851–9.

National Institute for Health and Care Excellence (NICE). (2017). *Nutrition Support for Adults: Oral Nutrition Support, Enteral Tube Feeding and Parenteral Nutrition: Clinical Guideline*. London: NICE.

NSW Ministry of Health. (2014). *Guidelines for the Inpatient Management of Adult Eating Disorders in General Medical and Psychiatric Settings in NSW*. North Sydney: NSW Ministry of Health.

Olmsted, M.O., MacDonald, D.E., McFarlane, T., Trottier, K. & Colton, P. (2015). Predictors of rapid relapse in bulimia nervosa. *International Journal of Eating Disorders*, 48(3), 337–40.

Palmer, B. (2014). *Helping People with Eating Disorders: A Clinical Guide to Assessment and Treatment*. Hoboken, NJ: Wiley-Blackwell.

Palmer, M., Matthews, K. & Owens, E. (2016). Consistency of Australian and New Zealand dietitians' identification of refeeding syndrome risk and comparison with refeeding guidelines and patient electrolytes and supplementation treatment. *Nutrition & Dietetics*, 73, 369–75. doi:10.1111/1747-0080.12227

Peterson, C.M., Baker, J.H., Thornton, L.M., Trace, S.E., Mazzeo, S.E., Neale, M.C., … Bulik, C.M. (2015). Genetic and environmental components to self-induced vomiting. *International Journal of Eating Disorders*, 49(4), 421–7.

Phillips, K., Keane, K. & Wolfe, B.E. (2014). Peripheral brain derived neurotrophic factor (BDNF) in bulimia nervosa: A systematic review. *Archives of Psychiatric Nursing*, 28, 108–13.

Rizk, M., Lalanne, C., Berthoz, S., Kern, L., EVHAN Group & Godart, N. (2015). Problematic exercise in anorexia nervosa: Testing potential risk factors against different definitions. *PLOS ONE*, 10(11), 1–18. doi:10.1371/journal.pone.0143352

Roux, H., Ali, A., Lambert, S., Radon, L., Huas, C., Curt, F., Berthoz, S., … EVHAN Group (2016). Predictive factors of dropout from inpatient treatment for anorexia nervosa. *BMC Psychiatry*, 16(339), 2–11.

Sharan, P. & Sundar, A.S. (2015). Eating disorders in women. *Indian Journal of Psychiatry*, 57(2), 286–95.

Stice, E., Shaw, H. & Nemeroff, C. (1998). Dual pathway model of bulimia nervosa: Longitudinal support for dietary restraint and affect-regulation mechanisms. *Journal of Social and Clinical Psychology*, 17(2), 129–49.

Thornton, L.M., Welch, E., Munn-Chernoff, M.A., Lichtenstein, P. & Bulik, C.M. (2016). Anorexia, major depression, and suicide attempts: shared genetic factors. *Suicide and Life-Threatening Behavior*, 46(5), 525–34. doi:10.1111/sltb.12235

Yom-Tov, E. & Boyd, D.M. (2014). On the link between media coverage of anorexia and pro-anorexic practices on the web. *International Journal of Eating Disorders*, 47(2), 196–202.

Vella-Zarb, R.A., Mills, J.S., Westra, H.A., Carter, J.C. & Keating, L. (2015). A randomized controlled trial of motivational interviewing + self-help versus psychoeducation + self-help for binge eating. *International Journal of Eating Disorders*, 48(3), 328–32.

White, E.K., Warren, C.S., Cao, L., Crosby, R.D., Engel, S.G., Wonderlich, S.A., Mitchell, J.E., … Le Grange, D. (2016). Media exposure and associated stress contribute to eating pathology in women with anorexia nervosa: Daily and momentary associations. *International Journal of Eating Disorders*, 49(6), 617–21.

Whiteway, A. (2015). Bulimia nervosa and the role of the dental professional. *Dental Health*, 54(3), 31–3.

Zeppegno, P. & Gramaglia, C. (2014). *New Developments in Anorexia Nervosa Research*. New York: Nova Biomedical Books.

CHAPTER 14

SUBSTANCE-RELATED AND ADDICTIVE DISORDERS

Desiree Smith and Glen Collett

LEARNING OUTCOMES

Upon completion of this chapter, you should be able to:

14.1 Outline the historical context of substance use and substance use disorders

14.2 Understand substance misuse and what defines illicit and psychoactive substances

14.3 Develop an understanding of addiction and dependence as well as familiarity with the appropriate terminology

14.4 Develop an understanding of the aetiology of substance use disorders and identify risk factors and high-risk populations as well as relevant comorbidities

14.5 Recognise the implications of substance use disorders on physical, mental and social health

14.6 Identify clinical course and characteristics and behaviours of each diagnostic criterion of substance use disorder

14.7 Develop an understanding of biopsychosocial assessment and how to screen, assess and support the consumer experiencing a substance use disorder

---

LEARNING FROM PRACTICE

My childhood was alright, it wasn't great, but it wasn't terrible, either, but the first time I took a drug of any kind was when me and my friends started drinking alcohol and smoking weed. I did okay at school and eventually went to university, where I liked to party and go out with my girlfriends. Back then, none of it seemed a problem, it was what I did, what everybody did. There were a few nights when I overdid it, blacked out and couldn't remember what happened, but we all have stories like that. Then, when I graduated, I got a job I really liked and life was good.

When I hit 28 – three years ago now – things changed. I got promoted at work and the hours got longer, so, to unwind I partied – booze, ecstasy, cocaine (I could afford that now) – and what was the occasional weekend bender, became every weekend. I'd start on a Friday night and go hard until the Sunday morning. And, to come down, I would smoke weed and when I could get it I'd take benzos – Valium – and it became the norm.

Everything spiralled; my anxiety was constant and I couldn't cope any more. I began drinking daily just to feel normal and began to miss days at work, stretching the tolerance of my boss. Then I fell over when I was wasted and injured myself – I can't remember it – and wound up in the emergency room. It was here that a doctor began talking to me about my habits, how much I drink and what I use, and suggested I get some help.

Ashleigh, a consumer living with an SUD

Substance use is described by some people as a 'rite of passage' for young people. Ashleigh's substance use behaviour commenced in adolescence and she feels her use was not out of the ordinary in comparison with her social group. What factors contribute to the change in substance use from episodic and social to problematic?

INTRODUCTION

People consume substances and engage in gambling pursuits for a number of reasons. For the majority of people, these activities are not problematic and do not have a negative impact on their lives. However, for some people their reliance on substances or high-risk behaviours such as gambling can result in a range of emotional, physiological, social and economic consequences. The *Diagnostic and Statistical Manual of Mental Disorders* (DSM-5) refers to these issues as substance-related and addictive disorders (APA, 2013). In this chapter, we focus on understanding the issues related to a consumer's experience of substance use disorder. In particular, we explore alcohol use disorder in more detail.

THE HISTORICAL CONTEXT OF SUBSTANCE USE AND MISUSE

It is believed that the use of substances may pre-date the beginning of recorded human history in human agricultural societies (Ritter, King & Hamilton, 2013). Attitudes, values and beliefs about substance use are influenced by complex social, cultural, environmental, political and economic factors. The relationship between these factors and their influences on attitudes, values and beliefs determine substance use behaviour and, as some people experience, the onset of problematic substance misuse. **Figure 14.1** depicts the historical global perspective of substance use and its influences at the time.

16th and 17th century – globalisation of psychoactive substances
European colonisation throughout Latin America globalised the use of psychoactive substances such as, tobacco, coffee, sugar (from which rum was derived) and cocoa.

19th century – industrial isolation of psychoactive components of plant products
Isolation of morphine from opium poppy and cocaine from the coca plant enabled highly potent compounds to be shipped in larger quantities. This led to increased use and subsequent recognition of morphine and cocaine addiction.

Earliest recorded human history
In agricultural societies, alcohol was derived seasonally from plants and crops and used by special social groups. Alcohol misuse was recorded but sustained heavy use was uncommon.

Opiates derived from the opium poppy were used for medicinal or religious purposes but only in oral form and it was not widely available. Risk of overdose and dependence, however, was recorded.

17th and 18th century – industrialisation of psychoactive production
Globalisation of psychoactive substances increased demand and drove production, sale and consumption. Psychoactive substance use moved from medicinal to recreational. Alcohol was the first psychoactive substance to become industrialised. The term 'addiction' emerged.

20th century – development of synthetic drugs by pharmaceutical companies
Substances such as amphetamines, anxiolytics, barbiturates, benzodiazepines and MDA (ecstasy) and synthetic opiates like methadone, pethidine and fentanyl were developed for medicinal purposes; however, by 1960/1970 they were available on the black market for recreational use.

SOURCE: ADAPTED FROM RITTER, KING & HAMILTON, 2013, PP. 29–31

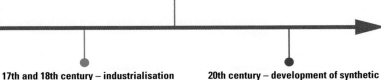

FIGURE 14.1
Chronological history of substance use

History of substance use in Australia

Substance use in Australia is recorded as occurring early in the Aboriginal and Torres Strait Islander populations and deviated significantly with European colonisation. Indigenous peoples fermented mild alcohol from honey and used a 'native form of tobacco called Pitjurri' (Ritter, King & Hamilton, 2013, p. 31). Early European settlement in Australia introduced a new form of alcohol and social and cultural practice of alcohol use. The introduction of distilled spirits to Indigenous populations has resulted in significant health, social and cultural effects that continue today.

Early settlers also introduced a cultural identity of alcohol use rooted in the social construct of mateship and working-class identities. Since this time, there have been an array of social-cultural, environmental,

political and economic factors that have influenced and shaped Australian society's values, beliefs around substance use and substance use behaviour (Ritter, King & Hamilton, 2013). Australian culture continues to have its own context of social-cultural, environmental, political and economic factors that shape attitudes, values and beliefs around substance use.

UNDERSTANDING SUBSTANCE MISUSE, AND DEFINING ILLICIT AND PSYCHOACTIVE SUBSTANCES

For many people, the engagement in 'substance use' occurs legally, within health recommendations and has positive outcomes such as pleasure and medicinal purposes; for example, drinking a cup of coffee, or taking prescription medication in response to an illness as prescribed by a doctor. However, when substance use deviates from these parameters and begins to cause harm the term **substance misuse** may be used. The World Health Organization (WHO, 2017, para. 1) defines psychoactive substance misuse as 'persistent or sporadic excessive drug use inconsistent with or unrelated to acceptable medical practice'. Substance misuse in this context has harmful effects and may involve the use of substances illegally or the use of substances that are, in Australia, classified 'illegal'.

Substances taken in harmful and illegal ways are referred to as *illicit substances* and can include illegal drugs – cannabis, heroin and amphetamines – over-the-counter and prescription **pharmaceuticals** that are used for non-medical purposes or taken in dosages or frequencies other than that prescribed (e.g. pain medications that are opioid based, benzodiazepines and steroids) and other psychoactive substances, such as

kava, synthetic cannabis and inhalants (AIHW, 2016). It is the misuse of illicit substances, alcohol, cannabis, stimulants (amphetamine/methamphetamines) and opioids that is the focus of this section on **substance use disorders (SUDs)**.

It is essential to remember that not all consumers with a history of substance misuse will develop a substance use disorder. The impact of substance misuse on a person's health and well-being includes a range of substance misuse behaviours. Substance misuse behaviours are presented here to demonstrate the progressive range of harm and onset of changes to neurobiological pathways and physiological adaptations related to the development of an SUD and onset of comorbidities associated with substance misuse behaviours. We now look at the range of substance misuse behaviour from hazardous, harmful, addiction and dependence. **Table 14.1** describes the range of substance misuse behaviours.

TABLE 14.1
Range of substance misuse behaviours

TYPE OF SUBSTANCE MISUSE	DEFINITIONS	DSM-5
Hazardous substance use	Substance use that has the potential for physical, psychological and social consequences; for example, risk of falls, motor vehicle accidents and violence	Mild, moderate, severe SUD DSM-5 does not use the term *addiction* in diagnostic clarification and uses the term *Substance Use Disorder* to describe a range of mild, moderate and severe substance use behaviours
Harmful substance use	A pattern of substance use that is damaging to health; for example, hepatitis from injecting, depression, liver disease	
Addiction	Substance use that causes changes in brain circuitry that persist after detoxification. These changes cause a 'chronic, relapsing brain disease that is characterised by compulsive drug seeking and use, despite harmful consequences' (NIDA, 2014, p. 5). Addiction is also associated with the physiological and psychological experience of cravings	
Dependence	Behavioural, cognitive, and physiological phenomena, developing after repeated use; including the urge to use substance (s), superseding other activities and responsibilities, difficulty controlling use, despite harmful consequences, increased tolerance and a physical withdrawal state	Severe SUD

SOURCE: APA, 2013, PP. 483, 485; NIDA, 2014; WHO 2016A, 2016B, 2017

The terms *addiction* and *dependence* can be used interchangeably, be given different definitions and, in more recent times, not used at all. Addiction is not applied as a diagnostic term in the DSM-5 classification of SUDs; however, some clinicians may choose to use the word addiction to denote a more serious substance use presentation (APA, 2013). For the purpose of demonstrating the neurobiological pathway and physiological changes that occur in SUDs, the terms addiction and dependence are used in this chapter. The term *substance use disorder*, however, is the preferred term in the DSM-5.

Categories of substances and their effects

The term *substance* refers to anything ingested that alters or affects mood, cognition, thinking,

perception, behaviour and consciousness. Referred to as *psychoactive*, these substances can be commonly categorised by their effect on the central nervous system (CNS), including the brain and spinal cord; and can be depressant, stimulant or hallucinogenic. **Table 14.2** provides examples of substances and their effects.

ADDICTION AND DEPENDENCE

The belief that those with an SUD choose to use and lack the willpower to 'just give up' impacts recovery and restricts therapeutic engagement. Naturally, choice is an element of any such activity. However, neurobiological factors strongly influence an

TABLE 14.2
Immediate physiological and psychological effects of substance use

SUBSTANCE	CNS EFFECT	PHYSIOLOGICAL EFFECT	PSYCHOLOGICAL EFFECT	EXAMPLES	METHOD OF USE
Alcohol	Depressant: suppresses, inhibits or decreases activity of the CNS	Impaired coordination, slurred speech, drowsiness, nausea and vomiting, low body temperature, sleep disturbances, blackouts, temporary loss of consciousness, coma, death	Euphoria, increased socialisation and confidence. Impairs problem solving, judgement and insight, memory and learning	Street names: booze, grog, piss, plonk, sauce	Orally
Cannabis	Depressant: suppresses, inhibits or decreases activity of the CNS	Increases heart rate, respiratory system complications related to smoking (e.g. bronchitis), bloodshot eyes, diminished psychomotor performance	Relaxation and euphoria, disinhibition, drowsiness, mild enhancement of senses, subtle changes in thought and expression, pain relief, decreased nausea. Increased appetite, impairs short-term memory and learning, ability to focus, confusion. Anxiety, panic, depression, dysphoria, depersonalisation. Increased risk of psychotic symptoms – hallucinations, delusions	Marijuana, hashish or hashish oil, synthetic cannabis Street names: grass, pot, hash, weed	Smoked, orally
Stimulants: amphetamines and cocaine	Stimulant: enhances or increases activity of CNS	Overstimulation, tachycardia and hypertension and cardiac complications, increased respiration, dry mouth, nausea, vomiting, jaw clenching and teeth grinding, increased body temperature and sweating, sleep disturbances, insomnia, rashes, dilatation of pupils, seizures and coma	Euphoria, feelings of confidence, increased energy, alertness and arousal (hypercognition), talkativeness and increased task orientation. Reduced sleep and appetite, impaired judgement and insight, anxiety, mood swings, greatly increased motor activity, compulsive repetitive actions, euphoric disinhibition and injury related to disinhibition. Increased risk of psychotic symptoms – delusions, hallucinations, thought disorders, bizarre behaviour, harm to self and others	Amphetamines, cocaine, phenethylamines (methylphenidate: Ritalin) Street names for amphetamines: Speed, go-ee, ice, whiz, crystal, base Street names for cocaine: blow, nose candy, charlie, rock, coke Street names for phenethylamines (MDMA, ecstasy): disco biscuits, Es, love drug, eckies	Smoking, snorting, orally, suppositories, injections
Opioids: Heroin and prescription opioids/codeine	Depressant	Decrease in pain, drowsiness and yawning, slurred speech (sedation), constricted pupils, decreased respiratory rate, hyper/hypo tension and arrhythmia, nausea, vomiting High risk – coma and death related to overdose	Euphoria and sense of tranquility. Apathy, dysphoria, attention and memory impairment, psychomotor agitation, sense of urgency and compulsion, hysteria, decreased libido	Street names: big H, beige powder, black tar, horse, MS contin, morph	Smoking, snorting, orally, injections

SOURCE: ADAPTED FROM CAMPBELL, 2001; RITTER, KING & HAMILTON, 2013, PP. 4–5

individual, leading to a disorder of volition. Addiction, cravings, tolerance and withdrawal involve changes in the brain (biochemical, functional and structural), affecting decision making and increasing compulsion, while restricting a consumer's ability to abstain from use despite the negative consequences. These neuroadaptations can give us valuable insight into how controlled, occasional substance use can progress into more chronic patterns of substance misuse and vulnerability of relapse in the absence of substance use (US Department of Health and Human Services, 2016).

Why don't people just STOP? The pathway to addiction and dependence

Addiction is a chronic condition and involves changes to the neurobiological pathways in a person's brain (see the 'Evidence-based practice' box). The brain reward system, or pathway, reinforces survival and adaptive behavioural patterns. Examples are sex and eating, which are geared towards survival, prompting the release of strong neurotransmitters (e.g. dopamine and endorphins) that create pleasurable sensations, thereby reinforcing behaviour for survival (Fraser, 2015). Substances of abuse (both licit psychotropic and illicit) 'hijack' this process, as the potency and method of administration overtly stimulates the reward pathway, notably dopamine and endorphins, creating euphoria and motivation. The hit of dopamine, however, is significantly faster and more intense than when released by survival activities, while positively reinforcing and leading to further, excessive use (NIDA, 2014). See **Figure 14.2**.

The mesolimbic dopamine reward pathway
Dr John Chow, consultant addiction medicine specialist describes the mesolimbic dopamine reward pathway as:

> a neural circuitry consisting of the Ventral Tegmental Area (VTA) in the brain where dopamine cell bodies are located, and the Nucleus Accumbens where the dopamine neurons project. There are connections between these areas and the amygdala where the dopamine-induced rewarding experience is learnt and reward cues are conditioned (associating cues with pleasure), and the prefrontal cortex where associative learning and regulation of emotions, impulses and behaviours and analysis take place (executive functioning).

SOURCE: DR JOHN CHOW, CONSULTANT ADDICTION MEDICINE SPECIALIST

Cravings, triggers and urges

Cravings, triggers and urges are common to all substance addictions and are characterised by the preoccupation with substance use and the development of drug associations in the absence of the substance. SUD prompts 'abnormal desire', associations and compulsive behaviours that are difficult to control and affect recovery. Pleasure associated with the reward system positively reinforces behaviour by creating a desire to experience that pleasure again. Abnormal desire occurs in response

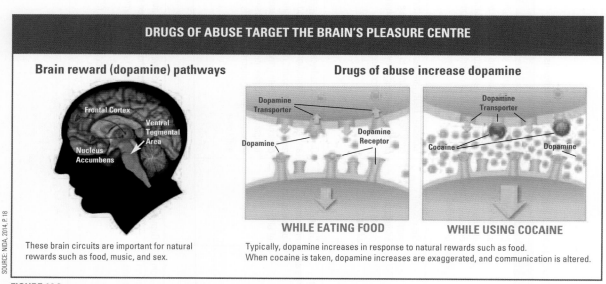

SOURCE: NIDA, 2014, P. 18

DRUGS OF ABUSE TARGET THE BRAIN'S PLEASURE CENTRE

Brain reward (dopamine) pathways

Frontal Cortex
Ventral Tegmental Area
Nucleus Accumbens

These brain circuits are important for natural rewards such as food, music, and sex.

Drugs of abuse increase dopamine

Dopamine Transporter
Dopamine
Dopamine Receptor

WHILE EATING FOOD

Dopamine Transporter
Cocaine
Dopamine

WHILE USING COCAINE

Typically, dopamine increases in response to natural rewards such as food. When cocaine is taken, dopamine increases are exaggerated, and communication is altered.

FIGURE 14.2
Drugs of abuse target the brain's pleasure centre

to overt stimulation of this feedback mechanism when the substance is not present and increases risk to use (Sinha, 2013). Associations occur when the reward pathway has been triggered by illicit substance use and an association is made with the behaviour, circumstance or place at the time it is triggered. For example, the association made between drug paraphernalia or internal states, such as stress or mood, can trigger an urge to use as it is associated with the substance-rewarding effects (Sinha, 2016; US Department of Health and Human Services, 2016). The experience of cravings can also be associated with impulsive behaviours that have negative outcomes. Strong urges or associations can override executive functioning, affecting choices and the ability to manage and override urges and associations (US Department of Health and Human Services, 2016). For example, cravings for the highly addictive substance methamphetamine (ice) can predispose people experiencing ice addiction to destructive behaviours; that is, criminal activity to get more ice and use it again.

Dependence
The experience of dependence in a person misusing substances may suggest a more severe SUD. The characterising difference between the two states of addiction and dependence is that the former is associated with a compulsion to use, and the latter with the body's physiological adaptation to long-term substance misuse. Where the body has adapted to the chronic misuse of a substance(s), tolerance and withdrawal syndrome will occur.

Dependence on a substance, however, can occur in the absence of addiction. It is important to be cognisant of avoiding a hasty assumption of an SUD where there is an experience of dependency, as further assessment is required; for example, the development of dependence from morphine use for pain management in terminal cancer. Here the patient will experience a withdrawal state if the morphine is abruptly ceased, but they do not experience the 'compulsion' to use the morphine and therefore are not addicted (NIDA, 2007).

Tolerance
Repeated chronic use of an illicit substance overtly stimulates the reward pathway and, over time, the body adjusts to the excessive dopamine production caused by the substance use, resulting in a decrease in pleasure or the 'high', and as a consequence, the person may require an increased dose and/or increased compulsion to use to achieve the same effect. Relative

to this is the effect of tolerance on the production of dopamine for natural survival behaviours such as food and sex. This means people experiencing tolerance may not only report a decrease in pleasure experienced by illicit substance use but also a decrease in the pleasure achieved from other once pleasurable, positive reinforcing activities (NIDA, 2014; US Department of Health and Human Services, 2016).

Withdrawal
A withdrawal syndrome may occur when substance use stops. Withdrawal syndrome is associated with the experience of a range of physiological and mental health symptoms that can be mild (e.g. withdrawal from caffeine) or in more severe cases, life-threatening (e.g. alcohol withdrawal and delirium tremens). See the section on 'Withdrawal' later in this chapter.

The neurobiological complexity of addiction perpetuates the cyclic nature of an SUD and must be understood and compensated for when educating people about SUDs and developing interventions to support consumers through recovery. Failure to do this will perpetuate the stigma that SUDs are a failure of moral nature and fail to recognise that recovery may be a lifelong process to prevent relapse.

Terminology: why does this matter?
The use of language can either advertently or inadvertently impact on therapeutic relationships and health outcomes for people experiencing substance use issues. Language that perpetuates stigma, stereotyping and/or defines a person by their behaviour or health status 'may actually induce implicit cognitive biases against those suffering addiction' (Kelly, Saitz & Wakeman, 2016, p. 117); and create significant barriers to seeking and accessing help, engagement with health workers, and recovery. For example, referring to a person as a 'junkie' or 'alcoholic' defines the whole person by their behaviour instead of identifying the behaviour itself as problematic, and may imply the need for 'punishment versus treatment' (Kelly, Saitz & Wakeman, 2016, p. 119).

The awareness of language used in the area of SUDs can promote a greater understanding of the complex pathological, biological and psychosocial nature of these disorders and potentially influence public understanding of SUDs. Using non-judgemental, rather than disapproving, terms encourages engagement and enhanced therapeutic relationships. **Table 14.3** identifies language that should be avoided and provides suggestions for alternative words and references.

TABLE 14.3

Language to avoid and alternatives to use when referencing substance-related and addictive disorders

LANGUAGE TO AVOID	RATIONALE	ALTERNATIVE LANGUAGE
Addict, abuser, junkie	These terms label the consumer. They are demeaning and deny dignity and humanity. They imply permanency to the condition.	Person in active addiction, person with substance misuse disorder, person experiencing drug/alcohol problems
Abuse	Negates that addictive disorders are medical conditions. Blames the individual for the illness and ignores aetiological factors. Absolves those selling or promoting addictive substances. Evokes implicit punitive biases. Feeds into stigma of not only people experiencing addictive disorders but also their family and the addiction treatment field.	Misuse, harmful use or hazardous use, inappropriate use, problem use or risky use
Clean, dirty (refers to drug test results)	Creates stigma as a positive test result which may indicate an illness is associated with filth. May decrease a person's sense of hope and self-efficacy for change. Evokes negative and punitive implicit cognitions.	Negative, positive or substance free
Habit or drug habit	Denies the medical nature of addictive disorders. Implies that to stop addictive behaviour is a matter of willpower.	Substance use disorder, alcohol and drug disorder, active addiction
A drug user, user or substance abuser	A stigmatising term, as it labels the consumer by their behaviour. Evokes punitive judgements and biases.	Use 'person first' language; for example, an individual with, or experiencing, a substance use disorder, person who misuses prescription drugs, harmful or hazardous alcohol use or a person who engages in risky substance use

SOURCE: ADAPTED FROM KELLY, SAITZ & WAKEMAN, 2016. PP. 118–20; NAABT, 2008

SUBSTANCE USE, MISUSE PROBLEMS AND SUBSTANCE USE DISORDERS

In the previous sections we explored the historical context of substance use, both generally and specific to Australia. In order to work with consumers experiencing a diagnosis of SUD, it is also necessary to understand some of the key terminology, the way in which substances are classified and their physiological and psychological effects. With this background in mind, we now explore factors related to the aetiology, incidence and impacts of SUDs.

Aetiology

No single causal factor leads to the development and progression of an SUD, with genetics, biology, social and environmental components impacting the initiation and progression of an SUD.

Genetic factors

It is estimated that genetic factors account for between 40–60% of a person's vulnerability for developing a substance use disorder. Twin studies have demonstrated genes themselves predispose a vulnerability to developing an SUD as much as they predispose a person to protective factors. According to Osborne and Thombs (2013, p. 35), 'genes do not determine destiny but shape parameters of risk as well as protections'. It is the influence of environmental factors, stages of development and other medical conditions that may 'trigger' a genetic predisposition. Genetic factors may also account for the different ways individuals metabolise substances, develop tolerances and sensitivities, experience intoxication and withdrawal, and experience side effects (Osborne & Thombs, 2013).

Biological factors

Biological factors, such as adolescence and gender, may increase a person's vulnerability to developing an SUD. In some cases, culture may also play a role, as outlined in the 'Cultural considerations' box.

CULTURAL CONSIDERATIONS

Culture-related substance use issues

Forty per cent of people from Asian countries such as Japan, China and Korea have a gene variation for the alcohol-metabolising enzymes alcohol dehydrogenase and aldehyde dehydrogenase. The impact of this is that the toxic by-product of alcohol is not broken down and instead builds up in the body (liver and blood). When alcohol is consumed, people will experience facial flushing, palpitations and severe reactions (APA, 2013).

Adolescence

Early childhood and adolescent experiences and exposure can greatly increase the vulnerability for substance use problems and their onset. Factors such as parents' substance use, exposure to substances and substance use, increased risk-taking behaviour, criminality, relationships and home environment, and peer drug-related behaviour can influence child and adolescent substance initiation and subsequent substance use behaviour. Substance use behaviour during adolescence can compromise the development of the area of the brain responsible for executive function, the pre-frontal cortex, which is responsible for functions such as planning, problem solving and decision making. According to the US Department of Health and Human Services (2016), adolescent brain development is not fully complete until approximately 21–23 years old in females and 23–25 years old in males, and the last part of the brain to develop is the pre-frontal cortex.

Gender

Differences in brain structure and functioning and social and cultural factors between men and women have been found to explain the differences in aetiological factors, clinical course and risks associated with an SUD (Becker & Koob, 2016; Lind et al., 2017). Prevalence of alcohol consumption and alcohol use disorder (AUD) is higher in males than females; however, women are more susceptible to alcohol-related harm due to biological factors, such as reduced ability to metabolise alcohol along with differences in physical make-up (smaller frame, higher body fat, different biochemical (hormonal) processes) and environmental influences (e.g. increased risk of vulnerability while intoxicated to sexual assault/violence). Women are also less likely to enter into treatment due to gender-specific issues, such as attitudes towards women drinkers,

depression, and concerns about children or fear of removal of children (NCETA, 2004).

Social and environmental factors

Social and environmental factors greatly influence the health and well-being of people globally. These factors include exposure to stress, cultural norms, political influences and legal system, socioeconomic status (SES), employment, education, where people live, the physical environment, availability of substances, relationships with family and friends, and access and use of health and social services. These factors have the potential to be either protective and/or risk factors. However, when they are risk factors, there may be an increased vulnerability for substance misuse behaviour. For example, it has been identified that there is a clear link between socioeconomic deprivation and risk of dependence on alcohol, nicotine and other drugs (Wilkinson & Marmot, 2003).

High-risk population groups within Australia

Certain population groups demonstrate a greater disparity in patterns of substance use and associated risks and harms. The Australian Institute of Health and Welfare (AIHW, 2013) has identified vulnerable populations within Australia; these include rural and remote communities, Aboriginal and Torres Strait Islander peoples, lesbian, gay, bisexual, transgender, transexual, queer, intersex, asexual and more (LGBTQ(IA+)) communities and prison populations.

Rural and remote communities

People who live in rural and remote communities within Australia were two times more likely to smoke, drink alcohol in risky quantities and use methamphetamines when compared with those who lived in major cities (AIHW, 2013). Factors that influence patterns of substance use include access to education and employment opportunities, unemployment, uncertainty about the future, isolation, lack of public transport and leisure activities, a culture of risk-taking behaviour, limited availability of services or difficulty accessing services (AIHW, 2013). These risk factors also perpetuate the health implications associated with SUDs.

Aboriginal and Torres Strait Islander peoples

Alcohol-related harm associated with alcohol consumption among Aboriginal and Torres Strait Islander peoples accounts for 8% of the total burden of disease and injury. It is the greatest burden of disease in Indigenous males aged 15–44 and is the leading cause of disease for Indigenous females aged 15–24 (AIHW, 2016, in AHMAC, 2017).

Patterns of alcohol consumption among Indigenous Australians indicate that there are a greater proportion of Indigenous Australians who abstain from alcohol consumption (1.6 times compared to non-Indigenous), but Indigenous people who do drink, drink at levels that exceed the single occasional guidelines and it subsequently causes greater harm. The prevalence of harmful alcohol use in Indigenous populations is twice as great as that in non-Indigenous populations (Wilson, Stearn, Gray & Saggers, 2010); and 2012–13 Health Survey data, based on 24-hour recall showed 'that the median amount of alcohol beverages consumed was more than twice as high among Indigenous consumers (equivalent to 1.2 bottles of beer or almost 5 glasses of wine) than non-Indigenous consumers' (AHMAC, 2017, p. 131) (see **Figure 14.3**).

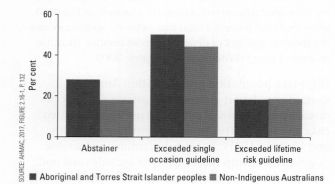

■ Aboriginal and Torres Strait Islander peoples ■ Non-Indigenous Australians

FIGURE 14.3
Alcohol risk levels by Indigenous status, persons aged 15 years and over, age-standardised, 2012–13

The harmful use of alcohol in Indigenous communities results from a complex relationship between the factors that contribute to the gap between social and health equalities (historical; i.e. colonialism, prohibition and dispossession, political, social and economic) and the consequences of harmful alcohol use in Indigenous communities compared with non-Indigenous communities perpetuating poorer health and social outcomes. Hence, harmful rates of alcohol consumption are both consequences and contributing factors to the health and social gap experienced by Indigenous people (Wilson et al., 2010).

The following points demonstrate the disparities of impact from harmful alcohol use between Indigenous and non-Indigenous Australians:

■ Male indigenous Australians are five times more likely to die from alcohol related causes than male non-Indigenous Australians. Indigenous women are six times more likely to die from alcohol-related causes. Refer to **Figure 14.4**.

■ Indigenous males and females were hospitalised for a diagnosis related to alcohol use at four times the rate of non-Indigenous males and females. Acute intoxication was the most common reason for admission (59%). Admission for acute intoxication

between 2013–15 was at 11 times the rate of non-Indigenous Australians.

■ Indigenous Australians died from mental and behavioural disorders due to alcohol use at six times the rate of non-Indigenous Australians.

■ Indigenous Australians are 3.6 times more likely to report family stressors related to alcohol problems (AHMAC, 2017, p. 131).

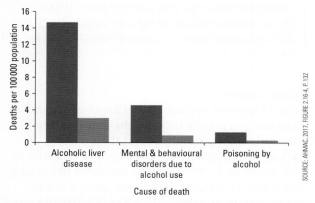

■ Aboriginal and Torres Strait Islander peoples ■ Non-Indigenous Australians

FIGURE 14.4
Age-standardised rates for deaths related to alcohol use, NSW, QLD, WA, SA and the NT, 2011–15

Gay, lesbian, bisexual, transgender and intersex LGBTQ(IA+)

While 'sexual orientation is not synonymous with greater risk or a causal factor for poor mental health' (Ritter, Matthew-Simmons & Carragher, 2012, p. 100), it is the greater experience of risk factors LGBTQ(IA+) communities face/encounter that increases vulnerability to harm related to substance use and SUDs. People who identify as LGBTQ(IA+) experience a disproportional percentage of other mental health conditions such as major depressive episode, anxiety disorders, mood disorders and are at higher risk of self-harm/non-suicidal self-injury and suicide behaviours than the general Australian population (National LGBTI Health Alliance, 2016). Ritter, Matthew-Simmons and Carragher (2012) identify that rates of alcohol consumption are higher in LGBTQ(IA+) communities, in particular among lesbian and bisexual women, than in non-LGBTQ(IA+) communities. There is also a higher prevalence of both problematic substance use and SUD in LGBTQ(IA+) communities, in particular among gay and bisexual men, than in non-LGBTQ(IA+) communities.

Prison populations

When exploring substance use in this marginalised at-risk group it is important to look at the demographic profile of the prison population to understand why substance use and SUDs are overrepresented and often chronic for this population. These demographics are consistent for men and women and include the following:

- lower SES
- poorer health
- lower levels of education
- higher proportions of Aboriginal and Torres Strait Islander peoples
- the diagnosis of a mental health condition
- have an intellectual disability
- have no stable family (Baldry & Russell, 2017).

In 2015, 67% of prison entrants reported using illicit substances in the previous 12 months before incarceration, of which 45% reported injecting drug use. Methamphetamine use was the most widely used illicit substance in most age groups apart from over 45 year olds, who mostly used cannabis. Thirty-nine per cent (2 in 5) prisoners consumed levels of alcohol that put them at high risk of health problems in the previous 12 months, findings that are statistically significant in comparison with the general population (AIHW, 2015).

Prevalence

In Australia, it is estimated that approximately 20% of the population experienced a mental health disorder in the previous 12 months, of which 5.1% experience an SUD. Women have a greater prevalence of anxiety and mood disorders; however, men are twice as likely to be diagnosed with an SUD and people in younger age groups have the highest prevalence of SUD (13% 16–24 years) (ABS, 2007). The prevalence of alcohol use disorders is significantly higher than that of illicit substances use disorders, including cannabis, stimulants, opioids and other psychoactive substance use (Kessler et al., 2005; WHO, 2010). The prevalence of alcohol use disorders in Australia is 5.0% for males and 2.1% for females (WHO, 2014).

The following data from the 2016 National Drug Strategy Household Survey (NDSHS) illustrates alcohol and substance use patterns in Australia. **Table 14.4** highlights some key points.

TABLE 14.4
Patterns of alcohol and substance use in Australia, 2016

ALCOHOL USE	OTHER SUBSTANCE USE
• Australians are drinking less in 2016 compared with 2013 and this is attributed to men changing their alcohol consumption behaviour. However, males were twice more likely than females to exceed lifetime risk guidelines, but this gap is narrowing due to fewer males drinking at risky levels. Overall lifetime risk rates are declining but single occasion use remains unchanged at 1 in 4 people. • Increase in the number of younger people (12–17 years old) abstaining from alcohol use. • Young adults (18–24 years old) have reduced their alcohol consumption. • Females in the 50–59-year age group are drinking in excess of the lifetime guidelines. • Significant increase in females in their 30s exceeding the single occasion risk. • Teenage males and young adult males reporting declines in single occasion use. • 3 in 10 males in their 40s, 50s and 60s are drinking in excess of the lifetime guidelines. However, this has not changed from previous years. • Men aged 40–49 are the age group most likely to exceed guidelines risk. • Increase in older people in their 50s and 60s exceeding the very high risk drinking guidelines. However people in their late teens and early 20s are still more likely to exceed the very high risk drinking guidelines.	• The number of Australians 14 years and older using illicit drugs is increasing over the long term; however, there have been some substances that have declined and stabilised between 2013 and 2016. • The average age at which people in Australia tried an illicit drug increased from 19.3 (2013) to 19.7 years (2016). • More people in their 40s used illicit substances in 2016 than 2013, particularly males. People in their 50s reported using cannabis and people in their 60s pharmaceuticals. Females 18+, especially females in their 30s, reported significant increase in illicit substance use, mainly cannabis, ecstasy and cocaine. • Cannabis is the most commonly used illicit substance in Australia both in lifetime and 12 months use measures. • Lifetime use of cocaine has increased and it is now the second-most commonly used illegal substance after cannabis. • Misuse of pharmaceuticals is the second-highest reported substance used in the past 12 months behind cannabis; 4.8% or 1 in 20 Australians had misused pharmaceutical drugs in the past 12 months. The most commonly misused substance are painkillers/opiates such as over-the-counter codeine products, for example, Nurofen plus. • Although meth/amphetamine use has declined in the last 3 years, ice continues to be the preferred form of meth/amphetamine used, with 57% (up from 22% in 2010) of users preferring this form of meth/amphetamine in the previous 12 months; 32% of ice users reported using ice at least weekly. Smoking ice is the most preferred method of administration for regular users. The proportion of regular users smoking ice has doubled from 20% to 40% (Healey, 2016). However, the proportion of ice users injecting has also increased. Meth/amphetamines are now perceived by the Australian public as the substance of greatest concern to the community (AIHW, 2017).

SOURCE: AIHW, 2016, 2017A, 2017B, 2017C; HEALEY, 2016

CLINICAL OBSERVATIONS

The Australian guidelines to reduce health risks associated with alcohol

To assist in the identification of potential substance misuse behaviour in Australia, the National Health and Medical Research Council (NHMRC) developed a set of evidence-based alcohol guidelines to reduce the health risk associated with drinking alcohol. These guidelines indicate levels of use and categorise them into levels of risk. These guidelines are helpful in interpreting levels of alcohol consumed with associated acute and chronic risk factors. Risky drinking in Australia is defined by the terms 'lifetime risk' and 'single occasion risk'. The familiarisation and use of these recommendations are important in the development of appropriate health promotion, brief intervention and referral to appropriate services for alcohol misuse behaviour. The NHMRC is currently revising these guidelines, which are scheduled for release in the first half of 2020.

The current guidelines are to reduce health risks associated with alcohol (see also **Figure 14.5**):

Guideline 1: Reducing the risk of alcohol-related harm over a lifetime

- The lifetime risk of harm from drinking alcohol increases with the amount consumed.
- For healthy men and women, drinking no more than two standard drinks on any day reduces the lifetime risk of harm from alcohol-related disease or injury.

Guideline 2: Reducing the risk of injury on a single occasion of drinking

- On a single occasion of drinking, the risk of alcohol-related injury increases with the amount consumed.
- For healthy men and women, drinking no more than four standard drinks on a single occasion reduces the risk of alcohol-related injury arising from that occasion.

SOURCE: NHMRC, 2009

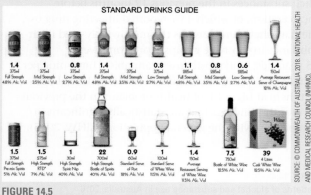

FIGURE 14.5
Australian recommendations of standard drinks

SOURCE: © COMMONWEALTH OF AUSTRALIA 2018. NATIONAL HEALTH AND MEDICAL RESEARCH COUNCIL (NHMRC).

Substance use disorder clinical course

A variety of social, cultural, psychological and economic factors can influence a person's decision to take substances. These factors can be static or dynamic and can influence attitudes towards substance use and substance use behaviour, including initiation and ongoing use. Factors that can influence initiation of and continuing use of substances include to:

- feel pleasure
- manage lives and emotions
- manage stress
- expand consciousness and provide a sense of enlightenment
- manage withdrawal and counteract other substances
- control pain
- control weight
- have something to do
- defy or rebel against parents
- fit into a social group
- manage shyness and lack of confidence
- be more creative (Centre for Addiction and Mental Health, 2010; Ritter, King & Hamilton, 2013).

Although substance use may appear to have advantages in the short term, ongoing substance use can create negative, unwanted effects that can quickly negate the advantages. Understanding the consumer's perspective, and why they use substances is important. The factors influencing use, unless identified, understood and addressed with appropriate interventions, will greatly impact a consumer's ability to change their substance use attitudes and behaviours (see **Figure 14.6**).

Initiation of substance use typically occurs during adolescence (but can occur at any age), with early onset of substance use, such as tobacco, alcohol and cannabis being a predictor of a progression into using other substances. Earlier adolescent use of alcohol and nicotine can progress into cannabis use and cannabis use is often regarded as a 'gateway' substance to other more socially regarded 'harder' substances such as stimulants, then opioids (Moran, 2010). According to the US Department of Health and Human Services (2016, p. 16), 'research now indicates that a majority of people who experience an SUD in their lifetime started using substances in their adolescence and had met the criteria for an SUD by the age of 20–25'. The progress of substance use to an SUD varies depending on the substance. **Table 14.5** identifies the clinical course for the development of alcohol, cannabis, stimulant and opioid use disorders.

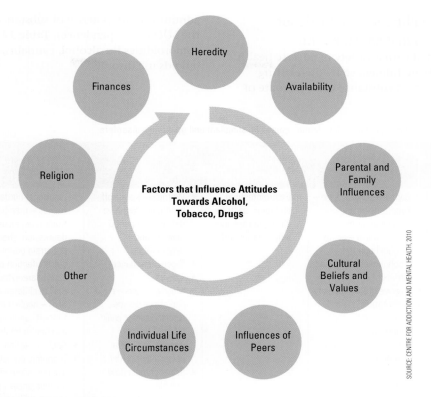

FIGURE 14.6

Factors that influence attitudes towards substances

Note: 'Other' factors would encompass specific individual factors as defined by individuals that do not fit into generalised themes.

TABLE 14.5

Clinical course for the development of alcohol, cannabis, stimulant and opioid use disorders

SUBSTANCE USE DISORDER	CLINICAL COURSE	OTHER CHARACTERISTICS
Alcohol use disorder (AUD)	Onset occurs in adolescents. 1st episode of intoxication occurs in mid-teens and may be accompanied by isolated alcohol-related problems. Late teens and early 20s progressing into early 30s increased problematic patterns of alcohol consumption and behaviour with increased occurrence of withdrawal. By age 40 diagnosis of AUD.	Over the course of AUD, consumers may experience periods of abstinence and relapse. After a period of abstinence, a relapse will often see a quick return to previous patterns of consumption and behaviour. AUD in older people is associated with increased risks due to changing neurobiology and co-occurrence of other health illnesses.
Cannabis use disorder (CUD)	Generally, onset is in late teens and early adulthood. Onset prior to 15 years is a predictor of onset of CUD and other substances use and mental health issues in adulthood. Pattern of use gradually increases in frequency and amount. Progression to using alone and through the day, interfering with functioning and social connectedness.	Onset of cannabis use is influenced by its medical use. Onset occurs more rapidly in adolescents with pervasive conduct disorders. Perceptions that cannabis use is less harmful than alcohol and tobacco likely contributes to increased use. Cannabis intoxication may be viewed as less disruptive, influencing use.
Stimulant use disorder (SUD)	Initiation of use influenced by desire to control weight, improve performance (school, work, sport). Onset of first regular use is between 23–31 years of age. Patterns of use are either episodic, binges or chronic use. Continued use is associated with tolerance.	Onset of first regular use for individuals in treatment is 23–31 years. SUD rate of progression is influenced by method of administration (intravenous (IV) and smoking).
Opioid use disorder (OUD)	Onset of use at any age. Onset of problematic use is first observed in late teens or early 20s. Once OUD is established, it continues for many years. Remission of symptoms may occur after age of 40 'maturing out'.	OUD is associated with a high mortality rate that impacts on prevalence rates.

SOURCE: CENTRE FOR ADDICTION AND MENTAL HEALTH, 2010

SOURCE: APA, 2013, PP. 493–565

Comorbidity: implications of SUDs for physical, mental and social health

SUDs are associated with a variety of adverse health conditions which are influenced by pre-existing conditions, the type of substance used, its route of administration, potency of substance and severity of the SUD (i.e. dependence). **Table 14.6** list common comorbidities for alcohol, cannabis, stimulants and opioids use disorders.

TABLE 14.6
Common comorbidities and complications for alcohol, cannabis, stimulant and opioid use disorders

SUBSTANCE	PHYSIOLOGICAL	ASSOCIATED WITH ROUTE OF ADMINISTRATION	MENTAL HEALTH	SOCIAL (NOTE: COMPLICATIONS CAN BE APPLIED TO ALL SUBSTANCES)
Alcohol	• Cardiovascular disease – hypertension and cardiomyopathy • Liver disease – acute alcohol hepatitis, alcoholic fatty liver and cirrhosis • Overweight and obesity • Pancreatitis • Bone marrow suppression • Peripheral neuropathy • Chronic infectious diseases – pneumonia and cancer – mouth, oesophagus, throat, liver, breast • Wernicke's encephalopathy	• Gastrointestinal problems, gastritis, ulcers, oesophageal inflammation, reflux	• Wernicke–Korsakoff syndrome, cognitive deficits – impaired memory and degeneration • Sleep disturbance • Trauma • Mood disorders – major depressive disorder, bipolar disorder, panic disorder, anxiety disorder, anti-social personality disorder • Schizophrenia (low prevalence) • Suicide and violence	• Emotional burden on career/families/friends – members may feel anger, frustration, anxiety, fear, worry, depression, shame and guilt that put strain on relationships (distress, dissatisfaction and instability) and cause career/family/friend burnout • Risk to children of parents affected by SUD – neglect and abuse that may lead to short- and long-term psychological and health implications • Social isolation • Economic burden related to substance use behaviour either by money spent on substances or impact of substance use on ability to work and maintain employment. This applies to both the consumer experiencing the SUD and the family who are endeavouring to support the consumer • Unemployment • Dependence on welfare • Housing instability • Homelessness • Criminal activity and violence • Domestic and family violence • Incarceration • Transmission of HIV due to IV drug use or high-risk sexual activity • The impact of acute and chronic substance use behaviour and health implications for substance use on communities and society as a whole; e.g. public safety and community spaces, crime, impact on health services, public welfare and road safety, community and workplace accidents
Cannabis	• Cardiovascular, immunity, neuromuscular, ocular, reproductive and respiratory, and cognitive and appetite problems • Chronic respiratory symptoms and lung cancer	• Smoking – respiratory complications including infections, cough, shortness of breath and wheezing	• Exacerbation of symptoms of pre-existing mental health issues, other SUDs, depression, anxiety disorder, bipolar disorder, obsessive compulsive disorder, conduct disorder, antisocial personality disorder, paranoid and personality disorder, attention-deficit/hyperactivity disorder, psychosis and suicide	

SUBSTANCE	PHYSIOLOGICAL	ASSOCIATED WITH ROUTE OF ADMINISTRATION	MENTAL HEALTH	SOCIAL (NOTE: COMPLICATIONS CAN BE APPLIED TO ALL SUBSTANCES)
Stimulants: amphetamine/ methamphetamines	• Cardiopulmonary problems – cardiotoxicity, medical complications caused by agents used to 'cut' the stimulant • Respiratory problems • Liver and kidney failure • Oral health problems – tooth decay	• Smoking – as above • Snorting – irritation to nasal mucosa, chronic rhinitis and nasal septum damage • IV use; blood-borne viruses (BBVs) and bacterial infections	• Other SUDs, anger, anxiety/panic, post-traumatic stress disorder, antisocial personality disorder, attention deficit/ hyperactivity disorder, gambling disorders, psychosis, violence	
Opioid	• Nausea • Constipation • Amenorrhea • Low bone density • Loss of libido • Cardiovascular and respiratory problems	• IV use – blood-borne viruses (BBVs), sclerosed veins, 'track marks' • Tuberculosis related to impaired immunity • Cellulitis related to skin popping • Bacterial infections – endocarditis, pneumonia, osteomyelitis, septic arthritis • Snorting – irritation to nasal mucosa and nasal septum damage	• Other SUDs • Depression (induced or exacerbated) • Antisocial personality disorder • History of conduct disorder • Post-traumatic stress disorder • Suicide (intentional and accidental)	

SOURCE: APA, 2013, PP. 492–567; CAMPBELL, 2001; KELLY & DALEY, 2013; PACE & SAMET, 2016, PP. 7–8

Physical complications

As highlighted in **Table 14.6**, chronic use of a substance, over the short and long term, can lead to various physical complications, due to the toxic effect on the human body and its systems. The following conditions may be encountered by mental health nurses in clinical practice and are, therefore, explored in more detail.

Wernicke's encephalopathy – Korsakoff syndrome

Wernicke's encephalopathy is an acute presentation, caused by an extreme deficiency in thiamine, or vitamin B1 (found in many foods including yeast, cereal grains, beans, nuts and meat), which is a nutrient essential for the functioning of the central nervous system. Depleted by excessive and prolonged alcohol misuse, it results in necrotic lesions on areas of the brain stem, and can be life-threatening, and only one symptom is required for diagnosis. Symptoms are:

■ confusional state
■ ocular disturbance – **horizontal nystagmus**
■ ataxia – wide-based, reeling steps.

This condition is reversible with the administration of intramuscular thiamine, with recovery being rapid.

Korsakoff psychosis, also caused by thiamine deficiency, is a chronic condition that can be characterised as a form of acquired brain injury and can require constant and prolonged care. It manifests with:

■ memory loss (**anterograde** and **retrograde**)
■ confusion

■ confabulation
■ normal intelligence quotient
■ Wernicke's symptoms.

Usually, this disorder cannot be completely reversed, with only 25% of patients making a full recovery, 25% of presentations being irreversible and others sitting on a spectrum of severity. The cessation of alcohol consumption will halt cognitive decline, but not reverse it (Lopatko et al., 2009; NCETA, 2004).

Delirium tremens (DTs)

The DTs are a severe form of alcohol withdrawal in a heavy user, characterised by a rapid onset confusional state, and are a medical emergency. Usually occurring within 1–5 days after cessation of alcohol (Manning et al., 2018), symptoms include:

■ disorientation
■ global confusion
■ agitation
■ auditory/tactile/visual hallucinations
■ paranoia
■ fluctuating blood pressure
■ sweating and nightmares.

Risk factors predisposing a person to develop this syndrome include:

■ history of withdrawal seizures and DTs
■ previous detoxification
■ concurrent illness and medical comorbidities
■ heavy and prolonged alcohol consumption; daily

- greater number of days since last drink
- intense cravings for alcohol
- severe withdrawal symptoms
- older age
- hypokalaemia and thrombocytopaenia
- presence of structural brain lesions (Burns, Lekawa & Price, 2018).

Treatment involves managing agitation, and preventing seizures and death. The use of benzodiazepines is a key medical component of managing DTs. Supportive interventions include monitoring vital signs, uses of an Alcohol Withdrawal Scale screen for withdrawal symptoms, managing sweating, tremors and anxiety, and reorienting the person to maintaining hydration (Manning et al., 2018; Schuckit, 2014).

High-risk complications for opioids

Intoxication and withdrawal syndromes from opioids are rarely life-threatening and risks tend to extend from means of use; for example, injecting practices or overdose.

Risks from injecting include:

- trauma to injection sites; scarring, thrombosis, thrombophlebitis, cellulitis
- bacterial and fungal infections
- septicaemia
- infective endocarditis
- osteomyelitis
- renal complications
- blood-borne infections, such as HIV, hepatitis B, hepatitis C.

Injecting opioids maximises their effects, and is the most dangerous route; taken orally, there are limited risks of adverse health effects, in appropriate dosages. Use, however, can lead to:

- suppression of the immune system
- change in hormone levels
- constipation
- malnutrition
- tooth decay
- menstrual problems
- decreased libido.

Many of these factors can also be exacerbated by the lifestyle accompanying drug use, such as poor dietary intake and self-neglect.

Opioid-related deaths result from a cessation of breathing. The drug causes CNS depression, affecting the part of the brain that regulates respiration. When too high a dose is taken, breathing slows and can stop, especially when combined with other drugs, such as benzodiazepines and alcohol.

Signs of overdose are:

- blue fingernails and lips (**cyanosis**)
- vomiting
- pinprick pupils
- slow respiration
- loss of consciousness
- pale colour and limp body.

In the clinical setting, naloxone is administered to prevent this leading to death (WHO, 2018).

High-risk complications for stimulants

The administration routes for stimulants – smoking and intravenous – tend to have similar risks as opioids.

Risks during intoxication can include tachycardia, dehydration, hyperthermia, seizures, stroke, cardiovascular events and death, with psychostimulant toxicity associated with myocardial infarction, ischaemia, arrhythmias and cerebral infarctions. Repeated use of methamphetamines leads to cumulative cardiac and coronary artery disease (Healey, 2016). Associated behaviours, such as fighting, driving, unsafe sex and risk taking, add additional elements to this risk profile (Healey, 2016; NCETA, 2004).

The potential risk of mental state deterioration, secondary to acute intoxication, and sleep deprivation are considerations. Onset of psychotic symptoms, including hallucinations and delusions, may be experienced.

Methamphetamine toxicity can occur at any stage (first, social or chronic use) and irrespective of dose, frequency or method of administration. Toxicity is associated with symptoms such as nausea and vomiting, chest pain, tremors, increased temperature and heart rate, breathing irregularities and seizure (Healey, 2016).

During the withdrawal phase, often called 'the crash', monitoring of physical and psychological health is crucial, with acute risks dissipating and psychosocial interventions becoming more appropriate.

Substance use and violence

Substance use can be linked to instances of violence across the spectrum of society, making it a significant public health issue. The presence of substance use increases the chances of being a victim or perpetrator, states that can, themselves, compound an SUD, leading to increased usage. In real terms, interpersonal violence can be categorised as youth violence, child maltreatment, intimate partner violence, elder abuse and sexual violence (Centre for Public Health, 2009).

In terms of severity, alcohol and methamphetamines are more likely to be associated with violent behaviour. Alcohol is by far the most prolific substance used in Australia, with an estimated 10 million people affected by another person's drinking. The negative effects vary in risk from annoyance and property damage to abuse, neglect, physical violence and death (Ritter, King & Hamilton, 2013). People who use methamphetamines (ice) are six times more likely to display interpersonal violence when using, as opposed to not using, ranging from altercations that lead to fights and seemingly unprovoked physical attacks. This can be influenced by the associated drug-using lifestyle and criminal behaviour (McKetin et al., 2014, in Healey, 2016). Use of ice is linked to increased risk taking behaviours, road deaths, crime, and assaults against frontline health workers, law enforcement and the public (Healey, 2016).

Substance use disorder and dual diagnosis

The presence of an SUD and co-occurring mental health condition is referred to as dual diagnosis. It is estimated that up to 50% of people experiencing a severe mental health condition will have a co-occurring SUD at some stage in their lifetime and approximately 35% of those experiencing an SUD will also experience a mental health condition (Andrews et al., 2013; Hunt et al., 2013).

The relationship between SUDs and mental health conditions is often complex, mutually influencing and, therefore, can be challenging to assess and treat. The co-occurrence of an SUD and mental health disorder can be 'through direct causal hypothesis or indirect causal relationship' (Marel et al., 2016, p. 7) and other common factors. The direct causal hypothesis suggests two pathways: first, that the mental health condition can be a consequence of substance use. For example, intoxication or withdrawal from a substance can induce a mental health disorder – alcohol withdrawal or intoxication can induce depression or anxiety, and intoxication from amphetamines and cannabis can induce psychotic symptoms. In the majority of cases, these presentations will subside in the absence of the substance, but for some people the mental health disorder continues for weeks, months and even years after the cessation of the substance. Second, a mental health condition can increase the vulnerability of developing an SUD; for example, the repeated use of alcohol to self-medicate symptoms of depression and anxiety. In this instance, both conditions tend to influence each other in their development and their severity (Marel et al., 2016). The indirect causal relationship suggests that one condition can have an effect upon an intermediary factor that leads to the onset of a secondary condition. This process is illustrated in **Figure 14.7**.

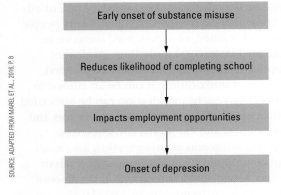

SOURCE: ADAPTED FROM MAREL ET AL., 2016, P. 8

FIGURE 14.7
Indirect causal relationship between an SUD and mental health condition

Other common factors relate to the risk factors that predispose an increased vulnerability for the onset of either an SUD or mental health disorder, such as biological, psychological, social and environmental factors (Marel et al., 2016). Regardless of the reason for the occurrence of a dual diagnosis, people experiencing dual diagnosis often experience 'greater negativity and have poorer health outcomes related to associated higher risk factors such as relapse, violence, homelessness, criminality and hospitalization' (Andrews et al., 2013, p. 290).

Substance use and suicide

There is a correlation between substance use and an increased rate of death by suicide with the risk further increasing in the presence of a mental health condition; for example, depression, post-traumatic stress disorder and bipolar disorder (Poorolajal, Haghtalab, Farhadi & Darvishi, 2016). A greater lifetime risk of death from suicide is associated with substance use than a mental health condition on its own. Substance use is a significant risk factor when assessing risk of suicide, and when combined with distress, anger and comorbid mental health conditions it contributes to increased impulsivity, potential to increase lethality of the suicide attempt, risk of accidental death, and unintentional suicide related to overdose. A previous history of suicide attempts is a risk factor and is an important component of any good risk assessment, especially when substance use is an issue. Of all deaths from suicide, 22% can be attributed to alcohol use. This statistic is higher in Indigenous Australian communities where alcohol is associated with 40% of male deaths from suicide and 30% of female deaths from suicide (Wilson, Stearn, Gray & Saggers, 2010). Opioid use is associated with accidental overdose and deliberate overdose, and risk increases especially when combined with other CNS depressants (e.g. alcohol).

Implications of substance use/misuse during pregnancy

Substances are known to impact the woman and the developing foetus during the perinatal period. Substance use, misuse or experiencing an SUD while pregnant has health implications for the developing foetus, birth complications, and increases risk of dependence and withdrawal in the newborn. SUDs are also associated with increased risk of poor prenatal and postnatal outcomes and care. Factors such as side effects of a substance – for example, nutritional deficits, mental health issues, social problems and economic disadvantage, lifestyle risks and effects – that impact on the woman will also have an impact on maternal and child bonding and infant and child outcomes (Gordon, Conley & Gordon, 2015). **Table 14.7** outlines the impacts of a range of substances on the woman and developing foetus/newborn/child during the perinatal period.

TABLE 14.7
Effects of substances during the perinatal period

SUBSTANCE	EFFECTS
Alcohol	There is no known safe level of alcohol consumption during pregnancy. The NHMRC recommendation for alcohol consumption while planning pregnancy, during pregnancy and breastfeeding is abstinence. Risks associated with alcohol consumption while pregnant include **foetal alcohol spectrum disorder (FASD)**, including **foetal alcohol syndrome (FAS)**, miscarriage, foetal growth problems, low birth weight, congenital abnormalities and abnormal infant neuro-behaviour. There is also evidence of long-term effects on growth, behaviour, cognition, language and achievement.
Methamphetamines	The use of methamphetamines during pregnancy has health implications for the mother and baby that cause both primary and secondary complications. These include gestational hypertension, pre-eclampsia, intrauterine foetal death, intrauterine growth restrictions, placental abruption, risk of preterm birth, neonatal death and infant death. Secondary to the direct effects of the methamphetamine use are those of prenatal nutritional deficits and mental health issues such as depression, anxiety and psychosis that impact on pregnancy health and outcomes.
Cannabis	There is increased risk of low birth weight, foetal growth restrictions, earlier gestational age, abnormal brain development and effects on nervous system function as evidenced by exaggerated startle response and poor habituation to stimuli, and altered sleep patterns in infants. Additionally, impacts on short-term and verbal reasoning at 3–4 years of age is affected by cannabis use during the first and/or second trimester and possibly deficits in higher cognitive function processors – executive functioning – in 9–12 year olds.
Opioids	Research indicates that with the increase in use and misuse of prescription opioids such as hydrocodone, codeine and oxycodone, 65% of infants with neonatal abstinence syndrome (NAS) were exposed to legally obtained opioids during pregnancy. Infants born with NAS were also more likely to experience birth complications such as preterm birth, low birth weight, meconium aspiration syndrome and respiratory distress, feeding difficulties and jaundice.

SOURCE: BEHNKE & SMITH, 2013; GORDON, CONLEY & GORDON, 2015; GORMA ET AL., 2014; PATRICK ET AL., 2015; WU, JEW & LU, 2011

DIAGNOSTIC CRITERIA

An SUD encompasses a range of substance use behaviours including harmful and hazardous use, addiction and dependence. The DSM-5 diagnosis of an SUD is based on a pathological pattern of behaviours related to the continued use and impaired control of the substance despite significant health consequences (APA, 2013).

Substance use disorder diagnostic criteria

The diagnostic criteria for SUD are applicable to all classes of substances identified in the DSM-5: alcohol, caffeine, cannabis, hallucinogens, inhalants, opioids, sedatives, hypnotics, anxiolytics, stimulants, tobacco and other substances. SUDs are classified according to a broad scale of severity; mild (two to three criteria), moderate (four to five criteria) and severe (six or more criteria) (APA, 2013). The level of severity a consumer is assessed as experiencing will relate to the number of diagnostic criteria they meet.

The DSM-5 states that all substance use disorders are based on a 'pathological patterns of behaviours related to use of the substance' (APA, 2013, p. 483). Diagnosis is facilitated by categorising these behaviours into four broad categories, which are impaired control over substance use; social impairment; risk use of the substance and pharmacological criteria (APA, 2013, p. 483). **Table 14.8** presents an example of this using 'Alcohol Use Disorder'.

The presence of tolerance and withdrawal are not required for a diagnosis of SUD; however, the presence or experience of tolerance and/or withdrawal is indicative of the severity of the substance use (APA, 2013). We now look at the manner in which substance use can progressively manifest into an SUD. Using these groupings as a framework, it is possible to identify the following behaviours that should be monitored for in clinical practice. **Table 14.9** outlines these behaviours.

Substance intoxication and withdrawal

Nurses may find themselves working with a consumer who is experiencing intoxication or withdrawal symptoms in any setting, be it on the general medical ward, in the emergency department or in a mental health unit. Assessment and implementing interventions for intoxication can be complex and challenging, as people can present differently despite having consumed the same substance and quantities. The DSM-5 outlines criteria for intoxication and withdrawal across a range of substances such as alcohol, cannabis and opiates, reviewed below, with a specific emphasis on alcohol and stimulants in this chapter.

Defining intoxication

Becoming intoxicated through the consumption of a substance such as alcohol has a number of potentially serious consequences for the individual. Many people have been intoxicated, or experienced someone in an intoxicated state, commonly through alcohol consumption. Depending on the person involved, and the level of intoxication, it can be an enjoyable experience. Conversely, intoxication can be associated with a host of risk-taking behaviours and factors and negative physical and emotional consequences.

Presenting symptoms of **intoxication** are caused by recent consumption, resulting in specific levels in the person's system, and it is reversible in the absence of further intake. Any syndrome associated with substance use will cause effects on the CNS, resulting in identifiable behavioural, psychological and physiological characteristics (Allen, 1996), as discussed previously.

DIAGNOSTIC CRITERIA

Characteristics and behavior for SUD

TABLE 14.8
Diagnostic criteria, alcohol use disorder

Alcohol use disorder

A problematic pattern of alcohol use leading to clinically significant impairment or distress, as manifested by at least two of the following, occurring within a 12-month period:

1. Alcohol is often taken in larger amounts or over a longer period than was intended.
2. There is a persistent desire or unsuccessful efforts to cut down or control alcohol use.
3. A great deal of time is spent in activities necessary to obtain alcohol, use alcohol, or recover from its effects.
4. Craving, or a strong desire or urge to use alcohol.
5. Recurrent alcohol use resulting in a failure to fulfill major role obligations at work, school, or home.
6. Continued alcohol use despite having persistent or recurrent social or interpersonal problems caused or exacerbated by the effects of alcohol.
7. Important social, occupational, or recreational activities are given up or reduced because of alcohol use.
8. Recurrent alcohol use in situations in which it is physically hazardous.
9. Alcohol use is continued despite knowledge of having a persistent or recurrent physical or psychological problem that is likely to have been caused or exacerbated by alcohol.
10. Tolerance, as defined by either of the following:
    a. A need for markedly increased amounts of alcohol to achieve intoxication or desired effect.
    b. A markedly diminished effect with continued use of the same amount of alcohol.
11. Withdrawal, as manifested by either of the following:
    a. The characteristic withdrawal syndrome for alcohol (refer to Criteria A and B of the criteria set for alcohol withdrawal, pp. 499-500).
    b. Alcohol (or a closely related substance, such as a benzodiazepine) is taken to relieve or avoid withdrawal symptoms.

Specify if:

In **early remission**: After full criteria for alcohol use disorder were previously met, none of the criteria for alcohol use disorder have been met for at least 3 months but for less than 12 months (with the exception that Criterion A4, "Craving, or a strong desire or urge to use alcohol," may be met).

In **sustained remission**: After full criteria for alcohol use disorder were previously met, none of the criteria for alcohol use disorder have been met at any time during a period of 12 months or longer (with the exception that Criterion A4, "Craving, or a strong desire or urge to use alcohol," may be met).

Specify if:

In a controlled environment: This additional specifier is used if the individual is in an environment where access to alcohol is restricted.

TABLE 14.9
Diagnostic clusters related to SUD and behaviour to monitor for

---

Impaired control over substance use (Criteria 1-4)

- Patterns of use, financial outlay for substance.
- Changes in pattern of use, triggers for use.
- Changes to daily/weekly routines, increased preoccupation with obtaining substance and using, physical illness associated with recovery and changes in patterns of use associated with relieving physical symptoms.
- Development of associations between situation, environment or emotions that trigger urge for substance.

Social impairment (Criteria 5-7)

- Repeated absences from work or poor work performance related to substance use, substance-related absences, suspensions or expulsions.
- Arguments with spouse/partner/family/friends about consequences of intoxication. Domestic violence.
- Changes in patterns of activities, changes in motivation and pleasure associated with activities.
- Collateral feedback from family/friends, motivation and pleasure associated with activities, changes in patterns of social activity and connections, social withdrawal and isolation.

Risky use of the substance (Criteria 8-9)

- Driving, operating machinery or engaging in some sporting activities when impaired by substance use.
- Deterioration in physical health and/or poor recovery from physical illness, deterioration in mental state and onset of comorbidities.

Pharmacological criteria (Criteria 10 and-11)

- Changes in pattern of use, increased money spent on substances, decreased pleasure from substance use.
- Physiological symptoms of withdrawal, changes in pattern of use; e.g. early morning drinking to alleviate onset of tremors.

Meeting the criteria for intoxication

To be considered intoxicated, the individual must be subject to the following diagnostic criteria, as described by the DSM-5:

- recent consumption of the substance; for example, by smoking, injecting or ingestion
- the manifestation of significant behavioural and psychological changes, usually problematic, and that develop following or during consumption

- the symptoms cannot be attributed to another causal agent, be it a medical condition or mental health disorder. The visible features will also have specific differences among the groups of intoxicants, thereby differentiating that presentation.

Table 14.10 presents the diagnostic criteria signs and symptoms for alcohol, cannabis, opioid and stimulant intoxication.

DIAGNOSTIC CRITERIA

Signs and symptoms of intoxication

TABLE 14.10
Diagnostic criteria signs and symptoms of intoxication

Alcohol Intoxication
A. Recent ingestion of alcohol.
B. Clinically significant problematic behavioral or psychological changes (e.g., inappropriate sexual or aggressive behavior, mood lability, impaired judgment) that developed during, or shortly after, alcohol ingestion.
C. One (or more) of the following signs or symptoms developing during, or shortly after, alcohol use: 　**1.** Slurred speech. 　**2.** Incoordination. 　**3.** Unsteady gait. 　**4.** Nystagmus. 　**5.** Impairment in attention or memory. 　**6.** Stupor or coma.
D. The signs or symptoms are not attributable to another medical condition and are not better explained by another mental disorder, including intoxication with another substance.
Cannabis intoxication
A. Recent use of cannabis.
B. Clinically significant problematic behavioral or psychological changes (e.g., impaired motor coordination, euphoria, anxiety, sensation of slowed time, impaired judgment, social withdrawal) that developed during, or shortly after, cannabis use.
C. Two (or more) of the following signs or symptoms developing within 2 hours of cannabis use: 　**1.** Conjunctival injection. 　**2.** Increased appetite. 　**3.** Dry mouth. 　**4.** Tachycardia.
D. The signs or symptoms are not attributable to another medical condition and are not better explained by another mental disorder, including intoxication with another substance. *Specify* if: **With perceptual disturbances:** Hallucinations with intact reality testing or auditory, visual, or tactile illusions occur in the absence of a delirium.
Opioid intoxication
A. Recent use of an opioid.
B. Clinically significant problematic behavioral or psychological changes (e.g., initial euphoria followed by apathy, dysphoria, psychomotor agitation or retardation, impaired judgment) that developed during, or shortly after, opioid use.
C. Pupillary constriction (or pupillary dilation due to anoxia from severe overdose) and one (or more) of the following signs or symptoms developing during, or shortly after, opioid use: 　**1.** Drowsiness or coma. 　**2.** Slurred speech. 　**3.** Impairment in attention or memory.
D. The signs or symptoms are not attributable to another medical condition and are not better explained by another mental disorder, including intoxication with another substance.

TABLE 14.10
(Continued)

Specify if:
With perceptual disturbances: This specifier may be noted in the rare instance in which hallucinations with intact reality testing or auditory, visual, or tactile illusions occur in the absence of a delirium.

Stimulant intoxication

A. Recent use of an amphetamine-type substance, cocaine, or other stimulant.

B. Clinically significant problematic behavioral or psychological changes (e.g., euphoria or affective blunting; changes in sociability; hypervigilance; interpersonal sensitivity; anxiety, tension, or anger; stereotyped behaviors; impaired judgment) that developed during, or shortly after, use of a stimulant.

C. Two (or more) of the following signs or symptoms, developing during, or shortly after, stimulant use:
   1. Tachycardia or bradycardia.
   2. Pupillary dilation.
   3. Elevated or lowered blood pressure.
   4. Perspiration or chills.
   5. Nausea or vomiting.
   6. Evidence of weight loss.
   7. Psychomotor agitation or retardation.
   8. Muscular weakness, respiratory depression, chest pain, or cardiac arrhythmias.
   9. Confusion, seizures, dyskinesias, dystonias, or coma.

D. The signs or symptoms are not attributable to another medical condition and are not better explained by another mental disorder, including intoxication with another substance.

Specify **the specific intoxicant** (i.e., amphetamine-type substance, cocaine, or other stimulant).

Specify if:

With perceptual disturbances: This specifier may be noted when hallucinations with intact reality testing or auditory, visual, or tactile illusions occur in the absence of a delirium.

Clinical presentation for alcohol intoxication

We now look at alcohol intoxication in more detail. Assessment of intoxication is a multidisciplinary team responsibility. For example, a medical officer should assess the consumer and take a comprehensive history, considering such aspects as differential diagnoses such as the presence of a head injury or infection that may explain the consumer's current behaviour and comprehension. Gathering collateral information from family members and friends, and previous records, can be crucial, along with previous contact with the individual. When interacting with a consumer who is intoxicated, it is essential to set aside presumptions and prejudices that may prevent further exploration of other potential causes. It is also crucial to assess the safety of the consumer and others in the clinical environment.

In addition to meeting the diagnostic criteria for indication as stated in **Table 14.10**, a consumer experiencing alcohol intoxication can also experience blackouts, where they are unable to consciously recall events despite being active. Blackouts are more likely to occur during rapid alcohol consumption, causing the blood alcohol level (BAL) to spike. Regular blackouts can lead to long-term cognitive deficits and contribute to degenerative brain disease. While experiencing a blackout, a person is more likely to participate in risk-taking behaviours, such as overspending, fighting, vandalism, casual and unprotected sex (Malone & Friedman, 2005).

Assessing level of alcohol intoxication

While it is important to ask a consumer how much alcohol they have consumed and when they last had any alcohol, establishing a person's **blood alcohol concentration (BAC)** or **level (BAL)** is always completed, as it provides an accurate measure of the alcohol concentration in a person's blood.

A BAL/BAC can be taken via a blood test or breath analysis; in the ward environment, the latter is preferred and is obtained through use of a blood alcohol monitor, a process by which the consumer provides a steady stream of breath into the device and a reading is calculated. It is not 100% accurate, but is adequate for the purposes of commencing treatment in a clinical setting.

Severe alcohol intoxication can be life-threatening and develops into toxicity; therefore, establishing the quantity of alcohol taken needs to be prompt.

With alcohol, other clinical points to consider are:
- time of last drink – if recently consumed, BAC may have increased, or withdrawal is beginning if significant time has passed

- period of consumption; for example, rapid binge drinking will affect intoxication
- quantity of alcohol consumed.

A BAL can increase over time, despite consumption having ceased, and regular checks are prudent following the initial screening. **Table 14.11**

identifies the clinical presentation of blood alcohol concentration and the effects on the non-dependent individual. **Table 14.12** outlines some common issues that present with intoxicated individuals within the mental health setting.

TABLE 14.11

Blood alcohol concentrations and effects on the non-dependent individual

BAC MG ALCOHOL/100 ML BLOOD%	SIGNS AND SYMPTOMS
20–30 mg/0.02–0.03%	Slight increases in talkativeness; relaxation.
50 mg/0.05%	Impairment in some tasks requiring skill.
60–100 mg/0.06–0.1%	Very talkative; speech is louder, acts and feels self-confident. Less cautious and inhibited than usual. Slowed reaction time.
200 mg/0.2%	Sedated rather than active, may be sleepy. Impairment now includes slurred speech, clumsiness, reduced responsiveness and marked intellectual impairment. Amnesia.
300–400 mg/0.30–0.40	Semiconscious or unconscious. Body functions are beginning to break down. Fatalities occur at and above these concentrations.

SOURCE: ADAPTED FROM MALONE & FRIEDMAN, 2005

TABLE 14.12

Common issues for individuals intoxicated in the mental health unit

POTENTIAL HEALTH RISK	NURSING INTERVENTION
Anxiety, agitation	Treat the person with respect and dignity. Approach the consumer calmly during all interactions. Provide reassurance and explain everything clearly. Speak slowly, simply and quietly, while avoiding being patronising and prescriptive. Minimise the number of people present to appear non-threatening. Provide a low stimulus environment.
Aggression	As above and in addition: • depending on the environment, manage the space to maintain self-protection • remain calm, checking your own body language, tone of voice, eye-contact • use the consumer's name, speak directly to them • acknowledge their feelings and levels of distress • be flexible in servicing their needs, while maintaining boundaries in terms of demands to protect the consumer, staff and other consumers • offer time out, reassuring them that you will return later, giving them time to calm down.
Physical complications	Take vital signs (blood pressure, temperature, pulse, oxygen saturation, respirations); repeat regularly. Ascertain blood alcohol concentration. Document and report to medical officer. Vomiting can occur when conscious, semi-conscious or unconscious, with inherent risks. If the consumer is unconscious, ensure they are laid in an appropriate position; should vomiting occur, this will limit the possibility of aspiration, the consequences of which can be severe and lead to death. Administer anti-emetic drugs, if appropriate, such as metoclopramide, prochlorperazine or domperidone.
Seizure	Likely to occur when BAC is dropping, risk increased if a person has a history of seizure during withdrawal, epilepsy, antipsychotic use. Maintain four-hourly observations. Administer benzodiazepines, as prescribed by a doctor when signs of withdrawal begin to appear or BAC drops to acceptable levels.
Coma	Maintain airway. If airway severely compromised, convey to an acute care facility (E.D.) for intensive treatment, as this is unlikely to be available on a mental health unit. Also, this is suitable when it is unclear as to the quantities consumed by the consumer.
Ataxia/gait	The consumer's ability to mobilise can be compromised, leading to falls and injury due to collision. It is important, therefore, to manage the environment where possible: • Remove dangerous objects from a consumer's room • Encourage rest and to remain in bed • Ensure access to call bell • Conduct regular visual checks.

CLINICAL **OBSERVATIONS**

Nursing interventions for the consumer experiencing intoxication

In addition to managing potential risks as described in **Table 14.12**, consumers require supportive interventions if they are experiencing the effects of intoxication. These interventions include:

- encouraging fluids, nutrition and rest;
- monitoring vital signs, and neurological assessment for level of consciousness;
- Record, document and report all observations as required by facility policies and processes.

Continue to assess the consumer's condition and provide supportive nursing care and manage the consumer's condition until stable and the effects of the acute stage of intoxication are mitigated.

SAFETY FIRST

PROVIDING EMERGENCY CARE FOR PEOPLE EXPERIENCING METHAMPHETAMINE INTOXICATION

Ice users usually present to emergency departments due to the nature of the psychological and physiological harms caused by intoxication; however, this can present safety concerns for health professionals. People experiencing ice intoxication may present with challenging behaviours such as aggression, lack of ability to be rational (secondary to experiencing psychotic features such as delusions and perceptual disturbances), and impaired insight and poor judgement that compromise safety for themselves and health professionals. Strategies need to be in place to support health professionals to feel safe and provide quality care in the least restrictive way that maintains the consumer's dignity. These strategies include:

- staff expertise in knowledge and experience working with people experiencing problematic ice misuse and disorder;
- the ability to recognise the potential for acute escalation;
- the need for additional resources such as security and police;
- the ability to maintain a calm and cautious demeanour;
- consideration of the context of practice when planning and taking action; that is, ward, ED or on the road;
- assessment and safety of others;
- identifying the stress and agitation that may occur in the people who accompany the ice-intoxicated person (Usher et al., 2017).

Defining withdrawal

The term **withdrawal** has several meanings. The *Oxford Dictionary* defines it as 'the unpleasant physical reaction that accompanies the process of ceasing to take an addictive drug' (Oxford Dictionaries Online, 2016). The WHO (2016a, 2016b) adds that the syndrome may also be accompanied by psychological disturbance and is an indicator of a more severe SUD/dependency.

Many people may have experienced withdrawal in one form or another, be it from alcohol (tremors and anxiety following a binge session), perhaps caffeine or sugar, or illegal or prescription drugs and medications. Withdrawal is the body's natural response to removal of a substance when it has developed a physical or emotional dependence over time. Psychological withdrawal can last much longer, and require more stringent intervention, than a physical dependence.

To be considered in withdrawal, the individual must meet the following diagnostic criteria, as asserted by the DSM-5.

1 The causal agent, following heavy and prolonged use, has been removed or reduced.
2 Clinically significant signs and symptoms, as a result, cause distress or impairment in social, occupational and other areas of functioning.
3 The consequent symptoms cannot be attributed to another causal agent, be it a medical condition or mental health disorder. The visible features will also have specific differences among the groups of intoxicants, thereby differentiating that presentation (APA, 2013).

It is important to accurately identify the presence of withdrawal symptoms and administer appropriate supportive care and interventions to manage their effects and prevent potentially life-threatening consequences.

Table 14.13 lists the diagnostic criteria for alcohol, cannabis, opioid and amphetamine withdrawal (APA, 2013).

Alcohol withdrawal and the alcohol withdrawal scale

Withdrawal occurs 6–48 hours after the last drink, and can persist for two to five days, depending on the severity of pre-admission consumption and historical pattern. Due to potential complications, such as grand mal seizures and delirium, pharmacological intervention is crucial to alleviate symptoms and prevent adverse events.

The Clinical Institute Withdrawal Assessment for Alcohol (CIWA or CIWA-Ar) consists of 10 items, each with a maximum score of 7, which is used for the assessment and management of withdrawal.

DIAGNOSTIC CRITERIA

Signs and symptoms of withdrawal

TABLE 14.13
Diagnostic criteria signs and symptoms of withdrawal

Alcohol withdrawal

A. Cessation of (or reduction in) alcohol use that has been heavy and prolonged.

B. Two (or more) of the following, developing within several hours to a few days after the cessation of (or reduction in) alcohol use described in Criterion A:
1. Autonomic hyperactivity (e.g., sweating or pulse rate greater than 100 bpm).
2. Increased hand tremor.
3. Insomnia.
4. Nausea or vomiting.
5. Transient visual, tactile, or auditory hallucinations or illusions.
6. Psychomotor agitation.
7. Anxiety.
8. Generalized tonic-clonic seizures.

C. The signs or symptoms in Criterion B cause clinically significant distress or impairment in social, occupational, or other important areas of functioning.

D. The signs or symptoms are not attributable to another medical condition and are not better explained by another mental disorder, including intoxication or withdrawal from another substance.

Specify if:

With perceptual disturbances: This specifier applies in the rare instance when hallucinations (usually visual or tactile) occur with intact reality testing, or auditory, visual, or tactile illusions occur in the absence of a delirium.

Cannabis withdrawal

A. Cessation of cannabis use that has been heavy and prolonged (i.e., usually daily or almost daily use over a period of at least a few months).

B. Three (or more) of the following signs and symptoms develop within approximately 1 week after Criterion A:
1. Irritability, anger, or aggression.
2. Nervousness or anxiety.
3. Sleep difficulty (e.g., insomnia, disturbing dreams).
4. Decreased appetite or weight loss.
5. Restlessness.
6. Depressed mood.
7. At least one of the following physical symptoms causing significant discomfort: abdominal pain, shakiness/tremors, sweating, fever, chills, or headache.

C. The signs or symptoms in Criterion B cause clinically significant distress or impairment in social, occupational, or other important areas of functioning.

D. The signs or symptoms are not attributable to another medical condition and are not better explained by another mental disorder, including intoxication or withdrawal from another substance.

Opioid withdrawal

A. Presence of either of the following:
1. Cessation of (or reduction in) opioid use that has been heavy and prolonged (i.e., several weeks or longer).
2. Administration of an opioid antagonist after a period of opioid use.

B. Three (or more) of the following developing within minutes to several days after Criterion A:
1. Dysphoric mood.
2. Nausea or vomiting.
3. Muscle aches.
4. Lacrimation or rhinorrhea.
5. Pupillary dilation, piloerection, or sweating.
6. Diarrhea.
7. Yawning.
8. Fever.
9. Insomnia.

TABLE 14.13
(Continued)

C.	The signs or symptoms in Criterion B cause clinically significant distress or impairment in social, occupational, or other important areas of functioning.
D.	The signs or symptoms are not attributable to another medical condition and are not better explained by another mental disorder, including intoxication or withdrawal from another substance.

Stimulant withdrawal

A.	Cessation of (or reduction in) prolonged amphetamine-type substance, cocaine, or other stimulant use.
B.	Dysphoric mood and two (or more) of the following physiological changes, developing within a few hours to several days after Criterion A: 1. Fatigue. 2. Vivid, unpleasant dreams. 3. Insomnia or hypersomnia. 4. Increased appetite. 5. Psychomotor retardation or agitation.
C.	The signs or symptoms in Criterion B cause clinically significant distress or impairment in social, occupational, or other important areas of functioning.
D.	The signs or symptoms are not attributable to another medical condition and are not better explained by another mental disorder, including intoxication or withdrawal from another substance. Specify the specific substance that causes the withdrawal syndrome (i.e., amphetamine-type substance, cocaine, or other stimulant).

Each item is scored, totalled and compared to the scale to establish severity. Additionally, physical observations are taken, which are directly affected by withdrawal.

The score informs the decision to administer benzodiazepines, and the appropriate dosage, alleviating withdrawal symptoms and decreasing the risk of seizure. Score ranges are: 15 or less – mild; 16 to 20 – moderate; greater than 20 – severe. There is a maximum score of 67.

Table 14.14 outlines the 10 items within an alcohol withdrawal scale that are assessed.

TABLE 14.14
Alcohol withdrawal symptoms and clinical signs

SYMPTOMS	CLINICAL QUESTIONS AND SIGNS
Nausea and vomiting	'Do you feel sick? Have you vomited?'
Tremor	Look for visual clues, ask to see the patient's extended arm/hands.
Paroxysmal sweats, perspiration	'Are you experiencing sweating?'
Anxiety	'Do you feel nervous?' Are there visual clues?
Agitation	Is the person restless, fidgety, pacing?
Tactile disturbances	'Have you any itching? Pins and needles? Numbness?'
Auditory disturbances	Sensitivity to sound? Hallucinations?
Visual disturbances	Sensitivity to light? Hallucinations?
Headache	'Does your head feel different?' 'Do you feel any dizziness?'
Orientation and clouding of senses	Presence of disorientation and confusion: time, place, person

SOURCE: MIRIJELLO ET AL., 2015

Clinical treatment for alcohol withdrawal

Based on current clinical guidelines (Manning et al., 2018), a consumer scoring below 10 is prescribed supportive nursing care; for a score over 10, diazepam – a long-acting benzodiazepine – is required for symptomatic relief. If the consumer has compromised liver function, a short-acting benzodiazepine (e.g. lorazepam) will prevent the build up of active metabolites (Manning et al., 2018). A tapering dose can be administered over a period of 2–6 days while the person detoxifies, and further doses administered in response to active symptoms, based on regular assessment by nursing staff and the treating medical officer (NSW Government, 2008).

With severe withdrawal, a loading dose regimen can be applied, where 20 mg doses of diazepam can be given every two to four hours, with pre-administration monitoring of the clinical condition undertaken, until the symptoms lessen (Manning et al., 2018; Sachdeva, Choudhary & Chandra, 2015). Managing dehydration is also essential, and the consumer will require monitoring of fluid intake and output through use of a fluid balance chart. In severe cases, intravenous fluid may be administered.

Further monitoring guidelines, and assessment questions, are outlined in **Table 14.14**.

Stimulant withdrawal

Methamphetamine withdrawal occurs in three stages: *the crash, acute* and *sub-acute phases*, with its severity dependent on pattern of use.

- *The crash* occurs between 1–3 days after use and is characterised by extreme fatigue and lethargy.
- *The acute* phase occurs between 7–10 days and includes depression, fatigue, vivid unpleasant

dreams, insomnia or hypersomnia, increased appetite, psychomotor retardation or agitation.

- *The sub-acute* stage follows a more extended period (Healey, 2016).

Focus of care should address re-establishing sleep, treating agitation, monitoring for psychological symptoms and promoting nutrition. Cognitive impairment can be significant in severe users.

BIOPSYCHOSOCIAL ASSESSMENT FRAMEWORK

Integration of mental health assessments and substance use assessments is necessary to ensure that the relationship between a mental health condition and substance use is identified early in treatment and a comprehensive integrated treatment plan reflects interventions addressing both conditions. Failure to address both conditions simultaneously could leave consumers vulnerable to substance use relapse and poor adherence to a mental health treatment plan (Marel et al., 2016; Munro & Edward, 2008).

Health implications and effects of SUDs are complex, multifaceted and intertwined, and it is the role of the clinician to facilitate the unravelling of this and identify risk and protective factors. Establishing a consumer's substance use, during a mental health assessment, requires the use of a biopsychosocial tool, ensuring that it is assessed within the context of their historical, social, religious and cultural practices, and not solely on substance use patterns. A nurse's role is to aid the consumer to tell their story, and through this process identify harmful, hazardous, addictive and dependent behaviours; thereby identifying whether their substance use is progressing to a chronic disease state, exists with a comorbid mental health condition (dual diagnosis) or other comorbid health conditions, and whether their presentation is associated with acute risks such as suicide, self-harm or harm to others.

Therapeutic engagement and assessment

The key to a rigorous and effective biopsychosocial assessment is positive therapeutic engagement, which is vital for engagement, assessment and collaboration with the consumer. SUD is a health issue, not a moral issue, and therefore it is essential that nurses adopt a non-judgemental approach, as they are assessing the pattern of substance use within the context of the patient's life and must not judge the behaviour. It is also essential to avoid labelling, as this creates and/or perpetuates stigma, as discussed earlier. Showing empathy and using sensitive questioning encourage the consumer to tell their story as they experience it and facilitate reflection. Understanding the neurobiological reward pathway involved in addiction, cravings, tolerance and withdrawal will help nurses to avoid the expectation that a person can 'just stop'. The nurse should work with the

individual at their pace and be flexible with goal setting. Maintaining a therapeutic connection with the consumer is essential to positive collaboration. Failure to work at the consumer's pace can make them feel unheard, not validated and set unrealistic expectations. This increases the risk of disengagement and poor adherence to the treatment plan. Employ a harm minimisation approach, as abstinence may not be the goal. Work with the consumer to identify realistic and attainable goals to minimise the harms associated with substance use.

Establishing trust with a consumer requires reflection on latent stigma about SUD, a shift in practice approach from 'doing' to 'facilitating' for the consumer, and having realistic expectations. A non-judgemental attitude will help in developing an understanding of the role of substance use in an individual's life. This process promotes a shared language and understanding of substance use behaviour, enhancing therapeutic engagement and adherence to treatment.

SAFETY FIRST

THERAPEUTIC ENGAGEMENT

It is essential that the nurse is aware of the level of appropriate therapeutic engagement during stages of intoxication or withdrawal. Substance use can often impair mental state and increase levels of risk to self and others. Nurses need to be mindful of the appropriate intervention to meet the level of risk. It would not be appropriate to engage a consumer in lengthy biopsychosocial assessments, harm minimisation or education when the consumer is aggressive, agitated, medically withdrawing or unable to engage due to altered level of consciousness. Interventions such as de-escalation, low stimulus environment, psychotropic administration, physiological observations and interventions are more appropriate at these stages.

Components of a biopsychosocial assessment

The identification and assessment of SUD require a set of robust screening and assessment tools. When used together, these facilitate a comprehensive holistic 'biopsychosocial' picture of a person's experience of SUD, identify risk and protective factors and identify comorbid physical or mental health conditions. The following sections identify the tools and components of robust assessment for comprehensive, strength-based and holistic integrated care planning.

Screening tools

As part of a biopsychosocial assessment framework, the CAGE-AID (**Table 14.15**) is a drug and alcohol screening tool that can be used in a variety of clinical settings to identify potential problematic substance use and suggest the need for a more comprehensive substance use assessment. Each letter in the acronym

CAGE (AID stands for 'adapted to include drugs') represents one of the four questions used in the screening tool, and a positive answer to any of the four questions indicates the need for a more comprehensive assessment.

TABLE 14.15
CAGE-AID questionnaire

CAGE-AID	QUESTIONS	ANSWER	
C	Cut down – have you ever felt that you ought to cut down on your drinking or drug use?	Yes	No
A	Annoyed – have people annoyed you by criticising your drinking or drug use?	Yes	No
G	Guilty – have you ever felt bad or guilty about your drinking or drug use?	Yes	No
E	Eye-opener – have you ever had a drink or used drugs first thing in the morning to steady your nerves or to get rid of a hangover?	Yes	No

A positive answer in the CAGE-AID questionnaire indicates a possible SUD and the need for further assessment using one of the following tools developed by the WHO:

- alcohol use disorders identification test (AUDIT; see http://auditscreen.org)
- drug use disorders identification test (DUDIT; see http://www.emcdda.europa.eu/attachements.cfm/att_10455_EN_DUDIT.pdf).

Alcohol, smoking, and substance involvement screening (ASSIST)

While screening tools provide important data in terms of working with the consumer to identify potential risk for problematic alcohol use, a comprehensive biopsychosocial assessment for SUD requires an understanding of the individual context of SUD. This understanding will facilitate formulation of person-centred care, identification of comorbidity and/or dual diagnosis and, above all, better health outcomes that may reduce **burden of disease**.

Assess the social and cultural context in which the individual lives

Often disclosure about substance use and substance use behaviour begins to occur during the assessment conversation. Encouraging a consumer to tell their story creates opportunities for clinicians to explore the consumer's world and understand what brings them to treatment. It also provides clinicians insight into a range of issues: identity, cultural identity, beliefs and practices, family history, family dynamics and relationships, family attitude to substance use, developmental history, social network and relationships with friends, friends' attitudes to substance use, premorbid personality, education and vocational history and situation, financial situation, living arrangements, religious practices and beliefs and

community group affiliations, hobbies and interest, the exploration of previous and/or current services provider involvement and any current or legal status or history (Victorian State Government, 2018).

The consumer's story and history provides opportunity to identify potential risk and protective factors, which need to either be addressed or built upon within the integrated treatment plan. Incorporating factors of the consumer's lived experience ensures that the treatment plan is consumer-centred, strengths- and recovery-focused, and allows prediction, with some degree of confidence, of any reduction of adverse patient outcomes in relation to clinical interventions.

Assess any medical history

Substance use, misuse and disorders are associated with a range of physical complications and comorbidities. It is imperative that these are identified during assessment and any existing treatment plan or medications are recorded and reconciled with other health professionals involved with the consumer's care. Any new onset of physical complaints or complications can be identified and interventions can be implemented.

Assess pattern of substance use and substance use behaviour

Initiating a conversation about a person's substance use can be delicate. It is helpful to start with a broad, normalising statement such as, 'We often see people who come here for help using substances for a variety of different reasons', followed by an open-ended question in relation to the consumer's substance use, such as, 'Could you tell me about your substance use?' This approach can be less confronting and judgemental, less stigmatising, and promote trust and rapport. From here, further questioning would focus on: history of substance use (including age of initiation of substance use, course of substance use, identification of problematic substance use); identification of poly substance use (use of more than one substance); patterns of substance use; and substance use behaviour. It is important to highlight that full disclosure of the extent of substance use may not occur in the initial assessment due to perceived or experienced stigma, discrimination, shame and guilt by the consumer. Therefore, the nurse should utilise the time to establish trust by actively listening in a non-judgemental way to the consumer's story or pathway to the service, as this will pay dividends in the development of therapeutic alliance and ongoing disclosure of substance use information. Also, gathering collateral information from alternative sources (carers, family, friends, other services) is invaluable if it is available and with consent from the consumer. **Table 14.16** is an extract of the alcohol and other drugs (AOD) comprehensive assessment framework for drug treatment providers to assess current patterns of substance use and behaviour.

TABLE 14.16
Assessing current levels of alcohol and other drugs

SUBSTANCE USE	AGE AT FIRST USE	AGE AT REGULAR USE	ROUTE OF USE	AVERAGE DAILY USE	DAYS USED IN PAST WEEK	DAYS USED IN PAST 4 WEEKS	DAYS INJECTED IN PAST 4 WEEKS	DATE OF LAST USE	SEEKING HELP FOR THIS DRUG
Tobacco products									
Alcoholic beverages									
Cannabis									
Cocaine									
Methamphetamine									
Other amphetamine type stimulants									
Inhalants									
Non-prescribed sedatives or sleeping pills									
Prescribed sedatives or sleeping pills									
Non-prescribed opioids									
GHB									
Prescribed opioids									
Other (steroids, caffeine, energy drinks, Phenergan, new and emerging drugs, etc.)									

SOURCE: DEPARTMENT OF HUMAN SERVICES, 2017

While assessing patterns of substance use, it is important to encourage the person to talk about their use in the context of impact within the biopsychosocial framework; for example, the impact of pattern of use on:

- functionality – work, school, activities of daily life
- relationships
- self-care – diet, sleep, hygiene
- mental state
- risky behaviours.

Assess for level of severity of SUD

The impact and severity of the SUD may require more intensive level of intervention, in consumer management and interdisciplinary involvement. Table 14.17 presents examples of questions that can be used to assess for the presence of comorbidities or serious complication as a consequence of SUD and may indicate the development of more severe SUD.

TABLE 14.17
Questions that can be used to assess for the presence of comorbidities and/or complications as a consequence of SUD

POSSIBLE COMORBIDITY AND/OR COMPLICATIONS	QUESTIONS TO ASK
Physical comorbidities	• Have you noticed any changes to your physical health? • Have you had this assessed? • How is it being managed? • Has your substance use changed as a consequence?
Severe substance use – presence of addiction, cravings, dependence, tolerance and withdrawal	Assess for patterns of substance use. • Do you use the same substance, at the same times and consume the same amount? • Are you finding that you are using more to get the same effect? • How often are you engaged in the activity of obtaining, using and recovering from the substance? • Do you feel a compulsion to take the substance? • What happens if you don't take the substance? • Have you ever experienced withdrawal? • Have you ever taken a substance to relieve withdrawal symptoms? • Have you had a period of abstinence and then a rapid return to previous substance use patterns?

SOURCE: ANDREWS ET AL., 2013, P. 293

CLINICAL PRESENTATION AND THE MENTAL STATE EXAMINATION

Before exploring the mental state examination (MSE) in relation to a person experiencing an SUD, it is important to note that the clinical presentation of a person experiencing an SUD can potentially be impacted by the presence of intoxication or withdrawal. Symptomatology within the MSE will therefore vary depending on the clinical presentation, and interpretation of all aspects of the MSE will be affected by substance intoxication or withdrawal. Identifying the presence of intoxication or withdrawal is crucial for an accurate screening, and assessment may need to occur at another time or in stages (dependent on risk).

In the absence of intoxication and withdrawal, the MSE facilitates exploration of attitudes and behaviours related to substance use. It also facilitates the identification of acute risks, such as harm to self and others related to impaired mental state caused by substance use or the development of insight into their SUD and its associated impacts. Furthermore, in the absence of intoxication and withdrawal, the MSE can provide evidence of the experience of other comorbid mental health conditions. The following MSE explores key areas in the *absence* of intoxication and withdrawal.

COMMONALITIES OF THE MSE

General appearance and behaviour

A person's willingness to engage in therapeutic communication and respond to the assessment itself can be impacted by the level of acknowledgement and acceptance they have in relation to their SUD.

The severity of substance misuse is associated with greater degrees of impairment to functioning and may include impaired self-care (e.g. dishevelled or unkempt) and impaired nutrition (e.g. malnutrition and looking gaunt). Agitation and distress may be evident by psychomotor hyperactivity and movement or the person's verbal account of distress and/or anxiety. Assessing a consumer's level of distress is important for formulation of risk, especially suicide, as distress is directly proportional to risk. It is also essential to gather the consumer's baseline measurement, observing for overt signs of distress, by asking, 'How is your level of distress today? Can you rate it 1–10?'. *Nursing interventions, tailored to de-escalating and containment, may need to be implemented where there is hyperarousal, activity, agitation and aggression, combined with poor insight.*

Speech

Fluctuations of speech can give the clinician insight into levels of distress and agitation; for example, fluctuating volume and increased rate. In the context of substance use, variations in speech can indicate level of intoxication – slurred or nonsensical – and agitation. Change in speech can be associated with mood variations; for example, monotone and quiet volume can indicate low mood and depression. Separating what is caused by a substance from an underlying mental state is crucial to providing appropriate treatment.

Mood

Assessing mood in the context of substance use can be suggestive of where the consumer is within the cycle of change, while identifying and highlighting comorbid mood or anxiety conditions, severity of use and their impact. The gradual development of insight into substance use behaviour can have an effect on mood and necessitate close monitoring, assessing for altered mood suggestive of suicide risk. Affective states that are low, flat, depressed, agitated, frustrated, hopeless, helpless, elevated, labile and easily irritated can be suggestive of increased risk to self and others.

Changes in sleep, appetite and libido are very common in SUDs. Sleep disturbances can easily exacerbate mental state deviations in mood, cognition, behaviour, thought content (rumination, intrusive thoughts) and judgement. Nutritional deficits related to substance use can compromise physical health and in severe alcohol use can cause serious neurological impairment related to vitamin B and thiamine deficiencies. Consequently, compromised physical health impacts cognition and a consumer's ability to engage in psychotherapy related to SUD. An altered libido can be a result of mood changes and be implicated with substance use, and impact intimate relationships.

Thought

Assessing a consumer's attitude, behaviour and impact on self and others, in relation to their substance use, is the focus in this section of the MSE. This provides an opportunity to explore, in depth, the patterns and behaviours of substance use and where the consumer is in the cycle of change. Exploration of triggers, preoccupations with substance use and presence of cravings can be identified here, which are essential to the management of an SUD, as they are factors that play an enormous role in potential lapse and relapse. Chronic substance use, intoxication and withdrawal can precipitate or exacerbate delusions of persecution, grandeur and/or paranoia and ideas of reference. For example, a chronic alcohol use condition can increase a person's vulnerability to paranoia and hallucinations. Particular attention needs to be paid to thinking, and the presence of themes such as guilt and shame, helpless and hopeless, anger and fear. These, coupled with the presence of distress, poor insight and judgement and/or co-occurring mental health condition, increase the level of risk.

Perceptual disturbances

The presentation of perceptual disturbances in someone experiencing SUD is indicative of intoxication, withdrawal, drug-induced psychosis or comorbid psychotic disorder.

Cognition

Impaired cognition can result from SUD, with severity related to chronicity of substance use. Problems associated with long-term, and persistent, memory deficits, rather than due to the presence of a substance, are noticeable even in its absence (e.g. Wernicke's encephalopathy – Korsakoff syndrome). Problems with level of consciousness, orientation of reality, attention and concentration and ability to process information and deal with abstract ideas will vary depending on severity of use, intoxication and withdrawal. A comorbid mental health condition will also compound these symptoms.

In the case of acute intoxication, using a Glasgow Coma Scale (GCS) will assess level of consciousness and appropriate physical interventions to be applied in response. A score of <8–9 is severe, 9–12 moderate and > or = to 13 is minor.

Judgement

The ability to make a rational/considered decision is generally compromised in a person experiencing an SUD. Assessing a consumer's decision-making capability, especially in relation to their substance use, is compounded by the pathology of addiction, cravings, tolerance and withdrawal, poor coping skills and sociocultural factors. The aetiology of SUD, and presence or exacerbation of comorbid mental disorders, increases a consumer's risk of making poor decisions and impulsive behaviours. Chronic substance use damages the brain's pre-frontal cortex (responsible for executive functioning), exacerbating cravings, inducing intoxication and withdrawal, thereby impacting impulse control and promoting harm and relapse; while also limiting the ability to engage in therapy.

Acute intoxication increases risk of impulsive behaviour; for example, alcohol consumption promoting suicidal ideation in a prone individual. Behaviours that may suggest impaired judgement can include sexual promiscuity, spending, violence and/or criminal activity.

Insight

Insight can vary, depending where the consumer is in relation to the cycle of change, and will develop as the consumer progresses through the cycle. In the early stages, developing insight – the impact on their own and other's lives – increases the propensity for guilt and shame. Nursing interventions must incorporate coping strategies to regulate and manage these emotions, mitigating risk.

SAFETY FIRST

SUBSTANCE-INDUCED PSYCHOSIS
The presence of positive symptoms such as delusions, thought disorder and/or perceptual disturbance need to be assessed in the context of potential drug-induced psychosis. This is where substance misuse, mainly misuse of stimulants, has induced a state of psychosis that can remain for days, weeks, months and even years after the drug use ceases.

Strengths and protective factors
Identification of protective factors and strengths within the biopsychosocial framework creates a basis upon which interventions can be built, encourages adherence and may decrease risk of lapse and relapse. The identification of protective factors, and working with people to build upon these, fosters self-efficacy, self-esteem and resilience, essential factors in primary, secondary and tertiary prevention and management of SUDs. Protective factors can include, but are not limited to, therapeutic relationships, engagement with services (irrespective of where the consumer is in relation to the cycle of change), work, school, family, friends, animals, hobbies, engagement in sporting and recreational activities, religion/spirituality and coping skills. Exploring and identifying strengths that can be built upon, and if there have been any previous strategies that have been helpful in the management of their substance use behaviour, can be incorporated in management and relapse prevention plans and positively reinforce strength and hope.

Assessing motivation for change and associated interventions
An important aspect of assessing a consumer's substance misuse is establishing their motivation to change their substance use behaviour. Prochaska, DiClemente and Norcross (1992) identified five stages through which consumers move to facilitate change in their substance misuse behaviour. The underlying premise of this assessment is to ensure that the right intervention is developed at the right time to optimise behaviour change. It is important to understand that this process is fluid and dynamic and consumers may 'recycle several times through the stages before achieving long-term maintenance' (Prochaska, DiClemente & Norcross, 1992, p. 1102). Understanding where consumers are within this cycle is important for the development of appropriate, targeted goals and interventions.

The five stages of change are: precontemplation, contemplation, preparation, action and maintenance. Clinicians can use motivational interviewing to support consumers through the stages of change –

refer to **Table 4.5** in Chapter 4 for a specific example on how the stages of change model and motivation interviewing are used in relation to working with a consumer who is experiencing an SUD.

Risk assessment
Assessing a consumer's risk related to their SUD includes assessing intoxication, withdrawal, lapse, relapse, associated risk related to substance use behaviour and dual diagnosis and/or co-occurring health implications. Assessing previous risk history and changes in pattern of substance use can also be a predictor of future risk. In this section, we identify risk in the context of substance use, risk-taking behaviours and lapse/relapse. Identifying specific risk factors can then be used to formulate interventions in collaboration with the consumer.

Potential risk issues related to SUDs may include:
- intoxication
- withdrawal
- toxicity and overdose
- increased impulsivity
- onset or exacerbation of a comorbid mental health condition
- presence and experience of distress
- onset or exacerbation of suicidal ideation or behaviours
- onset or exacerbation of self-harm/non-suicidal self-injury ideation or behaviours
- harm to others – aggression, violence, homicidality
- compromised care for others; for example, children
- presence and experience of perceptual and thought disorders – hallucinations and delusions
- presence and experience of fluctuations in mood and/or anxiety
- increased risk secondary to disinhibition: promiscuity, sexual assault, general vulnerability
- homelessness or unstable accommodation
- increased risk-taking behaviours – driving while intoxicated, criminality
- interpersonal violence
- physiological factors: exposure to BBVs, STIs
- use of other substances (poly substance use) – risk of accidental overdose, coma and death; for example, alcohol and opioids
- sleep disturbance
- nutrition deficits
- self-care deficits
- denial
- poor insight and impaired judgement
- ineffective coping
- relationship distress, dissatisfaction, conflict and instability
- vocational instability – risk of unemployment
- poor compliance with treatment plan
- shame and guilt.

Harm minimisation

Harm minimisation is an approach to substance use, misuse and SUD that focuses on the risks associated with substance use, rather than eliminating the substance, and how their harmful effects can be reduced (Haber & Day, 2014). Other than the physical consequences of substance use, harm minimisation also covers the social and economic impacts of SUD on the individual and the community (Department of Health, 2004). The three pillars of Australia's National Drug Strategy (NDS) harm minimisation strategy – a key policy of the federal government since 1985 – are harm, supply and demand reduction. The principles of harm minimisation in Australia were shaped by the 1980 human immunodeficiency virus (HIV) crisis, which impacted IV drug users, whose unsafe injecting practices increased the risk of exposure. **Table 14.18** provides a summary of interventions for each pillar of the Australian Government's harm minimisation strategy.

Treatment

Approaches to substance use, misuse and SUD from a population perspective require a public health framework that covers the spectrum of interventions required to address the progressive nature and harm related to substance use, misuse and SUD. Interventions specific to each level – primary, secondary and tertiary – ensure that consumers at risk of initiating substance use, engaging in substance use and misuse, developing an SUD, experiencing an acute episode of SUD or who are in active recovery from an SUD, receive the appropriate targeted treatment for positive health outcomes.

Table 14.19 summarises the appropriate interventions at each level.

TABLE 14.18
The three pillars of the harm minimisation strategy

PILLAR	RATIONALE	STRATEGIES
Harm reduction	Reduce harm associated from illicit substance use for both consumers and communities. Does not necessarily aim to stop substance use.	• Reducing risks associated with a particular context; e.g. safe injecting rooms • Protecting the community from infectious disease; e.g. needle syringe exchange programs • Methadone maintenance • Protecting children from another's substance use • Brief interventions • Peer education – reducing driving under the influence of alcohol and other drugs
Supply reduction	Prevent, stop, disrupt or reduce the production and supply of illicit substances and regulate the availability of legal drugs.	• Regulating retail and wholesale supply of substances • Enforcing age restrictions on purchasing substances; e.g. alcohol • Regulating or disrupting production and distribution • Real-time monitoring of prescription medications; e.g. opioids • Border patrol at ports and airports screening for illicit drug imports
Demand reduction	Prevent the uptake and/or delay onset of substance use; reduce substance misuse and support people to recover from SUD.	• Reducing availability and accessibility through price control (alcohol and tobacco) • Improving community understanding and knowledge, reducing stigma and promoting help seeking • Restrictions on marketing, including advertising and promotions • Programs focused on building protective factors and social engagement • Treatment services and brief interventions • Diversional initiatives • Targeted and culturally appropriate approaches to high risk populations • Addressing underlying social, health and economic determinants of substance use

SOURCE: BASED ON COMMONWEALTH OF AUSTRALIA. DEPARTMENT OF HEALTH, 2017, PP 7–14

TABLE 14.19
Summary of primary, secondary and tertiary interventions for substance use, misuse and SUD

LEVEL OF INTERVENTION	GOAL	INTERVENTIONS
Primary – prevention	Prevent people from developing SUD	• Educate people on the harms associated with SUD • Make laws that govern the sale and distribution of illicit substances • Build social capital • Provide positive role models • Build individual resilience • Develop safe environments
Secondary – early intervention	Directed towards people who are 'at risk' for developing an SUD and related harm or comorbidities	• Provide education programs for drink drivers • Screening for SUD • Offer counselling for people who use illicit substances at risky levels – motivational interviewing and brief intervention • Provide clean needles for people who inject substances
Tertiary – treatment and recovery	To help people with existing SUD overcome it, or to improve their quality of life	• SUD detoxification and withdrawal • Cognitive behavioural therapy • Relapse prevention and mindfulness-based relapse prevention • Pharmacotherapy • Twelve-step and other self-help programs • Residential rehabilitation • Therapeutic communities

SOURCE: AUSTRALIAN DRUG FOUNDATION, 2017

Approaches to treatment planning and processes for individuals who are experiencing an SUD need to be tailored to each person's presentation, history, where they are in the cycle of behavioural change and pattern of substance use. Approaches also need to address any co-occurring medical, psychiatric or social problems. They require a person-centred holistic approach where the person is at the centre of the decision making about their treatment plan to promote adherence and foster control to improve health outcomes. Approaches to treatment of SUDs need to factor in learning opportunities that are positively framed and normalised experiences of lapse and/or relapse for sustained recovery.

Treatment goals must link assessment to intervention. Points for consideration when formulating clinical goals include:

- the consumer's wants and needs even if these are in conflict with the health clinician's ideas of what is best
- personal circumstances (e.g. financial, family and social)
- where the consumer is in relation to stage of change
- type and severity of issues (social, cultural, physical and psychological)
- presence of comorbid mental or physical health conditions

- consumer safety
- the setting in which the intervention will occur (Andrews et al., 2013; NCETA, 2004).

Where appropriate, available and with the consumer's consent, involve the consumer's support network; this may include working with carers, family, friends, and coordination and collaboration with other service providers (mental health, medical providers and social services such as housing). Promoting and fostering relationships with a person's support network builds a unified and shared approach to treatment goals and provides essential support for those caring for someone with an SUD. Failure to involve, coordinate and support relevant people and services can create cracks in the treatment plan and increase risk of disengagement and/or poor adherence to the treatment plan. People experiencing SUD may find having to navigate services and work with and be supported by people with limited understanding of their experience of an SUD frustrating, disheartening and exhausting. Working closely and providing support for carers is also important, as caring for someone experiencing an SUD can create stressful life circumstances. Carers often also experience the stigma that creates barriers for them accessing support (Moriarty, Manthorpe, Cornes & Hussein, 2014).

CASE **STUDY**

A MENTAL HEALTH NURSE'S EXPERIENCE OF WORKING WITH THE CARER OF A PERSON WITH SUD

Working in mental health triage, I often become distraught when family members call in desperation for admission of their loved one into a service, as they are rightly concerned for their safety related to their substance misuse. What I find compounds the distress for the carer is not only the acuteness of their concern for the person experiencing substance misuse, but also the lack of knowledge of where and how to get help, the potential limitations of service provision if the person doesn't want help and their own mental health and well-being. There is despair; as one mother said to me, 'I'm just watching my son kill himself slowly and no one can do anything about it…I don't know what to do and I'm exhausted'. When this occurs, I spend time with the carer, listening and validating their distress and concern and where appropriate providing education, resources and linkages to services – not only for the person with the substance misuse issue, but also for the health and well-being of the carer.

Questions

1   Can you 'coerce or mandate' someone to engage or be admitted into an AOD service or mental health facility or program? If so, under what circumstance can you do so? If not, why?

2   What resources or services would you link this mother to?

Pharmacotherapy and psychological and behavioural approaches to substance use disorders

Treatment of SUDs can occur in a variety of settings, including the community or inpatient settings such as a medical ward in a general hospital, addictions unit in a mental health facility or a specialised drug and alcohol facility. Treatment for SUDs is multipronged and often involves intervention and treatment modalities that vary in accordance to the degree of severity of the SUD and different stages of recovery. The intervention process is often 'stepped' (step model of care), whereby the least invasive intervention is implemented first and then monitored to determine the progress after the initial intervention. Interventions are then realigned based on the outcome and adherence from the previous intervention. The following text looks at the pharmacological and psychological treatment approaches to SUD.

Pharmacotherapy treatment will depend on the substance used, intoxication, withdrawal or maintenance of SUD. **Table 14.20** lists the medications used for treatment of alcohol, cannabis, stimulant and opioid SUDs.

Psychological and behavioural therapies can be provided in group, family or individual sessions. They are designed to facilitate awareness of the impact of SUD behaviour and restore level of functioning to a 'healthy, safe and productive manner' (US Department of Health and Human Services 2016). Behavioural therapies such as cognitive behavioural therapy (CBT) are used to facilitate the development of insight, facilitate attitude and behaviour changes in relation to substance use, and develop skills in managing stress and strong emotions (see Chapter 4). Psychological and behavioural approaches can be used as stand-alone approaches, such as brief interventions, or used

TABLE 14.20
Pharmacotherapy use in alcohol, cannabis, stimulant and opioid use disorders

SUBSTANCE	MEDICATION	USES
Alcohol	Oral naltrexone	Maintenance
	IM naltrexone	Maintenance
	Acamprosate	Maintenance
	Disulfiram	Maintenance
	Benzodiazepines	Withdrawal
Stimulants	Antipsychotics	Intoxication
	Anxiolytics	Intoxication
	Hypnotics	Intoxication
Opioids	Methadone	Withdrawal and maintenance
	Buprenorphine – naloxone	Withdrawal and maintenance
	Buprenorphine	Withdrawal and maintenance
	Naltrexone	Maintenance

in combination with other treatment strategies. This is heavily dependent on the individual's presentation, circumstances and needs, and evidence of efficacy in the treatment of the specific substance(s) of use and pattern of use. Interventions are as follows:

■ *Brief interventions (BIs)* can be used in a variety of health settings, such as primary care, accident and emergency, hospital wards and antenatal settings. BIs are opportunities to engage the consumer in a conversation about their substance use behaviour and motivate them to think differently about it and reduce the risk associated with harmful use. BIs combine counselling and motivational interviewing to facilitate behaviour change and can be effective first-level treatment in a step model approach. BIs are effective for high-risk alcohol use (not for people who have more severe alcohol use disorders; i.e. dependence or more severe alcohol-related harm such as Wernicke's encephalopathy) and to a lesser extent amphetamines, dual diagnosis and mental health problems. BI involves three steps and can be a quick process (five to 30 minutes) as a one-off intervention; however, follow-up is advisable but not always practical (e.g. in accident and emergency). The three steps are:

a. Screen to identify at-risk alcohol or drug use (CAGE-AID).

b. Relate the consumer's symptoms, difficulties and risks to the use of substances (raise awareness and provide feedback).

c. Advise and facilitate the consumer to reduce consumption of substances to safe and responsible levels (harm reduction and minimisation) (Aldridge, Dowd & Bray, 2017; Andrews et al., 2013; NSW Government, 2008; Ritter, King & Hamilton, 2013).

- *Motivational interviewing* (see Chapter 4).
- *Cognitive behavioural therapy* (CBT; see Chapter 4).
- *Relapse prevention (RP)* works to identify and prevent those high-risk situations where the consumer is more likely to engage in substance use (McHugh, Hearon & Otto, 2010).
- *Mindfulness-based relapse prevention* builds on RP and incorporates the development of skills to accept and tolerate the internal discomfort and distress caused by cravings and risk situations that can cause relapse (Bowen et al., 2014).
- *Contingency management* uses positive reinforcement to foster engagement and compliance to treatment; for example, food vouchers.
- *Twelve-step programs* promote shared experiences and mutual support, such as Alcoholics Anonymous (AA) and Narcotics Anonymous (NA).
- *Family and couples counselling* to educate families about SUDs and facilitate changes in the family and home circumstances and dynamics that may perpetuate or increase risk for substance use.

Recovery and relapse prevention

When treated early, a consumer's likelihood of lapse and/or relapse is lessened, leading to a greater propensity for recovery. However, addiction is a chronic and relapsing condition, similar to other chronic disease processes such as asthma, and diabetes, prone to periods of stability and improvement, and recurrence. All consumers, despite dedication and commitment to recovery, may experience a lapse or relapse following a period of abstinence. The lapse is considered a brief episode, with the return to substance treatment goals, and not a re-initiation of

previous addictive behaviours; however, a lapse may prompt a relapse. **Relapse**, on the other hand, is when a person has recommenced using a substance, has not returned to their substance treatment goals and has returned to their former addiction patterns of substance use (Hendershot, Witkiewitz, George & Marlatt, 2011; Queensland Government Metro North Mental Health – Alcohol and Drug Services, 2013).

Table 14.20 identifies lapse and relapse and suggested interventions to address each.

Lapse and relapse should not be seen as a failure, as they are an important aspect in recovery and an opportunity for developing key insights into substance use behaviour. Should lapse or relapse occur, it is a prime opportunity for a consumer to take stock and reflect on their behaviour, identify triggers, develop insight and refine behaviour and intervention strategies. Engaging with supportive communities and services can be crucial at this time, and important in helping the consumer to reinforce existing skill sets. Precipitators of lapse and relapse may include:

- *acute triggers* – cravings, triggers or urges, withdrawal, lapse in substance use and the associated guilt and shame, relationship breakdown, interpersonal stress, social pressure, stress, loss of job or home, grief and negative emotional states
- *chronic and ongoing risk* – cravings, triggers or urges, living in remote communities, social isolation, poor connection to the community, unemployment, sexual abuse, bullying, unstable or inappropriate accommodation, financial difficulties, legal issues and mental health or physical comorbidities.

SAFETY FIRST

INCREASED RISK OF OVERDOSE
After periods of abstinence, a person's experience of tolerance to a substance may decline or stop altogether. This can pose a potential risk for overdose in the incidence of lapse as the person may return to previous amounts/quantities of substance use and their body cannot cope and unintentionally overdose and potentially die. For example, a person admitted into a detox/rehabilitation program will be abstinent for a period of time and when discharged, may use; however, they use the same amount of substance that had been used during an active stage of using.

With such factors in mind, developing a robust support network is essential and should be a key component of any care plan. Clinically, services such as outreach, day programs, along with specialist organisations such as AA or NA, should provide the backbone of any good support system, thereby reducing the risk of lapse or relapse. The consumer,

TABLE 14.20
Identifying lapse and relapse in recovery

STAGE	INDICATION	EVIDENCE	GOAL	INTERVENTION
Lapse	The consumer has used a substance in the short term and hasn't returned to prior substance use patterns. It is often referred to as a 'bust' or 'slip'. However, they continue to be committed to change.	'I bust on the weekend, I was doing so well. I just had a couple of beers but it's OK, tomorrow's a new day and I'll see my AOD counsellor first thing.'	To facilitate and support the use of coping strategies to deal with the consequences of lapse and assess the consumer's position in the cycle of change. Identify at-risk themes or mental state secondary to lapse.	• Ensure there is support in place. • Facilitate identification of trigger of lapse. • Explore the underlying thoughts and feelings that led to the lapse. • Reflect and readjust treatment goals and if required provide more intensive psychological support as lapses may be caused by an acute psychosocial stressor (prevention of lapse escalating to relapse). • Skill building – alternative coping, mindfulness, relaxation techniques or other stress-reducing techniques. • Identify and facilitate additional support. • Educate as to the importance of lapses for refinement of goals. • Monitor and support the consumer's mental state, as this stage may trigger guilt, remorse and failure.
Relapse	The return of the consumer's prior substance use patterns and behaviours	'I thought I could just use it like everyone else.' 'I can't believe I'm back in hospital.' 'I thought I could just stop.'	Identify potential for withdrawal and/or onset of physical complication related to relapse into substance use. To facilitate and support the use of coping strategies to deal with the consequences of relapse and assess the consumer's position in the cycle of change. Identify at-risk themes or mental state secondary to relapse.	• Supervised medical detox (and rehabilitation if necessary) or seek medical support. • Ensure support is in place. • Reflection of pattern of behaviour and risk factors leading up to relapse. • Explore the underlying thoughts and feelings that led to the relapse. • Skill building – alternative coping and mindfulness. • Readjustment of treatment goals and interventions. • Monitor and support the consumer's mental state as this stage may be associated with guilt, shame, helpless and hopeless themes or exacerbate or onset of deviations in perception/thought; i.e. hallucinations or delusions. • Above all, reinforce and normalise that relapse is an important component of recovery and an opportunity to identify risk, maladaptive coping strategies, negative thinking and refine goals and strategies.

their carers and families, and clinicians should see recovery from an SUD as a journey or process, rather than an end point. Lifestyle changes and adjustments, as with any illness, are essential, as are support and

reflection. Recovery involves a lifelong commitment, conscious monitoring, ongoing assessment and reflection, and identification and management of potential risk factors that may trigger lapse or relapse.

CASE STUDY

CASE 1: JACK

Jack is a 40-year-old male who first started drinking when he was 14 years old. He would hang out with his mates at weekends and drink 'whatever we could get our hands on', which remained a social activity and within the norms of teenage behaviour, although he would regularly become intoxicated.

Later, Jack found employment and married, and continued to drink socially until, due to chronic back pain, he lost his job and found it difficult to find another. Consequently, there were financial stressors and this caused him to drink more regularly, with his intake increasing to two bottles of wine daily, and sometimes more if he could afford it. This turned into a 15-year habit and resulted in the breakdown of his marriage and housing problems.

Jack currently lives in a boarding house, which isn't ideal, and recently had property stolen, leading to

further anxiety and stress. He has engaged with several detoxification and rehabilitation programs, and maintained periods of abstinence, but still struggles. In terms of his health, he has oesophageal ulcers and liver problems. Previously, when making a solo attempt at abstinence, Jack experienced a seizure, leading to admission to hospital.

Questions

1   Jack is being admitted to the detox unit and is intoxicated on arrival. What should be the first steps taken?

2   Given what you know of Jack's medical history, what risks might Jack present and what steps should be taken to mitigate these?

3   How might Jack's social situation impact his recovery?

CASE **STUDY**

CASE 2: MARY

Mary is a 63-year-old woman living alone, her two adult children having left home, and who has had a successful career for most of her adult life.

Mary suffered a back injury in her late 30s, which she initially managed with regular exercise, hydrotherapy and a small daily dose of a compound codeine product. However, as she aged, the condition worsened, causing her to increase her pain medication. Consequently, six months ago Mary became unable to continue working and this significantly impacted her life and sense of self, as she was no longer able to socialise as actively, exercise and became isolated. To cope, she used her prescribed medication over and above the recommended dosages while combining it with over-the-counter pain medications.

Mary came to the attention of services when she failed to show up for dinner with her daughter, and was subsequently found collapsed on the floor at home. She was taken to hospital with a suspected overdose and, once stable, admitted to taking over-the-counter pain medication and increased dosages of her prescription opiates; she denied an intentional overdose.

Questions

1 Given that Mary has been taking prescription opiates above the recommended dosages, how would opiate intoxication physically present itself?

2 Mary has experienced significant life changes recently, including the loss of her job and other activities. What concerns might you have regarding her mental health and what steps would you take as a first-line clinician?

3 What treatment options might you offer to her following discharge from hospital?

REFLECTION ON LEARNING FROM PRACTICE

The experience of detox was overwhelming. I laid in bed for those first few days, stunned that I was here, wondering where my life had taken me. I was in denial – this was a big mistake – I wasn't like the other patients here, they were all druggies and alcoholics.

I slept a lot, those first few days, and the nurses didn't harass me. They gave me pills when I needed them and reminded me to eat. I kept craving something, anything, to take the feeling away. The pills helped, sure, but they were getting less and less, but I needed that high, the feeling of relief. My anxiety was horrific and constant, and would push me to the edge of panic.

Then, they encouraged me to attend groups – insisted – and, initially, I was reluctant. I wasn't going to speak and I didn't want to listen to others whinging about their lives. But, then I did, I sat there in a circle, anxious, but listening to others talk. I heard myself in their stories, not lives of disrepair and desperation, but other human beings who made bad choices and were victims of circumstance. These were normal people – a mother with three children, a business owner, even a doctor – they had been brought here by the same problems I had.

I still didn't talk much, you know, but I listened. I analysed my behaviour, the excuses I'd been making, and the potential for loss and what I already had.

Before my discharge, I sat with the nurse while he talked about the next steps. I was booked in to see my treating doctor as an outpatient, and given information for support services, organisations who could help me along, but I wasn't sure. He talked about how I could occupy myself, of ways to 'self-soothe' and seek distraction, about what I should do when I felt the urges. This was in the name of relapse prevention and what to do should this happen.

When the 10 days were up, I still wasn't feeling great but I had more energy, I was thinking clearly and I wasn't craving the drugs in the same way. But, I had to go back to that job, and the pressure, and the thought filled me with dread. The urge to use hit me again – just a little bit, a drink or two and that would be all; I could cope with that.

Then I went home, and real life began again. I thought about going to this service, just to try, but I didn't. And my life has resumed again, and work is just as stressful. I haven't touched anything since my admission to hospital, but there is a work function that I am going to and, although I intend not to even drink, I'm scared I won't be able to say no.'

CHAPTER RESOURCES

SUMMARY

- Substance use has been present through the history of civilisation and is influenced by the beliefs, customs, economics, politics and values of the era. Substance use is categorised in the DSM-5 from mild to moderate and severe, with clear diagnostic criteria for each associated syndrome.
- The impact of substance misuse on a person's health and well-being occurs along a continuum of severity from hazardous, harmful, addiction and dependence. This continuum demonstrates the progression of harm related to the development of substance use disorders and onset of associated comorbidities. Drugs of abuse can be classified as depressants (suppressing/inhibiting the CNS), stimulants (enhancing/increasing CNS activity) or hallucinogens (altering perceptions, feelings and thinking processes).
- Addiction is a consequence of chemical changes in the brain, varying in each individual, and usually following a course from adolescent use to escalation in adulthood. A clear link exists between mental health conditions and substance use – comorbid and coexisting disorders – whether exacerbating each other or being a mutually causative factor. There are close links with stress, anxiety, depression and psychosis, with a high suicide rate among the group, as well as non-fatal attempts.
- Use is prevalent across genders, age groups and cultures, with a higher presentation of males and younger people likely to suffer from an SUD, whereas women are less likely to present to services yet are at a higher risk of comorbid complications with SUDs. High-risk populations include LGBTQ(IA+), prison populations, pregnant women, and Aboriginal and Torres Strait Islander peoples. The burden of disease and mortality across all illnesses, including physical and mental disorders, is exacerbated by the use of substances.
- Problematic substance use has both short- and long-term impacts on a person's physical health, leading to acute and chronic disease processes. Intoxication and withdrawal syndromes can lead to physically risky symptoms. Comorbid mental health disorders are commonplace among the substance-using community, with the drugs themselves being a causative, compounding and consequent factor. The impact on social well-being contributes to this (e.g. loss of job/career, impact on relationships, financial struggles and ostracism from society) and is a significant component of a treatment and rehabilitation plan.
- To receive a diagnosis of a substance use disorder, a consumer must meet specified criteria as outlined in the DSM-5. These criteria encompass behavioural, emotional, social and physiological features, such as tolerance and withdrawal syndromes.
- Screening, assessment and treatment options are understood within a biopsychosocial framework. Assessing and implementing treatment for intoxication and withdrawal exists within this, with further intervention prescribed for recovery and rehabilitation. Using tools to assess, such as the alcohol withdrawal scale, and other research-based markers, is essential for meeting the treatment needs of individuals. Treatment options for SUDs are based on a public health framework that covers the spectrum of screening, assessment and interventions. Brief interventions, assessing for readiness to change, motivational interviewing, harm minimisation principles and strategies, and pharmacological interventions are several treatment options. The experience of an SUD is a health issue, not a moral issue. Therapeutic engagement, non-judgemental attitudes and empathy are essential to create an environment where the consumer's lived experience can be heard and understood by the nurse. Only then can the multidisciplinary team, including the nurse, work collaboratively and effectively with a consumer.

REVIEW QUESTIONS

1   What are some of the factors that influence attitudes towards substances?
   a   Cultural beliefs and values
   b   Heredity
   c   Peers
   d   All of the above
2   What is meant by a biopsychosocial assessment of a person's substance use?
   a   Assessment of social and cultural context
   b   Assessment of the pattern of substance use and substance use behaviour

   c   Assessment approach which incorporates disease, medical, biological, psychological and social theories to understand the context of the person with the SUD
   d   An assessment approach that incorporates disease, biological, psychological and social theories to understand the context of the person with the SUD
3   What are some of the cognitive issues you might expect to see in acute alcohol intoxication?
   a   Poor judgement
   b   Poor attention and concentration
   c   Poor memory
   d   All of the above

4 When a consumer appears intoxicated, it is important to monitor for other possible causes: true or false?

5 The DTs are:
  a A symptom of Wernicke's encephalopathy – Korsakoff syndrome
  b A cluster of symptoms associated with withdrawal in a moderate drinker
  c A serious set of symptoms that require medical attention and result from acute intoxication in a heavy drinker
  d A serious set of symptoms that require medical attention and result from withdrawal in a heavy drinker

6 The three pillars of harm minimisation according to the National Drug Strategy are:
  a Harm reduction, supply cessation, demand reduction
  b Harm minimisation, supply reduction, demand reduction
  c Harm reduction, supply reduction, demand reduction
  d Harm reduction, legislation to stop supply, harsher penalties for users

7 You are assessing a consumer's motivation to stop their drug use. What statement(s) would make you suspect that they were in the 'contemplative' stage of change?
  a 'I don't have a problem.'
  b 'I like using, but I don't like the comedown.'
  c 'I want to cut down on how much I'm using.'
  d Both b and c

8 You have identified that a patient has a substance use issue. Would you:
  a Dismiss the issue as not relevant to their current presentation?
  b Tell the person to stop drinking?
  c Provide education on the harms of substance use as brief intervention?
  d Refer them to a detox program.

CRITICAL THINKING

1 In the clinical setting, what would indicate that a person was at risk of hazardous substance use, harmful substance use, addiction and dependence?

2 What is the difference between addiction and dependence?

3 What are the effects of alcohol, stimulants, cannabis and opioids on the CNS?

4 Why is the language we use so important when working with people who are experiencing substance use disorders?

5 What behaviours may indicate problematic substance use?

6 Why is it important to understand what influences people to use substances?

7 What is the impact of substance use during adolescence?

8 How can substance use lead to addiction, and progress into cravings, tolerance and withdrawal?

9 What risk factors contribute to the development of an SUD?

10 Who is at increased risk of harm related to SUD, and why?

11 Why is it important to conduct a holistic biopsychosocial assessment on someone presenting with physical complications from substance use?

12 What factors contribute to a safe environment when working with people affected by ice?

USEFUL WEBSITES

- 1800ICE Advice. Ice Action Plan: http://ice.vic.gov.au/facts-and-help
- Alcohol and Drug Foundation: http://www.adf.org.au
- Australian Government Department of Health – Alcohol: https://www.health.gov.au/health-topics/alcohol
- Australian Government Department of Health – About Drugs: https://www.health.gov.au/health-topics/drugs/about-drugs
- Australian Government Department of Health: National Drug Strategy: https://www.health.gov.au/resources/collections/national-drug-strategy
- Australian Government Department of Health: National Framework for Alcohol, Tobacco and Other Drug Treatment 2019–29: https://www.health.gov.au/resources/publications/national-framework-for-alcohol-tobacco-and-other-drug-treatment-2019-29
- Australian Institute of Health and Welfare: Alcohol, tobacco and other drugs in Australia: https://www.aihw.gov.au/reports/alcohol/alcohol-tobacco-other-drugs-australia/contents/about
- Centre of Research Excellence (CRE) in Mental Health and Substance Use: https://ndarc.med.unsw.edu.au/program/cre-mental-health-substance-use
- DirectLine: https://www.directline.org.au
- Drug and Alcohol Clinical Advisory Service (DACAS): https://www.dacas.org.au
- National Drug and Alcohol Research Centre: https://ndarc.med.unsw.edu.au
- National Institute on Drug Abuse: https://www.drugabuse.gov

SECTION 2

REFLECT ON THIS

Alcohol usage

As you have read in this chapter, people use substances such as alcohol for a variety of reasons. Reflect on your own use of alcohol, or that of someone you know.

1   How often would you/person you know consume alcohol?
2   In what situations would you most commonly consume alcohol?
3   When you/person you know were growing up, was the use of alcohol a regular activity in your/their household?
4   Why do you think the use of alcohol is such a strong part of many cultures?
5   If you/person you know do not consume alcohol, what are your reasons for this choice?

Also consider the following questions:

6   How would you explain the terms 'addiction' and 'dependence' to another person?
7   What supports/resources are available nationally, and in your state or territory, for people who are concerned about their alcohol use or believe they may have an alcohol use issue?
8   As a member of the multidisciplinary team, how can you work with your colleagues to support a consumer who has an alcohol use issue?

REFERENCES

Aldridge, A., Dowd, W. & Bray, J. (2017). The relative impact of brief treatment versus brief intervention in primary health-care screening programs for substance use disorders. *Addiction*, 112(S2), 54–64. doi:doi:10.1111/add.13653

Allen, K.M. (1996). *Nursing Care of the Addicted Client.* Lippincott Raven Publishers.

American Psychiatric Association (APA). (2013). *Diagnostic and Statistical Manual of Mental Disorders (DSM-5)* (5th edn). Washington, DC: APA.

Andrews, G., Dean, K., Genderson, M., Hunt, C., Mitchell, P., Sachdev, P. & Trollor, J. (2013). *Management of Mental Disorders* (5th edn). Sydney: School of Psychiatry, University of NSW.

Australian Bureau of Statistics (ABS). (2007). *National Survey of Mental Health and Wellbeing: Summary of Results.* Retrieved from http://www.ausstats.abs.gov.au/Ausstats/subscriber. nsf/0/6AE6DA447F985FC2CA2574EA00122BD6/$File/43260_2007.pdf.

Australian Drug Foundation. (2017). *Enquiry into Drug Law Reform by the Parliament of Victoria's Law Reform Road and Community Safety Committee.* Retrieved from https://www. parliament.vic.gov.au/images/stories/committees/lrrcsc/Drugs_/ Submissions/218_2017.03.31_-_ADF_-_submission.pdf.

Australian Health Ministers' Advisory Council (AHMAC). (2017). *Aboriginal and Torres Strait Islander Health Performance Framework 2017 Report.* Retrieved from https://www.pmc.gov. au/sites/default/files/publications/2017-health-performance-framework-report_0.pdf. © Commonwealth of Australia. Canberra. Released under CC BY 3.0 AU. Link to license: https:// creativecommons.org/licenses/by/3.0/au/.

Australian Institute of Health and Welfare (AIHW). (2015). *Alcohol and Other Drug Use and Treatment in Prison Populations.* Retrieved from http://www.aihw.gov.au/alcohol-and-other-drugs/data-sources/ aodts-nmds-2014.15/treatment/prisoners.

Australian Institute of Health and Welfare (AIHW). (2016). Australia's Health 2016. Australia's Health Series no. 15. Cat. no. AUS 199. Canberra: AIHW. *4.5 Illicit Drug Use.* Retrieved from https://www. aihw.gov.au/getmedia/e4f7cfc6-3cd5-4cf7-8c7e-dd77e83b8239/ ah16-4-5-illicit-drug-use.pdf.aspx. Released under CC BY 3.0. Link to license: https://creativecommons.org/licenses/by/3.0/au/.

Australian Institute of Health and Welfare (AIHW). (2017a). *2016 National Drug Strategy Household Survey Key Findings: Alcohol Use.* Retrieved from https://www.aihw.gov.au/reports/illicit-use-of-drugs/ndshs-2016-key-findings/contents/alcohol-use. Released under CC BY 3.0. Link to license: https://creativecommons.org/ licenses/by/3.0/au/

Australian Institute of Health and Welfare (AIHW). (2017b). *2016 National Drug Strategy Household Survey Key Findings: Illicit Use of Drugs.* Retrieved from https://www.aihw.gov.au/reports/illicit-use-of-drugs/ndshs-2016-key-findings/contents/illicit-use-of-drugs. Released under CC BY 3.0. Link to license: https://creativecommons. org/licenses/by/3.0/au/

Australian Institute of Health and Welfare (AIHW). (2017c). *National Drug Strategy Household Survey 2016: Detailed Findings. Drug Statistics series no. 31.* Cat. no. PHE 214. Canberra: AIHW. Released under CC BY 3.0. Link to license: https://creativecommons.org/ licenses/by/3.0/au/

Baldry, E. & Russell, S. (2017). The booming industry continued: Australian prisons. A 2017 update. ResearchGate. Retrieved from http://www.disabilityjustice.edu.au/wp-content/uploads/2015/10/ The-Booming-Industry-continued-Australian-Prisons-2017-.pdf.

Becker, J.B. & Koob, G.F. (2016). Sex differences in animal models: Focus on addiction. *Pharmacological Reviews*, 68(2), 242–63. doi:https://doi.org/10.1124/pr.115.011163

Behnke, M. & Smith, V. (2013). Prenatal substance abuse: Short and long-term effects on the exposed fetus. *American Academy of Pediatrics*, 131(3), e1009–e2014. Retrieved from http://pediatrics. aappublications.org/content/pediatrics/131/3/e1009.full.pdf.

Burns, M., Lekawa, M.E. & Price, J. (2018). Delirium tremens (DTs). Medscape. Retrieved from https://emedicine.medscape.com/ article/166032-overview.

Campbell, A. (2001). *The Australian Illicit Drug Guide.* Melbourne: Black Inc.

Centre for Addiction and Mental Health. (2010). *Addiction: An Information Guide.* Retrieved from https://www.camh.ca/-/media/ files/guides-and-publications/addiction-guide-en.pdf.

Centre for Public Health. (2009). *Interpersonal Violence and Illicit Drugs.* Liverpool: Centre for Public Health. Retrieved from https:// www.who.int/violenceprevention/interpersonal_violence_and_ illicit_drug_use.pdf.

Chau, S. (2016). Addiction to recovery: a biopsychosocial approach. Professional development. Lecture given at the Melbourne Clinic.

Commonwealth of Australia. Department of Health. (2017). *National Drug Strategy 2017–2026*. Retrieved from http://www.health.gov.au/internet/main/publishing.nsf/Content/ministerial-drug-alcohol-forum. © Commonwealth of Australia. Department of Health. (2017). Released under CC BY 4.0 International. Link to license: https://creativecommons.org/licenses/by/4.0.

Department of Health. (2004). Training Frontline Workers: Young People, Alcohol and Other Drugs. Module 9. 2.1 Harm minimisation. Retrieved from http://www.health.gov.au/internet/publications/publishing.nsf/Content/drugtreat-pubs-front9-wk-toc~drugtreat-pubs-front9-wk-secb~drugtreat-pubs-front9-wk-secb-2~drugtreat-pubs-front9-wk-secb-2-1.

Department of Human Services. (2017). *Victorian Alcohol and Other Drugs (AOD) Intake Tool*. Retrieved from https://www2.health.vic.gov.au/about/publications/FormsAndTemplates/victorian-aod-comprehensive-assessment-form.

Fraser, S. (2015). A thousand contradictory ways: Addiction, neuroscience, and expert autobiography. *Contemporary Drug Problems*, 42(1). Retrieved from http://search.proquest.com.ez.library.latrobe.edu.au/docview/1777909359?accountid=12001&rfr_id=info%3Axri%2Fsid%3Aprimo.

Gordon, A.J., Conley, J.W. & Gordon, J.M. (2015). Physical disease and addictive disorders: Associations and implications. In N. Sartorius, R.I.G. Holt & M. Maj (eds), *Comorbidity of Mental and Physical Disorders* (pp. 114–28). Basel: Karger. doi:10.1159/000365543

Haber, P.S. & Day, C.A. (2014). Overview of substance use and treatment from Australia. *Journal of Substance Abuse*, 35(3), 304–8. Retrieved from http://dx.doi.org.ez.library.latrobe.edu.au/10.1080/08897077.2014.924466

Healey, J. (2016). *Methamphetamine Use and Addiction*. Thirroul, NSW: The Spinney Press. Retrieved from http://ebookcentral.proquest.com/lib/latrobe/details.action?docID=4602925.

Hendershot, C.S., Witkiewitz, K., George, W.H. & Marlatt, G.A. (2011). Relapse prevention for addictive behaviors. *Substance Abuse Treatment, Prevention, and Policy*, 6, 17. http://doi.org/10.1186/1747-597X-6-17

Hunt, G.E., Siegfried, N., Morley, K., Sitharthan, T. & Cleary, M. (2013). Psychosocial interventions for people with both severe mental illness and substance misuse. *Cochrane Library*. doi:10.1002/14651858.CD001088.pub3

Kelly, J.F., Saitz, R. & Wakeman, S. (2016). Language, substance use disorders, and policy: the need to reach a consensus on an 'addiction-ary'. *Alcoholism Treatment Quarterly*, 34(1), 116–23. http://dx.doi.org/10.1080/07347324.2016.1113103

Kelly, T.M. & Daley, D.C. (2013). Integrated treatment of substance use and psychiatric disorders. *Social Work in Public Health*, 28, 388–406.

Kessler, R.C., Berglund, P., Delmer, O., Jin, R., Merikangas, K.R. & Walters, E.E. (2005). Lifetime Prevalence and Age-of-onset Distributions of DSM-IV Disorders in the National Comorbidity Survey Replication. *Archives of General Psychiatry*, 62(6) 593-602. DOI:10.1001/archpsyc.62.6.593.

Lind, K.E., Gutierrez, E.J., Yamamoto, D.J., Regner, M.F., McKee, S.A. & Tanabe, J. (2017). Sex disparities in substance abuse research: Evaluating 23 years of structural neuroimaging studies. *Drug and Alcohol Dependence*. 173, 92–8.

Lopatko, O., McLean, S., Saunders, J., Young, R., Robinson, G. & Conigrave, K. (2009). Chapter 10. Alcohol. In G. Hulse, J. White & G. Cape (eds), *Management of Alcohol and Drug Problems*. Melbourne: Oxford University Press (pp. 158–211).

Malone, D. & Friedman, T. (2005). Drunken patients in general hospital care. Their care and management. *Postgraduate Medical Journal*, 81(953), 161–6.

Manning, V., Arunogiri, S., Frei, M., Ridley, K., Mroz, K., Campbell, S., Lubman, D. (2018). *Alcohol and other Drug Withdrawal: Practice Guidelines*, 3rd ed. Richmond, Victoria: Turning Point. Retrieved from https://www.turningpoint.org.au/sites/default/files/inline-files/Alcohol-and-Drug-Withdrawal-Guidelines-2018.pdf

Marel, C., Mills, K.L., Kingston, R., Gournay, K., Deady, M., Kay-Lambkin, F., Baker, A. & Teeson, M. (2016). *Guidelines on the Management of Co-occurring Alcohol and Other Drugs and Mental Health Conditions in Alcohol and Other Drugs Treatment Settings* (2nd edn). Sydney: National Drug and Alcohol Research Centre, UNSW Australia. Retrieved from https://ndarc.med.unsw.edu.au/resource/guidelines-management-co-occurring-alcohol-and-other-drug-and-mental-health-conditions.

McHugh, R.K., Hearon, B.A. & Otto, M.W. (2010). Cognitive behavioral therapy for substance use disorders. *Psychiatric Clinics of North America*, 33(3), 511–25. doi:10.1016/j.psc.2010.04.012

McKetin, R., Lubman, D., Najman, J., Dawe, S., Butterworth. P. & Baker, A.L. (2014). Does methamphetamine use increase violent behaviour? Evidence from a prospective longitudinal study. *Addiction*, 109(5), pp. 798–806. doi:10.1111/add.12474

Mirijello, A., D'Angelo, C., Ferrulli, A., Vassallo, M.A., Caputo, F., Leggio, L., Gasbarrini, A. & Addolorato, G. (2015). Identification and management of alcohol withdrawal syndrome. *Drugs*, 75(4), 353–65.

Moran, R. (Florida Psychiatric Society) (2010). Late teen substance abuse [audio podcast]. Retrieved from http://www.katenagroup.org/expertsspeak/R_MORAN_MD_LATE_TEENAGE_SUBSTANCE_ABUSE_APRIL2010.mp3.

Moriarty, J., Manthorpe, J., Cornes, M. & Hussein, S. (2014). *Research Findings. Social Care Practice with Carers: What social care support is provided to family carers? What support do family carers want?* London: NIHR School for Social Care Research. Retrieved from http://www.kcl.ac.uk/sspp/policy-institute/scwru/pubs/2014/reports/NIHR-SSCR-Research-Findings-Carers-Nov-2014.pdf.

Munro, I. & Edward, K-L. (2008). Mental illness and substance use: An Australian perspective. *International Journal of Mental Health Nursing*, 17(4), 255–60. doi:10.1111/j.1447-0349.2008.00541.x

National Alliance of Advocates for Buprenorphine Treatment (NAABT). (2008). *The Words We Use Matter. Reducing Stigma through Language*. Retrieved from https://www.naabt.org/documents/NAABT_Language.pdf.

National Centre for Education and Training on Addiction (NCETA) Consortium. (2004). *Alcohol and Other Drugs: A Handbook for Health Professionals*. Canberra: Australian Government Department of Health and Ageing. Retrieved from http://nceta.flinders.edu.au/files/3012/5548/2429/EN199.pdf.

National Health and Medical Research Council (NHMRC). (2009). *Australian Guidelines to Reduce Health Risk from Drinking Alcohol*. Canberra: NHMRC. Retrieved from https://nhmrc.gov.au/about-us/publications/australian-guidelines-reduce-health-risks-drinking-alcohol. © Commonwealth of Australia 2018. Released under CC BY 3.0 AU. Link to license: https://creativecommons.org/licenses/by/3.0/au/.

National Institute on Drug Abuse (NIDA). (2007). *The Neurobiology of Drug Addiction 10: Addiction vs Dependence*. North Bethesda, MD: NIDA. Retrieved from https://www.drugabuse.gov/publications/teaching-packets/neurobiology-drug-addiction/section-iii-action-heroin-morphine/10-addiction-vs-dependence.

National Institute on Drug Abuse (NIDA). (2014). *Drugs, Brains, and Behavior: The Science of Addiction*. North Bethesda, MD: NIDA.

Retrieved from https://www.drugabuse.gov/sites/default/files/soa_2014.pdf.

National LGBTI Health Alliance. (2016). *Snapshot of Mental Health and Suicide Prevention Statistics for LGBTI People.* Sydney: National LGBTI Health Alliance. Retrieved from http://lgbtihealth.org.au/wp-content/uploads/2016/07/SNAPSHOT-Mental-Health-and-Suicide-Prevention-Outcomes-for-LGBTI-people-and-communities.pdf.

NSW Government. (2008). *Drug and Alcohol Withdrawal Clinical Practice Guidelines – NSW.* Sydney: Ministry of Health, NSW. Retrieved from https://www1.health.nsw.gov.au/pds/ActivePDSDocuments/GL2008_011.pdf.

Osborne, C.J. & Thombs, D.L. (2013). *Introduction to Addictive Behaviors* (4th edn). New York: Guilford Publishing.

Oxford Dictionaries online. Retrieved from http://www.oxforddictionaries.com.

Pace, C.A. & Samet, J.H. (2016). Substance use disorders. *Annals of Internal Medicine*, 164(7), ITC49–ITC64. doi:10.7326/AITC201604050

Patrick, S.W., Dudley, J., Martin, P.R., Harrell, F.E., Warren, M.D., Hartmann, E., Wesley, E., Grijalva, C.G. & Cooper, W.O. (2015). Prescription opioid epidemic and infant outcomes. *Pediatrics*, 135(5), 842–50. doi:10.1542/peds.2014.3299

Poorolajal, J., Haghtalab, T., Farhadi, M. & Darvishi, N. (2016). Substance use disorder and risk of suicidal ideation, suicide attempt and suicide death: A meta-analysis. *Journal of Public Health*, 38(3), e282–e291. https://doi.org/10.1093/pubmed/fdv148

Prochaska, J.O., DiClemente, C.C. & Norcross, J.C. (1992). In search of how people change. Applications to addictive behaviors. *American Psychologist*, 47(9), 1102–14. doi:10.1037/0003-066X.47.9.1102

Queensland Government Metro North Mental Health – Alcohol and Drug Services. (2013). Induction Module 6 Relapse Prevention and Management. Retrieved from http://insightqld.org/wp-content/uploads/2016/01/Relapse-Prevention-and-Management-Module.pdf.

Ritter, A., King, T. & Hamilton, M. (2013). *Drug Use in Australian Society*. Sydney: Oxford University Press.

Ritter, A., Matthew-Simmons, F. & Carragher, N. (2012). *Prevalence of and Interventions for Mental Health and Alcohol and Other Drug Problems amongst the Gay, Lesbian, Bisexual and Transgender Community: A Review of the Literature.* Sydney: National Drug and Alcohol Research Centre. Retrieved from https://ndarc.med.unsw.edu.au/sites/default/files/ndarc/resources/23%20Prevalence%20of%20%26%20interventions%20for%20mental%20health%20%26%20alcohol%20and%20other%20drug%20problems%20amongst%20the%20GLBT%20community%20-%20lit%20review.pdf.

Sachdeva, A., Choudhary, M. & Chandra, M. (2015). Alcohol withdrawal syndrome: Benzodiazepines and beyond. *Journal of Clinical and Diagnostic Research,* 9(9), VE01–VE07.

Schuckit, M. A. (2014). Recognition and management of withdrawal delirium (delirium tremens). *New England Journal of Medicine*, 371(22), 2109-2113. doi:10.1056/NEJMra1407298

Sinha, R. (2013). The clinical neurobiology of drug craving. *Current Opinion in Neurobiology*, 23(4), 649–54. http://doi.org/10.1016/j.conb.2013.05.001

US Department of Health and Human Services (HHS), Office of the Surgeon General. (2016). *Facing Addiction in America: The Surgeon General's Report on Alcohol, Drugs, and Health.* Washington, DC: HHS.

Usher, K., Jackson, D., Woods, C., Sayers, J., Kornhaber, R. & Cleary, M. (2017). Safety, risk, and aggression: Health professionals' experiences of caring for people affected by methamphetamine when presenting for emergency care. *International Journal of Mental Health Nursing*, 26(5), 437–44. doi:10.1111/inm.12345

Victorian State Government. (2018). *Clinician Guide to the Victorian AOD Intake and Assessment Tools.* Retrieved from https://www2.health.vic.gov.au/alcohol-and-drugs/aod-treatment-services/pathways-into-aod-treatment/intake-assessment-for-aod-treatment.

Wilkinson, R. & Marmot, M. (2003). *The Social Determinants of Health* (2nd edn). World Health Organization, Europe. Retrieved from http://www.euro.who.int/__data/assets/pdf_file/0005/98438/e81384.pdf.

Wilson, M., Stearne, A., Gray, D. & Saggers, S. (2010). The harmful use of alcohol amongst Indigenous Australians. *Australian Indigenous Health Bulletin,* 10(3).

World Health Organization (WHO). (2010). *ATLAS on Substance Use. Resources for the Prevention and Treatment of Substance Use Disorders.* Retrieved from http://apps.who.int/iris/bitstream/10665/44455/1/9789241500616_eng.pdf.

World Health Organization (WHO). (2014). *Australia: Alcohol Consumption: Levels and Patterns.* Retrieved from http://www.who.int/substance_abuse/publications/global_alcohol_report/profiles/aus.pdf.

World Health Organization (WHO). (2016a). *Hazardous Use. Definition.* Retrieved from http://www.who.int/substance_abuse/terminology/definition3/en.

World Health Organization (WHO). (2016b). *Harmful Use. Definition.* Retrieved from http://www.who.int/substance_abuse/terminology/definition2/en.

World Health Organization (WHO). (2017). *Management of Substance Abuse.* Retrieved from http://www.who.int/substance_abuse/terminology/abuse/en.

World Health Organization (WHO). (2018). Information sheet on opioid overdose. Retrieved from http://www.who.int/substance_abuse/information-sheet/en.

Wu, C.-S., Jew, C.P. & Lu, H.-C. (2011). Lasting impacts of prenatal cannabis exposure and the role of endogenous cannabinoids in the developing brain. *Future Neurology*, 6(4), 459–80. Retrieved from https://www.ncbi.nlm.nih.gov/pmc/articles/PMC3252200/www2.health.vic.gov.au/alcohol-and-drugs.

CHAPTER 15

NEURODEVELOPMENTAL DISORDERS

Gylo Hercelinskyj and Russell Fremantle

LEARNING FROM PRACTICE

As a baby, my grandson looked normal and seemed to be developing in line with other babies. It was only as he got older that we began to notice that he was not progressing like other children. At 10, he does not communicate verbally and he also shows other characteristics or behaviours associated with children diagnosed with autism spectrum disorder. But does he fit the picture so often portrayed in the media? No!

Last Christmas, after everyone had eaten and exchanged presents (which he participated in), my grandson came over and took my hand. He led me to the coffee table and pointed at a box sitting underneath – it was a box of Christmas crackers. I had forgotten to bring them out. I looked at my grandson and said, 'Well, we had better open them now!' He watched as I handed each bonbon out to family members and even helped break them with his parents. When we had finished he took himself off to his favourite 'chill out' spot in our house – the library. My grandson may not speak in the way we presume to be normal, but he communicates. He may not initiate interaction on every occasion, but he knew that those crackers were part of the tradition and he let me know this. He likes the beach, the colour yellow, bubble machines and having stories read to him. We know this because he communicates with us.

So, while he has a diagnosis of autism spectrum disorder, I can confidently say that autism is not an 'all or nothing' condition. There are degrees, or as the medical world would say, it is a spectrum disorder. My grandson shows us this every day.

Gyn, grandparent of a young boy diagnosed with autism spectrum disorder

After reading Gyn's story, does her description match your current understanding of autism spectrum disorder? Is it reasonable to expect that all communication between people must involve speaking? How can mental health nurses support individuals and families living with a diagnosis of ASD?

INTRODUCTION

In the opening vignette, Gyn has described some of the joys of being a grandparent. Yet Gyn's story is one that many people may not have experienced. There is an expectation that when a child is born, their development will follow a particular progression. Developmental milestones usually give an age range where certain physical, emotional and social skills and competencies will develop. Common examples include walking, speech development, and developing increasing complexity in thinking and reasoning abilities.

When a child does not meet the 'normal', anticipated milestones and demonstrates delays or deficits of behaviour, social skills and communication, families can be left searching for answers. Sometimes these answers can take time to find and families may be left to struggle on as best they can without information. When a diagnosis is confirmed, families will go through a period of transition. Diagnosis will impact on everyone, both individually and as a family group, and they will need information on accessing support and services.

This chapter explores a number of neurodevelopmental disorders that are classified in the *Diagnostic and Statistical Manual of Mental Disorders* (DSM-5; APA, 2013). The chapter describes the types of conditions, their aetiology, clinical course and management options, and explores some ways in which mental health nurses can support families and consumers, always keeping in mind the person with the diagnosis and their families.

NEURODEVELOPMENTAL DISORDERS

Broadly, neurodevelopmental disorders are conditions that result from impairments to the brain or central nervous system (CNS) development. This results in a failure to meet expected cognitive, behavioural or social developmental milestones. A narrower use of the term applies to disorders to brain function or the CNS that affect emotion, learning ability, self-control or memory, and that become apparent as a child grows. The DSM-5 (APA, 2013) classifies a number of neurodevelopmental disorders which typically become apparent as a child grows and develops, in particular prior to commencing formal education. Neurodevelopmental disorders include:

- attention deficit/hyperactivity disorder (ADHD)
- autism spectrum disorder (ASD)
- intellectual disability (intellectual developmental disorder; ID)

- tic disorder, incorporating Tourette's disorder, persistent (chronic) motor or vocal tic disorder, provisional tic disorder and other specified and unspecified tic disorders.

It is also known that the co-occurrence of neurodevelopmental disorders is common; for example, a child diagnosed with autism spectrum disorder can also have a diagnosis of an intellectual disability (intellectual developmental disorder) (APA, 2013).

ATTENTION DEFICIT/HYPERACTIVITY DISORDER

Essentially, ADHD is a condition in which a child experiences poor concentration and impulse control. The child demonstrates difficulty in concentration, impulsive behaviour and overactivity. This can impact significantly on educational outcomes, social skills and family functioning. ADHD is a condition where collaboration between health care professionals, family and educational providers is essential to promote best outcomes for children. Treatment strategies involve both behavioural strategies and pharmacological treatment (Caye, Swanson, Coghill & Rhode, 2019; Royal Children's Hospital, 2012b).

Aetiology and epidemiology

Capusan et al. (2019) drew upon twin analysis to determine the role of additive genetic and non-shared environmental factors and found a significant association between children of adults with alcohol dependence and a higher risk of ADHD. There is evidence that multiple genetic, neurobiological and environmental risk factors (such as foetal alcohol exposure) are linked with pathology and development of ADHD; that is, the aetiology of ADHD comprises a highly complex relationship between genetic and environmental factors.

Determining epidemiological data in relation to ADHD has been confounded by changes in DSM-5 (APA, 2013) criteria for ADHD. However, the Royal Australasian College of Physicians (2006) puts prevalence at 5–10% (Lawrence et al., 2015). One study, involving 6300 Australian families, found that ADHD was the number one prevalent mental health condition in children aged four to 17 years (Lawrence et al., 2015) (see also **Figure 15.1**).

Diagnostic criteria for ADHD

Lawrence et al. (2015) defined ADHD as a persistent pattern of inattention and/or hyperactivity-impulsivity that interferes with functioning or development. The DSM-5 (APA, 2013) diagnostic criteria for ADHD are outlined in **Table 15.1**.

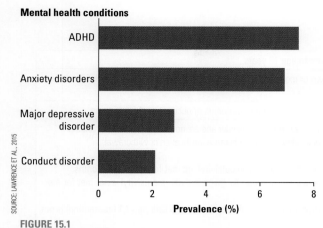

Mental health conditions

SOURCE: LAWRENCE ET AL. 2015

FIGURE 15.1
Prevalence of mental health conditions in any 12-month period in 4–17 year olds

Pharmacological management

Since the 1980s, amphetamines have become a standard treatment for children with ADHD with approximately 1–2% being prescribed stimulants.

One of the common amphetamines prescribed for ADHD in Australia is methylphenidate hydrochloride (Ritalin). These medications require a permit to prescribe and are among the most highly researched medications prescribed for children. Amphetamines are believed to improve concentration and impulse control and decrease overactivity in about 80% of children with ADHD. Nurses should be aware that there are short-acting (e.g. Ritalin 10) and long-acting variants (e.g. Ritalin LA).

The main side effects of amphetamines are decreased appetite and weight loss. Less common side effects include gastrointestinal (GI) upset, headaches, dizziness

DIAGNOSTIC CRITERIA

Attention deficit/hyperactivity disorder (ADHD)

TABLE 15.1
Diagnostic criteria attention deficit/hyperactivity disorder (ADHD)

A. A persistent pattern of inattention and/or hyperactivity-impulsivity that interferes with functioning or development, as characterized by (1) and/or (2):

1. Inattention: Six (or more) of the following symptoms have persisted for at least 6 months to a degree that is inconsistent with developmental level and that negatively impacts directly on social and academic/occupational activities:

Note: The symptoms are not solely a manifestation of oppositional behavior, defiance, hostility, or failure to understand tasks or instructions. For older adolescents and adults (age 17 and older), at least five symptoms are required.

  a. Often fails to give close attention to details or makes careless mistakes in schoolwork, at work, or during other activities (e.g., overlooks or misses details, work is inaccurate).

  b. Often has difficulty sustaining attention in tasks or play activities (e.g., has difficulty remaining focused during lectures, conversations, or lengthy reading).

  c. Often does not seem to listen when spoken to directly (e.g., mind seems elsewhere, even in the absence of any obvious distraction).

  d. Often does not follow through on instructions and fails to finish schoolwork, chores, or duties in the workplace (e.g., starts tasks but quickly loses focus and is easily sidetracked).

  e. Often has difficulty organizing tasks and activities (e.g., difficulty managing sequential tasks; difficulty keeping materials and belongings in order; messy, disorganized work; has poor time management; fails to meet deadlines).

  f. Often avoids, dislikes, or is reluctant to engage in tasks that require sustained mental effort (e.g., schoolwork or homework; for older adolescents and adults, preparing reports, completing forms, reviewing lengthy papers).

  g. Often loses things necessary for tasks or activities (e.g., school materials, pencils, books, tools, wallets, keys, paperwork, eyeglasses, mobile telephones).

  h. Is often easily distracted by extraneous stimuli (for older adolescents and adults, may include unrelated thoughts).

  i. Is often forgetful in daily activities (e.g., doing chores, running errands; for older adolescents and adults, returning calls, paying bills, keeping appointments).

2. Hyperactivity and **impulsivity:** Six (or more) of the following symptoms have persisted for at least 6 months to a degree that is inconsistent with developmental level and that negatively impacts directly on social and academic/occupational activities:

Note: The symptoms are not solely a manifestation of oppositional behavior, defiance, hostility, or a failure to understand tasks or instructions. For older adolescents and adults (age 17 and older), at least five symptoms are required.

  a. Often fidgets with or taps hands or feet or squirms in seat.

  b. Often leaves seat in situations when remaining seated is expected (e.g., leaves his or her place in the classroom, in the office or other workplace, or in other situations that require remaining in place).

  c. Often runs about or climbs in situations where it is inappropriate. (**Note:** In adolescents or adults, may be limited to feeling restless.)

  d. Often unable to play or engage in leisure activities quietly.

  e. Is often "on the go," acting as if "driven by a motor" (e.g., is unable to be or uncomfortable being still for extended time, as in restaurants, meetings; may be experienced by others as being restless or difficult to keep up with).

  f. Often talks excessively.

  g. Often blurts out an answer before a question has been completed (e.g., completes people's sentences; cannot wait for turn in conversation).

  h. Often has difficulty waiting his or her turn (e.g., while waiting in line).

  i. Often interrupts or intrudes on others (e.g., butt's into conversations, games, or activities; may start using other people's things without asking or receiving permission; for adolescents and adults, may intrude into or take over what others are doing).

TABLE 15.1
(Continued)

B.	Several inattentive or hyperactive-impulsive symptoms were present prior to age 12 years.
C.	Several inattentive or hyperactive-impulsive symptoms are present in two or more settings (e.g., at home, school, or work; with friends or relatives; in other activities).
D.	There is clear evidence that the symptoms interfere with, or reduce the quality of, social, academic, or occupational functioning.
E.	The symptoms do not occur exclusively during the course of schizophrenia or another psychotic disorder and are not better explained by another mental disorder (e.g., mood disorder, anxiety disorder, dissociative disorder, personality disorder, substance intoxication or withdrawal).

Specify whether:
- **Combined presentation:** If both Criterion A1 (inattention) and Criterion A2 (hyperactivity-impulsivity) are met for the past 6 months.
- **Predominantly inattentive presentation:** If Criterion A1 (inattention) is met but Criterion A2 (hyperactivity-impulsivity) is not met for the past 6 months.
- **Predominantly hyperactive/impulsive presentation:** If Criterion A2 (hyperactivity-impulsivity) is met and Criterion A1 (inattention) is not met for the past 6 months.

Specify if:

in partial remission: When full criteria were previously met, fewer than the full criteria have been met for the past 6 months, and the symptoms still result in impairment in social, academic, or occupational functioning.

Specify current severity:
- **Mild:** Few, if any, symptoms in excess of those required to make the diagnosis are present, and symptoms result in no more than minor impairments in social or occupational functioning.
- **Moderate:** Symptoms or functional impairment between "mild" and "severe" are present.
- **Severe:** Many symptoms in excess of those required to make the diagnosis, or several symptoms that are particularly severe, are present, or the symptoms result in marked impairment in social or occupational functioning.

and sleep disturbance; irritability and emotional lability are also known. Side effects are often dose related and in many circumstances can be managed by changing the dose or timing of administration; fortunately, dexamphetamine can be ceased without weaning. Children taking amphetamines should be regularly monitored by their doctor (APA, 2013).

Non-pharmacological management

Collaborative care planning and management is made through observation of behaviour and reports from parents and/or teachers. Caye and colleagues (2019) outline a number of non-pharmacological strategies, including behavioural and psychosocial approaches, cognitive training and even dietary modifications. While taking into account and giving due consideration to third-party reports, it is essential to perform an extensive nursing assessment in order to identify issues and formulate nursing care plans with consumers and their families. Due to the complex nature of ADHD, individualised care planning is essential and will result in varied plans and strategies.

CASE STUDY

A CARE PLAN FOR JAMES

James is nine years old and has recently been diagnosed with ADHD. James' behaviour has always been described as erratic and impulsive. His progress at school has been poor. Teachers describe that he has difficulty concentrating and is not reading or writing at the expected standard for his age. Socially, James is described as disruptive in class and regularly gets into fights with other children. His parents also indicate that when James becomes frustrated he behaves aggressively by either biting, hitting out or throwing objects.

Based on the case study, **Table 15.2** outlines a possible nursing care plan for James.

Questions

1. How can the school nurse support James' family?
2. What other treatments might be helpful for James?
3. What are the potential impacts for James related to his schooling and social interactions?

TABLE 15.2
ADHD care plan for James

ASSESSMENT	NURSING DIAGNOSIS	PLAN	IMPLEMENTATION	EVALUATION
Cannot remain still, frequently moving. Unable to concentrate.	Risk of injury related to hyperactivity secondary to ADHD.	Provide a safe area to play and discuss management with a parent.	Cleared room, relocated sharps container, provided soft toys and spoke with child's mother.	The child played with toys with occasional direction from mother. Ability to concentrate and follow mother's directions improved.

Examples of other behavioural strategies that can be useful when developing care plans are outlined in **Table 15.3**.

TABLE 15.3
Useful behavioural strategies for developing nursing care plans for people with ADHD

AIM	STRATEGIES
Communication skills	• Clear communication using short concise words • Maintain eye contact • Ensuring understanding of communication by asking the child to repeat instructions
Reduce over-stimulation and fatigue	• Ensure appropriate rest times throughout the day. Ensure there is a balance between academic activity with exercise
Build self-esteem	• Provide opportunities where the child can experience success. • Set achievable goals. Often it helps to break down a task into smaller components (particularly if it is a complex task).
Develop social skills	• Provide opportunities to build skills in smaller group activities. • Implement programs that teach interactions skills. • Provide positive reinforcement when social interactions are successful.

SOURCE: ADAPTED FROM ROYAL CHILDREN'S HOSPITAL, 2018

INTELLECTUAL DISABILITY (INTELLECTUAL DISABILITY DISORDER)

Key characteristics of intellectual disabilities (also referred to as intellectual disability disorder in the DSM-5) are deficits in general mental abilities such as reasoning, problem-solving, planning, abstract thinking, learning and learning from doing (APA, 2013). Various definitions of intellectual disability focus on deficits in intellectual functioning and behaviour, which are apparent by the age of 18. The impact of these deficits is seen in the difficulty that consumers have in achieving independence and taking on social responsibilities. This includes difficulties in communication, social participation, employment and personal independence.

While intelligence quotient (IQ) can be used as a measure of intellectual functioning, it is not viewed as a useful measure of adaptive functioning. Measurements of adaptive functioning are best achieved through assessing an individual's competency and social interaction functioning, understanding and capacity to pick up on social cues and performance of tasks associated with activities of daily living (Sadock, Sadock & Ruiz, 2015). The DSM-5 (APA, 2013) also refers to global developmental delay, which is diagnosed when a person does not meet expected developmental milestones in several areas of intellectual functioning. This term is used particularly when a child is too young to undertake comprehensive systematic assessment.

Aetiology and epidemiology

In an Australian Bureau of Statistics study, 2.9% of the Australian population was identified as having an intellectual disability in 2012 (ABS, 2014). This equates to approximately 670000 people. Data published in 2019 states that 1 in 5 (22%) of the Australian population have a 'mental or behavioural disorder as their main disabling condition' of which 6.3% have an intellectual or developmental disability (AIHW, 2019, p. 2). In a breakdown of these figures, intellectual disability was most commonly seen at both ends of the lifespan (the young and the old), with children from birth to 14 years of age having a prevalence rate of approximately 4% and older people (75 years of age and older) accounting for approximately 10%. The lifetime prevalence for adults aged 15–64 years is 1.3% (AIHW, 2003).

In terms of comorbid (or co-occurring) disorders, between 60–70% of children and adults who have a diagnosis of intellectual disability also have a co-occurring mental health condition (AIHW, 2008; Munir, 2016). Examples of mental health conditions include schizophrenia, mood disorders, ADHD and conduct disorder. Autism spectrum disorder (ASD), which is discussed later in the chapter, is another common co-occurring condition. Neurological disorders such as epilepsy also occur more frequently in consumers who have a diagnosis of intellectual disability. Andrews et al. (2013) also state that life expectancy is dependent on the level of severity; that is, a person with a severe level of intellectual disability can be expected to have a shorter lifespan. The Australian Institute of Health and Welfare (2008) also identified that 57% of people aged under 65 years with a diagnosis of intellectual disability disorder also had a diagnosed mental health condition. Speech problems were the most common problems reported by people with intellectual disability in 2003.

Intellectual disability can be a consequence of physical, genetic, psychosocial or environmental factors such as infection, trauma and genetic syndromes or the consequence of **teratogenic effect** of a specific pharmacological agent. These factors include:

■ Rubella is linked with the development of intellectual disability, particularly if a pregnant woman contracts rubella in the first trimester of pregnancy.

- Down syndrome and Fragile X syndrome are two genetic disorders associated with intellectual disability. Prader-Willi syndrome is also associated with intellectual disability, although this condition is less common than either Down syndrome or Fragile X syndrome.

- The human immunodeficiency virus (HIV) is also associated with intellectual disability, with some children developing seizures and showing intellectual/cognitive disability in the first 12 months following birth.

- Foetal alcohol syndrome, which results from exposure to alcohol during the antenatal period, can result in a number of consequences for the child. Beside characteristic physical features, the child can also experience learning difficulties and ADHD. Some children will also have an intellectual disability. **Cardiovascular** development is also commonly adversely affected. Perinatal influences such as drug use (other than alcohol), sustained during foetal development, and extreme premature birth can increase risk of cognitive impairment and later learning difficulties.

- Infections such as encephalitis and meningitis are associated with significant negative effects on cognitive development. Traumatic brain injury and asphyxia (e.g. near drowning) are also associated with the development of intellectual disability. Long-term exposure to lead is associated with cognitive impairment and learning difficulties (Sadock, Sadock & Ruiz, 2015).

Andrews et al. (2013) identify that there are a range of biopsychosocial determinants pertinent to the mental health of people who have a diagnosis of intellectual disability. **Figure 15.2** illustrates those factors that are relevant.

Other theories related to the aetiology of intellectual disabilities focus on genetic abnormalities, while approximately 60% of diagnoses have no attributable cause or aetiology (Ellison, Rosenfeld & Shaffer, 2013). Sadock, Sadock and Ruiz (2015) identify that very common single gene causes of intellectually disability can be identified in a mutation found in the FMR1 gene, which causes Fragile X syndrome. It is the most common and first X-linked gene to be identified as a direct cause of intellectual disability. Visible and submicroscopic abnormalities are also associated with intellectual disability (Sadock, Sadock & Ruiz, 2015).

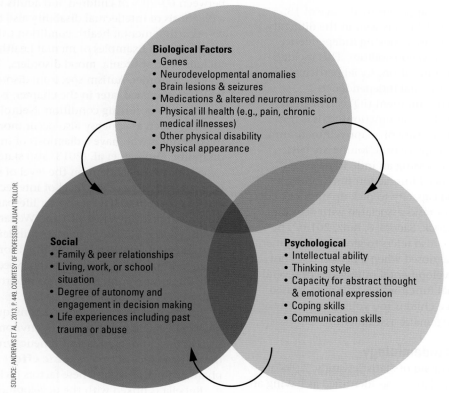

SOURCE: ANDREWS ET AL., 2013. P. 449. COURTESY OF PROFESSOR JULIAN TROLLOR.

Biological Factors
- Genes
- Neurodevelopmental anomalies
- Brain lesions & seizures
- Medications & altered neurotransmission
- Physical ill health (e.g., pain, chronic medical illnesses)
- Other physical disability
- Physical appearance

Social
- Family & peer relationships
- Living, work, or school situation
- Degree of autonomy and engagement in decision making
- Life experiences including past trauma or abuse

Psychological
- Intellectual ability
- Thinking style
- Capacity for abstract thought & emotional expression
- Coping skills
- Communication skills

FIGURE 15.2
Factors influencing the mental health of consumers diagnosed with an intellectual disability (intellectual developmental disorder)

Diagnostic criteria for intellectual disability (intellectual developmental disorder)

The DSM-5 (APA, 2013) outlines the diagnostic criteria for intellectual disability (intellectual developmental disorder) and includes three criteria. The first relates to deficits in intellectual functioning, which must be confirmed by a thorough assessment and intelligence testing. Second, there are deficits in adaptive functioning, which are seen in the person's inability to achieve the developmental and sociocultural standards required for independence and social responsibility. Finally, the onset of the intellectual and adaptive deficits occurs during the developmental period. Intellectual disability (intellectual developmental disorder) is also coded in terms of the severity of the deficit identified. Severity is classified as mild, moderate, severe or profound (APA, 2013). The degree of severity is judged by the individual's adaptive capacity, and the level of support required in order to achieve personal independence and social responsibility. The greater the level of severity, the more complex issues there are related to the consumer's intellectual disability.

The full diagnostic criteria for intellectual disability are shown in **Table 15.4**.

Table 15.5 provides an overview of factors used to specify the level of severity in intellectual disability.

DIAGNOSTIC CRITERIA

Intellectual disability (Intellectual developmental disorder)

TABLE 15.4
Diagnostic criteria intellectual disability

Intellectual disability (intellectual developmental disorder) is a disorder with onset during the developmental period that includes both intellectual and adaptive functioning deficits in conceptual, social, and practical domains. The following three criteria must be met:
A. Deficits in intellectual functions, such as reasoning, problem solving, planning, abstract thinking, judgment, academic learning, and learning from experience, confirmed by both clinical assessment and individualized, standardized intelligence testing.

B. Deficits in adaptive functioning that result in failure to meet developmental and sociocultural standards for personal independence and social responsibility. Without ongoing support, the adaptive deficits limit functioning in one or more activities of daily life, such as communication, social participation, and independent living, across multiple environments, such as home, school, work, and community.

C. Onset of intellectual and adaptive deficits during the developmental period.
Specify current severity:
- **Mild**
- **Moderate**
- **Severe**
- **Profound.**

TABLE 15.5
Factors used to specify level of severity in intellectual disability

LEVEL OF SEVERITY	CONCEPTUAL DOMAIN	SOCIAL DOMAIN	PRACTICAL DOMAIN
Mild	Greater support is required to achieve skills in reading. Thinking tends to be more concrete.	Social relationships are more concrete than would be expected at a particular developmental level. Children are often quite vulnerable and there can be increased risk of exploitation by others.	Children and adults can maintain independence in personal care and other activities of daily living. Support in making more complex decisions related to health and legal concerns and raising a family is required.
Moderate	Conceptual skills such as reading, writing and abstract thinking for a while, are behind other people.	Consumers maintain close relationships with family and others. Support and assistance is required for life decisions. Significant support required to achieve occupational success.	Consumers maintain independence in personal care, although they may require more intense repetitive support and teaching to achieve this. Strategies to assist in retention and recall are often required.
Severe	Achieving skills in reading, writing, mathematics and so forth require extensive support as the person has extreme difficulties with problem solving.	Verbal speech is limited and is more likely to involve single words or phrases as opposed to complex communication. Consumers understand speech that is simple and clear. Individuals benefit from using additional communication strategies to complement verbal communication and they enjoy communicating with familiar people.	While the consumer may be able to participate/assist in activities of daily living, they are dependent on others for aspects of personal care, health and safety. Acquiring daily living skills requires ongoing teaching and support.
Profound	Very limited development of conceptual skills.	The individual may understand simple words and gestures from others but has limited verbal capacity. The individual will communicate by non-verbal means.	The consumer is fully dependent on others for achievement of daily living tasks. The person may be able to participate and assess activities if they are not experiencing physical impairments.

Assessment and management of consumers who have a diagnosis of intellectual disability (intellectual developmental disorder)

In general, consumers with co-occurring intellectual disability and a mental health condition will be treated within a mental health service for a small percentage of the time. The primary goal is to link consumers with appropriate primary health care and community mental health (Andrews et al., 2013). The degree to which specialist services can enhance individual treatment plans will depend on the level of severity of the consumer's intellectual disability, the presence of co-occurring mental health conditions, and contact, liaison and collaboration between all parties who provide care and support to the individual.

Andrews et al. (2013) acknowledge that one of the difficulties in accurately assessing the occurrence of the mental health condition is when symptoms are inaccurately assumed to be part of the individual's intellectual disability. This is referred to as **diagnostic overshadowing** (a term that is also used in relation to the presence of physical symptoms being mistakenly presumed to be the result of a consumer's mental health condition) and highlights the need for mental health clinicians to have appropriate knowledge and experience in working with consumers who have a co-occurring intellectual disability and mental health condition. Important strategies to remember when involved in the assessment include:

- A person-centred/recovery-oriented approach is essential. Principles such as obtaining consent (in situations where this is not possible then obtaining consent from the appropriately designated person), maintaining the consumer's dignity and respect, providing real choices, and collaborating with the consumer to the greatest extent possible are crucial.
- Adapt the assessment as required, which can include assessment being conducted over several sessions.
- Adapt communication to the needs and capacity of the consumer. Keeping language clear, avoiding jargon, being concise and offering a choice of responses may be useful strategies.
- Access other sources of information if required, such as school records, residential facility feedback or information from families/carers (adapted from Andrews et al., 2013).

Non-pharmacological management for a consumer who has a diagnosis of intellectual disability

Chapter 3 explored the requirements of informed consent and capacity. A person with an intellectual disability must be involved in conversations and the decision-making process to a level where their capacity enables them to be involved. If a consumer does not demonstrate capacity, then appropriate appointed persons as identified under the relevant legislation would be involved.

One area that requires a multidisciplinary approach is **challenging behaviours**. Challenging behaviours are defined later in this chapter under the discussion of autism spectrum disorder (ASD). Examples of challenging behaviours include non-suicidal self-injury, aggression towards others and property, socially inappropriate behaviours, repetitive behaviour such as excessive rocking, and withdrawal from specific activities (Woods, 2011). Ali, Blickwedel and Hassiotis (2014) identify a number of common causes for challenging behaviours. **Table 15.6** lists a number of causes of challenging behaviour and some examples of them.

TABLE 15.6
Causes and examples of challenging behaviour

CAUSES OF CHALLENGING BEHAVIOUR	EXAMPLES
Physiological factors	• Constipation • Dental pain • Menstruation • Headache
Mental health conditions	• Mood disorders • Anxiety disorders • Autism spectrum disorder • Psychotic disorder
Behavioural phenotypes	• Fragile X syndrome • Prader-Willi syndrome
Psychosocial factors	• Traumatic events • Stress
Meeting needs	• To gain attention from carers • To avoid tasks or activities

SOURCE: ALI, BLICKWEDEL & HASSIOTIS, 2014

While behaviours may be labelled as challenging, it is essential to understand that all behaviours, including those behaviours defined as challenging, serve as a means of communication and represent the interaction of the individual with their social and physical environment (Ali, Blickwedel & Hassiotis, 2014). The main principles of managing challenging behaviours include the assessment of underlying causative factors, such as communication difficulties, triggering factors and physiological factors. All of this information becomes integrated into what is referred to as a behavioural management plan. Psychological therapies are also preferred first-line management approaches for consumers with a diagnosis of intellectual disability. Adaptations of cognitive behavioural therapy (CBT), dialectical behaviour therapy, mindfulness, positive behavioural support and environmental adaptation are some approaches cited in the literature (Ali et al., 2014; Crossland, Hewitt & Walden, 2017; Trollor, Salomon & Franklin, 2016).

Pharmacological treatment

There are no specific pharmacological treatments for intellectual disability. The use of medications is considered when a consumer experiences either a co-occurring physical and/or mental health condition. Andrews et al. (2013) state that the use of psychotropic medications should be limited to situations where the consumer demonstrates clear symptoms of a mental health condition. Trollor, Salomon and Franklin (2016) also state that psychological and behavioural interventions such as mindfulness and CBT are the most commonly preferred first-line methods of treatment. When the decision is made to administer psychotropic medications, this should only be done after a thorough assessment is completed. Particular attention needs to be paid to the high number of co-occurring conditions that the consumer with a diagnosis of intellectual disability may have. For example, some psychotropic drugs lower the seizure threshold, and therefore they should not be prescribed to a consumer who has a co-occurring diagnosis of epilepsy. From a nursing perspective, it is essential that mental health nurses understand that the diagnosis of intellectual disability can be associated with a range of other complex neurodevelopmental, physical and/or congenital disorders, and adverse reactions can occur due to the heightened sensitivity to psychotropic medication. Understanding and the ability to recognise adverse reactions is a key nursing responsibility.

AUTISM SPECTRUM DISORDER

Autism spectrum disorder (ASD) is identified by persistent deficits in social interaction and social communication. Also key to a diagnosis of ASD is the presence of restricted, repetitive patterns of behaviour interests or activities. ASD is conceptualised as being on a continuum (or spectrum), with the manifestations of the disorder varying depending on the consumer's developmental level, age and the severity of the disorder. Parents will often become aware that their child's responses to them and other family members does not fit with what is expected. Diagnosis requires information from multiple sources, including formal assessments and family feedback. Verbal and non-verbal communication difficulties exist to varying degrees. For example, some consumers diagnosed with ASD have no verbal communication in terms of recognisable speech, but they may communicate verbally with a range of sounds, while other consumers will have delayed speech development. The DSM-5 also states that even when formal speech has been developed, it is not used in the context of social interaction (APA, 2013).

The DSM-5 diagnostic criteria for ASD are listed in **Table 15.7**.

DIAGNOSTIC CRITERIA

Autism spectrum disorder (ASD)

TABLE 15.7
Diagnostic criteria autism spectrum disorder (ASD)

A. Persistent deficits in social communication and social interaction across multiple contexts, as manifested by all of the following, currently or by history (examples are illustrative, not exhaustive; see text):
   1. Deficits in social-emotional reciprocity, ranging, for example, from abnormal social approach and failure of normal back-and-forth conversation; to reduced sharing of interests, emotions, or affect; to failure to initiate or respond to social interactions.
   2. Deficits in nonverbal communicative behaviors used for social interaction, ranging, for example, from poorly integrated verbal and nonverbal communication; to abnormalities in eye contact and body language or deficits in understanding and use of gestures; to a total lack of facial expressions and nonverbal communication.
   3. Deficits in developing, maintaining, and understanding relationships, ranging, for example, from difficulties adjusting behavior to suit various social contexts; to difficulties in sharing imaginative play or in making friends; to absence of interest in peers.

B. Restricted, repetitive patterns of behavior, interests, or activities, as manifested by at least two of the following, currently or by history (examples are illustrative, not exhaustive; see text):
   1. Stereotyped or repetitive motor movements, use of objects, or speech (e.g., simple motor stereotypes, lining up toys or flipping objects, echolalia, idiosyncratic phrases).
   2. Insistence on sameness, inflexible adherence to routines, or ritualized patterns of verbal or nonverbal behavior (e.g., extreme distress at small changes, difficulties with transitions, rigid thinking patterns, greeting rituals, need to take same route or eat same food every day).
   3. Highly restricted, fixated interests that are abnormal in intensity or focus (e.g., strong attachment to or preoccupation with unusual objects, excessively circumscribed or perseverative interests).
   4. Hyper- or hypo reactivity to sensory input or unusual interest in sensory aspects of the environment (e.g., apparent indifference to pain/temperature, adverse response to specific sounds or textures, excessive smelling or touching of objects, visual fascination with lights or movement).

TABLE 15.7
(Continued)

C.	Symptoms must be present in the early developmental period (but may not become fully manifest until social demands exceed limited capacities, or may be masked by learned strategies in later life).
D.	Symptoms cause clinically significant impairment in social, occupational, or other important areas of current functioning.
E.	These disturbances are not better explained by intellectual disability (intellectual developmental disorder) or global developmental delay. Intellectual disability and autism spectrum disorder frequently co-occur; to make comorbid diagnoses of autism spectrum disorder and intellectual disability, social communication should be below that expected for general developmental level.

Note: Individuals with a well-established DSM-IV diagnosis of autistic disorder, Asperger's disorder, or pervasive developmental disorder not otherwise specified should be given the diagnosis of autism spectrum disorder. Individuals who have marked deficits in social communication, but whose symptoms do not otherwise meet criteria for autism spectrum disorder, should be evaluated for social (pragmatic) communication disorder.
Specify if:
- **With or without accompanying intellectual impairment**
- **With or without accompanying language impairment**
- **Associated with a known medical or genetic condition or environmental factor**
- **Associated with another neurodevelopmental, mental, or behavioral disorder**
- **With catatonia.**

CLINICAL **OBSERVATIONS**

Changes to the classification of Asperger's disorder and developmental delay

With the release of the DSM-5 (APA, 2013), there has been a great deal of debate regarding the incorporation of Asperger's disorder and developmental delay into a broader diagnostic classification of ASD. One of the major concerns relates to funding of services for consumers previously diagnosed with Asperger's syndrome or pervasive developmental delay-not otherwise specified (PDD-NOS). In practice, consumers previously diagnosed with Asperger's syndrome or PDD-NOS retain this diagnosis for practical purposes, but from a diagnostic classification perspective they come under the role of ASD. Consumers newly diagnosed are done so under the classification. Children previously diagnosed with PDD-NOS would in most instances continue to meet the criteria for a diagnosis of ASD.

Aetiology and epidemiology

Approximately 164000 Australians have a diagnosis of ASD according to the ABS (2017), but the Australian Medical Association has suggested that the actual number of people diagnosed with autism is well over 200000 (AMA, 2016). Autism spectrum disorders are more common in males than females. **Figure 15.3** shows the prevalence of ASD diagnosis according to age in 2009, 2012 and 2015.

Theories related to the aetiology of ASD include genetic and epigenetic factors, prenatal and perinatal factors, hormonal and immunological factors (Sadock, Sadock & Ruiz, 2015). Approximately 20% of individuals who have a diagnosis of ASD have an identified genetic aetiology. These include chromosomal abnormalities and other genetic disorders which are associated with ASD, including Fragile X syndrome, Down syndrome and Prader-Willi syndrome (Betancur & Coleman, 2013). Researchers in 2010 looked at identifying common risk factors for ASD and identified five common **alleles** for ASD across a sample of 1558 families. Overall, the evidence suggests that ASD results from a constellation of genetic factors rather than one single genetic cause (Giarelli & Gardner, 2012). A range of risk factors have also been associated with ASD. These risk factors include being older parents, pre-term birth, foetal exposure to valproate, and low birth weight.

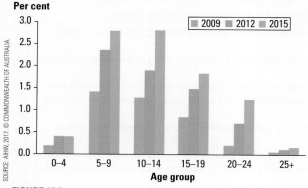

FIGURE 15.3
Prevalence of autism according to age

Research dating from the 1970s has also identified a strong hereditary component in ASD. The concordance rate for ASD is shown to be much higher in **monozygotic twins** than **dizygotic twins**. Concord rates have varied between 37–90% in a number of studies completed; the key points being that in all studies the rate was much higher in monozygotic twins compared with dizygotic twins (APA, 2013).

Clinical course

ASD is a lifelong condition and parents can notice some of the behavioural features associated with ASD early in their child's development. ASD is diagnosed in boys more frequently than girls (APA, 2013). Many parents notice delayed speech development in their child. However, it is not uncommon for children, particularly boys, to have delayed speech up until approximately two years of age, so parents will often wait, thinking that their child may in fact be a slow talker. The DSM-5 (APA, 2013) states that symptoms are generally recognised between 12 and 24 months of age. Symptoms can also be recognised earlier or later, usually reflecting the severity of the symptoms (APA, 2013). Delayed language development is usually the first indication of the possibility of a diagnosis of autism or the child may also demonstrate a lack of social interest in other people. Autism spectrum disorder is not a degenerative condition, although as parents journey through the process of recognising their child's development is not meeting milestones and adjusting to a diagnosis of ASD, it may seem that the child will not be able to move forward in their development. However, the child with a diagnosis of ASD will continue to learn and adapt to their environment. Symptoms are most obvious in early childhood and school years, with improvements in areas such as social interaction being seen in later school. In adulthood, it is more realistic to expect a person with ASD will need varying degrees of support. Social and occupational independence is usually only likely for consumers who have high-level language and intellectual abilities (APA, 2013).

Comorbidity

Comorbid (or co-occurring) conditions associated with ASD include a number of developmental psychiatric and neurological diagnoses. Examples include ADHD, intellectual disability, epilepsy, Fragile X syndrome (as mentioned previously), anxiety disorders and depression.

Management of ASD

Management options and strategies for a consumer who has received a diagnosis of ASD focus on non-pharmacological and pharmacological interventions where required. Key to effective management is a multidisciplinary approach between clinicians, other service delivery organisations (such as schools or disability services), family, carers and the consumer.

Non-pharmacological management

Accurate diagnosis of ASD is crucial to effective management and support of consumers and their family. Non-pharmacological approaches to management involve educational and behavioural interventions. Because ASD is such a diverse condition, it is not possible to say that one approach will meet the needs of an individual. And because a person diagnosed with ASD lives within their family context, the family will have developed their own unique way of traversing the challenges associated with ASD. Therefore, management must be an integrated approach that involves the consumer, their family, education providers and health care professionals. No one treatment plan will work for every person.

The core feature of any management plan is to build on the individual's strengths and abilities, promote confidence, and build self-esteem and resilience. The approaches described here are central to working with consumers and families. Educational interventions include specialist schools for children and older students with ASD. Education is provided through a structured curriculum, aimed at expanding children's knowledge and skills as well as their understanding of the broader community. Additional support and learning opportunities are integrated as required for students and are developed to meet the specific learning needs of the child who has a diagnosis of ASD.

Managing challenging behaviours

Challenging behaviours include aggression, self-harm or harm towards other people. It may appear that this type of behaviour is spontaneous, having no identifiable cause; however, challenging behaviour always occurs because of some underlying reason. Interventions for addressing challenging behaviours have been reframed as positive behaviour support by Autism Spectrum Australia (2017) and this refers to a range of strategies based on learning theory. Ideas around positive behaviour support are outlined below.

As members of the multidisciplinary team, mental health nurses will contribute to the overall care planning and support for consumers and families living with a diagnosis of ASD. This begins with a thorough assessment relevant to the consumer's developmental level (Giarelli & Gardner, 2012). In Raine's story (see the 'Clinical observations' box), the nurse and psychologist would meet with Raine's parents and ask them to document each event of challenging behaviour, identifying the activity that Raine was involved in prior to the event, any triggers (antecedents), Raine's specific behaviours, and the response of her parents and sibling. Collecting this type of information in a clear, objective manner can help families, the nurse and the psychologist identify the reasons for Raine's 'meltdowns' and look at specific strategies for each behaviour. This process follows the principles of CBT, as discussed in Chapter 4.

CLINICAL **OBSERVATIONS**

Addressing challenging behaviours: Raine's story

Raine, who is nine years old, lives with her parents and three-year-old brother. Raine is non-verbal and uses Picture Exchange Communication cards to communicate. Over the past several weeks, Raine has become increasingly agitated, having what her parents describe as 'meltdowns'. Raine scratches, bites and screams and her parents have resorted to isolating Raine in her bedroom at these times, which is difficult. Her parents have no explanation for this change in Raine's behaviour. They are struggling to find ways to manage it.

Autism Spectrum Australia (Aspect) refers to the process of positive behaviour support (Autism Spectrum Australia, 2017). Positive behaviour support is a strategy based on learning theory, which states that all behaviour has a purpose and is in fact a form of communication (particularly for a person who is non-verbal). Positive reinforcement is used to increase the likelihood of, and strengthen, positive behaviours as well as to build in strategies to prevent challenging behaviours occurring in the first place. This increases the likelihood that other people will be proactive rather than reactive. For further information regarding positive reinforcement, refer to Chapter 2.

Pharmacological management

There is no specific medication to treat ASD. The use of medication may be of benefit in helping consumers manage comorbid anxiety and/or depression. As mentioned previously, anxiety disorders are a commonly occurring condition for a consumer who has a diagnosis of ASD (MIMS Online, 2018). Tonge and Brereton (2011) also identified that depression can be experienced during adolescence as a young person gains more insight in relation to the condition. Risperidone, an atypical antipsychotic, has demonstrated a positive effect in managing disruptive and aggressive behaviour (aggression towards others and non-suicidal self-injury) in low doses. In Raine's

story, her paediatrician commenced her on a low dose of risperidone of 0.4 mg/day based on her weight of 48 kg. Raine's parents were advised to monitor her diet as one of the common side effects that children on risperidone can experience is weight gain. They also found that administering her dose in the morning helped to manage meltdowns throughout the day and did not make her overly sleepy (another common side effect of risperidone – more likely at higher doses).

Improving quality of life for consumers and families

Behavioural strategies such as positive behaviour support, specialist educational opportunities, support groups and appropriate use of medications have done much to improve the quality of life for a person with a diagnosis of ASD. Raine's parents commented on how much more settled and happier at home and school she was after she commenced on risperidone. Raine's parents also explored strategies for helping Raine to identify and communicate her emotions.

Consumers and their family living with a diagnosis of ASD need opportunities to create family memories. Recreational activities that may be common for others, such as going to the movies, eating out or shopping, can be extremely stressful occasions for the consumer with ASD. A consumer's difficulty with changes in routine and/or new environments, and disapproving looks and comments from other people, can make activities like these traumatic for the entire family. However, opportunities are increasingly being made available to families to ensure they can experience social and family activities that many others take for granted. Cinema companies are increasingly holding a sensory friendly screening of movies. Families may also have the opportunity to experience live theatre through autism-friendly performances of musical theatre productions. For example, in Australia there have been recent performances of major musicals, which provide family and consumers of all ages the opportunity to enjoy family time in a safe and non-judgemental environment.

Like all children, child consumers with ASD will work through the physical, emotional and social stages of each developmental level. However, depending on the complexity of their needs, parents (and other family members) may well experience additional challenges. Education and support from educational and health care providers as well as support groups will be vital during these times. Referring back to the scenario presented above, Raine's parents will also benefit from regular updates and education on Raine's development and transition through various developmental milestones.

COMMONALITIES OF THE MSE: NEURODEVELOPMENTAL DISORDERS

The following sections outline some features of neurodevelopmental disorders which can be seen in the context of the mental state examination (MSE). This list is not exhaustive, but provides some key examples in order to help you integrate a range of clinical observations into the assessment framework of the MSE.

Appearance and behaviour

For consumers with limited to no verbal capacity, changes in appearance and behaviour can provide important information.

While certain behaviours can be associated with a particular neurodevelopmental disorder (e.g. repetitive behaviours associated with ASD), any changes in normal behaviour patterns need to be investigated further; for example, increased agitation.

Speech

For a consumer who is non-verbal, assessing speech may be inappropriate. However, for consumers who have verbal capacity, any changes to usual speech patterns should be noted.

Mood and affect

Collateral information from family/carers can provide important information regarding a person's mood, particularly if a consumer is unable or unwilling to describe their mood. Providing visual aids to describe mood may be useful. Asking about changes to sleep and appetite also provides important information

related to the individual's experience as all are impacted by changes in mood.

Thought (content and stream)

Abnormal experiences in thought are more likely to be associated with the experience of psychotic symptoms. Disturbances in thought can also be associated with distress. However, talking to oneself may be a usual behaviour for the individual, so changes from usual behaviour patterns needed to be identified. Information from families/carers will be important.

Perception

Hallucinations can be experienced but it is important to distinguish the experience of perceptual disturbance from usual communication patterns such as talking to oneself. The knowledge family/carers have about the individual is important collateral information. The experience of distress is thought to be associated with disturbances in perceptions

Cognition/memory

As with any consumer, premorbid level of functioning must form the baseline against which changes in cognition and memory are compared.

Insight

Insight will be assessed within the context of the consumer's level of cognitive functioning and communication skills (adapted from Radhakrishnan, 2011).

CASE **STUDY**

SAMPLE MENTAL HEALTH ASSESSMENT INCORPORATING AN MSE

Consumer's name: Connor
Gender: Male
Age: 12 years
Medical history: Diagnosed with ASD at three years of age. Parents describe Connor's development as an infant to be 'what we expected. He was our first child and he seemed to fit the picture of what we thought was usual development'. At approximately 12–15 months of age, Connor increasingly displayed repetitive behaviours such as walking on the tips of his toes and flapping his arms when he was excited. Connor also had limited eye contact with people and would spend excessive amounts of time staring at specific objects such as the ceiling fans. Connor was formally diagnosed with ASD at three years of age.
Family/social history: Oldest of three children. Lives at home with parents (mother and father) and two siblings,

Peter aged seven years and Toni aged three years. Neither sibling has ASD. Attends local autism specialist school and recently commenced Year 7. Connor responds to people he knows well but will withdraw from contact with people he is unfamiliar with or when he is agitated.

History of present symptoms

Connor is reported to have become increasingly withdrawn even with people he is comfortable around. He becomes agitated when encouraged to come and sit with the family at meal times and has shown increased resistance to attending school or going on outings. He is also more agitated by any changes to his routine at home and has been insisting even more on his established routines.

Question

Using the information provided, complete an MSE for Connor.

RISK ASSESSMENT FOR PEOPLE DIAGNOSED WITH A NEURODEVELOPMENTAL DISORDER

Because of the impact of neurodevelopmental disorders on consumers' intellectual and adaptive functioning, social interactions and interpersonal relationships, it is essential that assessment of potential risk is always part of the assessment and care planning processes for consumers and their families.

Assessment of risk includes assessment for risk of harm to self, harm to others, property, and assessment of risk for exploitation (financially, socially, sexually and interpersonally) by others. Risk of harm to self can be assessed in terms of the risk of non-suicidal self-injury (e.g. head banging/self-injury/aggressive behaviour towards self). Risk assessment should also involve accurate documentation of any previous risk behaviour and include triggers, specific behaviours, outcomes and strategies that were implemented. Vulnerability and risk of exploitation and/or abuse by others must also be assessed.

THE IMPACT OF CARING FOR A PERSON WITH A DIAGNOSIS OF A NEURODEVELOPMENTAL DISORDER: WHO CARES FOR THE CARERS?

The responsibility of caring for a family member with a diagnosis of a neurodevelopmental disorder such as ASD on a daily basis can have an impact on the physical, psychological and social health and well-being of individual family members (Rogers, Ozonoff & Hansen, 2012), as well as impacting on the family's overall quality of life (Green et al., 2016). From the growing realisation that their child is perhaps not meeting milestones that other children are, or that a child who was previously meeting all the milestones suddenly seems to be regressing, families must come to terms with a new reality. Families will encounter the need to rethink direction and goals for their family member. This does not mean that a child with a diagnosis of ASD, for example, will not have a fulfilling life and that all families do not experience challenges and need to adapt to change. However, in the case of caring for a family member with a neurodevelopmental disorder, there are different layers of complexity that will impact on the daily care of, and interactions with, their family member, as well as affect priorities and goals for the future. Emotional expression and reciprocity are often experienced in contradictory ways. For example, while a child can and will respond to a parent's reassurance in times of stress or when in an unfamiliar environment, they are less likely to respond to parents consistently, particularly when it comes to expressing and regulating emotions (Keenan, Newman, Gray & Rinehart, 2017).

EVIDENCE-BASED PRACTICE

Coping with challenging behaviours

Title of study
Coping strategies in mothers of children with intellectual disabilities showing multiple forms of challenging behaviour: Associations with maternal mental health

Authors
D. Adams, J. Rose, N. Jackson, E. Karakatsani and C. Oliver

Background
Knowledge exists on the impact of caring for a child with a diagnosis of intellectual disability on maternal mental health and well-being. However, there is little documented evidence related to the coping strategies used by mothers in managing challenging behaviours and their effectiveness.

Aim
To explore the coping strategies used by a group of mothers in managing challenging behaviours of their children and impact of these strategies on their mental health and well-being.

Method
89 mothers completed a range of questionnaires that assessed maternal mental health and coping strategies. These questionnaires were the Hospital Anxiety and Depression Scale, Positive and Negative Affect Scale and the Brief COPE Scale.

Results
The use of coping strategies was not associated with child age or ability, but was associated with maternal mental health. The most frequently used coping strategies were acceptance, planning, active coping and positive reframing. These types of coping strategies were associated with higher positive mental health and well-being. Substance use, religion and behavioural disengagement were the least used coping strategies. Actively avoiding coping strategies (such as self-blame, self-criticising and substance use) were associated with higher levels of anxiety and depression.

Implications
Supporting mothers to develop and use positive coping strategies in order to maintain positive health and well-being is a crucial area of future professional work.

SOURCE: ADAMS, D., ROSE, J., JACKSON, N., KARAKATSANI, E. & OLIVER, C. (2018). COPING STRATEGIES IN MOTHERS OF CHILDREN WITH INTELLECTUAL DISABILITIES SHOWING MULTIPLE FORMS OF CHALLENGING BEHAVIOUR: ASSOCIATIONS WITH MATERNAL MENTAL HEALTH. *BEHAVIOURAL AND COGNITIVE PSYCHOTHERAPY*, 46(3), 257–75.

REFLECTION ON LEARNING FROM PRACTICE

Gyn's experience as a grandparent highlights the complexity of living with an individual who has a diagnosis of a neurodevelopmental disorder. Understanding the disorder and being able to understand that a diagnosis of ASD is not the same for every child is part of the process of coming to terms with it and being able to move forward. Gyn's appreciation of her grandson's capacity to communicate in ways that work for him and his family illustrates the importance of not having a stereotypical view of the person who has a diagnosis of ASD.

CHAPTER RESOURCES

SUMMARY

- Neurodevelopmental disorders are conditions that result from impairments to the brain or central nervous system (CNS) development. This results in a failure to meet expected cognitive, behavioural or social developmental milestones. Consumers who have a diagnosis of a neurodevelopmental disorder also have an increased possibility of diagnosis of a comorbid mental health condition. Promoting quality of life and social inclusion for consumers who have a diagnosis of a neurodevelopmental disorder is an essential feature of working with consumers, families and carers.
- Attention deficit/hyperactivity disorder (ADHD) is a condition in which a child demonstrates difficulty in concentration, impulsive behaviour and overactivity. This can impact significantly on educational outcomes, social skills and family functioning. A multidisciplinary approach between health care professionals, the consumer, family and educational providers is essential to promote best outcomes for children. Treatment involves both behavioural strategies and pharmacological treatment. ADHD is noted to be a prevalent mental health condition in children aged four to 17 years.
- Intellectual learning disability focuses on deficits in intellectual functioning (including planning, executive functioning and problem solving) and behaviour, which are apparent by the age of 18. The impact of these deficits is seen in the difficulty that consumers have in achieving independence and taking on social responsibilities. This

includes difficulties in communication, social participation, employment and personal independence. It is identified that approximately 3% of the Australian population have a diagnosis of intellectual disability.
- Key features of autism spectrum disorder (ASD) involve persistent deficits in social interaction and social communication and the presence of restricted, repetitive patterns of behaviour interests or activities. ASD is conceptualised as being on a continuum (or spectrum) with the manifestations of the disorder varying depending on the consumer's developmental level, age and severity of the disorder. Management strategies involve non-pharmacological interventions such as positive behaviour support, providing opportunities for social interactions and where necessary pharmacological interventions.
- Undertaking a mental state examination (MSE) is a key component of a thorough mental health assessment. Adaptation may be required to ensure that it is completed in a person-centred manner and the use of collateral information can be important. Risk assessment must also be undertaken in order to maximise consumer safety and safety of others.
- Families, carers and support organisations play a pivotal role in supporting consumers with a diagnosis of a neurodevelopmental disorder, on both a daily and long-term basis. Ensuring support services are available is essential in promoting ongoing health and well-being.

REVIEW QUESTIONS

1 The most common medication to manage challenging behaviour associated with autism spectrum disorder is:
   a Sertraline
   b Carbamazepine
   c Lithium
   d Risperidone

2 What type of theory is positive behavioural support (PBS) based on?
   a Learning
   b Genetic
   c Behavioural
   d All of the above

3   The core features associated with intellectual disability are:
    a   Deficits in intellectual functioning, adaptive functioning and onset after puberty
    b   Normal intellectual functioning, deficits in adaptive functioning and onset during the development period
    c   Moderate deficits and adaptive functioning onset at any time
    d   Deficit intellectual and adaptive functioning, and onset during the developmental period

4   Communication skills, reducing overstimulation and fatigue and developing social skills are useful strategies in working with a consumer who has a diagnosis of:
    a   Autism spectrum disorder
    b   Attention deficit/hyperactivity disorder
    c   Anxiety disorder
    d   All consumers even if they do not have a diagnosis

5   A teacher reports that he has concerns regarding a new student in his class. The student has trouble maintaining attention on class activities, becomes disruptive when asked to complete an activity or task, is easily distracted, seems to have trouble waiting their turn and is increasingly disruptive towards other children, often interrupting their activities. The teacher has spoken with the student's parents, who say this behaviour is also apparent at home. The parents and teacher think the child may have:
    a   Anxiety disorder
    b   Intellectual disability
    c   Attention deficit/hyperactivity disorder
    d   Conduct disorder

CRITICAL THINKING

1   A number of films representing people with a neurodevelopmental disorder have been produced over the years. Choose one of the following films (below) to view. Reflect on the questions and discuss them with your colleagues or classmates:
    a   Having worked through this chapter, how accurate is the representation of the individual in the selected movie?
    b   What issues/challenges did the protagonist encounter?
    c   What does the selected movie communicate about the community's views of neurodevelopmental disorders?
    d   How will you educate friends and the wider community regarding neurodevelopmental disorders? What would be your key message?
        •   *I am Sam* (2001; director Jessie Nelson in association with Avery Picks, the Bedford Falls Company and Red Fish Blue Fish Films)

•   *Rain Man* (1988; director Barry Levinson, United Artists; the Guber-Peters Company, in association with Star Partners II Limited and Mirage Entertainment)
•   *What's Eating Gilbert Grape?* (1993; director Lasse Hallström, Paramount Pictures)

2   While Gyn, in the 'Learning from practice' vignette at the start of the chapter, has known her grandson for 10 years, health care clinicians may not have the same length of relationship with consumers and families. As a nurse meeting Gyn and her grandson for the first time, what communication strategies would you adopt when trying to communication with her grandson? What do you see as some of the potential challenges?

3   What areas of risk assessment are pertinent to the case study of Connor presented earlier?

USEFUL WEBSITES

■   Amaze (Autism Victoria): http://www.amaze.org.au
■   Autism Spectrum Australia – Positive Behaviour Support: https://www.autismspectrum.org.au/pbs

■   FIND – Further Inform Neurogenetic Disorders: http://www.findresources.co.uk

REFLECT ON THIS

Home schooling and mental health support

The COVID-19 pandemic has seen the lives of people turned upside down in many ways: socially, emotionally, economically, psychologically as well as physiologically. The need for remote learning has been one obvious way in which people's lives have been impacted upon. During the pandemic, remote learning in the form of home schooling became a way of life for countless families in Victoria. Home schooling children has been a challenge for families, with parents balancing work (or lack of it), financial considerations and maintaining their usual parental role and responsibilities. Added to this has been the requirement for parents to take on the role of educator of their children. It is not surprising that many parents have felt overwhelmed by this task. The following website provides a range of resources that have been available for families to access and use during the pandemic: https://www.education. vic.gov.au/school/teachers/teachingresources/Pages/ coronavirus-home-learning.aspx

Go to this website and look through some of its resources. In particular, make sure you view the resources related to mental health support. Thinking about the information you have read, reflect on the following questions:

1   Identify someone you know who has been involved with remote learning. Specifically, try to identify some who has primary or secondary aged children. This could be your own family, another relative or friend.

2   What are the challenges they have experienced in relation to remote learning?

3   What resources were they provided access to?

4   What other support might they have found useful?

Now turn your attention to children who are diagnosed on the autism spectrum. During the pandemic, children attending autism specialist schools, as well as those in mainstream schools, have been required to isolate at home and parents asked to take on the role of educating their child/children.

5   Given your understanding from the information provided in this chapter, what do you think are some of the unique challenges that families may have been faced with in home schooling a child who has a diagnosis of ASD?

6   What resources are available for these families?

7   What emotional and mental health support do you think these families might find beneficial?

To help you explore these questions, the following websites will be useful:

■   Learning from Home in a School Setting: https:// www.education.vic.gov.au/school/teachers/ teachingresources/Pages/coronavirus-home-learning. aspx

■   Supporting Individuals with Autism through Uncertain Times: https://afirm.fpg.unc.edu/sites/afirm.fpg.unc.edu/ files/covid-resources/Supporting%20Individuals%20 with%20Autism%20through%20Uncertian%20Times%20 Article%20Only.pdf

REFERENCES

Adams, D., Rose, J., Jackson, N., Karakatsani, E. & Oliver, C. (2018). Coping strategies in mothers of children with intellectual disabilities showing multiple forms of challenging behaviour: Associations with maternal mental health. *Behavioural and Cognitive Psychotherapy*, 46(3), 257–75.

Ali, A., Blickwedel, J. & Hassiotis, A. (2014). Interventions for challenging behaviour in intellectual disability. *Advances in Psychiatric Treatment*, 20(3), 184–92. doi:10.1192/apt.bp.113.011577

American Psychiatric Association (APA). (2013). *Diagnostic and Statistical Manual of Mental Disorders (DSM-5)* (5th edn). Washington, DC: APA.

Andrews, G., Dean, K., Genderson, M., Hunt, C., Mitchell, P., Sachdev, P. & Trollor, J. (2013). *Management of Mental Disorders* (5th edn). Sydney: School of Psychiatry, University of NSW.

Australian Bureau of Statistics (ABS). (2014). *Disability in Australia: Intellectual Disability*. Retrieved from http://www.abs.gov.au/ ausstats/abs@.nsf/Lookup/4433.0.55.003main+features102012.

Australian Bureau of Statistics (ABS). (2017). *Autism in Australia. 2015 Survey of Disability, Ageing and Carers (SDAC). Summary of Findings, 2015*. Retrieved from http://www.abs.gov.au/AUSSTATS/abs@.nsf/ Lookup/4430.0Main+Features902015?OpenDocument.

Australian Institute of Health and Welfare (AIHW). (2003). *Disability Prevalence and Trends*. AIHW cat. no. DIS34. Retrieved from https://www.aihw.gov.au/getmedia/08fa900b-559a-4af9-9466-b3c200e99bd5/dpt.pdf.aspx?inline=true.

Australian Institute of Health and Welfare (AIHW). (2008). *Disability in Australia: Intellectual Disability*. Bulletin 67, November. Retrieved from http://www.aihw.gov.au/WorkArea/DownloadAsset. aspx?id=6442452891.

Australian Institute of Health and Welfare (AIHW). (2017). *Autism in Australia*. Retrieved from https://www.aihw.gov.au/reports/disability/ autism-in-australia/contents/autism. © Commonwealth of Australia. Released under CC BY 3.0. Link to license: https://creativecommons. org/licenses/by/3.0/au/.

Australian Institute of Health and Welfare (AIHW). (2019). People with disability in Australia 2019: In brief. Cat. no. DIS 74. Canberra: AIHW. Retrieved from https://www.aihw.gov.au/getmedia/3bc5f549-216e-4199-9a82-fba1bba9208f/aihw-dis-74.pdf.aspx?inline=true.

Australian Medical Association (AMA). (2016). *Autism Spectrum Disorder 2016 AMA Position Statement*. Retrieved from https://ama. com.au/position-statement/autism-spectrum-disorder-2016.

Autism Spectrum Australia. (2017). *What is PBS?* Retrieved from https://www.autismspectrum.org.au/content/what-pbs.

Betancur, C. & Coleman, M. (2013). Etiological heterogeneity in autism spectrum disorders: Role of rare variants. In J.D. Buxbaum & P.R. Hoff (eds), *The Neuroscience of Autism Spectrum Disorders* (pp. 113–44). Burlington, NJ: Elsevier Science.

Capusan, A.J., Bendtsen, P., Marteinsdottir, I. & Larsson, H. (2019). Comorbidity of adult ADHD and its subtypes with substance use disorder in a large population-based epidemiological study. *Journal of Attention Disorders*, 3(12), 1416–26. doi:doi:10.1177/1087054715626511

Caye, A., Swanson, J.M., Coghill, D. & Rohde, L.A. (2019). Treatment strategies for ADHD: An evidence-based guide to select optimal treatment. *Molecular Psychiatry*, 24(3), 390–408. https://doi.org/10.1038/s41380-018-0116-3

Crossland, T., Hewitt, O. & Walden, S. (2017). Outcomes and experiences of an adapted dialectic behaviour therapy skills training group for people with intellectual disabilities. *British Journal of Learning Disabilities*, 45(3), 208–16. doi:10.1111/bld.12194

Ellison, J.W., Rosenfeld, J.A. & Shaffer, L.G. (2013). Genetic basis of intellectual disability. *Annual Review of Medicine*, 64, 441–50. doi:10.1146/annurev-med-042711-140053

Giarelli, E. & Gardner, M. (2012). *Nursing of Autism Spectrum Disorder: Evidence-Based Integrated Care across the Lifespan*. New York: Springer Publishing.

Green, J.L., Rinehart, N., Anderson, V., Efron, D., Nicholson, J.M., Jongeling, B., … Sciberras, E. (2016). Association between autism symptoms and family functioning in children with attention-deficit/hyperactivity disorder: A community-based study. *European Child and Adolescent Psychiatry*, 25(12), 1307–18. doi:10.1007/s00787-016-0861-2

Keenan, B.M., Newman, L.K., Gray, K.M. & Rinehart, N.J. (2017). A qualitative study of attachment relationships in ASD during middle childhood. *Attachment and Human Development*, 19(1), 1–21. doi:10.1080/14616734.2016.1246580

Lawrence, D., Johnson, S., Hafekost, J., Boterhoven, De Haan, K., Sawyer, M., Ainley, J. & Zubrick, S.R. (2015). *The Mental Health of Children and Adolescents. Report on the Second Australian Child and Adolescent Survey of Mental Health and Wellbeing*. Canberra: Department of Health. Retrieved from https://www.health.gov.au/internet/main/publishing.nsf/Content/9DA8CA21306FE6EDCA257E2700016945/%24File/child2.pdf.

MIMS Online. (2018). *Monthly Index of Medical Specialties Online*. St Leonards: MIMS Australia. Retrieved from https://www.mimsonline.com.au/Search/Search.aspx.

Munir K.M. (2016). The co-occurrence of mental disorders in children and adolescents with intellectual disability/intellectual developmental disorder. *Current Opinion in Psychiatry*, 29(2), 95–102. https://doi.org/10.1097/YCO.0000000000000236

Radhakrishnan, V. (2011). Principles of assessing the mental health of people with learning disabilities. In S. Bonell, T. McInerny & J. O'Hara (eds), *Neurodevelopmental Psychiatry: An Introduction for Medical Students* (pp. 13–18). London: Kings Health Partners South London and Maudsley NHS Foundation Trust. Retrieved from https://www.rcpsych.ac.uk/docs/default-source/members/faculties/intellectual-disability/id-neurodevelopmental-psychiatry—an-introduction-for-medical-students.pdf?sfvrsn=5d1898c5_2.

Rogers, S.J., Ozonoff, S. & Hansen, R.L. (2012). Autism spectrum disorders. In R.L. Hansen & S.J. Rogers (eds), *Autism and Other Neurodevelopmental Disorders* (pp. 1–28). Washington, DC: American Psychiatric Publishing.

Royal Children's Hospital (2012). *ADHD: Stimulant Medication. Factsheet*. Centre for Community Child Health and General Paediatrics. Retrieved from http://www.rch.org.au/kidsinfo/fact_sheets/ADHD_Stimulant_medication.

Sadock, B.J., Sadock, V.A. & Ruiz, P. (2015). *Kaplan & Sadock's Synopsis of Psychiatry. Behavioral Sciences/Clinical Psychiatry* (11th edn). Philadelphia, PA: Wolters Kluwer.

The Royal Children's Hospital Melbourne (2018). ADHD – Ways to help children at school and home. Retrieved from https://www.rch.org.au/kidsinfo/fact_sheets/ADHD_ways_to_help_children_at_school_and_home/.

Tonge, B. & Brereton, A. (2011). Autism spectrum disorders. *Australian Family Physician*, 40, 672–7. Retrieved from http://www.racgp.org.au/download/documents/AFP/2011/September/201109tonge.pdf.

Trollor, J.N., Salomon, C. & Franklin, C. (2016). Prescribing psychotropic drugs to adults with an intellectual disability. *Australian Prescriber*, 39(4), 126–30. doi:10.18773/austprescr.2016.048

Woods, R. (2011). Behavioural concerns: Assessment and management of people with intellectual disability. *Australian Family Physician*, 40, 198–200.

CHAPTER 16

NEUROCOGNITIVE DISORDERS

Gylo (Julie) Hercelinskyj

LEARNING OUTCOMES

Upon completion of this chapter, you should be able to:

16.1 Understand the demographics of the older population in Australia and the prevalence of neurocognitive disorders in the community

16.2 Explore the concept of healthy ageing and its application to working with older people living with mental health issues

16.3 Reflect on the issue of elder abuse in the community

16.4 Identify the expected changes related to the ageing process against conditions that are not considered part of the normal ageing process

16.5 Understand delirium, including its aetiology, risk factors, diagnostic criteria and management

16.6 Understand major neurocognitive disorder (dementia), including its aetiology, risk factors, diagnostic criteria and management

16.7 Reflect on the impacts of neurocognitive disorders for families

LEARNING FROM PRACTICE

When my grandmother passed away in 2008, I remember my cousin telling me that in a way he was relieved. When I asked why he felt this, he said that the woman who had died was not really his grandmother. He had watched his grandmother die slowly over the previous seven years or so. He had watched her go from a vivacious person who was always the centre of attention even well into her seventies, to a person who could not remember his name, looked blankly into space as though trapped in some long-forgotten memory, needed full-time care and eventually did not communicate at all. 'Dementia stole her from us Eleni,' he said. For my cousin, the tragedy was that his last memories of her were her final months, not the person he grew up calling Baba. Dementia stole our Baba from us.

Eleni, Baba's granddaughter

Eleni gives a picture showing two sides of her grandmother – the person she was before dementia and the person she became afterwards. There is a sense that dementia took away her grandmother's identity and her cousin's comments reflect the sense of grief that families often experience when they care for a relative with dementia. What do you think are some of the feelings that families can experience?

INTRODUCTION

If you speak to a gardener, they will invariably talk about how plants are nurtured and grown. You will hear comments about planting seedlings, providing the right nutrients and environmental conditions for the plant to thrive and grow to maturity. A mature plant will be admired (and often judged) for its bloom and fragrance. This life cycle is painstakingly followed by the gardener, who will care for the plant for as long as possible to ensure a thriving plant that contributes to the satisfaction of people's lives. But environmental conditions, the amount and consistency of nurturing and the inevitable ageing of the plant will see the petals drop off a tulip or rose, the grass turn brown and die, or a bush not grow to its full potential. It can often be the case that in those last growing seasons, a bloom will still be produced that reminds us that plants have the capacity to keep giving and keep contributing if only we will look, listen and care.

People also require conditions that promote optimum growth and development. Our parents, teachers, extended family and others will all contribute to our development. Youth and adulthood are seen in many cultures as the most important and valued times in a person's life. But, just like a plant, all people will age. In fact, we begin ageing from the moment we are born. The necessity to value people across their lifespan is integral to the professional practice of mental health nurses. This chapter explores ageing through a review of the contemporary trends and issues related to older people in Australia. Major mental health conditions

as identified in the *Diagnostic and Statistical Manual of Mental Disorders* (DSM-5; APA, 2013) are considered, together with implications for mental health nursing practice. Issues related to elder abuse and healthy ageing are also introduced.

AGEING IN AUSTRALIA TODAY: CONTEMPORARY TRENDS AND ISSUES

While the proportion of people in the 15–64-year age bracket remains relatively steady, statistics indicate that in the last two decades the proportion of the Australian population aged 65 and over has increased from 12.0% to 15.3% (ABS, 2016; **Figure 16.1**). The ABS states that the percentage of the Australian population over the age of 65 years is expected to increase more rapidly in the next decade as more **baby boomers** turn 65.

Older people are generally living longer and healthier lives than experienced by people in previous generations (AIHW, 2017). Recent data predicts that girls born in 2013 have a life expectancy of 84 years and that boys have a life expectancy of 81 years. These increases in life expectancy are related to higher standards of living and better access to social support and health care services (AIHW, 2017). However, statistics also show increasing rates of mental health issues for older people. The DSM-5 classifies a number of these mental health conditions, including dementia (APA, 2013). **Figure 16.2** shows the changes in life expectancy over the next 40-plus years.

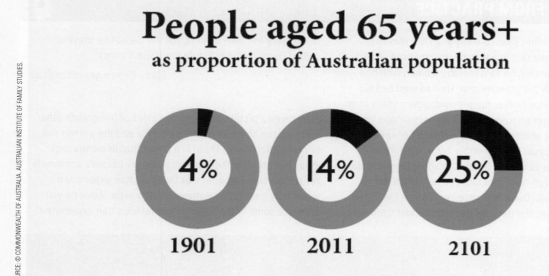

SOURCE: © COMMONWEALTH OF AUSTRALIA. AUSTRALIAN INSTITUTE OF FAMILY STUDIES.

FIGURE 16.1
Proportion of population aged 65 years and over

Growth rates of the oldest is set to dramatically increase over the next 20 years

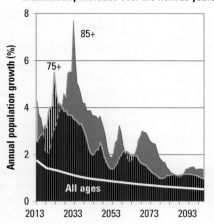

The age structure becomes more uniformly distributed across ages

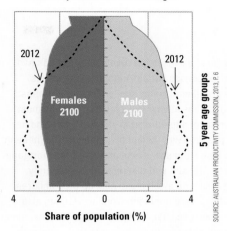

FIGURE 16.2
Australian life expectancy distribution until the 22nd century

HEALTHY AGEING

The preceding sections clearly show that Australia is an ageing nation. People are living longer and more likely to stay in their own homes for a greater length of time. Therefore, before delving into the mental health issues that are associated with living longer, it is essential to frame these issues in the context of contemporary government policy regarding older people. The idea of healthy ageing not only encompasses good physical health, it also looks at how the environment and socioeconomic determinants of health impact on a person's experience of ageing. This includes physical and emotional safety, social and cultural inclusion, and community participation. Healthy ageing is defined by the World Health Organization (WHO, 2015, p. 41) as 'the process of developing and maintaining the functional ability that enables well-being in older age'. Closely aligned with this is the concept of active ageing defined by the WHO as 'optimizing opportunities for health, participation and security in order to enhance quality of life as people age' (WHO, 2002, p. 12). Taken together, these two concepts demonstrate the way in which physical, emotional and social domains of living need to be recognised and addressed as a whole in order to facilitate emotional health and well-being for older people. For example, Guure, Ibrahim, Adam and Said (2017) identified through a meta-analysis of the literature that physical activity can be beneficial in reducing the risk of Alzheimer's disease, particularly for men.

Healthy ageing incorporates physical, emotional and social domains. Governments are implementing a healthy and active ageing agenda through policy directives. Healthy ageing requires clinicians, the older person and their family or carers to work together.

ELDER ABUSE

Elder abuse is understood to be any act that causes harm to an older person (Seniors Rights Victoria, n.d.). Elder abuse can be physical, emotional, sexual, financial or psychological in nature and can involve either mistreatment or neglect. Elder abuse occurs within the context of a trusted relationship with another person such as a partner or an adult child. However, it can also involve the relationship between an older person and a care provider in the case where a person lives in supported living arrangements. Financial abuse towards older people is particularly common. Elder abuse is a difficult topic to discuss openly, as it challenges ideas regarding the meaning of families and relationships, as well as the status of older people in the community generally.

Residential aged care facilities are bound by legislation under the *Aged Care Act 1997* regarding compulsory reporting related to assaults of older people living in residential care. However, there is no requirement for compulsory or mandatory reporting for other forms of elder abuse, with the law not making any distinction between older people and other adults. Organisations such as Seniors Rights Victoria play a pivotal role in raising community awareness of elder abuse, providing both community and professional education and acting as a resource for older people if they require information and/or support.

The following Case Study illustrates two examples that could be regarded as elder abuse.

CASE **STUDY**

SIGNS OF ELDER ABUSE

Case 1: Polina

Polina is widowed and lives in her own home. She has two children, one of whom has serious mental health issues and a drug use problem. Coming from an Eastern European background, Polina has always believed that parents must help their children get a good start in life. At 72, she and her husband (who passed away 12 months ago) had bought each child their own home and she is also paying off the mortgage on her own place. Her son and daughter-in-law recently demanded that Polina be available to pick up their children from school as they were now both working. Her son also demanded that Polina sell her house so he and his wife could choose a more suitable residence closer to their children's school. Polina felt coerced into selling her house and then depositing the money into her son's bank account. The new house was bought in her son's name, not Polina's, and Polina also contributes towards the rent as she has been told she is responsible for half of the mortgage repayments. This money comes from Polina's pension, leaving little spare cash for her daily living expenses and requirements. Polina does not know who to turn to and feels trapped.

Case 2: Eric

Eric recently moved to supported living in a residential care facility. At 83, his children felt he was no longer able to care for himself independently and their busy lives left little time for them to make regular visits to their father. The care facility was some distance from where Eric had lived previously and was not even that close to his children, but they felt this was the best option for him. Eric could attend to his own activities of daily living, but occasionally needed reminding to do so. There was one carer who Eric first met several weeks after he had moved to the care facility. This carer became increasingly agitated and verbally demeaning towards Eric if he felt that Eric was taking too long to get dressed in the morning. He would often roughly grab the electric razor or comb out of Eric's hands and say, 'For God's sake, I'll do that.' He would call Eric names and repeatedly tell him how lucky he was to be at this particular care facility because they didn't usually take 'retards' like him. One day as Eric was trying to dry himself after his shower, the carer ripped the towel out of his hands and began towelling him down roughly. Eric repeatedly asked him to stop, when the carer rolled up the towel and threw it at Eric's face. Eric only just managed to keep his balance and not fall. Eric did not know who he could talk to.

Questions

1   Are there any signs of elder abuse in these scenarios? What are the signs?
2   What type of elder abuse are Polina and Eric experiencing?
3   What support services would be helpful for Polina and Eric?

MENTAL HEALTH ISSUES AND OLDER PEOPLE

While this chapter looks specifically at neurocognitive disorders, it is important to understand that older people, as part of the overall adult population, can experience any type of mental health issue. While the onset of mental health conditions most commonly occurs in middle adolescence to early adulthood, an older person can experience a mental health condition in older age or have lived with a diagnosis of a mental health condition over the course of their life. However, a person with no previous lived experience of a mental health condition can experience onset in older age (AIHW, 2015).

The impact on older people of mental health, other than major and minor neurocognitive disorder and delirium, can be summarised as follows:

■   Anxiety affects approximately 10% of older people.
■   Depression affects between 10–15% of older people.
■   Suicide rates for both males and females over the age of 85 are higher than for any other age group. (Issues related to depression and suicide for older people are discussed in Chapters 10 and 20.)

■   While illicit drug use is less common among older adults, dependence on prescription medications is more prevalent. Drugs such as alcohol are also commonly consumed by people, but binge drinking is less common in this age group (AIHW, 2014; beyondblue, 2009; VAADA, 2011).

In the DSM-5 (APA, 2013), neurocognitive disorders are described within the following categories: delirium major neurocognitive disorder (NCD) and minor neurocognitive disorder (NCD). The term 'dementia' is now subsumed under the heading of major NCD (APA, 2013), but is still used extensively in clinical practice as well as in contemporary literature. Therefore, **dementia** will be used in this chapter for clarity and consistency. When a diagnosis of a neurocognitive disorder is made, it is based on changes in a number of cognitive areas. These domains are attention, executive function, learning and memory, language, perceptual motor and social cognition (APA, 2013).

Prevalence of neurocognitive disorders

Dementia is *not* a normal part of the ageing process. While the rate of dementia does increase as people age, dementia can develop and impact on a person and their loved ones at any age. Worldwide, there are more than 46.8 million people with dementia and 131.5 million people predicted to have dementia by 2050 (Alzheimer's Disease International, 2015). Just over 400 000 people were estimated to be living with a diagnosis of dementia in 2016, with over 50% of these people being women. Projections indicate that by 2056 this number will increase to over 1 000 000 (Brown, Hansnata & La, 2017). In Australia, the term 'younger onset dementia' has been used to describe a person under the age of 65 years being diagnosed with any type of dementia. Dementia has been diagnosed in people in their 40s and 50s and even diagnosed in younger people in their 30s. Alzheimer's Australia identifies that currently just over 25 000 younger people have been affected by the onset of dementia (AIHW, 2012; Alzheimer's Australia, n.d).

The prevalence of delirium is highest among older persons who are hospitalised. The actual rate will vary depending on the personal characteristics of the individual, as well as where they are residing (e.g. a residential aged care facility as opposed to living at home); the overall prevalence of delirium for older people living in the community is low but increases with age. The reported prevalence rates for delirium vary from 10–31% for older people admitted to hospital. However, the prevalence rate of delirium has also been reported to be as high as 80% for older people admitted to an intensive care environment (Vasilevskis, Han, Hughes & Ely, 2012).

DSM-5 classification of neurocognitive disorders

The major feature of neurocognitive disorders described in the DSM-5 is related to changes in **cognitive functioning** (APA, 2013). These cognitive changes are related to aspects such as memory, language, and frontal executive or visuospatial functioning (Andrews et. al., 2013). The DSM-5 (APA, 2013) lists several domains used to classify neurocognitive disorders. These domains are attention executive functioning, which relates to the capacity to plan, make decisions, respond to others and demonstrate mental flexibility; learning and memory; language such as the capacity to express oneself clearly; perceptual-motor, which involves tasks that require hand–eye coordination; and social cognition, which involves things such as the ability to recognise one's own emotions as well as the emotions of other people (Andrews et al., 2013). Unlike many mental health conditions, it is possible to identify the underlying pathology for neurocognitive disorders such as dementia and delirium (APA, 2013). The DSM-5 uses the categories of major and minor neurocognitive disorders, which include the various sub-types of dementia as well as neurocognitive disorders due to conditions such as Parkinson's disease, traumatic brain injury and Huntington's disease (APA, 2013). Delirium exists as its own specific disorder. The DSM-5 (APA, 2013) also

specifies mild neurocognitive disorder, which refers to forms of cognitive impairment that are less severe than major neurocognitive disorder (dementia).

While there are a number of other neurocognitive disorders identified in the DSM-5, in this chapter we focus on delirium and dementia, and spend some time considering the different types of dementia, which the DSM-5 classifies according to aetiology (APA, 2013). We also consider the distinctions between dementia, delirium and depression, remembering that depression is not classified as a neurocognitive disorder; however, a person experiencing a major depressive episode can experience some cognitive changes.

DELIRIUM

Delirium is considered a medical emergency and is common in older people admitted to acute care facilities. Rates of delirium have been reported to vary from 10–31% on admission and between 3–29% during admission for medical treatment. Rates are reported to be much higher for older people following surgery with rates of between 47–53% being reported (Travers et al., 2013). The study by Travers et al. (2013) identified that older people experiencing delirium while in hospital experience longer hospital admissions, more falls and higher mortality rates up to 28 days following discharge.

A person who has been diagnosed with delirium will need to meet the diagnostic criteria outlined in **Table 16.1** (see also the 'Clinical observations' box for more information on the subtypes of delirium).

DIAGNOSTIC CRITERIA

Delirium

TABLE 16.1
Diagnostic criteria delirium

A. A disturbance in attention (i.e., reduced ability to direct, focus, sustain, and shift attention) and awareness (reduced orientation to the environment).
B. The disturbance develops over a short period of time (usually hours to a few days), represents a change from baseline attention and awareness, and tends to fluctuate in severity during the course of a day.
C. An additional disturbance in cognition (e.g., memory deficit, disorientation, language, visuospatial ability, or perception).
D. The disturbances in Criteria A and C are not better explained by another preexisting, established, or evolving neurocognitive disorder and do not occur in the context of a severely reduced level of arousal, such as coma.
E. There is evidence from the history, physical examination, or laboratory findings that the disturbance is a direct physiological consequence of another medical condition, substance intoxication or withdrawal (i.e., due to a drug of abuse or to a medication), or exposure to a toxin, or is due to multiple etiologies.

SECTION 2

Risk factors for delirium

There are certain factors that can predispose a person or increase the risk of them experiencing delirium, and it is essential to be familiar with these. The factors that increase the risk of experiencing delirium include:

- infection (e.g. urinary tract infection, respiratory infection)
- previous history of delirium
- depression
- dehydration
- being older
- postoperatively due to the effects of anaesthesia or pain relief medication
- **polypharmacy** (the use of multiple medications)
- pre-existing dementia
- renal failure
- abnormal sodium, potassium or glucose levels

- substance withdrawal including drugs and alcohol (alcohol withdrawal can lead to delirium tremens) (DeLaune et al., 2016; Hunt, 2017).

SAFETY FIRST

RISK ASSESSMENT FOR DELIRIUM

Risk assessment for delirium is an essential component of caring for the person at risk of experiencing delirium. It should be completed on admission and as required during a person's admission to a facility. Knowledge of the risk factors will help you identify a person at risk. The Cognitive Decline Partnership Centre outlines the Delirium Risk Assessment Tool (DRAT) as one tool that can be used easily. Details of this tool are available at: aci.health.nsw.gov.au

CLINICAL OBSERVATIONS

Types of delirium

TYPE OF DELIRIUM	WHAT WILL THE NURSE SEE	EXAMPLES
Hyperactive	The nurse will see an individual who has a significantly increased level of psychomotor activity. The person may also experience a labile mood, be agitated and refuse to cooperate with care.	• Sadie Brown is brought to the ED in an agitated state. She is very distractible and highly agitated when asked to sit still to have her vital signs taken. • This change in her behaviour commenced over the past 12 hours. Her family describe her as usually very calm, able to follow directions and sleeps well.
Hypoactive	A person experiencing hypoactive delirium will have a significantly reduced level of psychomotor activity. They may also feel sluggish and lethargic to the point of stupor.	• Enver's family are concerned. Over the past 24 hours he has appeared increasingly sluggish and unable to respond to his family. • They describe him as seeming confused and uninterested, and unable to concentrate on normal activities.
Mixed	Mixed delirium sees the individual experiencing a normal level of psychomotor activity; however, attention and awareness are disturbed and a person may also experience rapid fluctuations in activity levels.	• The care staff are concerned about Walter's erratic behaviour. Over the past 12 hours he has demonstrated erratic behaviour fluctuating from severe agitation and confusion to being extremely sluggish in his movements and behaviour and uninterested in everything around him. He was confused about where he was and who the staff were.

The implications of delirium are significant. For example, delirium related to substance withdrawal such as alcohol withdrawal is a medical emergency. Thorough assessment and medical and nursing management are required. Substance intoxication and withdrawal are covered in Chapter 14.

Additionally, people who develop delirium have an increased mortality risk, an increased risk of falls, a higher chance of being discharged to higher dependency care facilities and an increased risk of dementia. Even though delirium is a commonly occurring condition, it continues to be poorly recognised and therefore poorly managed (ACSQHC, 2017).

Management of delirium

The main aim of management is to identify and treat the underlying cause of the delirium. This will usually involve a range of diagnostic tests; for example, blood assays to check level urea and electrolyte levels, drug levels, full blood count, wound cultures and stool cultures.

However, it is essential that interventions are implemented that support the person's dignity, safety and emotional and physical well-being during an episode of delirium. Specific strategies include:

- assessment of risks (e.g. falls)
- management of any underlying physical conditions

- maintaining rest and sleep
- ensuring adequate nutrition and hydration
- maintaining safety in relation to preventing falls/other injury; for example, if a person is experiencing delirium postoperatively
- minimising the use of restraints if delirium occurs post-operatively, as restraints can exacerbate delirium and increase risk of falls
- reorientation strategies such as family being present, the use of cue cards, clocks, family photos
- environmental considerations; for example, a well-lit and ventilated room during the day. The use of a night light at night particularly if the person is experiencing perceptual disturbances, appropriate sensory stimulation such as a family member reading the newspapers, or a radio
- low dosage risperidone may also be prescribed to manage extreme agitation that has not been successfully managed through non-pharmacological interventions (ACSQHC, 2014).

MAJOR NEUROCOGNITIVE DISORDERS: DEMENTIA

The easiest way to describe dementia is as a series of disorders involving progressive decline in brain function. This progressive deterioration results in a loss of memory, intellect, rationality, social skills and what would be considered normal emotional reactions (Westerby & Howard, 2011). People living with early stages of dementia continue to live in the community with the need for residential care coming into play as people develop higher levels of cognitive loss. The major features of any dementia involve changes in cognitive function in language, previously learned motor skills, the ability to recognise people and objects, and higher executive functions such as problem solving and planning.

Dementias fall under the classification of neurocognitive disorders in the DSM-5 (APA, 2013). The diagnostic criteria for dementia are outlined in **Table 16.2**.

The DSM-5 (APA, 2013) also requires that the type of dementia be specified. The DSM-5 specifies a number of types of dementia; however, four common types of dementia are:
- dementia – Alzheimer's disease
- dementia – vascular type
- Lewy body dementia
- fronto-temporal dementia (APA, 2013).

It is also important to note that people can develop dementia as a result of traumatic brain injury; substance/medication use; HIV infection; and conditions such as Parkinson's disease and Huntington's disease, or from multiple aetiologies (APA, 2013).

DIAGNOSTIC CRITERIA

Major neurocognitive disorder (dementia)

TABLE 16.2
Diagnostic criteria major neurocognitive disorder (dementia)

A. Evidence of significant cognitive decline from a previous level of performance in one or more cognitive domains (complex attention, executive function, learning and memory, language, perceptual-motor, or social cognition) based on: 1. Concern of the individual, a knowledgeable informant, or the clinician that there has been a significant decline in cognitive function; and 2. A substantial impairment in cognitive performance, preferably documented by standardized neuropsychological testing or, in its absence, another quantified clinical assessment.
B. The cognitive deficits interfere with independence in everyday activities (i.e., at a minimum, requiring assistance with complex instrumental activities of daily living such as paying bills or managing medications).
C. The cognitive deficits do not occur exclusively in the context of a delirium.
D. The cognitive deficits are not better explained by another mental disorder (e.g., major depressive disorder, schizophrenia). *Specify* current severity: **Mild:** Difficulties with instrumental activities of daily living (e.g., housework, managing money). **Moderate:** Difficulties with basic activities of daily living (e.g., feeding, dressing). **Severe:** Fully dependent.

Dementia is seen to follow a particular trajectory or course. It is a progressive disorder with the average course of the disorder being approximately 10 years. Dementia – Alzheimer's disease is generally identified in three categories:

1 *Mild/early stage:* Changes in cognitive function are noticed, particularly in areas such as personal care and memory, but the individual can maintain independence with minimal support.

2 *Moderate:* At this stage the person needs increasing assistance and supervision in order to remain independent in the community.

3 *Severe/late stage:* At this stage the person requires constant supervision and assistance. It is at this point that many people transition to residential facilities for continuous care (adapted from Andrews et al., 2013).

Aetiology

Dementia results in the death of brain cells, leaving the person with fewer connecting and functioning brain cells. Dementia – Alzheimer's disease is characterised by the formation of plaques and tangles. Plaques are clumps of a protein called beta-amyloid that may damage and destroy brain cells in several ways, including interfering with cell-to-cell communication. Brain cells depend on an internal support and transport system to carry nutrients and other essential materials throughout the long extensions. This system requires a normal structure and functioning of a specific protein called tau. For a person diagnosed with Alzheimer's disease, these threads of tau protein twist into abnormal tangles inside brain cells, leading to failure of the transport system. Dementia – vascular type broadly refers to dementia that is a consequence of inadequate, intermittent or problematic cerebral blood flow. One of the most common types of vascular dementia is multi **infarct** dementia. This type of dementia is the result of a person experiencing multiple small strokes (infarcts). **Table 16.3** outlines some of the major features of all four types of dementia.

Risk and protective factors for dementia

A number of risk and protective factors have been identified for dementia. The main risk factor for most types of dementia is increasing age; this can be seen clearly in the increasing rate of diagnoses of dementia in older people. Many of the other risk and protective factors pertain primarily to Alzheimer's disease and vascular dementia. Other risk factors associated with these two types of dementia include a family history of dementia, a diagnosis of Down syndrome and cerebro-vascular accidents (also referred to as a stroke).

TABLE 16.3
Features of different types of dementia

DEMENTIA TYPE	AETIOLOGY	MAJOR FEATURES
Vascular dementia	The result of any condition that causes blockages of the blood supply to the brain. This blockage results in destruction of brain cells. This process is known as infarction.	Symptoms vary with the degree or extent of memory loss experienced, dependent on whether the reduced blood flow has impacted on that area of the brain. Other symptoms include confusion, impaired memory and planning capacity, loss of social skills in situations previously addressed well and decreased attention and concentration.
Alzheimer's disease	The characteristic feature is the development of amyloid plaques and tangles. These structures result in the death of brain cells and is progressive in nature, impacting on increasing areas of the brain.	Irreversible and progressive disease that affects the person's memory, problem-solving, social and interpersonal skills such as communication. A consumer may repeatedly ask the same questions, misplace possessions, become disoriented and lost in places that they have previously been familiar with, forget words or be unable to take part in conversations, and not recognise family members. Concentration, abstract thinking and ability to undertake multiple tasks is increasingly difficult for a person with a diagnosis of dementia – Alzheimer's disease. The person can also experience increasing difficulty with completing daily tasks and responding to unexpected situations. Other changes associated with this diagnosis include depression, social withdrawal, changes in sleeping patterns, wandering, agitation and disturbed thought content (delusions).
Dementia with Lewy bodies	Occurs when protein deposits in the brain disrupt normal brain functions.	Major features include difficulties in concentration and attention, confusion, visual hallucinations, parkinsonism and fluctuations in mental state.
Fronto-temporal dementia	Results from the progressive degeneration of the frontal lobes of the brain. Picks disease is one type of fronto-temporal dementia.	A consumer with a diagnosis of fronto-temporal dementia experiences progressive damage to the frontal and temporal lobes of the cerebral cortex. Frontal lobe damage can result in changes to mood, emotions and behaviour. A consumer may have difficultly adapting to new situations, have difficulty expressing emotions, become disinhibited and easily distracted. Damage to the temporal lobe is associated with understanding and processing auditory information. A person may experience increasing difficulty in understanding messages and communicating with others. Difficulties in reading and comprehension, and recognising people they previously knew are experienced.

SOURCE: ADAPTED FROM ALZHEIMER'S ASSOCIATION, 2017; ALZHEIMER'S AUSTRALIA, N.D.A; APA, 2013; GOODE & BOOTH, 2012

Referred to as the three Ds, dementia, delirium and depression are three discrete clinical conditions but can also share some symptoms, and a person may have symptoms of more than one of these conditions. **Table 16.4** outlines some of these key distinctions as well as commonalities.

TABLE 16.4
The three Ds

	DEMENTIA	DELIRIUM	DEPRESSION
Definition	A gradual and progressive decline in cognitive functioning. Short-term memory, language, judgement, reasoning and abstract thinking are all affected.	A medical emergency. Acute onset and fluctuating course of confusion, disorganised thinking and/or declining consciousness.	Depression is a condition where an individual experiences symptoms that meet the criteria for depressive illness (see Chapter 10). Depression affects the person's thinking, feelings, behaviour and physical health.
Onset and duration	Gradual onset over months to years. The clinical course is slow, chronic and irreversible.	Delirium has a sudden onset and can usually occur over hours to several days.	There are changes in the person's mood that persist for a period of at least two weeks. Depression can last weeks to years (particularly if undiagnosed).
Changes in cognition	Progressive cognitive decline with problems in memory. Also, person experiences one of the following: **aphasia**, **apraxia**, **agnosia** and/or deterioration in executive functioning.	There are fluctuations in the person's level of alertness, cognition, perceptions and thought processes.	Impaired memory, concentration and thinking. Low self-esteem identified through poor sense of self-concept.
Changes in mood	Depressed mood may be evident in early dementia.	Significant fluctuations in mood; e.g. anger, crying, being fearful.	Depressed mood, anhedonia, appetite changes (under- or over-eating), feelings of hopelessness.
Sleep and appetite	Sleep cycle can be impacted. Loss of appetite and nutritional deficits.	Sleep disturbance is experienced.	Disturbance to the sleep–wake cycle.
Thought and perception	Disturbed thought content, such as delusion; e.g. objects or money being stolen.	Confused thought processes. Visual hallucinations can be present.	Suicidal thought/ideas/plan.
Clinical course	Slow, progressive and irreversible.	Short (often frequent) variations in symptoms.	Variations in mood over the course of the day. Mood is often lowest in the morning.

SOURCE: ADAPTED FROM MUIR-COCHRANE, BARKWAY & NIZETTE, 2014; HUNT, 2017

Aspects of mental health assessment and the MSE relevant to older people with neurocognitive disorder

As outlined in earlier chapters, the mental health assessment/mental state examination (MSE) relies heavily on the interaction between the clinician and the consumer. Information from other sources such as general practitioners (GPs), family or friends is also useful, but is not relied on as the primary method of gaining assessment information. When interacting with older consumers, the use of what a **collateral history** (Plakiotis & O'Connor, 2012) may be an important additional source of information, particularly if the consumer is experiencing cognitive impairment.

Information will be obtained under headings such as presenting complaint; history of presenting illness; past psychiatric history; alcohol and drug history; and premorbid personality. A mental health assessment of the older person will also look at the extent of any cognitive decline and the person's capacity to carry out their activities of daily living. The combination of physical frailty and cognitive decline can affect an older person's ability to maintain independent levels of functioning. Therefore, it is essential that a mental health assessment considers any changes noticed by the consumer and carers in this area (Plakiotis & O'Connor, 2012).

Assessment of cognitive function will look at the person's orientation, and long-term and short-term memory executive functioning. Changes in these facets of cognitive function can impact on an individual's safety; for example, wandering off, forgetting where they are and forgetting to turn off household items (e.g. iron, stoves or heating). An assessment will also review the older person's capacity to maintain activities of daily living such as personal hygiene and grooming as well as the capacity to live independently in such areas as cooking and finances (APA, 2013; Hunt, 2017). Interviewing family and friends will also provide information regarding increasing responsibility for helping older relatives to meet activities of daily living. Changes in the older person's behaviour, such as agitation and increasing aggression (e.g. as part of developing dementia), is also important information to gather.

The MSE will not only look at changes in cognitive function. Other aspects of the MSE will need to be assessed for and this will depend on the reasons for the older person presenting for assessment, such as depression (see Chapter 10). The following section provides some useful information on specific aspects of the MSE for older people.

COMMONALITIES OF THE MSE: OLDER PEOPLE

Appearance and behaviour
Appearance and behaviour can be impacted by a range of conditions such as dementia, depression or physical health problems. Psychomotor agitation is commonly seen in older people experiencing a depressive episode.

Speech
Lack of speech is seen in depression and dementia. Aphasia is a key feature of dementia but not of depression or delirium.

Mood and affect
Anxiety can be a prominent feature of depression. Mood depression will likely be seen in older persons with depression, and elevation in mood in those experiencing mania. Mood and affect also incorporates appetite, sleep and libido. Sleep disturbances, such as **sundowning**, can be experienced by a person with dementia.

Thought
Delusions are often experienced by older people with dementia. They are not usually as complex as those experienced by people with a psychosis. Delusions are more commonly centred on theft of personal items or incorrectly identifying other people.

Perception
Perceptual disturbances such as hallucinations can be experienced in delirium, and major neurocognitive disorder such as Alzheimer's disease.

Cognition
As with any disorder in the neurocognitive classification, changes to cognition are a key feature of changes to an older person's mental state. However, an older person who retains social skills may not appear to have issues with cognition.

Deficits in cognitive functioning such as short-term memory often appear. **Confabulation** is a commonly assessed symptom. Attention is impacted; for example, difficulty sustaining attention in an environment with multiple stimuli occurring, which can be seen in major NCD or taking longer to complete regular tasks and needing to go back and check frequently.

Executive function is altered; for example, when a person cannot concentrate on more than one task at a time or requires increased effort to complete multiple tasks.

Insight and judgement
An older person will retain varying degrees of insight, particularly when they are in the earlier stages of dementia. As dementia progresses, insight is increasingly reduced.

Poor insight can lead to issues in judgement. An example of this is an older person who continues to drive a motor vehicle even when it is clear to family and friends they are unable to do so (adapted from APA, 2013; Plakiotis & O'Connor, 2012).

Other important areas of assessment of older people diagnosed with major neurocognitive disorder
In addition to the comprehensive mental health assessment, other areas of assessment that need to be undertaken relate to physiological health and well-being, pain, social functioning and spiritual matters.

Physiological assessment considers the individual's past and present physical health state and includes a physical examination, physical functioning, pain assessment and review of past and current medications. For example, polypharmacy is common in older people and one of the key considerations is the potential for adverse interactions between different medications as older people often experience increased sensitivity to medications. Therefore, it is important to document all medications, including over-the-counter medications, vitamins and/or herbal supplements as well as prescribed medications.

Assessment of physical functions includes an assessment of mobility, nutrition, eating and sleeping patterns. Specific areas to be assessed under these domains include:
- **functional status** such as bathing, toileting, dressing and mobility
- weight loss

- dysphasia
- sleep changes that may be reflective of an underlying disorder such as insomnia, as opposed to the age-related reduction in the number of hours slept that is commonly experienced by older people.

Experiencing unrelieved pain should not be a normal part of a person's life at any age, yet there appears to be a belief that pain is an expected part of growing older (Douglas, Hayden & Wollin, 2016). The experience of pain is often under-recognised and undertreated for people experiencing neurocognitive disorder. This is particularly evident as a condition like dementia progresses and the person loses the capacity to verbalise pain. Often non-verbal (including vocal) cues of pain are not adequately identified, assessed and appropriately managed (Australian Pain Society, 2005).

Assessment of social functioning includes the following areas:

- *Social support*: Areas include the degree to which older people are socially connected and participate in family and community activities, or the degree to which the older person experiences feelings of isolation, hopelessness and helplessness.
- *Social systems*: This refers to the degree to which an older person is connected to community resources as well as factors such as income sources; for example, whether the older person is a self-funded retiree and/or a recipient of an age pension.
- *Legal status*: This considers such factors as the older person's capacity (as defined by law – refer to Chapter 3) to advocate on their own behalf. It is also important to recognise the signs of ageism.
- **Instrumental activities of daily living**: These include the ability to shop or use the telephone.
- *Quality of life*: An assessment of quality of life considers:
  1 the presence or absence of distressing physical symptoms
  2 a sense of emotional well-being
  3 the degree of independence the older person maintains in their functional status
  4 the quality of their relationships with other people such as family and friends
  5 the extent to which they can access, participate in and enjoy social activities
  6 the extent to which they can express their sexuality, continue to enjoy intimate relationships and experience positive self-esteem.

Management of major neurocognitive disorder

There are several principles that are important in positively and effectively helping consumers who are diagnosed and living with major neurocognitive disorder. These principles encompass:

- person-centred care practices
- implementing appropriate management and treatment options, including managing the behavioural and psychological symptoms of dementia
- managing co-occurring medical conditions
- coordinating care using a multidisciplinary approach
- maintaining social connectedness through appropriate support groups, social activities and other relevant support services (adapted from Alzheimer's Association, 2012).

The importance of a person-centred approach when working with consumers diagnosed with dementia must not be underestimated. A person-centred approach to practice treats all people as unique individuals, and is aimed at building trust and understanding through therapeutic engagement. It requires nurses to work with the person's beliefs and values.

Principles of effective communication with the person who has major neurocognitive disorder (dementia)

A question often asked by students is, 'How do I communicate with a person who has dementia?' The principles for effective communication are no different for a person with dementia from any other person. First, this means communication is based on respect, being non-judgemental and genuineness. Second, effective communication is based on responding to the cues that the person gives us. In working and communicating with a person who has a diagnosis of dementia, this same principle applies; it is the strategies we use in responding that are important. Goode and Booth (2012) provide a comprehensive framework that can guide the nurse's interactions when communicating with the person with dementia. **Table 16.5** considers each of these ideas.

Behavioural and psychological symptoms of dementia

Based on the assessment outlined above, there is a range of behavioural and psychological symptoms (BPSD) that a person diagnosed with dementia can experience. Loi, Westphal, Ames and Lautenschlager (2015) identify a number of neurocognitive manifestations of dementia. These are aggression, depression, apathy, psychosis and agitation. Depression and apathy are the most commonly experienced symptoms. These are known collectively as behavioural and psychological symptoms of dementia (BPSD). **Table 16.6** outlines the different types of BPSD.

TABLE 16.5
Guide to communicating with a person with dementia

PRINCIPLE	RATIONALE	EXAMPLES
Understand the relationship and impact of dementia on language use	Altered communication capacity is one of the most noticeable symptoms of dementia. It is essential to remember that just because a person cannot communicate verbally, they can communicate in other ways.	Aphasia and dysphasia are two common symptoms that can result from memory loss.
Know the person's preferred ways of communicating	When we understand and have information regarding a person's preferred way of communicating, it becomes easier to identify different ways of engaging. Understanding the family and close friends' experience of living with/caring for their relative can provide important information about the way in which the consumer interacts with others, their hobbies and dislikes.	Knowing the person's preferred first language enables the nurse to work collaboratively with relevant support services such as interpreters and culturally appropriate liaison workers. Use visual devices/flip charts to aid in communication. Knowledge of any sensory issues allows the nurse to implement appropriate referral pathways.
Communication is based on an understanding of the individual abilities and needs of the person	Be aware of any barriers to communication. Use active listening skills. When a person communicates, they tell a story verbally and non-verbally. Look at all parts of the message. Remember that communication is verbal and non-verbal. Where someone cannot communicate verbally, the nurse must be careful not to disregard subtle, non-verbal messages. Allow time for communication. Do not overwhelm a person with too many messages or stimuli. Be observant.	Barriers to communication include pain, noise, visual and or hearing loss. Non-verbal communication can provide important information (e.g. grimacing in pain, clenching their mouth when they do not wish to eat, or squeezing your hand in response to you taking it to communicate acceptance of this gesture.) Go at the person's pace. If they are walking, walk with them. Look for consistent behaviours and track them against the verbal/non-verbal cues given.
Consider specific strategies that could be implemented	Knowing the person you are working with enables you to adopt a range of possible strategies.	Observe for non-verbal signs to work out what the person may be feeling. Memory loss does not mean the person cannot hear; keep your voice at a normal speaking level, as speaking loudly can actually increase anxiety and escalate a challenging situation. Be clear and concise in communication. Long explanations or too much information can increase confusion. Listen for the emotion that is underpinning what the person says and what they are thinking, rather than whether what they are saying seems to be true or not. Learn to respond to the person's behaviour and emotions in the moment. For example, if they are singing, join in with them. If a person is folding washing, talk to them about what aspects of housekeeping they may enjoy.

SOURCE: ADAPTED FROM GOODE & BOOTH, 2012

TABLE 16.6
Types of behavioural and psychological symptoms of dementia (BPSD)

TYPE OF SYMPTOM	EXAMPLES
Disinhibited behaviour	Socially inappropriate behaviour, uncontrolled eating, removing clothing
Restless/agitated behaviour	Aggression, agitation, wandering, verbally disruptive behaviours, sleep disturbances, sundowning
Psychotic symptoms	Delusions, hallucinations
Mood symptoms	Apathy, depression, anxiety

SOURCE: LOI, WESTPHAL, AMES & LAUTENSCHLAGER, 2015

Non-pharmacological management of BPSD

Non-pharmacological strategies available to work with BPSD are based on pragmatic interventions that aim to respond to the factors contributing to BPSD (Loi et al., 2015) and are the first line of management for the consumer experiencing BPSD. The key elements in working with BPSD non-pharmacologically involve maintaining the person's safety, modifying the environment and activities, and implementing specific treatments (NSW Health & RANZCP, 2013). There is a risk that a person presenting with dementia and BPSD may be labelled as 'difficult' or a 'management problem'. Labels such as these dehumanise the person diagnosed with dementia and experiencing BPSD, rather than seeing them as someone requiring support and a coordinated approach to care. There are some key principles of caring for a person experiencing BPSD:

- *Ensure a person-centred approach to care:* This sees the consumer as someone to work with, not as a problem to be managed. This philosophy is at the centre of the multidisciplinary team approach where the consumer, carers and health staff work together. It is a holistic approach to practice rather than a task and/or deficit style of practice. Person-centred care requires that the mental health nurse 'knows' that person.

- *Care should be provided through a multidisciplinary team approach:* This means it is more likely that the appropriate clinicians and/or support staff will be involved in helping to address the specific consumer's needs. Care planning and implementation are more likely to reflect a holistic approach and provide clear guidelines if staff need to implement strategies rapidly. This multidisciplinary approach must involve the family who have knowledge and understanding of their loved one. Family can provide essential information on aspects such as:
  - triggers that increase the likelihood of certain behaviours such as changes to routines or shower times. A consumer with dementia can be sensitive to non-verbal communication. If they are responding to the behaviour of others, then it is essential that the mental health nurse presents a calm and reassuring presence
  - when symptoms of BPSD occur
  - what strategies help their loved one.

- *Ensure that legal and ethical responsibilities are adhered to by all care staff:* Maintaining one's legal and ethical responsibilities in relation to caring for someone experiencing BPSD means that principles of beneficence – such as least restrictive practice, clear communication, assessing the capacity of the individual, ensuring procedures for gaining consent (in line with the level of capacity the individual

displays at that point in time) – are adhered to. It is also essential that the multidisciplinary team have knowledge of any advance care directives or statements or whether there are appointed powers of attorney in place (adapted from NSW Ministry of Health & RANZCP, 2013).

Validation therapy and doll therapy

To feel validated is to feel accepted for who you are and cared about by others, and to have this care and respect communicated. The need for validation is important for all people. Validation therapy is a way of communicating with a person who, as a consequence of their diagnosis of dementia or Alzheimer's, is unable to communicate verbally. Developed by Naomi Feil (1992), validation therapy places greater emphasis on the emotional aspect of communication as opposed to the verbal content of a message. The aim is to be respectful of a person's beliefs and feelings. Listening without judging, without trying to convince a person with dementia their ideas or thoughts are incorrect, but to accept that the ideas they are expressing are real for them, validation therapy assumes to increase empathy, promote dignity and reduce anxiety.

Validation therapy recognises that people are unique individuals at any age, and that there is a reason for the way a person with dementia is behaving. This can be linked, meeting basic human needs such as being appreciated, to be listened to or feeling safe. In this way validation therapy is a person-centred and focused therapeutic activity. Communication strategies that the nurse can use in implementing validation therapy include:

- Being prepared to listen and putting preconceptions and judgements to one side
- Reminisce with the person to promote dignity and focus on strengths
- Maintain eye contact (that is culturally appropriate)
- Avoid arguing, which will only increase a person's agitation (Feil, 1992).

Doll therapy provides a structured opportunity for an older person with dementia to engage in a purposeful and satisfying activity. A number of benefits have been identified, such as stress reduction and increased interactions with others. Mitchell and Templeton (2014) believe there are ethical considerations in the use of such a strategy. While the use of such a strategy can promote an individual's well-being (beneficence), there is a concern that it can cause distress for family members and impact negatively on a person's dignity. Several principles have been identified that must be considered prior to the use of doll therapy. Involving the family in any discussions regarding the possible use of doll therapy, and not forcing the older person to hold a doll, are two important principles that must be adhered to by clinicians.

There is also little theoretical basis for the use of doll therapy in dementia, where it is poorly understood and morally questionable (Mitchell & Hugh, 2013; Mitchell & Templeton, 2014). Mitchell and Hugh identify that the advent of doll therapy stems from Bowlby's work on attachment. Much

evidence is anecdotal, with the first empirical study done in the mid-2000s. A critical review of the literature by Mitchell, McCormack and McCance (2014) argues that further research is required to clearly identify best practice, and ongoing education for clinicians and carers.

Priorities of care focus on one or more of the domains seen in **Table 16.7**.

TABLE 16.7
Care priorities and examples

MANAGEMENT OF PHYSICAL CARE NEEDS	BEHAVIOURAL AND ENVIRONMENTAL MANAGEMENT STRATEGIES	PSYCHOLOGICAL ENGAGEMENT	USE OF PSYCHOTROPIC MEDICATION	CARING FOR THE CARER
Use bed baths as opposed to full showers.	Use music to assist with agitation and verbal aggression, and aromatherapy (e.g. lavender oil) to assist with agitation and mood. Avoid too many staff crowding around the consumer. If possible have a clinician whom the consumer responds to as the primary contact. Do not respond personally to disturbed delusions or hallucinations (e.g. if they say you have stolen their clothes). Having a familiar environment, care staff and routine are important to engender feelings of safety and security. Consider use of validation/doll therapy.	Use multisensory interventions (e.g. Snoezelen therapy). Implement emotion-oriented care. This incorporates a person-centred approach. Specific strategies include: • acknowledge situations/events that increase the person's anxiety • provide appropriate and meaningful reassurance • identify the trigger(s) for increasing anxiety so that it can be addressed.	Specific use in the management of persistent agitation related to behavioural and psychological symptoms of dementia for consumers with a diagnosis of Alzheimer's dementia (see **Table 16.8**). Acetylcholinesterase inhibitors can be used in the treatment of mild to moderately severe Alzheimer's dementia (see **Table 16.9**).	Ensure staff and family education (e.g. behaviour management techniques, problem solving).

SOURCE: ADAPTED FROM GUURE, 2015; HEALTH.VIC, 2018; LOI ET AL., 2015; NSW MINISTRY OF HEALTH & RANZCP, 2013

Pharmacological management of BPSD

The aim of supporting individuals with BPSD is to adapt the environment to meet the person's unique needs. However, there are instances when the experience of the BPSD can pose a risk to the safety

and well-being of the individual and/or others. In this situation, the use of a low dose of Risperidone (an atypical antipsychotic) can be used to manage the symptoms of aggression, psychosis and agitation.

TABLE 16.8
Provides information on risperidone

MEDICATION	INDICATION	DOSE	PRECAUTIONS/SIDE EFFECTS/ CONTRAINDICATIONS
Risperidone	Indicated where an older person is experiencing persistent agitation/aggression that has been unresponsive to non-pharmacological approaches.	Administered as two divided doses. Dosage is increased with a starting dose of 0.5 mg/day in the first instance. This can be increased to a maximum dose of 1.5 mg/day. Use of Risperidone is for a maximum of 12 weeks.	Side effects include: • parkinsonism • headache • insomnia • agitation • anxiety • infection including URTI, UTI, sore throat • pneumonia • weight gain • appetite change • extrapyramidal symptoms • dizziness • tremor • lethargy

MEDICATION	INDICATION	DOSE	PRECAUTIONS/SIDE EFFECTS/ CONTRAINDICATIONS
			• **somnolence** • blurred vision • tachycardia; arrhythmia • GI upset • fatigue • pyrexia • rash • tardive dyskinesia, neuroleptic malignant syndrome • cerebrovascular problems such as stroke and transient ischaemic attacks • hypersensitivity, including anaphylaxis (very rare). Contraindicated where there has been a known hypersensitivity.

SOURCE: ADAPTED FROM MIMS ONLINE, 2018

Pharmacological management of major neurocognitive disease (dementia)

A number of pharmacological agents are available and used in the treatment of dementia. In particular, there are several medications used in the treatment of Alzheimer's type dementia. Acetylcholinesterase inhibitors are used in the treatment of mild to moderately severe Alzheimer's type dementia. **Table 16.9** reviews these medications.

TABLE 16.9
Pharmacological agents used in the management of major neurocognitive disorder (dementia)

DRUG NAME	DOSE	CONTRAINDICATIONS/PRECAUTIONS	SIDE EFFECTS/ADVERSE REACTIONS
Rivastigmine	1.5–6 mg per day titrated	Known hypersensitivity. If treatment is interrupted for more than three days then the person should be recommenced on the lowest daily dose to avoid possible adverse reaction. Weight needs to be monitored. Can cause **bradycardia**.	Include: • GI upsets • nausea, vomiting, diarrhoea • anorexia, weight loss. Central nervous system: • dizziness, headache • somnolence. Rare: • GI haemorrhage • pancreatitis • hallucinations • arrhythmias.
Donepezil	5 mg/day–max. 10 mg/day after 1 month	Monitor for GI bleeding if there is a history of peptic ulcers. Monitor cardiac function. Precautions are necessary for consumers who have a history of respiratory and/or pulmonary conditions such as asthma and pneumonia.	• Gastrointestinal: nausea, vomiting, diarrhoea • Fatigue • Insomnia • Muscle cramp • Asthenia • Weight loss • Infection • Influenza • Seizure • Syncope • Bradycardia • Headache • Dizziness • Aggression • Neuroleptic malignant syndrome (very rare)

DRUG NAME	DOSE	CONTRAINDICATIONS/PRECAUTIONS	SIDE EFFECTS/ADVERSE REACTIONS
Galantamine (prolonged release) Galantamine (immediate release)	4 mg twice daily (immediate release or 8 mg per day (prolonged release)	Known sensitivity. Increased risk of peptic ulcers. Consumers with a history of respiratory/ pulmonary disorders such as severe asthma or obstructive or active pneumonia. Can cause bradycardia.	• Gastrointestinal: irritation, anorexia, weight loss. • CNS: dizziness, headache, somnolence, fainting, blurred vision. • Depression, fatigue, asthenia.

SOURCE: ADAPTED FROM ANDREWS ET AL., 2013; MIMS ONLINE, 2018

Co-occurring dementia and depression

Depression, mood and affective disorders and bipolar disorders have been reported as co-occurring conditions for 33% of people with dementia (AIHW, 2012). Alzheimer's Australia indicates that this figure is between 40–50% for people diagnosed with dementia (Alzheimer's Australia, n.d.), with older people in residential care being at a higher risk. Experiencing symptoms of depression is common in the early stages of the dementia. A person can experience major interference with their ability to function and participate in regular activities. While antidepressants may be used in the treatment of depression for a person with dementia, there is debate regarding their efficacy versus the impact of side effects. If antidepressants are prescribed, selective serotonin reuptake inhibitors (SSRIs) would be the medication of choice (Chi, Yu, Tan & Tan, 2014; Leong, 2014). ECT has also been indicated as safe in older persons who may not be able to tolerate the side effects of antidepressant mediations, or may be impacted by polypharmacy.

Non-pharmacological approaches to managing depressive symptoms are strongly recommended with strategies such as physical exercise, promoting a regular daily routine and maintaining social connections (Chong, 2012).

EVIDENCE-BASED PRACTICE

Dementia and suicide

Title of study

A complex relationship between suicide, dementia and amyloid: A narrative review

Authors

Ismael Conejero, Sophie Navucet, Jacques Keller, Emilie Olié, Philipe Courtet and Audrey Gabelle

Background

Neurocognitive disorders are associated with high rates of suicide in older adults. However, the authors noted that analysis of the relationships between dementia and suicidal behaviors showed conflicting results.

Method

A narrative review of original studies published between 2000 and 2017 on the links between suicidal behaviours, dementia and amyloid load. Additionally, the authors explored the role of depression in these relationships.

Results

The study results showed that late stage dementia may be a protective factor against thoughts of suicide and attempts to end one's life by suicide. On the other hand, there is an increased risk of older people dying by suicide in the early stages of cognitive decline.

Implications

Further research is required in order to develop prevention programs that appropriately meet the needs of older people in the early stages of dementia. Multidisciplinary team members play a vital role in working with consumers and their families/carers in the early stage of a diagnosis of dementia in relation to education, support and assessment of risk addressing specific health-related issues.

SOURCE: CONEJERO, I., NAVUCET, S., KELLER, J., OLIÉ, E., COURTET, P. & GABELLE, A. (2018). A COMPLEX RELATIONSHIP BETWEEN SUICIDE, DEMENTIA, AND AMYLOID: A NARRATIVE REVIEW. *FRONTIERS IN NEUROSCIENCE*, 12, 371. DOI: 10.3389/FNINS.2018.00371

Minor neurocognitive disorder

The DSM-5 (APA, 2013) outlines the diagnostic criteria for minor neurocognitive disorder including evidence of modest cognitive decline of previous level performance in one or more cognitive domains. This is a key distinction from major neurocognitive disorder, which specifies a significant cognitive decline. The other key element of the diagnosis of minor neurocognitive disorder is that the cognitive deficits experienced in everyday activities such as managing medications and paying bills can still be undertaken by the person while often requiring additional supports, strategies and adjustments (APA, 2013). The specific types of minor neurocognitive disorder include Alzheimer's disease, vascular disease, Lewy body disease and fronto-temporal lobar degeneration. As with major neurocognitive disorder, there are a number of other conditions that also contribute to minor neurocognitive disorders, such as traumatic brain injury, Parkinson's disease, Huntington's disease and substance/medication use (APA, 2013).

THE IMPACT OF NEUROCOGNITIVE DISORDERS ON FAMILIES

When a person is diagnosed with a neurocognitive disorder such as dementia, the entire family unit is impacted. Research clearly demonstrates the impact on families through increased levels of distress, physical and emotional burden and increased experience of depression as well as financial and social impacts (Ching-Tzu, Hsin-Yun & Yea-Ing Lotus, 2014; Grano, Lucidi & Violani, 2017).

Family members of people with dementia face a unique set of challenges and consequent high levels of distress when caring for their family member (Hungerford, Jones & Cleary, 2014). Older carers experience a range of possible adverse outcomes arising from their caring role, including stress-related illness and feelings of weariness, worry, anger and depression (Alzheimer's Australia, 2015). Other issues include the physical impact of care-giving, changes to family and social relationships, and the lack of resources to support carers (Flynn & Mulcahy, 2013). One reason for the high levels of stress experienced by family carers of people with dementia is the older age of spousal carers; another reason is the behavioural and psychological symptoms of dementia that the carer may be struggling to manage (Hungerford, Jones & Cleary, 2014).

One way of beginning to understand the impact of a diagnosis of dementia on a family is through the idea of 'grieving the losses'. In broad terms, loss refers to the absence of something, either in the present or the future. Each person will place a different value on the current or anticipated loss, the meaning and value of which is mainly determined by the individual experiencing that loss. Therefore, loss is unique to each person, as well as being a universal experience. Loss is a fact of life and encompasses grief, but also the opportunity for growth. Grief is most commonly thought of as the emotional experience associated with a loss, but grief will also encompass physical and social dimensions as well.

Table 16.10 identifies a range of potential losses that families as well as their relatives can experience when faced with a diagnosis of dementia.

TABLE 16.10
The experience of loss by families of a person diagnosed with dementia

DOMAIN OF LOSS	EXAMPLE
Physical	Increased burden of care, fatigue, role strain
Social	Loss of social connections contributing to increased isolation
Emotional	Guilt, anger, depression
Financial	Restricted employment opportunities, prospects, increased medical costs

How can mental health nurses support families as they experience their own journey with their loved one diagnosed with a major neurocognitive disorder? First, it is important to consider how families are coping and what strategies are more or less useful. Gallagher et al. (2011) look at the way in which family caregivers used emotion-focused, task-focused and ineffective coping strategies and the impact on their feelings of self-efficacy and experience of depression. Examples of these coping strategies are outlined in **Table 16.11**.

TABLE 16.11
Coping strategies

EMOTION COPING STRATEGIES	TASK-FOCUSED COPING STRATEGIES	INEFFECTIVE COPING STRATEGIES
Seeking emotional support Being socially connected to support networks Controlling upsetting thoughts Positive reframing	Seeking practical assistance Education on dementia	Denial Self-blame Disengaging from emotional connection with their loved one

There are a variety of different ways in which families can be supported to increase their feelings of self-efficacy in caring for family members, contributing to their ongoing care and maintaining a personal sense of health and well-being. These include information-based psychoeducation sessions, role transition, mindfulness-based interventions, emotion management, continuity of care through a case management model provided by the facility, and being involved in conversations regarding the ongoing support and management of their relatives (Tang & Chan, 2015).

A diagnosis of dementia does not automatically mean that a person is admitted to a residential aged care facility. However, if the older person's capacity to maintain their independent living means that increasing levels of support will be required, ultimately this can result in admission to a residential aged care facility.

This transition can often result in a further sense of loss for both the person and their family, in terms of a further loss of identity, control, status and choice for the individual affected. While independence may no longer be reflected by remaining independent in their own home, it is essential to promote continued personal independence in a supported environment like a residential aged care facility. There are other ways to maintain personal independence while living within a supported care environment.

NURSING CARE PLAN

PLAN 1: LISA'S DIAGNOSIS OF VASCULAR DEMENTIA

Lisa is an 87-year-old woman whose second husband passed away 20 years earlier. Lisa emigrated to Australia from Europe following World War II with her first husband. They were small business owners and had two sons. Lisa had started working with children with special needs following her divorce and had worked in this area for 25 years prior to her retirement. She had contributed to the childcare of her grandchildren and had been actively involved in family life. Lisa had also been actively involved in the local day program for older people in her community, where she had been a volunteer, received several commendations for her work and featured in the local newspaper.

Her sons had noticed subtle changes in Lisa's behaviour over the past three years, with Lisa seeming to become more forgetful and less able to complete regular activities. For example, Lisa had always been completely independent with her finances and was never late paying bills. Recently, her younger son had seen a reminder notice from the local utility company. This was unusual, and when he questioned Lisa about it, she claimed not to have known the bill had arrived and said she couldn't work out how to organise the payment.

Lisa was diagnosed with type 2 diabetes several years earlier. Given her recent forgetfulness, her sons were concerned that she was not eating regularly and taking her medication. Lisa assured them that she was and went to great lengths to explain her daily eating habits. However, when asked about her medication, Lisa became vague and progressively agitated, telling her sons to stop 'treating her like a child'. They asked to see her medication and could only find one bottle of prescribed medication that had been dispensed approximately six months earlier and which was still three-quarters full. Lisa had also stopped showering on a regular basis and again became agitated when her sons attempted to question her about this. Lisa complained the bathroom was too cold, so her sons fitted the bathroom out with appropriate heating. This had little impact, with Lisa still not showering sometimes for several weeks at a time. When the suggestion was made to have some personal help Lisa became increasingly agitated and distressed.

Socially, Lisa had stopped volunteering at the local day program in the past six months, saying she had too much to do and it was too hard to get up in the mornings. She no longer went on her daily walks or visited the local club with her neighbour. She appeared increasingly frail and would often start crying when her sons came to visit, saying that she was so lonely and she had no one to talk to.

After a great deal of persuasion, Lisa agreed to see the GP with her sons. Following a series of investigations, which showed the presence of a number of small strokes, together with the reported changes in her behaviour and daily living routine, Lisa was diagnosed with vascular dementia. As she was still living independently, it was essential that she be supported in maintaining this for as long as possible. However, Lisa was adamant that she did not want strangers in her house and was perfectly capable of looking after herself. Over the next few months Lisa continued to have difficulties managing her blood sugar levels effectively and was not attending to her activities of daily living or eating or drinking properly. In this time, she was also diagnosed with renal failure, only having 25% of renal function left.

Her sons were able to institute some support services when her older son informed Lisa that he was going overseas on an extended holiday with his family, something that he had to explain to her several times. Based on this, Lisa reluctantly agreed to have the district nursing service attend on a daily basis to administer her insulin and ensure she was caring for herself. She was also referred to a podiatrist for foot care and saw her GP again prior to her son going away. However, she continued to refuse assistance with meals or housework. Her younger son visited her twice weekly to take her shopping and spend time with her. These support measures have remained in place since her older son's return from his holiday and Lisa now seems to accept the daily visits from the district nurses as part of her routine. While Lisa's sons are keen for their mother to remain in her own home for as long as possible and are both providing increased support and family socialisation opportunities for her during the week, they are starting to feel the strain of the caring role. They are currently investigating care options for their mother.

PLAN 2: MARY AND TONY: A STORY OF EARLY ONSET DEMENTIA

Mary P, 63 years of age, was admitted to a dementia-specific care unit three months ago. Prior to this she had been living at home with her husband, Tony, and one of her three adult children. Tony had given up full-time work 12 months previously in order to care for Mary, who had been diagnosed with early onset dementia Alzheimer's type at the age of 59. Tony assisted with meals and personal hygiene, and spent a great deal of time attempting to maintain Mary's connections with extended family and friends.

In the past six months, Tony had noticed a rapid deterioration in Mary's memory, problem-solving capacity, social interaction skills and ability to assist with her activities of daily living. She had become increasingly verbally abusive towards Tony and had also started hitting out when he tried to engage her in social activities or assist with personal hygiene. Mary was eating less and spent most of her day in the sunroom of the house staring into the garden.

Following lengthy discussions with his GP and an assessment by the aged care assessment team in his local area, Tony reluctantly recognised he could no longer care for Mary in the way that he wanted to. Tony's health was also not good, as he has been recently diagnosed with hypertension and was experiencing symptoms of anxiety. On admission, a team meeting was called to consider priority areas of care for Mary, in particular in relation to her behaviour. In addition to the information above, Mary's children also reported that their mother was sleeping poorly and often found wandering through the house. Tony also acknowledged that Mary became increasingly agitated, restless and resistive at night, often shouting out at something Tony could not see or hear. He also confirmed the changes in sleeping patterns. As part of her admission, the unit manager asked the care staff to obtain a urine sample and complete a urinalysis, which showed negative results. In consultation with Mary's family, the care staff completed a thorough assessment of Mary's behaviour over the course of the day, specifically looking for situations that triggered changes in Mary's behaviour. Further discussion with Mary's family revealed that she was normally a very social person, had previously worked as an artist and was involved in many community activities. She knitted and played the piano and always enjoyed listening to music. This collateral information from Mary's family enabled other members of the multidisciplinary team, such as the occupational therapist, to look at a range of activities that Mary could potentially engage in.

Mary was encouraged to join in the regular music appreciation activity that was held twice weekly. Her favourite music was played each morning prior to showering and dressing and also prior to retiring for the night. A soft nightlight was left on overnight to help orient Mary to where she was upon waking. At mealtimes, Mary was seated at a table with a smaller number of other residents. Her family were encouraged to visit and bring in items from home that Mary valued and would find enjoyable. Tony was also provided with additional support from the welfare worker and was able to join a carers support group. Tony found this strategy particularly beneficial because it helped him connect with other carers and their family members in a social and supportive environment.

REFLECTION ON LEARNING FROM PRACTICE

Eleni's recollection of her cousin's experience of dementia is one that resonates with many people. It is a story of loss, a battle a person will ultimately never win. This experience of loss is felt by all people in a family with the care-giving role assumed by many partners and/or children having a potentially significant impact on their own health and well-being. The role of the nurse as a member of the multidisciplinary team is to ensure that they work with consumers and carers/families to promote dignity, maximise strengths and provide opportunities for ongoing positive life experiences.

CHAPTER RESOURCES

SUMMARY

- Neurocognitive disorders are prevalent worldwide and nationally. The defining feature of neurocognitive disorder is changes in cognitive functioning.
- Healthy ageing is a framework for maximising older people's functional capacity and quality of life. It is increasingly being implemented through government policy and health care reforms.
- Elder abuse is a reality for older people in the community. It can take many forms and is still seen as a taboo subject as it challenges many of the ideas communities associate with families and attitudes towards older people.
- The DSM-5 (APA, 2013) classifies a number of neurocognitive disorders. Major neurocognitive disorders, minor neurocognitive disorders and delirium are three groups of conditions.
- Delirium is considered a medical emergency and is common in older people admitted to acute care facilities. Management of delirium combines both non-pharmacological and pharmacological interventions in a person-centred approach.
- Management of neurocognitive disorders such as dementia requires a person-centred, multidisciplinary approach. Management of dementia combines both non-pharmacological and pharmacological interventions. Neurocognitive disorders such as dementia occur concurrently with a range of physical and other mental health conditions. Depression is one notable example.
- Caring for a loved one with a diagnosis of neurocognitive disorder can have a profound impact on families and carers emotionally, physically, socially and financially. Education, support and recognition of the vital role families and carers play in the care of a person with a neurocognitive disorder is essential. Support aims to offer respite when necessary and build resilience.

REVIEW QUESTIONS

1 How would you explain the difference between delirium and dementia to a family member?
2 The nursing care plans in this chapter follow the stories of Lisa and Mary. Lisa was diagnosed with vascular dementia, and Mary with Alzheimer's, and the plan outlines key aspects of each woman's experience and that of their families. As you read through the care plans, identify what aspects of your reading relate to each story in terms of the journey to diagnosis, the impact on each family and strategies used in working with Lisa and Mary.
3 Pharmacological agents used in the management of dementia include:
   a Olanzapine
   b Rivastigmine
   c Lithium
   d St John's wort

4 Attending a support group for family members of an older person diagnosed with dementia is an example of:
   a Emotion-focused coping
   b Just surviving
   c Not realising the impact of caring for a person diagnosed with dementia
   d Task-focused coping
5 Dementia that results from numerous small strokes is referred to as:
   a Lewy body dementia
   b Delirium
   c Dementia – Alzheimer's type
   d Vascular dementia – multi-infarct type

CRITICAL THINKING

1 Reflect on a recent clinical experience where you cared for a person diagnosed with dementia.
   a Did the person experience any difficulties in communicating with others?
   b What strategies were useful in facilitating communication with this person?

   c How did registered staff intervene if the person was experiencing BPSD?
   d What involvement did family and friends have in their ongoing care?
2 Reflect on the first time you met a friend. What information helped you get to know that person better? How did you use this knowledge to help you get to know them?

USEFUL WEBSITES

- COTA for Older Australians: https://www.cota.org.au
- Dementia Australia: https://www.dementia.org.au
- Seniors Rights Victoria: https://seniorsrights.org.au
- World Health Organization: Ageing: Healthy ageing and functional ability: http://www.who.int/ageing/healthy-ageing/en

REFLECT ON THIS

COVID-19 in residential aged care
While Australia stood out in 2020 as having a strong (and overall successful) response to the COVID-19 pandemic, there is one clear area where this claim cannot be made: the residential aged care sector. Read the following article by Cousins (2020) and reflect on the questions that follow: https://www.thelancet.com/journals/lancet/article/PIIS0140-6736(20)32206-6/fulltext
1 What are the major factors that contributed to a surge of deaths in residential aged care facilities as outlined by Cousins?
2 One point made in the article is that there were not enough staff working in residential aged care and many staff were inadequately educated for this role. What are

your thoughts on why it may be difficult to attract health care staff, such as registered nurses, to this sector? What knowledge and skills do staff need?
3 If we consider the human impact of COVID-19 on aged care residents and their families (both in Australia and internationally), it is clear that people have been significantly affected, including those residents living with a diagnosis of dementia. Conduct some research into the range of experiences that families have encountered when restrictions prevented them from seeing family members with dementia. What are the main themes you found in your research? Look for the positive stories as well as examples of stressful or negative experiences.

REFERENCES

Alzheimer's Association. (2017). Vascular dementia. Retrieved from https://www.alz.org/dementia/vascular-dementia-symptoms.asp.

Alzheimer's Australia. (n.d.a). Lewy body disease. Retrieved from https://www.fightdementia.org.au/about-dementia/types-of-dementia/lewy-body-disease.

Alzheimer's Australia (n.d.b). What is younger onset dementia? Retrieved from https://www.fightdementia.org.au/about-dementia/what-is-younger-onset-dementia.

Alzheimer's Australia. (2015). Caring for someone with dementia: The economic, social and health impacts and evidence based supports for carers. Retrieved from https://www.dementia.org.au/files/NATIONAL/documents/Alzheimers-Australia-Numbered-Publication-42.pdf.

Alzheimer's Disease International. (2015). *World Alzheimer Report 2015: The Global Impact of Dementia – An Analysis of Prevalence, Incidence, Cost and Trends*. Retrieved from https://www.alz.co.uk/research/WorldAlzheimerReport2015.pdf.

American Psychiatric Association (APA). (2013). *Diagnostic and Statistical Manual of Mental Disorders (DSM-5)* (5th edn). Washington, DC: APA.

Andrews, G., Dean, K., Genderson, M., Hunt, C., Mitchell, P., Sachdev, P. & Trollor, J. (2013). *Management of Mental Disorders* (5th edn). Sydney: School of Psychiatry, University of NSW.

Australian Bureau of Statistics (ABS). (2016). *4430.0 – Disability, Ageing and Carers, Australia: Summary of Findings, 2012*. Retrieved from http://www.abs.gov.au/ausstats.

Australian Commission on Safety and Quality in Health Care (ACSQHC). (2014). *A Better Way to Care: Safe and High-Quality Care for Patients with Cognitive Impairment (Dementia and Delirium) in Hospital – Actions for Health Service Managers*. Sydney: ACSQHC. Retrieved from https://www.safetyandquality.gov.au/our-work/cognitive-impairment/better-way-to-care.

Australian Commission on Safety and Quality in Health Care (ACSQHC). (2017). *Delirium Clinical Care Standard*. Retrieved from https://www.safetyandquality.gov.au/our-work/clinical-care-standards/delirium-clinical-care-standard.

Australian Institute of Family Studies. (2013). Retrieved from Australia's ageing population: Special series. https://aifs.gov.au/facts-and-figures/ageing-australia. © Commonwealth of Australia. Released under CC BY 4.0. Link to license: https://creativecommons.org/licenses/by/4.0/.

Australian Institute of Health and Welfare (AIHW). (2012). *Dementia in Australia*. Cat. no. AGE 70. Canberra: AIHW. Retrieved from http://www.aihw.gov.au/WorkArea/DownloadAsset.aspx?id=10737422943.

Australian Institute of Health and Welfare (AIHW). (2014). *National Drug Strategy Household Survey. Detailed Report 2013. Drug Statistics Series No. 28*. Cat. No. PHE183. Canberra: AIHW. Retrieved from http://www.health.nsw.gov.au/mentalhealth/publications/Publications/opdap-fullreport.pdf.

Australian Institute of Health and Welfare (AIHW). (2015). *Australia's Welfare 2015. Australia's Welfare Series no. 12*. Cat. no. AUS 189. Canberra: AIHW. Retrieved from https://www.aihw.gov.au/getmedia/692fd1d4-0e81-41da-82af-be623a4e00ae/18960-aw15.pdf.aspx?inline=true.

Australian Institute of Health and Welfare (AIHW). (2017). Dementia. Retrieved from http://www.aihw.gov.au/dementia.

Australian Productivity Commission. (2013). *Overview – An Ageing Australia: Preparing for the Future*. Retrieved from https://www.pc.gov.au/research/completed/ageing-australia/ageing-australia-overview.pdf. p. 6. © Commonwealth of Australia. Released under CC BY 3.0 AU. Link to license: https://creativecommons.org/licenses/by/3.0/au/.

beyondblue (2009). *Depression in Older Age: A Scoping Study. Final Report*. Melbourne: National Ageing Research Institute. Retrieved from https://www.beyondblue.org.au/docs/default-source/research-project-files/bw0143---nari-2009-full-report---minus-appendices.pdf?sfvrsn=4.

Brown, L., Hansnata, E. & La, H.A. (2017). *Economic Cost of Dementia in Australia 2016–2056. Report for Alzheimer's Australia*. NATSEM at the Institute for Governance and Policy Analysis, University of Canberra. Retrieved from DEH.0001.0001.0001.pdf (http://royalcommission.gov.au).

Chi, S., Yu, J.-T., Tan, M.-S. & Tan, L. (2014). Depression in Alzheimer's disease: Epidemiology, mechanisms, and management. *Journal of Alzheimer's Disease*, 42(3), 739–55. doi:10.3233/JAD-140324

Ching-Tzu, Y., Hsin-Yun, L. & Yea-Ing Lotus, S. (2014). Dyadic relational resources and role strain in family caregivers of persons living with dementia at home: A cross-sectional survey. *International Journal of Nursing Studies*, 51(4), 593–602. doi:10.1016/j.ijnurstu.2013.09.001

Chong, S. (2012). Feature – mental health: Depression and dementia. *Australian Journal of Pharmacy*, 93(1105), 34–6, 38, 40.

Conejero, I., Navucet, S., Keller, J., Olié, E., Courtet, P. & Gabelle, A. (2018). A complex relationship between suicide, dementia, and amyloid: A narrative review. *Frontiers in Neuroscience*, 12, 371. DOI: 10.3389/fnins.2018.00371

DeLaune, S.E., Ladner, P.K., McTier, L., Tollefson, J. & Lawrence, J. (2016). *Australian and New Zealand Fundamentals of Nursing*. South Melbourne: Cengage Learning Australia.

Douglas, C., Hayden, D. & Wollin, J. (2016). Supporting staff to identify residents in pain: A controlled pretest–posttest study in residential aged care. *Pain Management Nursing*, 17(1). doi:10.1016/j.pmn.201.08.001

Feil, N. (1992). Validation therapy. *Geriatric Nursing*, 13(3), 129–133. Retrieved from https://www.sciencedirect.com/science/article/pii/S0197457207810214.

Flynn, R. & Mulcahy, H. (2013). Early-onset dementia: The impact on family care-givers. *British Journal of Community Nursing*, 18(12), 598–606.

Gallagher, D., Ni Mhaolain, A., Crosby, L., Ryan, D., Lacey, L., Coen, R. F., … Lawlor, B.A. (2011). Self-efficacy for managing dementia may protect against burden and depression in Alzheimer's caregivers. *Aging & Mental Health*, 15(6), 663–70. doi:10.1080/13607863.2011.562179

Goode, B. & Booth, G. (2012). *Dementia Care. A Care Worker Handbook*. London: Hodder Education.

Grano, C., Lucidi, F. & Violani, C. (2017). The relationship between caregiving self-efficacy and depressive symptoms in family caregivers of patients with Alzheimer disease: A longitudinal study. *International Psychogeriatrics*, 29(7), 1095–1103. doi: 10.1017/S1041610217000059

Guure, C.B., Ibrahim, N.A., Adam, M.B. & Said, S. (2017). Impact of physical activity on cognitive decline, dementia, and its subtypes: Meta-analysis of prospective studies. *Biomed Research International*. doi:10.1155/2017/9016924

Health Vic. (2013). Managing behavioural and psychological symptoms of dementia. Retrieved from https://www2.health.vic.gov.au/

SECTION 2

hospitals-and-health-services/patient-care/older-people/cognition/dementia/dementia-bpsd.

Hungerford, C., Jones, T. & Cleary, M. (2014). Pharmacological versus non-pharmacological approaches to managing challenging behaviours for people with dementia. *British Journal of Community Nursing*, 19 (2), 72–7.

Hunt, S. (2017). Working with older people. In J. Crisp, C. Douglas, G. Rebeiro & D. Waters (eds), *Potter and Perry's Fundamentals of Nursing* (5th edn, pp. 393–421). Chatswood: Elsevier Australia.

Leong, C. (2014). Antidepressants for depression in patients with dementia: A review of the literature. *The Consultant Pharmacist*, 29(4), 254–63. doi:10.4140/TCP.n.2014.254

Loi, S.M., Westphal, A., Ames, D. & Lautenschlager, N.T. (2015). Minimising psychotropic use for behavioural disturbance in residential aged care. *Australian Family Physician*, 44(4), 180–4. Retrieved from http://search.informit.com.au/documentSummary;dn=051002572749424;res=IELHEA.

MIMS Online. (2018) *Monthly Index of Medical Specialties Online*. St Leonards: MIMS Australia. Retrieved from https://www.mimsonline.com.au/Search/Search.aspx.

Mitchell, G., McCormack, B., & McCance, T. (2014). *Therapeutic use of dolls for people living with dementia: A critical review of the literature*. 15(5), 976–1001.

Mitchell, G. & O'Donnell, H. (2013). The therapeutic use of doll therapy in dementia. *British Journal of Nursing*, 22(6), 329–334. Retrieved from http://ezproxy.acu.edu.au/login?url=http://search.ebscohost.com/login.aspx?direct=true&db=ccm&AN=108011266&site=ehost-live&scope=site.

Mitchell, G. & Templeton, M. (2014). Ethical considerations of doll therapy for people with dementia. *Nursing Ethics*, 21(6), 720–30. doi:http://dx.doi.org/10.1177/0969733013518447.

Muir-Cochrane, E., Barkway, P. & Nizette, D. (2014). *Mosby's Pocketbook of Mental Health* (2nd edn). Chatswood: Mosby Elsevier.

NSW Health & Royal Australian and New Zealand College of Psychiatrists (RANZCP). (2013). *Assessment and Management of People with Behavioural and Psychological Symptoms of Dementia (BPSD). A Handbook for NSW Health Clinicians*. Retrieved from

https://www.ranzcp.org/Files/Resources/Reports/A-Handbook-for-NSW-Health-Clinicians-BPSD_June13_W.aspx.

Plakiotis, C. & O'Connor, D.W. (2012). Psychiatric disorders affecting the elderly in Australia. In G. Meadows, J. Farhall, E. Fossey, M. Grigg, F. McDermott & B. Singh (eds), *Mental Health in Australia: Collaborative Community Practice* (3rd edn, pp. 615–46). Melbourne: Oxford University Press.

Seniors Rights Victoria. (n.d.). Homepage. https://seniorsrights.org.au.

Tang, W.K. & Chan, C.Y.J. (2016). Effects of psychosocial interventions on self-efficacy of dementia caregivers: A literature review. *International Journal of Geriatric Psychiatry*, 31(5), 475–93. doi:10.1002/gps.4352

The Australian Pain Society. (2005). *Pain in Residential Aged Care Facilities: Management Strategies*. Retrieved from http://www.apsoc.org.au.

Travers, C., Byrne, G. J., Pachana, N. A., Klein, K. & Gray, L. (2013). Delirium in Australian hospitals: A prospective study. *Current Gerontology and Geriatrics Research*, 8. doi:10.1155/2013/284780

Vasilevskis, E.E., Han, J.H., Hughes, C.G. & Ely, E.W. (2012). Epidemiology and risk factors for delirium across hospital settings. *Best Practice and Research. Clinical Anaesthesiology*, 26(3), 277–87.

Victorian Alcohol and Drug Association (VAADA). (2011). *Responding to Older AOD Users*. Collingwood: VAADA.

Westerby, R. & Howard, S. (2011). Early recognition and diagnosis of dementia. *Practice Nurse*, 42(16), 42–7.

World Health Organization (WHO). (2002). *Active Ageing: A Policy Framework*. Retrieved from http://apps.who.int/iris/bitstream/10665/67215/1/WHO_NMH_NPH_02.

World Health Organization (WHO). (2015). *World Report on Ageing and Health*. Geneva: WHO. Retrieved from http://apps.who.int/iris/bitstream/10665/186463/1/9789240694811_eng.pdf?ua=1.

World Health Organization (WHO). (2017). Ageing and life course: What is active ageing? Retrieved from http://www.who.int/ageing/active_ageing/en.

CHAPTER 17

OBSESSIVE COMPULSIVE AND RELATED DISORDERS

Louise Alexander and Scott Trueman

LEARNING OUTCOMES

Upon completion of this chapter, you should be able to:

17.1 Develop an understanding of obsessive-compulsive disorder, including its aetiology and how the mental state examination may appear

17.2 Understand hoarding disorder, identify its diagnostic features, aetiology and treatment

17.3 Develop an understanding of trichotillomania its diagnostic features, aetiology and treatment

17.4 Understand excoriation disorder, identify its diagnostic features, aetiology and treatment

---

LEARNING FROM PRACTICE

I was 15 years old and it was the height of the AIDS epidemic. Overnight I was horrified that I had AIDS and was spreading it everywhere I went. I was convinced I was infected. I started constantly telephoning the AIDS hotline, informing them that I had given someone AIDS who had either sat on a toilet seat after me, or that I might have accidentally gotten some saliva on someone and in that way transferred the AIDS virus. The hotline reassured me that people couldn't get AIDS from toilet seats or saliva. I would feel better for a while and then I would get anxious again and recommence telephoning the hotline seeking reassurance.

I started to wash my hands until they bled. I didn't want anyone to get sick because of me. I just couldn't get the idea out of my head. I refused to use my towels or soaps more than once. I tried my best not to touch people. I began to avoid leaving the house unless absolutely necessary. If I was going socialise with people, I would make sure to wash my hands to rid my contamination. If I ate, I used disposable cutlery and plates whether at home or when out.

I didn't know such behaviour was enabling the OCD because I didn't know I had OCD.

A friend referred me to a therapist who saved my life. When I told them about the thoughts I was having, they said that they could help me but that it would involve a lot of 'hard work'. I have been seeing her for over a year and my life is completely different than it used to be. I have learned through cognitive behaviour therapy (CBT) and have learned how to resist doing rituals and compulsions despite my brain sending faulty signals. I have learned that OCD is not who I am. OCD is something that I have.

Jane, a consumer living with OCD

Jane's experiences highlight the distress caused by OCD, and the lengths to which a person will go when experiencing such heightened anxiety. As well as frequent handwashing, what other behaviours does Jane describe that could be detrimental to her mental health?

INTRODUCTION

You may have heard the term obsessive-compulsive disorder, or OCD. You may have even used it to describe someone who likes their house to be kept clean, or dislikes the idea of germs on them. It is in fact a term that is frequently misused to describe people who are probably simply fastidious or particular. OCD in its true diagnostic form is a distressing and debilitating condition that significantly impacts on the lives of consumers who have it. Imagine being unable to leave the house because you have rituals that require you to check on the door locks 20 times while saying a prayer; or needing to wash your hands so many times that you make them bleed. OCD is a condition with a foundation in anxiety.

This chapter explores OCD in detail, looking at the causes, symptoms and treatments of the condition. This chapter also explores other OCD-related conditions such as hoarding, and the lesser known trichotillomania, and excoriation condition.

OBSESSIVE-COMPULSIVE DISORDER

Obsessive-compulsive disorder (OCD) is a misunderstood mental health condition that can result in significant impairment in an individual's ability to work, study and share time with friends and family. As the name suggests, OCD is characterised by both **obsessions** and **compulsions**. Obsessions result in intrusive and unwanted thoughts that are repetitive, which usually result in anxiety and distress (APA, 2013). These obsessions may comprise images, thoughts or urges, and usually result in feelings of danger for the individual. Obsessions may include things such as being overly concerned about germ contamination, doors being unlocked or food being contaminated. Compulsions (sometimes called rituals) are behaviours that are repetitive and help the consumer to alleviate their anxiety. Compulsions include *behaviours* or *mental acts* and these are undertaken to alleviate the distressing anxiety that the person feels (APA, 2013). Some examples of OCD compulsive behaviours include washing hands (repeatedly and vigorously); sorting or ordering objects (e.g. by colour); and continuous checking (e.g. checking the doors are locked, the oven is off, the gate is locked).

Mental acts include counting (e.g. concern with odd or even numbers); praying (e.g. repeating 'The Lord's Prayer' or 'Hail Marys' in succession) (see **Figure 17.1**). The compulsive mental acts undertaken by someone with OCD can be very preoccupying, and the individual often feels compelled by their obsessive thoughts. Many people with OCD will have

rules around their behaviours and obsessions, and the individual will usually have rigid beliefs around how precise their rituals need to be. If, for example, they do not recite a prayer perfectly, their system of rules may compel them to begin again, in order to properly comply with their obsessive thoughts and alleviate anxiety. It is not hard to imagine the impacts that these behaviours and mental acts can have on an individual's ability to function.

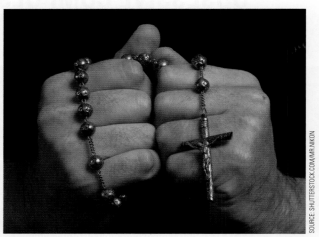

SOURCE: SHUTTERSTOCK.COM/MR.NIKON

FIGURE 17.1
Reciting prayers can form the basis of compulsions for individuals with OCD

Incidence

OCD affects around 1.2% of individuals in the United States and documented rates internationally are between 1.1–1.8% (APA, 2013). In Australia, rates of OCD have been reported at 1.9% (Slade et al., 2009). While males are understood to have higher rates in childhood, females have marginally higher rates in adulthood (APA, 2013). Males are also more likely to experience a comorbid tic condition (such as Tourette's).

Experiences of obsessions and compulsions may differ between genders too. Males may be more likely to experience thoughts which are 'forbidden' (e.g. sexualised thoughts or thinking about masturbation), and they may also require symmetry (e.g. with numbers), while females may present with symptoms necessitating cleaning (such as handwashing). For many people with OCD, symptoms will usually begin when they are children; however, a common time for diagnosis or investigation is during adolescence. While most individuals with OCD will have both obsessions *and* compulsions, in children compulsions are more easily identified because such behaviours are able to be observed by parents, teachers and peers (APA, 2013).

Aetiology

Given that OCD has some foundation in anxiety, it is not uncommon that individuals with OCD may have a close family member with anxiety. This section will explore the causes of OCD.

Genetic factors

OCD remains a condition that is poorly understood. In the limited number of twin studies that have been conducted, a correlation between heredity and the development of OCD has been noted in approximately 45–65% of cases (Krebs & Heyman, 2014). Rates of OCD are higher in those who have a parent with the condition (APA, 2013).

Biological factors

Complex neuroimaging has also yielded some interesting results suggesting that OCD may be associated with front cortex abnormalities (APA, 2013; Krebs & Heyman, 2014). The orbitofrontal cortex of the brain is responsible for mediating thoughts of threat and harm, and hyperactivity of this cortex may be responsible for an increase in symptoms of OCD (Krebs & Heyman, 2014).

REFLECT ON THIS

OCD and COVID-19

Unsurprisingly, the COVID-19 pandemic, which was caused by an initially poorly understood contagion, has resulted in worsening mental health for many people. We have all been inundated with advice to practise social distancing and frequent handwashing to guard against this threat. One of the groups of people hardest-hit by COVID-19 are those with OCD, who are affected by germ obsessions; although, paradoxically, their extreme concern about germs and personal hygiene is also more likely to prevent them catching COVID-19. Despite the infancy of COVID-19, there are already many research articles about its impact on those with OCD.

Using the Google Scholar function, type in 'OCD and COVID-19'. Choose one article and review the recommendations made for working with consumers with OCD during the pandemic.

Environmental factors

Environmental factors associated with the development of OCD have been inconsistently reported. Rates of childhood physical and sexual abuse in addition to traumatic experiences are thought to be related to the development of OCD (APA, 2013). It is important to note, however, that other studies have refuted such suggestions (Krebs & Heyman, 2014). A number of more recent studies have explored the experiences of children who developed OCD suddenly after becoming unwell with streptococcal infections (APA, 2013; Krebs & Heyman, 2014).

Clinical course

In the event that OCD is left untreated, the course will typically become chronic with some acute exacerbations (APA, 2013). Chronic OCD will typically result in significant impairment in everyday functioning (Krebs & Heyman, 2014). OCD may result in increases in other mental health conditions, such as depression, and this is thought to be more common when OCD develops in childhood.

Diagnostic criteria OCD

Table 17.1 outlines the diagnostic criteria for OCD. These criteria include an evaluation of the individual's insight. In order to understand the diagnostic criteria better, it is important to look at examples of different compulsions and obsessions.

Common obsessions include:

- feelings of contamination
- sexual (such as feeling disgust at sexual activity)
- religious (e.g. intrusive, blasphemous thoughts)
- perfectionism
- aggression and harm (e.g. fear of being assaulted or victimised)
- concerns about safety.

Common compulsions include:

- checking and counting (e.g. rearranging and counting objects, arranging by colour/shape)
- seeking reassurance
- repetition
- arranging and reordering
- washing/cleaning
- touching, aligning or tapping objects
- safety checking (e.g. doors locked, oven turned off).

DIAGNOSTIC CRITERIA

Obsessive-compulsive disorder (OCD)

TABLE 17.1
Diagnostic criteria obsessive-compulsive disorder (OCD)

A. Presence of obsessions, compulsions, or both:
- Obsessions are defined by (1) and (2):
1. Recurrent and persistent thoughts, urges, or images that are experienced, at some time during the disturbance, as intrusive and unwanted, and that in most individuals caused marked anxiety or distress.
2. The individual attempts to ignore or suppress such thoughts, urges, or images, or to neutralize them with some other thought or action (i.e., by performing a compulsion).
- Compulsions are defined by (1) and (2):
1. Repetitive behaviors (e.g., hand washing, ordering, checking) or mental acts (e.g., praying, counting, repeating words silently) that the individual feels driven to perform in response to an obsession or according to rules that must be applied rigidly.
2. The behaviors or mental acts are aimed at preventing or reducing anxiety or distress, or preventing some dreaded event or situation; however, these behaviors or mental acts are not connected in a realistic way with what they are designed to neutralize or prevent, or are clearly excessive.

B. The obsessions or compulsions are time-consuming (e.g., take more than 1 hour per day) or cause clinically significant distress or impairment in social, occupational, or other important areas of functioning.

C. The obsessive-compulsive symptoms are not attributable to the physiological effects of a substance (e.g., a drug of abuse, a medication) or another medical condition.

D. The disturbance is not better explained by the symptoms of another mental disorder (e.g., excessive worries, as in generalized anxiety disorder; preoccupation with appearance, as in body dysmorphic disorder; difficulty discarding or parting with possessions, as in hoarding disorder; hair pulling, as in trichotillomania [hair-pulling disorder]; skin picking, as in excoriation [skin-picking] disorder; stereotypies, as in stereotypic movement disorder; ritualized eating behavior, as in eating disorders; preoccupation with substances or gambling, as in substance-related and addictive disorders; preoccupation with having an illness, as in illness anxiety disorder; sexual urges or fantasies, as in paraphilic disorders; impulses, as in disruptive, impulse-control, and conduct disorders; guilty ruminations, as in major depressive disorder; thought insertion or delusional preoccupations, as in schizophrenia spectrum and other psychotic disorders; or repetitive patterns of behavior, as in autism spectrum disorder).

Specify if:
- **With good or fair insight:** The individual recognizes that obsessive-compulsive disorder beliefs are definitely or probably not true or that they may not be true.
- **With poor insight:** The individual thinks obsessive-compulsive disorder beliefs are probably true.
- **With absent insight/delusional beliefs:** The individual is completely convinced that obsessive disorder beliefs are true.

CASE **STUDY**

LIVING AND WORKING WITH OCD

Adam is a 44-year-old high school maths teacher. He leaves for work at 7.55 am every morning. He only lives six minutes from the school, but he has a series of rituals he must complete in order to successfully leave the house, as he is very anxious that his home might burn down or be burgled.

Adam must check the stove and oven five times each before he leaves to confirm that they are both turned off. He recites particular passages from the Bible while doing this. Once he is out the front door, Adam feels compelled to check his lock exactly 12 times *every* time he leaves the house. While doing this, he must also recite 'The Lord's Prayer' in his head. If Adam is not turning his front door handle at the exact time he finishes reciting the prayer, then he will have to start all over again…from the beginning, even if he was up to the 11th check. Adam will do this until he has checked 12 times, in the correct prayer succession. This process can

take him a very long time, and sometimes he is even late for work. When Adam arrives at work, he must check the doors of his car six times by walking in an anticlockwise direction, while reciting 'The Lord's Prayer', because he is worried that if he doesn't complete the ritual, his car will be broken into.

Adam understands that he has OCD, and has good insight into his condition. He is, however, compelled to undertake these rituals, because the anxiety he feels is overwhelming, and the rituals alleviate his anxiety.

Questions

1. What impacts on Adam's interpersonal relationships may result from his experience of OCD?
2. How might Adam's diagnosis of OCD affect his work as a high school teacher?

Treatment of OCD

While OCD is obviously a distressing condition, it is important to note that treatment is available. For some individuals with OCD, there may be particular prominence to their symptoms. For example, obsessions may be more of an issue, while for others, the focal issue may be compulsions. Individuals who have prominent compulsive rituals may benefit from exposure therapy (see Chapter 11) while those with obsessions may require more specialised treatment with a clinician who is skilled in this area (Andrews et al., 2013).

First-line treatment is usually cognitive behavioural therapy (CBT; see Chapter 4); however many individuals will receive adjunct therapy. Many individuals with OCD will benefit from the addition of a selective serotonin reuptake inhibitor (SSRI) medication (see Chapter 10) such as fluoxetine, sertraline, paroxetine or citalopram, and studies have indicated good responses in individuals receiving an SSRI (Krebs & Heyman, 2014).

Clinical presentation and the mental state examination

Because OCD has a strong association with anxiety and a comorbidity with depression, there are some similarities between the MSE presentations between these conditions. It is important to note that delusions are not a normal progression of OCD, and therefore distinguishing between delusional thoughts and OCD behaviours is important. For example, the individual who is overly concerned with their safety should not be mistaken for paranoid. There will be an absence of thought disorder and hallucinations (as seen in psychosis), which will help with diagnosis.

Supportive mental health nursing interventions are based on a person-centred approach to practice. Being empathic, supportive and non-judgemental are central components of this approach at all times, from assessment through implementation of therapeutic interventions, and supporting the consumer. Examples include:

1 acknowledging the consumer's anxiety response to thinking and rituals/compulsions in a non-judgemental way
2 working with the consumer to identify situations that increase anxiety
3 assisting the consumer to implement stress management strategies
4 psycho-education related to the condition, and if prescribed medications, appropriate education related to its use
5 where appropriate and consented to by the consumer, involve their family/other support networks.

COMMONALITIES OF THE MSE: OBSESSIVE-COMPULSIVE DISORDER

General appearance and behaviour

There may be prominent issues with behaviour, particularly if the individual feels compelled to undertake their rituals during the interview. The individual with OCD who has obsessions regarding contamination may have prominent contact dermatitis caused by frequent hand-washing (see **Figure 17.2**). Individuals with OCD may also demonstrate stereotyped behaviours that are similar to those seen in autism spectrum disorder (such as tapping or touching). These behaviours may be complex, such as sequential taps of the index finger onto the left wrist eight times, followed by six taps of the right ear. In some individuals you may notice muttering and distraction (e.g. religious compulsions and prayer reciting). Approximately 31% of individuals with OCD will also have a tic disorder and, as such, conditions such as Tourette's disorder may be responsible (APA, 2013). Tics in Tourette's disorder tend to be uncomplicated (such as brief tapping), while tics associated with OCD are more complex (as mentioned earlier).

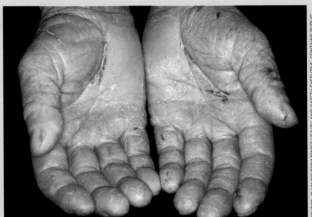

FIGURE 17.2
Contact dermatitis caused by frequent handwashing

Mood

OCD has a strong correlation with anxiety and depressive conditions and therefore it is important to consider this when evaluating mood. Generally, individuals with OCD may be more anxious, distressed and fearful. In those who have good insight, the impacts on their everyday life may result in depressed mood. Consider the impacts that OCD may have on intimate relationships, in addition to their ability to achieve enough rest every day. For individuals with OCD who have contamination fears, consider the impacts this may have on their diet.

Thought

Individuals with OCD will have intrusive and persistent thoughts (or images) that continue to plague them and result in distress. These thoughts may be constant, all-encompassing and result in rumination. It is important to consider the impacts of suicide on individuals with OCD as research suggests that around half have had suicidal thoughts and about one in four individuals with OCD will try to die by suicide (APA, 2013). If comorbid depression is evident, then this risk increases.

Insight

OCD is a condition where insight is often present, yet the intensity of obsessions and compulsions is so overwhelming and distressing that this may not make responses to treatment any easier; it can be even more distressing for the individual to understand they have a mental health condition, but feel unable to control their thoughts and behaviours. Insight may, however, make *engagement* in treatment more likely.

HOARDING DISORDER

Hoarding disorder (HD) is a condition that is new to the *Diagnostic and Statistical Manual of Mental Disorders* (DSM-5; APA, 2013), and has seen an increase in interest, both from the general public and researchers, in the last few years. Imagine never being able to throw anything away, or collecting items that others might consider rubbish. Then imagine accumulating these items in your house, filling one room up at a time, but feeling incredibly distressed by the thought of throwing the items away (see **Figures 17.3** and **17.4**). This is the life of someone with hoarding disorder. Hoarding disorder is characterised by both *acquisition of* and difficulty in *parting with* possessions (an individual may have one or both of these symptoms) (APA, 2013). Individuals who acquire possessions may collect items such as broken items (e.g. broken furniture, lawn mower, a broken television, etc.) that other people have left out as

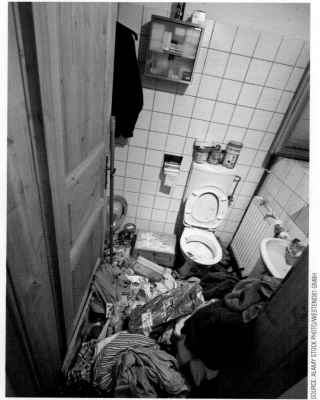

FIGURE 17.4
The bathroom of an individual with hoarding disorder

SOURCE: ALAMY STOCK PHOTO/WESTEND61 GMBH

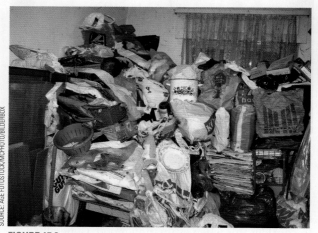

SOURCE: AGE FOTOSTOCK/MCPHOTO/BILDERBOX

FIGURE 17.3
Individuals with hoarding disorder experience heightened anxiety at the thought of throwing out even trivial items

rubbish; or they may purchase multiple items in bulk, or when on sale. For those who experience only the difficulty in parting with possessions, this may include difficulty in discarding household rubbish, such as empty food containers, boxes or empty cans.

Individuals with HD will have unrelated items that clutter and occupy a room; for example, bags of rubbish, a lawn mower, birdcages and cereal boxes in the living room. Eventually, these items begin to fill up the person's house, rendering living spaces inhabitable and unhygienic. As seen in **Figure 17.3**, the kitchen is unusable, making preparation and storage of food impossible. Hygiene can become a serious issue for an individual with HD, as shown in the bathroom in **Figure 17.4**. HD is often characterised by unsanitary conditions that resemble squalor, pose serious risks to health from unhygienic conditions, and injury from an inability to navigate clutter (Kyrios et al., 2018).

Not all hoarding relates to the accumulation of rubbish or acquisition of objects. Animal hoarders are known to collect animals such as dogs or cats (see **Figure 17.5**). These animals may be starving, devoid of veterinary care and living in squalid, unsanitary conditions that impact on everyone living in the house. Animals will often remain lying where they die, contributing to the squalor. Animal hoarding may attract more attention, as the noise, smell and squalor may result in complaints from neighbours.

Impacts of hoarding disorder

The impacts of HD are often severe and can result in significant impairment to everyday functioning.

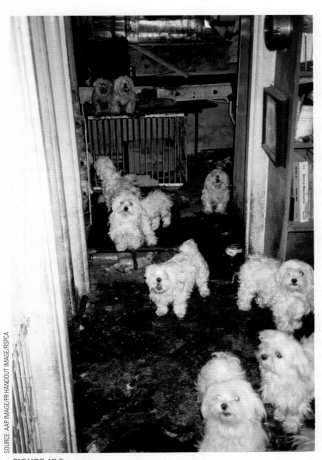

SOURCE: AAP IMAGE/PR HANDOUT IMAGE/RSPCA

FIGURE 17.5
Animal hoarding results in particular unsanitary and squalid conditions

The presence of clutter poses a serious fire risk and seriously impacts on an individual's ability to:
- maintain personal hygiene
- cook
- clean
- wash
- navigate areas within the house
- sleep (as beds are often covered in items)
- maintain collegial relationships with neighbours.

Many individuals with HD may have their utilities (such as electricity, gas and water) disconnected due to failure to pay bills, and many face eviction and/or legal action from their neighbours or municipality (APA, 2013).

Due to its recency as a recognised mental health condition, there is a considerable lack of empirical research on HD. However, rates of the condition in Europe and the United States are understood to be between 2–6%, with a higher presence in males (APA, 2013). HD appears to occur in older persons (55–94 years) more frequently at rates approximately three times higher than those seen in other adults (APA, 2013).

Motivations for hoarding behaviours

Individuals with HD are often motivated by similar urges to collect and hoard items, and these include:
- difficulty with decision-making and processing
- avoidant behaviours, such as avoiding cleaning, washing, checking mail, etc.
- inherent issues with emotional attachments to objects (that to others may seem inanimate or waste)
- poor memory of where they placed items (and therefore replacing items frequently)
- feeling that they need to keep items in case they need them no matter how 'trivial' they may be
- fear of waste.

Aetiology

Hoarding disorder is a condition with varying contributing factors. However, there is a strong genetic association and very high comorbidity with major depressive disorder and anxiety (APA, 2013). This section explores the causes of HD in more detail.

Genetic factors

There are strong links between family members and hoarding behaviours. Approximately 50% of individuals with HD have a family member who also hoards (APA, 2013).

Individual factors

Like most mental health conditions, temperament is understood to play a role in the development of HD. An inability to commit to a decision (or indecisiveness) is a common feature in individuals experiencing the condition (APA, 2013). Other characteristics of individuals with HD include:

- a tendency towards perfectionism
- propensity to demonstrate avoidant behaviours
- poor memory
- a strong attachment to objects/items/things
- procrastination.

Environmental factors

Research suggests that early childhood traumatic experiences and deprivation may play a role in the development of HD. For some, the condition will develop after a traumatic experience, but this is usually realised retrospectively when they seek (or are made to seek) help (APA, 2013). There also are shown to be links with a lack of warmth in the families of individuals with HD, which may suggest that people with the condition seek comforts from 'things' rather than people (Kyrios et al., 2018). Therefore, both material and physical deprivation may play a role in this condition.

Clinical course

The pattern of HD is progressive and for many with the condition, symptoms begin early in life, and reach more critical, disruptive stages later in life. One way to understand the condition is to consider the time it takes to accumulate items. This may take years, so it is perhaps not surprising that the condition is seen more frequently in older people. For every decade an individual lives, symptoms of HD become worse (APA, 2013). Symptoms may begin in childhood, begin to interfere with functioning in the person's 20s, and become significantly problematic in their 30s. Contact with services may occur in the 50s, or earlier if the family intervenes.

Diagnostic criteria hoarding disorder

There are a number of specific features of hoarding disorder that are described in the diagnostic criteria in **Table 17.2**.

DIAGNOSTIC CRITERIA

Hoarding disorder

TABLE 17.2
Diagnostic criteria hoarding disorder

A.	Persistent difficulty discarding or parting with possessions, regardless of their actual value.
B.	This difficulty is due to a perceived need to save the items and to distress associated with discarding them.
C.	The difficulty discarding possessions results in the accumulation of possessions that congest and clutter active living areas and substantially compromises their intended use. If living areas are uncluttered, it is only because of the interventions of third parties (e.g., family members, cleaners, authorities).
D.	The hoarding causes clinically significant distress or impairment in social, occupational, or other important areas of functioning (including maintaining a safe environment for self and others).
E.	The hoarding is not attributable to another medical condition (e.g., brain injury, cerebrovascular disease, Prader-Willi syndrome).
F.	The hoarding is not better explained by the symptoms of another mental disorder (e.g., obsessions in obsessive-compulsive disorder, decreased energy in major depressive disorder, delusions in schizophrenia or another psychotic disorder, cognitive deficits in major neurocognitive disorder, restricted interests in autism spectrum disorder).

Specify if:
- **With excessive acquisition:** if difficulty discarding possessions is accompanied by excessive acquisitions of items that are not needed or for which there is not available space.

Specify if:
- **With good or fair insight:** the individual recognizes that hoarding-related beliefs and behaviors (pertaining to difficulty discarding items, clutter, or excessive acquisition) are problematic.
- **With poor insight:** the individual is mostly convinced that hoarding-related beliefs and behaviors (pertaining to difficulty discarding items, clutter, or excessive acquisition) are not problematic despite evidence to the contrary.
- **With absent insight/delusional beliefs:** the individual is completely convinced that hoarding-related beliefs and behaviors (pertaining to difficulty discarding items, clutter, or excessive acquisition) are not problematic despite evidence to the contrary.

Treatment

Like other conditions that have anxiety as a feature, individuals may be prescribed SSRI medication; however, this should be an adjunct to therapeutic interventions such as CBT (see Chapter 11). CBT has a number of goals, and these include:

- assisting the individual to reduce clutter

- helping them to make appropriate decisions about what to throw away and what to keep
- assisting the individual to organise their belongings
- assisting in managing anxiety associated with 'letting go' of items
- assisting the individual to increase their opposition to hoard items.

Managing hoarded items is incredibly overwhelming for an individual with HD and the clinician should try to understand the enormity of the task of cleaning and the impact this has on the individual's motivation to change. Individuals with HD may be encouraged to commence a daily routine of cleaning or washing, and sorting through their mail. A small start may be placing a 'no junk mail' sign on the mail box to prevent the urge to hoard advertisements.

TRICHOTILLOMANIA

Trichotillomania is a condition that is characterised by recurrent hair-pulling. Pronounced *trick-o-til-o-mania*, this condition results in considerable hair loss and causes significant social and occupational dysfunction (see **Figure 17.6**). This distress often presents as shame and embarrassment. Individuals with trichotillomania usually pull hair out of their scalp (72%), but they may also remove hair from the eyebrows (56%), eyelids or pubic and peri-rectal areas (50%) (APA, 2013; Grant & Chamberlain, 2016). Individuals with trichotillomania will often vary the regions of their body where they pull their hair out. Some individuals with this condition may pull single hairs out of their body, making the signs less obvious (APA, 2013).

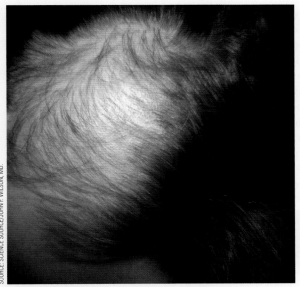

FIGURE 17.6
Trichotillomania results in significant hair loss and is most commonly associated with scalp pulling

Behaviours associated with trichotillomania
Individuals with trichotillomania will often demonstrate some similarities in their behaviours such as the rituals that are associated with hair pulling. These similarities include:

- hair-pulling which is associated with particular mood states, such as when feeling anxious or bored
- only pulling certain types of hair (because of the length, colour, texture, location, etc.)
- pulling out the hair root to examine it
- playing with the pulled follicle, such as placing the hair between their teeth, pulling it into pieces or ingesting the hair
- an unconscious pulling of hair
- hair-pulling in private.

SAFETY FIRST

TRICHOPHAGIA
Approximately 20% of individuals with trichotillomania will eat their hair and this is called trichophagia (Grant & Chamberlain, 2016). Consumption of hair can result in serious medical issues that cause gastrointestinal obstruction that can be life-threatening. The hairballs, called trichobezoars, often need to be surgically removed (see **Figure 17.7**). Therefore, care must be taken in alerting individuals with trichotillomania of the potential complication of the condition in the event they also ingest their hair.

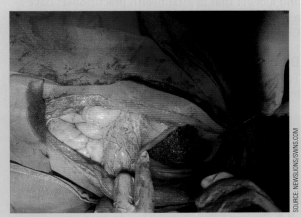

FIGURE 17.7
Trichobezoars (or hairballs) are a potentially life-threatening complication of trichophagia (which is the ingestion of pulled hair) and occurs in about 20 per cent of individuals with trichotillomania

---

Incidence
Trichotillomania is more commonly seen in females at a ratio of 10:1, and affects between 1–2% of the population (APA, 2013). Trichotillomania is not widely researched and it can be difficult to accurately determine the likely prevalence. Some studies have put the prevalence rates between 0.1–3.9% (Grant & Chamberlain, 2016).

Aetiology
As noted, trichotillomania has not been extensively researched, and as such obtaining an understanding of the causes of the condition is difficult. This section explores the genetic factors of trichotillomania and the clinical course the condition usually takes.

Genetic factors

Trichotillomania is more commonly seen in individuals with a relative with the condition, and is more frequently seen in individuals with OCD (APA, 2013). Relatives of individuals with trichotillomania may also demonstrate an increase in rates of depression and anxiety (Grant & Chamberlain, 2016).

Clinical course

Typically, trichotillomania presents at around 10 to 13 years, although some degree of hair-pulling is often seen in young children who do not go on to develop the condition (APA, 2013; Grant & Chamberlain, 2016). Hair loss can result in lowered self-esteem and social withdrawal and anxiety (Grant & Chamberlain, 2016). Aside from trichophagia, skin infections and other dermatological complications from pulling hair may bring the individual to the attention of medical personnel. Help-seeking behaviours are uncommon in individuals with trichotillomania and reticence to seek help may be due to shame, embarrassment and a belief that mental health practitioners have a poor understanding of the condition (Grant & Chamberlain, 2016).

Diagnostic criteria trichotillomania

The specific features of trichotillomania are described in the diagnostic criteria in **Table 17.3**.

DIAGNOSTIC CRITERIA
Trichotillomania (Hair-pulling disorder)
TABLE 17.3   Diagnostic criteria trichotillomania
A. Recurrent pulling out of one's hair, resulting in hair loss.
B. Repeated attempts to decrease or stop hair pulling.
C. The hair pulling causes clinically significant distress or impairment in social, occupational or other important areas of functioning.
D. The hair pulling or hair loss is not attributable to another medical condition (e.g., dermatological condition).
E. The hair pulling is not better explained by another mental disorder (e.g., attempts to improve a perceived defect or flaw in appearance in body dysmorphic disorder).
SOURCE: REPRINTED WITH PERMISSION FROM THE *DIAGNOSTIC AND STATISTICAL MANUAL OF MENTAL DISORDERS*, FIFTH EDITION. (COPYRIGHT ©2013). AMERICAN PSYCHIATRIC ASSOCIATION. ALL RIGHTS RESERVED.

Treatment

The role and need for treatment is significantly increased in individuals who ingest their hair due to the potential life-threatening complications of this, and assertive treatment is recommended in these instances (Grant & Chamberlain, 2016). Individuals who eat their hair need to be mindful of:

- abdominal pain
- alterations to stools (colour change from dark green to black)
- weight loss
- constipation
- diarrhoea (Grant & Chamberlain, 2016).

Behavioural therapy is indicated in the treatment of trichotillomania and usually comprises a therapy called 'habit reversal', but may also include dialectical behaviour therapy (DBT) and acceptance and commitment therapy (ACT) (Grant & Chamberlain, 2016; see also Chapter 4). Habit reversal is a therapy that was initially developed to help people with nervous tics and it may be helpful for individuals with trichotillomania. Habit reversal encourages the individual to monitor their hair pulling (e.g. by keeping a diary) and develop awareness and control over their urges (Grant & Chamberlain, 2016). Currently, there are no medications clinically indicated for trichotillomania; however, with high rates of comorbid conditions such as depression and anxiety, antidepressant medication may be used. Some studies have indicated positive results using low dose olanzapine (see Chapter 8); however, the potential side effects such as metabolic syndrome need to be mitigated against the possible benefits (Grant & Chamberlain, 2016).

EXCORIATION

Excoriation, also known as skin-picking, is most commonly associated with picking on the arms, face and hands. Individuals who have excoriation will pick at scabs or sores on the skin until they bleed, causing pain, scarring and even infection (see **Figure 17.8**). People who have this condition will spend large periods of their day picking their skin and have scars from this behaviour. The scars and damage to their skin are often a further source of upset, and can result in social withdrawal and avoidance behaviours. When they are not picking their skin, they are often thinking about it, and resisting their urge to

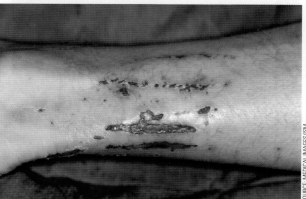

SOURCE: MEDICAL IMAGES/ISM

FIGURE 17.8
Excoriation results in significant skin damage to individuals who continually pick at their skin

pick. Unlike many mental health conditions in this textbook, the diagnostic criteria for excoriation are quite self-explanatory.

Diagnostic criteria excoriation

The specific features of excoriation are described in the diagnostic criteria in **Table 17.4**.

Incidence

Excoriation affects 1.4% of the population and is more common in persons with obsessive-compulsive disorder and their first-degree family members (APA, 2013; Grant et al., 2012). This condition is highly gender specific, with females constituting 75% of the people affected. Although onset may occur at any age, most frequently it coincides with the onset of puberty and may begin with a dermatological condition such as acne, and may increase in time spent and rituals.

Little is understood about excoriation, making exploration into its aetiology difficult. The condition's recent inclusion into the DSM-5 also results in a lack of empirical research on the condition. What is understood about the condition, is that individuals

with excoriation have higher rates of OCD (APA, 2013).

DIAGNOSTIC CRITERIA

Excoriation

TABLE 17.4
Diagnostic criteria excoriation

A.	Recurrent skin picking resulting in skin lesions.
B.	Repeated attempts to decrease or stop skin picking.
C.	The skin picking causes clinically significant distress or impairment in social, occupational or other important areas of functioning.
D.	The skin picking is not attributable to the psychological effects of a substance (e.g., cocaine) or another medical condition (e.g., scabies).
E.	The skin picking is not better explained by symptoms of another mental disorder (e.g., delusions or tactile hallucinations in a psychotic disorder, attempts to improve a perceived defect or flaw in appearance in body dysmorphic disorder, stereotypies in stereotypic movement disorder, or intention to harm oneself in nonsuicidal self-injury).

REFLECTION ON LEARNING FROM PRACTICE

Jane's experiences are reflective of the significant distress that is caused by OCD and the lengths that consumers with this condition will go to in order to manage their increasing anxiety. There is hope, however, and as Jane has indicated, contact with a therapist can be helpful in controlling the intrusive and recurrent thoughts associated with OCD.

CHAPTER RESOURCES

SUMMARY

- Obsessive-compulsive disorder is a distressing condition with a complex aetiology and involves specific attention to various sections of the MSE. This and other conditions discussed in this chapter have a foundation in anxiety, and as such anxiety-alleviating therapies and SSRIs may be helpful.

- Hoarding disorder is a relatively new condition that results in the collection and inability to part with innate objects and often rubbish.
- Trichotillomania is a condition associated with distressing hair pulling.
- Excoriation is a poorly understood condition associated with skin picking.

REVIEW QUESTIONS

1 Obsessive-compulsive disorder is a condition associated with high levels of:
   a Stress
   b Serotonin
   c Anxiety
   d Psychosis

2 A consumer with hoarding disorder will:
   a Buy and throw out useless items
   b Collect and store items, resulting in an unsafe living environment
   c Breed and sell animals
   d Dislike keeping their house tidy

3 One of the potentially fatal complications of trichophagia is:
   a Trichobezoars
   b Trichotillomania
   c Trichomonas
   d Trichomoniasis

4 Describe the differences between obsessions and compulsions in OCD.

5 A possible complication of excoriation may be:
   a Wound infections
   b Trichobezoars
   c Rituals
   d Unhygienic living conditions

CRITICAL THINKING

1 What is the difference between obsessions and compulsions in OCD? In your response, provide examples of each.

2 Hoarding disorder is often not diagnosed until the individual is older. Discuss why this may be the case.

3 What do you think some of the potential physiological risks associated with excoriation may be?

REFLECT ON THIS

OCD pandemic resources

It is easy to speculate about what living with OCD during COVID-19 would be like, but most of us can only imagine. A number of mental health services have developed web resources in response to the COVID-19 pandemic that are specific to consumers with OCD.

1 Explore the internet for credible resources that consumers living with OCD could access during the pandemic. How helpful do you think these resources are for people with OCD?

2 Reflect on what it would be like living with OCD during a global pandemic. What do you think are the barriers and facilitators to consumers with OCD accessing appropriate health care during this time? Do you think health care will change permanently in response to the pandemic?

REFERENCES

American Psychiatric Association (APA). (2013). *Diagnostic and Statistical Manual of Mental Disorders (DSM-5)* (5th edn). Washington, DC: APA.

Andrews, G., Dean, K., Genderson, M., Hunt, C., Mitchell, P., Sachdev, P. & Trollor, J. (2013). *Management of Mental Disorders* (5th edn). Sydney: School of Psychiatry, University of NSW.

Grant, J.E. & Chamberlain, S.R. (2016). Trichotillomania. *American Journal of Psychiatry*, 173(9), 868–74. Retrieved from https://ajp.psychiatryonline.org/doi/full/10.1176/appi.ajp.2016.15111432.

Grant, J., Odlaug, B., Chamberlain, S., Keuthen, N., Lochner, C. & Stein, D.J. (2012). Skin picking disorder. *American Journal of Psychiatry*, 169(11), 1143–9.

Krebs, G. & Heyman, I. (2014). Obsessive-compulsive disorder in children and adolescents. *Archives of Disease in Childhood*, 100, 495–9. Retrieved from https://adc.bmj.com/content/archdischild/100/5/495.full.pdf.

Kyrios, M., Mogan, C., Moulding, R., Frost, R.O., Yap, K. & Fassnacht, D.B. (2018). The cognitive-behavioural model of hoarding disorder: Evidence from clinical and non-clinical cohorts. *Clinical Psychology & Psychotherapy*, 25, 311–21. Retrieved from https://onlinelibrary.wiley.com/doi/epdf/10.1002/cpp.2164.

Slade T., Johnston A., Teesson, M., Whiteford, H., Burgess, P., Pirkis, J. & Saw, S. (2009). *The Mental Health of Australians 2: Report on the 2007 National Survey of Mental Health and Wellbeing*. Canberra: Department of Health and Ageing. Retrieved from https://immunise.health.gov.au/internet/publications/publishing.nsf/Content/mental-pubs-m-mhaust2-toc.

CHAPTER 18

TRAUMA AND STRESS-RELATED DISORDERS

Melody Carter and Louise Ward

LEARNING OUTCOMES

Upon completion of this chapter, you should be able to:

18.1 Introduce trauma and the principles of trauma-informed care

18.2 Describe trauma and stress-related disorders

18.3 Develop an understanding of the assessment of people with trauma and stress

18.4 Develop an individualised plan of care for a person experiencing a mental health condition because of trauma/stress

18.5 Develop knowledge and skills to support family/carers

18.6 Apply knowledge to support clients on the recovery journey

LEARNING FROM PRACTICE

My name is Henry (not my real name). I am 15 years old. I came from Sierra Leone last year. It was a long journey. My uncle was going to meet me but I couldn't find him for a long time when I got here. I had all my stuff stolen and it took a long time to sort out. My mum and my brothers and sisters died in the epidemic so I was sent to join my uncle and his kids but I just feel terrible inside. I was told I should feel grateful (I survived) but I don't, I just feel scared all the time, I can't sleep. I have new clothes and a phone and stuff but I need to keep everything with me in my bag. I need to keep checking it – where I go, my bag goes. It gets me into arguments with people but they don't understand what it's like. I don't go to places where I can't keep my bag with me.

Henry, Sierra Leone refugee and trauma survivor

There are symptoms of Post Traumatic Stress Disorder (PTSD) evident in Henry's narrative. How do you think these symptoms and behaviours will impact on Henry's daily living and personal development?

INTRODUCTION

Think about your own personal experience and or that of your family and friends coping with the effects of trauma, stress, and anxiety. Are your stories similar? Do they recount the same signs and symptoms? What treatment have they engaged? What worked and what didn't? We know that people who have experienced trauma, and are living with stress and anxiety, have different and highly individual experiences. Trauma, stress and anxiety can be highly debilitating and distressing for the person and for their families and caregivers. Recognising this, nurses are encouraged to take a person-centred and personally reflective approach to their learning in relation to this cluster of mental health diagnoses.

The rise in the incidence of non-suicidal self-injury and suicide in Australia and in other parts of the world is of great concern. Trauma and stress-related disorders are increasingly recognised as factors precipitating suicide, particularly among adolescents, young adults and the Indigenous community (Australian Government Department of Health, 2015). It is therefore critical to understand how to provide high-quality nursing assessment, care and treatment. Finally, reporting of unrest and violent acts overseas and at home can create feelings of terror and cause physical and psychological trauma. Nurses and other health professionals are present in the frontline and in the aftermath of such events and need to recognise the short- and long-term impact of these public events, as well as responding to people whose trauma may be historical and has been hidden from view.

UNDERSTANDING TRAUMA AND STRESS-RELATED DISORDERS

Trauma and stress-related disorders include **post-traumatic stress disorder (PTSD)**, adjustment disorders, reactive attachment disorder, disinhibited social engagement disorder and acute stress disorder (APA, 2013). Trauma can include childhood sexual abuse, neglect, witnessing violence, social disadvantage, hardship due to war, and catastrophic events such as experiencing torture and being involved in natural disasters (Courtois & Ford, 2009; Isobel & Edwards, 2016).

Attempting to understand trauma and stress-related disorders can be difficult, as each person's definition of their own trauma and experience of stress will be different. Trauma can also affect people in different ways. People can experience a range of physical symptoms such as headaches, sleeping problems, nightmares, night sweats, change of appetite, increased weight gain or rapid weight loss. To cope with these symptoms, people may choose to use alcohol or other drugs that can in turn create further problems and comorbidities (Afzali et al., 2016; Evans, Nizette & O'Brien, 2017; Phoenix Australia, 2013). Further to this, researchers report that, 'In addition to complexities arising from comorbidity, health practitioners working with more chronic cases of PTSD often find themselves having to work with a myriad of psychosocial problems that have evolved secondary to the core disorder' (Australian Centre for Posttraumatic Mental Health, 2007, p. 16). Experiencing, adjusting to and recovering from trauma across the lifespan can impact on every aspect of an individual's life. Childhood development, social relationships, attachment to others, education and employment can all be affected. The overarching effect of trauma on an individual results in a complex picture and presentation that can challenge nurses' skills of assessment and the planning of effective care (Phoenix Australia, 2013).

Treating trauma requires maintaining a strong focus on the consumer's lived experience. Their life story must be central to the therapeutic relationship (Evans, Nizette & O'Brien, 2017). Effective treatment must respond to the person's immediate needs, be person-centred and based on the principles of a recovery framework (VicHealth, 2017). Caring for someone who has experienced trauma requires the mental health nurse to be present and to work alongside them. Most importantly, the nurse needs to be accepting of the time it may take the consumer to disclose their experience and its impact, if they choose to do so at all. A trauma-informed approach or trauma-informed care recognises that the symptoms of trauma are adaptive behaviours that can form the primary focus of care planning (Isobel & Edwards, 2016). The way in which a person copes with trauma may, however, directly inform their care planning and treatment options (Evans, Nizette & O'Brien, 2017).

It is important to remember that the actual experience of even routine health care can, if inappropriately or insensitively provided, accentuate or re-traumatise the individual (Reeves, 2015). Nurses and other professionals wishing to help and support survivors of trauma need to recognise that a collaborative and compassionate approach is essential; for example, coercive interventions, as well as being unethical, can re-traumatise the person and should be avoided (Evans, Nizette & O'Brien, 2017). The actual trauma may be secondary to the reason a person presents to the health care service. Subsequent care provided to an individual could therefore result in the consumer 're-experiencing' the event; for example, in maternal care, during invasive diagnostic procedures or in sexual health care screening. Therefore, caring for someone who has experienced trauma requires a non-judgemental approach that is supportive and based on effective communication skills such as active listening, being present, patient and empathic. Establishing a therapeutic relationship within which the individual feels safe is central to effective trauma-informed care (Chandler, 2008; Fallot & Harris, 2009).

The principles of trauma-informed care

Many mental health care organisations have now adopted a trauma-informed care approach (Isobel & Edwards, 2016) that is underpinned by a number of key principles. These principles include supporting:

1 relationships that are focused on empowering the consumer to identify their strengths and build on their learning (Fallot & Harris, 2009)
2 comprehensive treatment plans based on professional assessments of a consumer's experience with trauma (Isobel & Edwards, 2016)
3 close collaboration with agencies and multidisciplinary experts in the provision of specialised advice
4 education and training for staff on the prevalence and impacts of trauma, violence and victimisation among people accessing mental health care services (Bloom, 2010)
5 ensuring appropriately trained staff are available in the health care setting, to provide staff who are fully aware of the potential for re-traumatisation and the reality that ongoing trauma may still be present in the consumer's life experience
6 the assumption that everyone accessing the service has potentially experienced trauma, and the need to adopt trauma-informed approaches in all aspects of the service's treatment and care (Bloom, 2010).

TRAUMA AND STRESS-RELATED DISORDERS

Based on current statistics, anxiety and depression are considered the leading causes of Australia's non-fatal disease burden (AIHW, 2016). While a person can experience anxiety symptoms following a traumatic event, trauma- and stress-related disorders are identified separately in the DSM-5. This recognises the diversity in the individual experience of, and response to, stressful/traumatic events, which may or may not include anxiety-based symptoms.

This highlights the importance of mental health nurses being competent in the recognition, assessment, planning, care of and appropriate referral to specialist mental health practitioners for patients with these disorders.

Post-traumatic stress disorder

The essential feature of PTSD is the development of characteristic symptoms following exposure to one or more traumatic events. The *Diagnostic and Statistical Manual of Mental Disorders* (DSM-5) diagnosis outlines traumatic events as including exposure to death, the threat of death, serious injury and sexual violence (APA, 2013). PTSD can develop in anyone who has been through or witnessed a traumatic event, or had their safety and/or life threatened (Forbes et al., 2007). This condition has received more prominence in recent years as the effects of combat have been better understood through the reported experience of servicemen and women, medical, nursing and volunteer workers and, in particular, civilians working and living in war zones and in areas where natural disasters have occurred (NICE, 2018).

CASE **STUDY**

CARING FOR SOMEONE WHO EXPERIENCED TRAUMA

For the last three years I have been caring for my 24-year-old son (John) who was involved in a hostage situation. He was held at gunpoint for four hours during a robbery. He witnessed a colleague being assaulted and his life was threatened a number of times during the incident. He has not been able to work since the event. He had to move back home because he could not afford to live independently. He does not sleep, he is irritable and hard to talk to. At times,

I think he is opening up and then he ends up in tears and retreats to his room. At times, I worry he will do something stupid. I am worrying about him all of the time.

Questions
1 What symptoms of PTSD does John appear to exhibit?
2 What support could the mental health care team offer John's mother?

Supporting John's recovery would include providing his family and friends with the adequate skills and knowledge to help him. John appears to have lost his sense of safety. He will need to regain his trust in the world before he can move forward. It is important for families and others caring for someone who is experiencing PTSD to learn to identify the triggers that may precipitate feelings of distress.

These may include sights and sounds, conversations and/or media coverage about the event. John may feel more vulnerable when discussing money, as this may trigger thoughts of returning to work, and these thoughts may remind him of the assault. John appears to be experiencing strong emotions of helplessness and a sense of being out of control. Based on the account in the case study, a suicide risk assessment is essential. John requires immediate follow-up by his general practitioner (GP) and/or the mental health care team.

Providing the opportunity for John to connect with other family members and/or a community group may support his recovery and reduce the strain on the mother–son relationship. Further treatment options for John could include cognitive behaviour therapy (CBT), involving working with a therapist to identify negative thought and behaviour patterns. There are also a number of online CBT programs to work from home. Medication could also be prescribed and may include:

- *antidepressant medication:* fluoxetine, sertraline, paroxetine and escitalopram
- *antipsychotic medication:* olanzapine, quetiapine, clozapine and risperidone
- *hypnosedative medication:* diazepam, temazepam, alprazolam (Phoenix Australia, 2013).

Risk factors

Risk factors for developing PTSD include a history of trauma or previous mental health issues. Ongoing stressful life events after the trauma and an absence of social supports increase the risk of developing PTSD (Phoenix Australia, 2013). For this reason, recognition of the importance of early skilled interventions for those who have experienced trauma is essential, as is including this phenomenon in civil disaster planning by governments. This may include support for service personnel, people who are immigrants and refugees who have been exposed to war.

Most people experience a psychological reaction to trauma. Feelings of fear, sadness, guilt and anger are common. PTSD is usually diagnosed if symptoms persist for at least one month after a traumatic experience. Symptoms include experiencing trauma-intrusive memories/'flashbacks'. People with PTSD will often avoid new situations, will have increased fear, hyper-vigilance, anger, irritability and often report trouble sleeping and problems concentrating (Dixon, Ahles & Marques, 2016). They may be easily startled or exhibit depression. They may also report generalised anxiety and to have misused/be dependent on drugs and/or alcohol. Refer to Chapter 11 for further information about generalised anxiety signs and symptoms and the effect this condition can have on an individual's life.

Adjustment disorder

The DSM-5 (APA, 2013) classifies attachment disorders as two distinct disorders:

1 reactive attachment disorder (RAD)
2 disinhibited social engagement disorder (DSED).

A child with DSED may reflect the signs and symptoms of attention-deficit/hyperactivity disorder (ADHD). They may demonstrate an inability to establish appropriate social boundaries and or present with a dampened affect, similar to anxiety disorder or depression (APA, 2013).

Adjustment disorder is a response to a stressful life event, a change in circumstance or a situation that causes distress. Stressful life events may include relationship breakdown, transitional life events such as childbirth, retirement and experiencing a serious illness. Adjustment disorder is common with 5–20% of people diagnosed worldwide (APA, 2013; Craske & Stein, 2016). An individual with a diagnosis of adjustment disorder will demonstrate a response to the stressor that is out of proportion to the event within three months and lasts no longer than six months. Symptoms include low mood, increased worry and inability to cope with daily life, resulting in social withdrawal. The difference between what we

---

CASE **STUDY**

MARY'S STORY

My name is Mary. I am just an ordinary person and everything was fine until my husband died. We did not have children (which made us sad) but we had each other and loved doing things together; especially after we retired, we had lots of friends and we travelled all over the world. We used to have loads of friends and we had a lot of respect, now I hardly see anyone. I keep the house nice and clean but nobody seems to come around except a few 'old faithfuls', but they seem to get on my nerves, and we always seem to be falling out. They used to take my advice but now they don't listen to me and say that I have changed; well, of course, I have! I don't cry as much now, but I miss my husband more than ever. I do go around to see them sometimes but quite often have to walk out and go home early and besides, there are lots of things I used to do that I just can't face any more. They say that there are five stages to grief, but I would say the main one I am stuck with is anger. I think it's so unfair to be left like this. I feel so lonely and disconnected. It feels pointless now; in fact, I think I might as well be dead. In the end, everyone leaves you to it, they say they will stand by you, but they don't mean it. I often wish something would just 'happen' to me so that it would all be over.

Questions

1 As a student nurse, what could you offer Mary? What interventions would you consider might be useful for her recovery?
2 Why do you think her friends (except for the 'old faithfuls') may have abandoned her?

might consider to be normal stress and a diagnosis of adjustment disorder is defined by the severity, duration and intensity experienced and the level of impairment. Mary, in the 'Case study' below, is experiencing adjustment disorder after the death of her husband. She appears to be struggling to cope with her loss and is experiencing the signs and symptoms of an adjustment disorder. Treatment for Mary should include support and guidance on how to manage stress.

CBT and relaxation techniques such as mindfulness-based therapy (Evans, Nizette & O'Brien, 2017) are commonly used with positive effect. Supporting Mary through the grieving process and helping her to regain functioning and a sense of purpose is critical. Mary requires a suicide risk assessment based on her withdrawn appearance, irritability and lack of concentration. Diagnosing Mary with an adjustment disorder is likely because she has experienced psychological or behavioural symptoms within three months of an identifiable stressor in her life – the death of her husband – and she has experienced stress that has caused issues with her relationships and significantly affected her quality of life.

Reactive attachment disorder

Reactive attachment disorder (RAD) and disinhibited social engagement disorder present in childhood. Both can affect a person's ability to develop relationships. RAD is recognised as a clinical disorder that limits a child's social abilities, emotional regulation and cognitive functioning (Pritchett et al., 2013). RAD is a potential consequence of insecure attachment due to pathogenic care. Pathogenic care can result in a child's inability to socially and emotionally engage with others. Pathogenic care is described as a primary caregiver's persistent neglect of a child's physical and emotional needs (Dahmen, Putz, Herpertz-Dahlmann & Konrad, 2012; Schwartz & Davis, 2006).

Inhibited RAD and disinhibited RAD

Two distinct presentations of the disorder have been identified. **Inhibited RAD** refers to a child who is detached socially and emotionally (Gleason et al., 2011; Pritchett et al., 2013). **Disinhibited RAD** refers to a child displaying 'indiscriminate sociability' (Gleason et al., 2011). The child is not highly selective in their choice of attachment figures and is more likely to express attachment and friendliness towards a stranger/new acquaintance than their own primary caregiver (Gleason et al., 2011; Pritchett et al., 2013). RAD and DSED both present in early childhood. Both disorders can have an impact on a person's ability to develop appropriate, trusting, short- and long-term relationships. Both disorders can have significant, long-term health, safety and social consequences (O'Connor & Zeanah, 2003). Research reports that the most effective treatment for attachment disorder is the provision of a safe, predictable, stable environment over a long period of time (Chaffin et al., 2006).

CASE **STUDY**

REACTIVE ATTACHMENT DISORDER RESULTING FROM NEGLECT

My partner and I adopted Caitlin when she was three years old. She had been looked after in the care system since she was six months old; we were told that she experienced severe neglect. She had moved several times to different foster homes and although she found it difficult to settle we had hoped that she would become attached to us and start to develop 'normally; you know, playing and talking. She is now seven years old and still has very little language and communicates her wishes by shouting and rattling or throwing things. She is always 'jumpy' and anxious. She gets up early in the morning and dresses herself to go out. She is unable to wait for anything, tends to grab and snatch things. She runs to the door in a panicked way whenever the door bell sounds and runs to the phone when it rings. She has real problems at school too. She doesn't play with others but does enjoy being outside with a scooter or bicycle; indoors she is jumpy and nervous all the time. It's also hard to get her to sit up at the table and eat. I have to get her to eat

snacks on the go as she is underweight. One of the things we worry about all the time is how impulsive she is. When I am cooking in the kitchen, she runs to the stove and will grab at the saucepans. It's a real challenge keeping her out of danger – one of us has to be with her all the time and she's like a highly mobile baby! At night she goes to bed quite well but often cries out in the night. We go to her and she is asleep but with big tears rolling down her cheeks. We wonder how long this will go on and have no idea how to help her. We know she is frightened and unhappy most of the time.

Questions

1 Consider the impact of past experience on Caitlin's development. What specialist services might help to address her needs?

2 Reflect on the impact of Caitlin's needs on family life. How could you support her parents to sustain their care for her in the immediate situation and in the long term?

In the case study, Caitlin appears to present with RAD. Her parents have identified the risks she poses to herself due to her impulsive behaviours. Caitlin will require significant support as she learns to regain a sense of trust and love in those around her. Family therapy, play therapy, counselling and parenting education would support Caitlin's recovery. There is a need to ensure her living environment is safe, that she develops positive interactions with others and can improve her peer relationships.

Presentation and treatment

The presentation of individuals and recognising the symptoms they present with is a complex process. For example, Caitlin is presenting with signs and symptoms of RAD. She appears to be in a persistent state of fear. She is said to be 'jumpy' and 'anxious' and is having difficulty forming friendships. Her behaviour is erratic and inappropriate at times, making it difficult for her to make meaningful connections with others and develop alongside her peers. Mental health care and treatment would follow a family therapy focus with the primary goal being to ensure Caitlin's immediate environment remains stable and safe (Chaffin et al., 2006). This sustained high level of anxiety will affect every aspect of her childhood development and her experience as a young person and as an older adult.

Her family will need support to help Caitlin regain or establish trust in human relationships through a guided therapeutic process with a multidisciplinary team of highly trained clinicians and professionals; for example, speech and language, occupational therapists, social work and psychology support. Nurses and others working with the family can support Caitlin's parents to establish rules within the family unit to allow Caitlin space and understanding as she learns how to self-regulate her emotions. Her parents will need advice and guidance to help Caitlin to develop effective communication with her parents, any siblings and peers. As the development of language has been delayed, the development of language that Caitlin can use when she is feeling unsafe is essential. It is important that Caitlin's school has a full understanding of Caitlin's disorder and appropriate support has been put in place to ensure her safety at all times, including a safe space at school where Caitlin can go if she is feeling threatened. All those involved with Caitlin's care will need to be educated about the risk of Caitlin forming inappropriate relationships with strangers and wandering. As well as responding to Caitlin's needs, it is important to offer separate counselling for Caitlin's parents and ensure they have the adequate coping strategies to

manage Caitlin's complex behaviours. This might include encouraging them to attend a support group and learning to monitor Caitlin for signs of increased anxiety and/or signs and symptoms of depression. Careful coordination of care is essential, as it can involve so many professionals and agencies and may continue as Caitlin transitions to adolescence and adult life.

Disinhibited social engagement disorder

Disinhibited social engagement disorder (DSED) is a trauma and stress-related disorder that develops because of severe neglect during the first two years of life (McLaughlin, Espie & Minnis, 2010). DESD involves a pattern of inappropriate overly familiar behaviour with strangers. A diagnosis of DESD should not be made before the age of nine months. The DSM-5 defines DSED as 'a pattern of behavior in which a child actively approaches and interacts with unfamiliar adults' (APA, 2013). Symptoms include a lack of discretion with strangers and indiscriminate friendships.

Acute stress disorder

The essential feature of **acute stress disorder** is the development of characteristic symptoms lasting from three days to one month following exposure to one or more traumatic events (APA, 2013). Traumatic events that are experienced directly may include exposure to war, threatened or actual violent personal assault (e.g. sexual violence, physical attack, active combat, mugging, childhood physical and/or sexual violence, being kidnapped, being taken hostage, terrorist attack, torture), natural or human-made disasters (e.g. earthquake, hurricane, aircraft crash), witnessing severe trauma or the sudden death of others (e.g. motor vehicle collisions) (APA, 2013).

Acute stress disorder may also be a condition that resolves within one month of exposure to the traumatic event or it may result in a diagnosis of PTSD if signs and symptoms persist for longer than one month. In about 50% of people who eventually develop PTSD, the initial presenting condition was acute stress disorder. Symptoms of acute stress disorder include:

- regular, intrusive memories
- dreams or flashbacks that cause great distress
- avoiding reminders of the traumatic event
- hyper-vigilance
- problems concentrating
- problems sleeping
- being easily startled and/or having a negative mood
- separation anxiety (APA, 2013).

ASSESSMENT AND TREATMENT OF TRAUMA AND STRESS-RELATED DISORDERS

The approach to a nursing assessment for people experiencing trauma and stress-related disorders should follow best practice guidelines and be in accordance with the local policy of the organisation you are working within. It is important to remember that nurses are working as part of a multidisciplinary team; the approach to assessment must allow the individual's voice to be heard and their experiences expressed, and allow for your record of the assessment to be coherent and understood by both the patient and other professionals.

Consider how you will prepare for an interview or conversation with the patient:

- What preparation will you undertake?
- How will you create a 'safe space' for the conversation to take place?
- Will the consumer find discussing their concerns and experiences straightforward?
- Is your language also their first language; will you need the presence of an interpreter or a chaperone, or in the case of a child or young person, a responsible adult?

In general, the assessment activity will follow a three-stage approach:

1 Convene and conduct a clinical interview.
2 Elicit and identify the consumer's and carer's concerns.
3 In partnership with the consumer and appropriate others, develop a personalised, evidence-based treatment plan.

The aim of the assessment and development for a plan of care and treatment is to:

- reduce the negative impact the traumatic or stressful event is having on the person's thoughts, feelings and behaviours – identifying the way in which individuals are managing their day-to-day activities can provide insight into where they may require support and or resource
- improve daily functioning – supporting the consumer to maintain quality of life or make appropriate changes to support recovery
- implement strategies – developing opportunities for the consumer to engage in therapeutic processes
- improve coping skills – encouraging a strengths-based approach to care.

Listening and effective communication

When approaching the consumer who has experienced stress and/or trauma, it is important to introduce yourself and explain your role in the team, the purpose of the conversation you hope to have and the observations you may make and record. The person may demonstrate poor attention and concentration (due to anxiety); therefore, speaking in short, easy-to-understand sentences will help to reduce any further stress. Attending, observing, perceiving, interpreting and recalling are the essential skills associated with effective listening (Stein-Parbury, 2018). The team will need to consider whether the spoken language might be a barrier to effective communication and whether there are developmental or cognitive impairments that act as a barrier to the exchange of information or interpretation (Arnold & Underman Boggs, 2016). If an interpreter or a caregiver needs to speak on behalf of the person, this will have implications for the accuracy of the assessment as well as confidentiality and dignity.

A person's informal account of what has distressed, or is distressing, them when you first meet or speak with them and the accounts of family or friends accompanying them are of great importance. It is essential that this information is included in the information gathering that supports assessment and decision making, for ensuring the person's safety and recovery as a care plan is implemented. Successful assessment will depend on effective and functional communication and must be principally based on active listening and recording of what the individual wants to tell you at a particular time about themselves, their experiences, their strengths and their hopes for the future (Arnold & Underman Boggs, 2016).

The nursing team should have a clear plan to ensure that there are people available to listen as the person and their carers need to talk or ask questions. Best practice would include regular updates, effective handover within the multidisciplinary team, and regular case meetings. Shared decision making is an important and effective element that ensures that the patient and their carers know what is happening, when things will happen and why, and continue to feel included and valued in this process.

Using an ethical approach

Nurses in Australia follow a human rights and person-centred approach, meaning an approach that recognises the uniqueness of the individual and their right to receive the best available care. This care is focused on the current priorities and preoccupations of the distressed individual. Listening and communicating honestly and helpfully is of great importance in the first and subsequent encounters. Carl Rogers (1951) has used the terms 'genuineness', 'congruency' and 'unconditional positive regard' to support the development of a therapeutic relationship. We stress the importance of focusing and acting on the risk factors and of tuning into the mood and temperament of the person. There are often very complex and variable events/factors that have precipitated the occurrence or situation; nurses and other health care professionals must avoid prejudgement and be mindful of avoiding a stigmatising response to aspects that may offend or affront them.

Practical physical care
Nurses are concerned for the whole person and it is important to take note of the physical condition of the individual. Intense experience of symptoms related to trauma and/or stress-related disorders may include the disruption of sleeping patterns, eating and other activities of daily living. Other symptoms may include palpitations, chest pain, faintness, flushing, sweating, shortness of breath (SOB), hyperventilation, dry mouth, nausea, vomiting and diarrhoea. An individual may report being thirsty (to the point of dehydration) and hungry and even malnourished. They may be unkempt in their personal appearance or their hygiene may be neglected. The behavioural expressions of their fears and anxieties may mean that they are physically trembling, pacing or repeating a series of actions or gestures.

It is important to ensure that nutritional needs are met, that physical comfort is available and that these immediate, very human and ordinary everyday needs are met in the context of supporting the person as appropriate. Baseline observations of the vital signs should also be taken and recorded (including temperature, heart rate, respiratory rate and blood pressure). These objective measurements are important in understanding any underlying physical health risks and the impact of the person's mental health state on their physical well-being (Alvares et al., 2013).

Systematic mental health assessment
The formal or systematic assessment of mental health should include the mental state examination (MSE) and other tools such as a suicide risk assessment and a clinical risk assessment (Hungerford et al., 2018). Ideally, these would be undertaken early in the care episode and then regularly reviewed. The MSE is concerned with assessing and documenting the person's current mental state. It can be repeated and comparisons made as the individual's care plan is implemented and the person's progression towards recovery evaluated. Mary's account from the case study earlier in the chapter is used as an example.

COMMONALITIES OF THE MSE: ADJUSTMENT DISORDER

Appearance, behaviour and attitude
I observe that Mary is very smartly dressed and given it is winter she is wearing a coat and boots. Her hair is neatly cut, she is not wearing makeup. I offer her a chair to sit in or the sofa if she prefers. She chooses the chair first, then decides on the sofa, and then immediately changes her mind and returns to the chair. She keeps her bag on her lap and says she prefers to keep her coat on as 'this is pretty pointless and won't take long'. I introduce myself and explain the MSE and roughly how long it will take; I ask if she has any questions. She replies very irritably that she hopes it will not take long, and adds that these things are a waste of time.

Mood and affect
Mary is not openly hostile to me but she is apparently tense and her replies are abrupt. When I ask her about what has been happening with her in the last few weeks she complains about her GP, who she says has been 'no help at all', is 'ignorant' and 'unkind'. She says that her niece, who has brought her here today, 'thinks she is mad'. I ask her if she and her niece are close, and she says, 'She's like a daughter because I

have always helped her so much'. I observe Mary's face and gestures during this discussion; she is very still and does not quite make eye contact with me. Her face does not show emotion.

Speech
Mary's speech is rapid and abrupt. It sounds harsh, with short sentences and audible sighs in the gaps. When she speaks, her voice is louder than mine is, louder than is necessary as we are sitting a metre or so from each other.

Thought
Process and form
Mary's ideas seem logical in sequence. When she describes events and her husband's death, she uses appropriate words and describes her loneliness, grief and increasing isolation.

Content
Mary describes her hope that it will soon all be over for her. She talks about the ways she has tried to put herself 'in harm's way'. She says there is 'no point in carrying on'. I ask her to tell me more about these thoughts and intentions.

Perception

I ask Mary about what she sees, feels and hears when she is alone at home; she says she feels complete loneliness and desolation. She says she sometimes imagines her husband is in another room but that she knows this is not possible. She tells me that she dreams about him often and when she wakes, she remembers he is gone. She says that she visits the grave most days, but that the graveyard is not looked after properly, so she takes a bag to collect the litter that other people leave behind.

Cognition

Mary is very alert to the time and date and is clear about the series of events that have brought her to the assessment. I do not consider that she has any cognitive or sensory deficit; she appears alert and orientated to the events and the discussion.

Insight and judgement

I ask Mary if she is able to talk to me about her husband. Mary speaks at length about her husband's illness and death, and during this part of the discussion she seems to be more focused, relaxed but not tearful. I ask about the other people that were mourning him. She becomes irritated and says, 'They have no idea what it means to lose a husband'. She says that she has lost many friends over it, 'which is just as well' and besides 'they will be glad when I'm gone'. At this point, the discussion ends and she says she has to leave.

This MSE illustrates the kinds of observations and details the mental health nurse needs to pay attention to in an assessment. The nurse must also consider how, given Mary's mistrust of other professionals resulting in social isolation, it is imperative to develop a partnership with her or encourage her to talk more about her distress and her desire to be helped to recover.

Reflection on the MSE

After conducting the MSE, the nurse will need to prepare and write a summary of the assessment findings, update the team about the initial discussion and document the details carefully in their record. While reflection does not form part of formal assessment documentation, it is a worthwhile personal process for the mental health nurse to undertake. Indeed, it may be something that can later be shared during supervision (see Chapter 5). The reflection in this instance could be framed as follows:

> I might in future create a safer and more relaxed space/situation and whether I would open the conversation differently next time. The amount of information I collected was very much determined by what she wanted to share. I was focusing on encouraging her to speak and telling her story in her own way. I wanted to stay attentive and 'tuned in' to her mood and priorities. A future conversation might elicit more facts about her life and experience, and the history of her family, her relationship and her vulnerability/resilience to previous grief experiences. She has expressed a desire to die and says she does not have a plan for this now, but described an accident she had on the stairs where she received a head injury and her reckless approach to activities where she has described that she hopes something might happen. Her suicidal intentions are recorded and then reported to the team. It will be important to explore these in future meetings.

Supporting family and other caregivers

Knowing who is important in an individual's life, their strengths and whom they rely on to get through the day is essential in understanding lived experience, personalised approaches and supporting recovery. It is also important to remember that people other than family may have more significance to an individual than the next of kin (Arnold & Underman Boggs, 2016). Recognising who is providing support is an important aspect of care. Consider, for example, the way that the prevalence of anxiety disorders peaks in the population between the ages of 14 and 24; the significance for family caregivers, parents, partners, siblings and grandparents cannot be understated.

Episodes of non-suicidal self-injury and the impact on education and physical well-being will in turn cause distress to loved ones. Effective listening, communication about what has been happening, and the creation of a safe space is an important dimension of effective care. Family and other caregivers need to know that their concerns are being recognised and that communication is regular and effective. Allowing them to tell their story, share their concerns and experiences, and be helped to understand what is happening to their loved one, are important steps in building a recovery plan for the person and in building confidence and resilience in their caregivers.

DEVELOPING AN INDIVIDUALISED PLAN OF CARE FOR A PERSON EXPERIENCING A DISORDER AS A RESULT OF TRAUMA/STRESS

Treatment plans must be prepared for each individual using a person-centred approach, but will often include elements of the following:

- cognitive behaviour therapy
- exposure therapy

- anxiety programs
- resilience group programs.

Cognitive behaviour therapy

As described in Chapter 4, cognitive behaviour therapy (CBT) is a treatment option for many mental health conditions, and it is commonly used in the treatment of trauma and stress-related disorders. CBT proposes that our thoughts, beliefs and memories can both positively and negatively affect our behaviour. CBT provides the trauma/stress consumer with an opportunity to identify thoughts and beliefs that trigger their distress. It also provides a process of exploration of alternative, more constructive behavioural responses (Phoenix Australia, 2013). CBT clinicians aim to link current ways of being in the world to past memories and experience (VicHealth, 2017).

Exposure therapy

Exposure therapy challenges consumers to confront the situation that elicits fear in an attempt to reduce the feelings or symptoms associated with the experience (Mills et al., 2016). This may involve looking at a picture, listening to a sound or entering a public space. The idea is to desensitise the consumer to the fear, reducing the anxiety associated with the trigger response. Initial sessions can last one to two hours (Phoenix Australia, 2013).

Anxiety programs

Treatment for anxiety consists of inpatient and community group therapy. Group therapy supports participants to develop strategies to cope with the symptoms of stress, through strategies such as relaxation or breathing exercises, in an attempt to reinterpret stimuli considered threatening. The therapeutic response focuses on individual strengths and the aim is to replace safety seeking and avoidance with coping behaviours. Experienced mental health nurses, allied health care practitioners and psychologists facilitate anxiety programs (Craske & Stein, 2016) and resilience group programs. Resilience group programs encourage the development of problem-solving skills, positive thinking, understanding emotional responses and the ability to negotiate difficult life experiences.

NURSING CARE PLAN

POST-TRAUMATIC STRESS DISORDER

The mental health nurse must be mindful that talking and retelling the story of the events can be a traumatic event in itself. It is important that an assessment interview is planned in such a way that a safe space/situation is guaranteed. It is also important to put a time limit on the conversation so that when it is time to end the conversation the individual does not feel cut off or dismissed, but knows that they can return to the story later. Ensuring that the interview is not interrupted or overheard is an important consideration. Remember, not all information and details need to be collected and documented, but it is important that the nurse has enough information to ensure that the consumer does not have to keep repeating the story to every new professional they encounter. Using a systematic approach (i.e. the MSE) will ensure the nurse covers all the key areas and is able to carefully observe a number of elements and identify any important risk factors or key information.

Effective listening is key; traumatic stories do not necessarily have a logical sequence in retelling. The story can sometimes begin with a long preamble and set of explanations and seemingly tangential elements. It is important to let the person tell their story in the way that feels comfortable to them. This may be a very vulnerable time for the consumer and the retelling may evoke the fears and emotions that they experienced at the time. It is a very intimate context and it is important to focus on the listening and on the first telling to note important elements that might need following up later.

If the story is flowing, keep interruptions to a minimum. If the individual is struggling to describe what occurred, use open questions to encourage them to move forward.

Reassurance of the safety of the present time and the commitment to help the individual to recover may be important aspects of the conversation. Key elements to observe will be assessment data based on information about flashbacks, insomnia, nightmares and recurrent dreams, difficulty in expressing emotions about ordinary everyday life, as well as guilt and remorse about aspects of the traumatic event. Be attentive and attuned to the individual as they talk. Allow time at the end of the conversation to share your thoughts on what they have told you and the impression you have gained about their concerns. Acknowledge any feelings of guilt about their experience, their survival and sadness for the effect their illness is having on those they love/care about. Ensure they have the opportunity to summarise or emphasise what is most important to them. Tell them what the next steps will be and ask how they plan to spend the next hours, day or week. Remember that hearing firsthand stories of trauma can have an effect on the nursing professional. It is important that the listener also attends team debriefings appropriate to the situation, and that any remaining anxieties or distress from the impact of listening is shared with a supervisor.

Using John's case study as an example (see p. 353), a nursing care plan would involve consideration of the following potential issues.

PROBLEM	NURSING GOAL 1	NURSING THERAPEUTIC PRIORITIES AND INTERVENTIONS
The individual may be experiencing altered personal relationships related to: • a lack of trust • feelings of anger • difficulty expressing feelings • the experience of sexual problems.	To rebuild and maintain personal relationships	Prevent the person from causing harm to self or others Develop a therapeutic relationship that is mindful of cultural safety needs Enable rest, sleep and activity Facilitate therapeutic interventions to decrease anxiety Psychological treatment as first-line treatment Medication after non-response to psychological treatment Treatment for PTSD specialty area Disclosure of traumatic event within structured framework Management of avoidance Social skills groups Review nutrition and hydration Review general health
PROBLEM	**NURSING GOAL 2**	
The individual may be experiencing a disturbance in sleep related to: • nightmares • insomnia • early wakening.	To establish a healthy sleep/activity pattern	
PROBLEM	**NURSING GOAL 3**	
Fear and anxiety related to: • unresolved grief • feelings of helplessness • lack of control.	To reduce the levels of fear and anxiety and regain a sense of control	
PROBLEM	**NURSING GOAL 4**	
The individual may be experiencing depressive behaviour related to: • unresolved grief • internalised blame • internalised anger.	To achieve a more comfortable, stable mood, and recognise the triggers for these feelings	
PROBLEM	**NURSING GOAL 5**	
The individual may be experiencing poor physical health due to: • poor dietary/fluid intake • recent neglect of physical health.	To achieve a healthy nutrition and fluid intake To ensure physical health problems are resolved or investigated	

CLINICAL OBSERVATIONS

Trauma

Nurses contribute to care in a number of ways and these include observing the consumers, collecting and collating relevant information. The purpose of the clinical observations is to:

■ safeguard the individual to ensure that any signs of risk of non-suicidal self-injury are identified and reported so that the individual and those around them are kept safe

■ establish a therapeutic relationship through talking and listening to understand their immediate needs for support, their hopes and fears as well as cultural and/or spiritual needs

■ monitor the patient's mental and physical status and well-being

■ inform safe decision-making and review.

Trauma interventions and preventing re-traumatisation

One of the key features of trauma-informed care is to avoid re-traumatising the person through the practices of the service. For many people, being admitted to a mental health service places them at risk of witnessing or experiencing a traumatic event and hence being re-traumatised (Mills et al., 2016). Some of these traumatising events may include:

■ physical assault

■ sexual assault

■ witnessing traumatic events

■ being around frightening or violent patients

■ being secluded

■ being restrained

■ feeling medications are used as a threat or punishment

■ unwanted sexual advances

■ inadequate privacy (Robins et al., 2005).

The challenges of safeguarding vulnerable people in a hospital, clinical or community setting are significant. There have been many reports of institutional failings including in the mental health system, structures and in matters of professional conduct (Arbuckle, 2013). Nurses have a particular professional responsibility to ensure that any risks are identified and that systems for observing, supporting and safeguarding individuals in their care are their priorities (NMBA, 2016).

The setting for trauma screening and assessment

Advances in the development of simple, brief and public-domain screening tools mean that at least a basic screening for trauma can be done in almost any setting. Not only can clients be screened and assessed in behavioural health treatment settings, they can also be evaluated in the criminal justice system, educational settings, occupational settings, physicians' offices, hospital medical and trauma units, and emergency rooms. Wherever they occur, trauma-related screenings and subsequent assessments can reduce or eliminate wasted resources, relapses and, ultimately, treatment failures among clients who have histories of trauma, mental illness and/or substance use disorders.

SAFETY FIRST

ASSESSING RISK OF SUICIDE OR NON-SUICIDAL SELF-INJURY

Take account of any aspects of your assessment that highlight a risk of suicide and non-suicidal self-injury. The evidence for good practice (Phoenix Australia, 2013) tells us to:

- treat talk of suicide and non-suicidal self-injury as serious
- always complete and review an assessment of risk
- be supportive
- actively listen
- be non-judgemental – show understanding and acknowledge distress
- be prepared to use crisis intervention
- always seek help if a concern is unresolved or beyond your scope of practice.

EVIDENCE-BASED PRACTICE

Sensitivity and avoiding re-traumatisation

Trauma-informed care recognises many individuals experiencing a mental health disorder have also experienced trauma. Therefore, trauma-informed nursing care must be sensitive and avoid re-traumatisation at all costs. This can be achieved by providing a space of safety and respect in a calm environment. Inpatient mental health units can be busy, stressful and chaotic environments (Ward, 2011) that have been considered detrimental to recovery practices. It is important to recognise this so as to support consumers appropriately. It is also relevant to consider the number of people who do not actively seek out ongoing treatment based on past experience with service providers.

Research continues to focus primarily on treatments that are person-centred and recovery-focused. An emphasis on teaching coping skills to build resilience (without revisiting the traumatic memory) is considered best practice (Mills et al., 2016).

New treatments and interventions are evolving, including the use of creative arts for mental health and well-being. These include the visual arts, dance, music and writing (Daykin & Joss, 2016). As well as having application in the clinical setting, these approaches are increasingly emerging as community-based interventions that are focused on prevention, enabling recovery, enhancing dignity and reducing social isolation. The evidence for the benefit of these kinds of interventions is not always easily accessible, but new frameworks are emerging for evaluation and to increase their sustainability (Clift, 2012).

SUPPORTING FAMILY AND OTHER CAREGIVERS

Most consumers will be receiving some support from family, caregivers or friends. Often recovery and coping will be dependent on this informal support, more than on professional support. It is essential that mental health nurses are mindful of the need to show respect and understanding to the people on whom the consumer relies. It is also important to be mindful of the impact that care-giving in stressful and distressing circumstances can have on those who live alongside the person experiencing a mental health condition.

In the case studies earlier in this chapter, the caregivers of Caitlin and John are central to their lives and Caitlin and John are often wholly dependent on them for everything they need both to develop and thrive as young people and adults. In the case study about Mary, the mental health nurse might consider the situation of Mary's friends, who are experiencing the difficult behaviours and the change in Mary because of her mental health condition.

SUPPORTING CLIENTS ON THE RECOVERY JOURNEY

For people experiencing trauma and stress-related mental health conditions, there is now an expectation that recovery can happen even when illness/symptoms persist and this is not dependent upon appropriate support, although support is hugely helpful. There is increasing evidence that people who have anxiety-related and post-traumatic stress disorders can make a recovery, although more research is needed on interventions to help young people, for example (Simonds et al., 2014). The National Institute of Care Excellence Guidance (2018) places emphasis on the use of non-pharmacological therapeutic interventions such as a series of sessions of trauma-focused CBT and other therapeutic interventions.

It is important to be mindful of the need for specialist mental health oversight of therapeutic interventions, including the use of medication; for example, in the context of comorbidities such as alcohol and drug misuse. There is a great deal more that nurses working in wider health care settings can do to support individuals experiencing anxiety and stress – in the immediate period after a traumatic event, during the experience of long-term/chronic health problems and in prevention through disaster planning and management. Using a trauma-informed approach is just one way in which nurses can anticipate the accentuated anxiety that certain procedures and interventions and also clinical situations can provoke. When the nurse invites or welcomes the consumer to an appointment, they need to:

- ensure privacy and be open to questions or concerns
- be able to clearly and honestly explain what will happen and why in a way that is appropriate and relevant to the consumer of any age or intellectual ability

- have the skills and abilities to use appropriate language and terminology and be open and ready for questions and challenges.

It is for these reasons that the consumer's consent is required for even what may seem to the nurse to be the simplest or most basic procedures; for example, looking at, touching or holding the other person. The nurse must be mindful of the potential impact of such contact on the consumer and allow time for them to recover or compose themselves and ask further questions, taking the time to provide useful information in different formats and mediums once the appointment or procedure is concluded. Just like the professionals, consumers may find a debriefing session helpful. On a broader scale, health care professionals will be involved in the work that governments and states do to prepare for major disasters; for example, the effects of extreme weather, large-scale human trauma arising from pandemics, or aircraft or road traffic collisions. These events create psychological as well as physical trauma that is sometimes complicated by grief, disability, loss of income and housing. Planning for such events is an essential function of authorities and many nurses have experience and expertise to contribute to this planning, at home and in service overseas. They use their clinical skills but also their communication, listening and therapeutic counselling skills to assist people in their recovery.

Alongside individual psychological therapies, there is increasing value placed on activities that support people at a local community level. Nurses working in community and primary care settings are working with other disciplines and agencies to facilitate recovery through community groups, where individuals support each other via mediums such as creative arts, for example. For the nurse assisting or supporting a person who has a mental health condition, recognising the nature of recovery for that individual is an essential starting point for effective care.

REFLECTION ON LEARNING FROM PRACTICE

Henry has moved to a new country and needs to establish new relationships and a safe community in which to recover from his traumatic experiences. His trauma experiences affect his relationships, community and connectedness.

CHAPTER RESOURCES

SUMMARY

- Trauma and stress-related disorders include post-traumatic stress disorder (PTSD), adjustment disorders, reactive attachment disorder, disinhibited social engagement disorder and acute stress disorder, and all respond to the principles of person-centred, trauma-informed care.

- Trauma and stress-related disorders occur as a result of the experience of something traumatic, such as witnessing an accident, experiencing abuse.
- Individualised care plans are essential to ensure the mental health team is working to the needs of the consumer.

Nursing care needs to be in collaboration with the consumer so that their strengths are recognised and built on.

- Acknowledging the needs of family/carers is imperative and the student nurse's knowledge of how to assist should be always developing. Engaging consumers, family and carers in the recovery process ensures a person-centred, trauma-informed approach to care.
- The case studies in this chapter outline the support required for recovery to commence, but are not prescriptive to all situations. Consumers will all present their experience of trauma differently and each individual assessment and care plan will differ. Recognising that most people will have experienced trauma in some way should now inform your nursing care and ensure that the possibility of re-traumatisation is minimised.
- Individual lived experience is shared through attentive and effective listening. Nurses need to be cognisant of what is being said, and how it is being said. Assessment must respond to the consumer's account and care and treatment must be reflective of their needs.

REVIEW QUESTIONS

1 What kind of experiences and situations might give rise to PTSD?
2 What is the likely impact of severe neglect on childhood development?
3 What are the key skills that mental health nurses need to develop to assess, support and assist people who have experienced trauma and stress?

4 What do you understand by the term 'trauma-informed care'?
5 What are the likely therapeutic interventions that can be applied for people who are experiencing PTSD?

CRITICAL THINKING

1 Consider three of the trauma and stress-related disorders outlined in this chapter. Conceptualise a brief description of each and reflect on the significance of the lived experience of consumers with these disorders. Choosing one of the case studies in the chapter, or an example from your own experience, write a short, reflective summary of the key issues that impact on their daily life and those around them.
2 Develop an understanding of the assessment of people with trauma and stress. List 10 of the key considerations for planning a safe assessment of a person presenting with a history of stress, anxiety or trauma. Identify key areas of risk for the person, and identify areas of understanding that require further knowledge/skills development in practice. Discuss your findings with your colleagues and classmates.

3 Create an individualised plan of care for a person experiencing a disorder as a result of trauma/stress. Choose one of the case studies or an example of your own and identify the key elements of a safe plan of care, including the sources of support that might be available.
4 Explore your knowledge and skills to support family/carers. Choose two of the case studies. What nursing skills will you draw upon to support the carers in these examples? What barriers or challenges do you foresee?
5 Apply your knowledge to support clients on the recovery journey. Choose one of the case studies and describe the key elements of recovery. How will you increase your understanding of the individual's perspective on their recovery?

USEFUL WEBSITES

- Mental Health Australia: https://mhaustralia.org/general/trauma-informed-practice
- Mind Australia: https://www.mindaustralia.org.au/resources/recovery

- Phoenix Australia – Centre for Posttraumatic Mental Health: http://phoenixaustralia.org
- Save the Children Australia: https://www.savethechildren.org.au/About-Us/Issues/Emergency-Response

REFLECT ON THIS

Responses to stress and trauma

The COVID-19 pandemic is a health crisis on a global scale. A crisis can be thought of as an unexpected event leading to feelings of distress and anxiety. The individual finds that their usual coping strategies do not help in managing their anxiety and distress. Read the following article and reflect on the questions that follow: Madanes, S.B, Levenson-Palmer, R., Szuhany, K.L., Malgaroli, M., Jennings, E.L., Anbarasan, D. & Simon, N.M. (2020). Acute stress disorder and the COVID-19 pandemic. *Psychiatric Annals*, 50(7), 295–300, https://doi.org/10.3928/00485713-20200611-01

1 What are some of the psychosocial stressors identified by the authors?

2 The authors speak of the importance of building resilience. What does this mean to you? How is resilience discussed in this textbook (in particular, look at the discussion on resilience in Chapter 21).

3 How can nurses in any context, including mental health, support consumers and families to build resilience?

REFERENCES

Afzali, M.H., Sunderland, M., Batterham, P.J., Carragher, N., Calear, A. & Slade, T. (2016). Network approach to the symptom-level association between alcohol use disorder and posttraumatic stress disorder. *Social Psychiatry and Psychiatric Epidemiology*, 1–11.

Alvares, G.A., Quintana, D.S., Kemp, A.H., Van Zwieten, A., Balleine, B.W., et al. (2013). Reduced heart rate variability in social anxiety disorder: Associations with gender and symptom severity. *PLOS ONE*, 8(7), e70468. https://doi.org/10.1371/journal.pone.0070468

American Psychiatric Association (APA). (2013). *Diagnostic and Statistical Manual of Mental Disorders (DSM-5)* (5th edn). Washington, DC: APA.

Arbuckle, G.A. (2013). *Humanizing Health Care Reforms*. London: Jessica Kingsley.

Arnold, E.C. & Underman Boggs, K. (2016). *Interpersonal Relationships: Professional Communication Skills for Nurses* (7th edn). St Louis, MO: Elsevier Saunders.

Australian Bureau of Statistics (ABS). (2008). Prevalence of Mental Disorders. Cat. 4326.0. Canberra: ABS. Retrieved from http://www.abs.gov.au/ausstats/abs@.nsf/Latestproducts/4326.0Main%20Features32007.

Australian Government Department of Health. (2015). *The Mental Health of Children and Adolescents: Report on the Second Australian Child and Adolescent Survey of Mental Health and Wellbeing*. Canberra: Commonwealth of Australia. Retrieved from https://www.health.gov.au/internet/main/publishing.nsf/Content/9DA8CA21306FE6EDCA257E2700016945/$File/child2.pdf.

Australian Institute of Health and Welfare (AIHW). (2016). *Australia's Health 2016. Australia's Health Series* no. 15. Cat no. AUS 199. Canberra: AIHW.

Bloom, S.L. (2010). Organizational stress as a barrier to trauma-informed service delivery. In M. Becker & B. Levin (eds). *A Public Health Perspective of Women's Mental Health* (pp. 295–311). New York: Springer. Retrieved from http://www.sanctuaryweb.com/PDFs_new/Bloom%20Organizational%20Stress%20as%20a%20Barrier%20to%20Trauma%20Chapter.pdf.

Chaffin, M., Hanson, R., Saunders, B.E., Nichols, T., Barnett, D., Zeanah, C., Berliner, L., ... Miller-Perrin, C. (2006). Report of the APSAC task force on attachment therapy, reactive attachment disorder, and attachment problems. *Child Maltreatment*, 11(1), 76–89. doi:10.1177/1077559505283699

Chandler, G. (2008). From traditional inpatient to trauma-informed treatment: transferring control from staff to patient. *Journal of*

the American Psychiatric Nurses Association, 14(5), 363–71. doi:10.1177/1078390308326625

Clift, S. (2012). Creative arts as a public health resource: Moving from practice-based research to evidence-based practice. *Perspectives in Public Health*, 132(3). Retrieved from http://journals.sagepub.com/doi/pdf/10.1177/1757913912442269.

Courtois, C.A. & Ford, J.D. (eds) (2009). *Treating Complex Traumatic Stress Disorders: An Evidence-Based Guide*. New York: Guilford Press.

Craske, M.G. & Stein, M.B. (2016). Anxiety. *The Lancet*, 388(10063), 3048–59.

Dahmen, B., Putz, V., Herpertz-Dahlmann, B. & Konrad, K. (2012). Early pathogenic care and the development of ADHD-like symptoms. *Journal of Neural Transmission*, 119(9), 1023–36.

Daykin, N. & Joss, T. (2016). *Arts for Health and Wellbeing: An Evaluation Framework*. London: Public Health England. Retrieved from https://www.gov.uk/government/uploads/system/uploads/attachment_data/file/496230/PHE_Arts_and_Health_Evaluation_FINAL.pdf.

Dixon, L.E., Ahles, E. & Marques, L. (2016). Treating posttraumatic stress disorder in diverse settings: Recent advances and challenges for the future. *Current Psychiatry Reports*, 18(12), 108.

Elliott, D.E., Bjelajac, P., Fallot, R.D., Markoff, L.S. & Reed, B.G. (2005). Trauma-informed or trauma-denied: Principles and implementation of trauma-informed services for women. *Journal of Community Psychology*, 33(4), 461–77. doi:10.1002/jcop.20063

Evans, K., Nizette, D. & O'Brien, A.J. (2016). *Psychiatric and Mental Health Nursing*. Chatswood: Elsevier Australia.

Fallot, R. & Harris, M. (2009). Creating cultures of trauma-informed care (CCTIC): A self-assessment and planning protocol. *Community Connections*, 2(2), 1–18.

Forbes, D., Creamer, M., Phelps, A., Bryant, R., McFarlane, A., Devilly, G.J., Matthews, L. ... Newton, S. (2007). Australian guidelines for the treatment of adults with acute stress disorder and post-traumatic stress disorder. *Australian & New Zealand Journal of Psychiatry*, 41(8), 637–48. Retrieved from https://journals.sagepub.com/doi/pdf/10.1080/00048670701449161.

Gleason, M.M., Fox, N.A., Drury, S., Smyke, A., Egger, H.L., Nelson, C.A. & Zeanah, C.H. (2011). Validity of evidence-derived criteria for reactive attachment disorder: Indiscriminately social/disinhibited and emotionally withdrawn/inhibited types. *Journal of the American Academy of Child and Adolescent Psychiatry*, 50(3), 216–31.e3.

Hodas, G.R. (2006). *Responding to Childhood Trauma: The Promise and Practice of Trauma Informed Care*. Pennsylvania Office of Mental Health and Substance Abuse Services. Retrieved from http://www.dhs.pa.gov/cs/groups/public/documents/manual/s_001585.pdf.

Hungerford, C. & Fox, C. (2014). Consumers' perceptions of recovery orientated mental health services: An Australian case-study analysis. *Nursing and Health Sciences*, 16, 209–15.

Hungerford, C., Hodgson, D., Murphy, G., de Jong, G., Ngune, I., Bostwick, R. & Clancy, R. (2018). *Mental Health Care* (3rd edn). Hoboken, NJ: Wiley Blackwell.

Isobel, S. & Edwards, C. (2016). Using trauma informed care as a nursing model of care in an acute inpatient mental health unit: A practice development process. *International Journal of Mental Health Nursing*, 26(1), 88–94.

Madanes, S.B, Levenson-Palmer, R., Szuhany, K.L., Malgaroli, M., Jennings, E.L., Anbarasan, D. & Simon, N.M. (2020). Acute stress disorder and the COVID-19 pandemic. *Psychiatric Annals*, 50(7), 295–300, https://doi.org/10.3928/00485713-20200611-01

McLaughlin, A., Espie, C. & Minnis, H. (2010). Development of a brief waiting room observation for behaviours typical of reactive attachment disorder. *Child and Adolescent Mental Health*, 15(2), 73–9.

Mills, K.L., Barrett, E.L., Merz, S., Rosenfeld, J., Ewer, P.L., Sannibale, C., Baker, A.L., Hopwood, S., Back, S.E., Brady, K.T. & Teesson, M. (2016). Integrated exposure-based therapy for co-occurring post traumatic stress disorder (PTSD) and substance predictors of change in PTSD symptom severity. *Journal of Clinical Medicine*, 5(11), 101.

National Institute for Health and Care Excellence (NICE). (2018). *Post-traumatic Stress Disorder*. Retrieved from https://www.nice.org.uk/guidance/ng116.

Nursing and Midwifery Board of Australia (NMBA). (2016). *Registered Nurse Standards for Practice*. Retrieved from https://www.nursingmidwiferyboard.gov.au/Codes-Guidelines-Statements/Professional-standards/registered-nurse-standards-for-practice.aspx.

O'Connor, T.G. & Zeanah, C.H. (2003). Attachment disorders: Assessment strategies and treatment approaches. *Attachment & Human Development*, 5(3), 223–44. doi:10.1080/14616730310001593974

Phoenix Australia – Centre for Posttraumatic Mental Health. (2013). *Australian Guidelines for the Treatment of Acute Stress Disorder and Posttraumatic Stress Disorder*. Melbourne: Phoenix Australia.

Pritchett, R., Pritchett, J., Marshall, E., Davidson, C. & Minnis, H. (2013). Reactive attachment disorder in the general population: A hidden ESSENCE disorder. *Scientific World Journal*, Art. ID 818157, 1–6.

Reeves, E. (2015). A synthesis of the literature on trauma-informed care. *Issues in Mental Health Nursing*, 36(9), 698–709.

Robins, C.S., Sauvageot, J.A., Cusack, K.J., Suffoletta-Maierle, S. & Frueh, B.C. (2005). Consumers' perceptions of negative experiences and 'sanctuary harm' in psychiatric settings. *Psychiatric Services*, 56(9), 1134–8.

Rogers, C.R. (1951). *Client-Centered Therapy*. Boston, MA: Houghton-Mifflin.

Schwartz, E. & Davis, A.S. (2006). Reactive attachment disorder: Implications for school functioning. *Psychology in the Schools*, 43(4), 471–9.

Simonds, L.M., Pons, R.A., Stone, N.J., Warren, F. & John, M. (2014). Adolescents with anxiety and depression: Is social recovery relevant? *Clinical Psychology and Psychotherapy*, 21, 289–98.

Stein-Parbury, J. (2018). *Patient and Person: Interpersonal Skills in Nursing*. St Louis, MO: Elsevier Saunders.

VicHealth. (2017). Trauma – Understanding and treating. Retrieved from https://www2.health.vic.gov.au/mental-health/practice-and-service-quality/safety/trauma-informed-care/trauma-understanding-and-treating.

Ward, L. (2011). Mental health nursing and stress: Maintaining balance. *International Journal of Mental Health Nursing*, 20, 77–85. doi:10.1111/j.1447-0349.2010.00715.x

CHAPTER 19

OTHER DISORDERS OF CLINICAL INTEREST

Louise Alexander

LEARNING OUTCOMES

Upon completion of this chapter, you should be able to:

19.1 Explore conduct disorder, and develop an understanding of its clinical presentation, aetiology and treatment

19.2 Develop an understanding for oppositional defiant disorder, its clinical presentation, diagnostic criteria and treatment

19.3 Consider the diagnostic criteria, aetiology and presentation of dissociative identity disorder

19.4 Understand gender dysphoria and consider the perspective of the lived experience of this condition

19.5 Explore conversion disorder, and develop an understanding of its presentation and aetiology

19.6 Develop an understanding of factitious disorders

LEARNING FROM PRACTICE

After a difficult delivery, my child was born a beautiful, healthy girl. We coasted along, meeting developmental milestones either on schedule or slightly ahead. During childcare, my child was always referred to as the 'tom boy', never liked dresses to the point of meltdowns and blatant refusal to wear them, and always liked the trucks or what was deemed gender stereotypical boy toys. At around three years, my child was calmly playing in her bedroom when I went to check in and found her trying to cut off her labia with some safety scissors. I screamed stop, took the scissors away and asked 'what are you doing?' Her response was 'I'm a boy, I don't want a vagina'. This was the beginning of a rocky few years. The intensity of my child hating her body and wanting it to change grew. Every year the Santa letter would have 'penis' as a request. Clothes shopping became a battle. The start of primary school saw the most challenging time we faced come to a head. My child never had an accident once toilet trained, then all of a sudden it was becoming a weekly occurrence and no matter how we tried to get to the bottom of it, we couldn't, until we brought in the school psychologist. We found out that our child wanted to use the boys' toilet because he was a boy, but the boys wouldn't let him in and he was worried

he would get into trouble, so he was holding on all day and sometimes he couldn't hold on any longer.

I was starting to hear more and more stories of children with gender dysphoria. Even though I knew logically it described my child perfectly, it took my child coming to me and saying, 'Mum I am not a girl, I am a boy. God made me wrong and I want it fixed', before I was ready to accept it. I confided in a flood of tears to a friend, who calmly said, 'Your child is transgender and unless you get on board you know what can happen.' Unfortunately, I knew the suicide statistics; I knew the detrimental effects of an unsupportive environment.

We went through the process of socially transitioning at age seven. This entailed changing name and pronouns, and that is it. When your child transitions you almost grieve as if you have lost a child. It is one of the hardest things to explain. Grieving the loss of someone who isn't actually gone is surreal. I struggled to look at baby photos, I became acutely aware of things that had his birth name on them. I also learned quickly how people can become unsupportive and about the discrimination you face.

My days now are filled with a happy, thriving son who was once shy and reserved. I am often asked what I think about the future. I worry about what sort of discrimination my son will face. He is, luckily, unaware of the medical battles we will go through to get him cross-hormonal treatment when he is a teenager. He hasn't witnessed the fights I have had with medical staff in hospitals and clinics who cannot get their head around someone his age being transgender and the inappropriate questions I am asked like, 'Are you sure it's not a phase?' and 'You must have always wanted a son'.

Leigh, mother to a child with gender dysmorphia

Leigh's experiences of having a child with gender dysmorphia are not uncommon. Consider the discrimination laws of your state or territory. How are they posed to support individuals whose sexual or gender identity is outside what society may deem as 'the norm'? As a nurse, how do you think you can practise in a gender- and sexuality-sensitive manner?

INTRODUCTION

This chapter explores conditions that may not necessarily be clinically *common*, but consist of conditions that are interesting, and those which often capture people's attention. We explore a number of conditions that cross the expanse of many different sections within the *Diagnostic and Statistical Manual of Mental Disorders* (DSM-5; APA, 2013) and you will see an array of diverse conditions, with different symptoms and aetiology. Some of these conditions are emerging in society, and becoming more widely understood. In this chapter, we consider conduct disorder, oppositional defiant disorder, dissociative identity disorder, gender dysphoria, conversion disorder and factitious disorders.

CONDUCT DISORDER

Conduct disorder (CD) is a condition seen in childhood and adolescence and falls under the category of disruptive, impulse-control and conduct disorders within the classification system of the DSM-5. CD and behaviours of conduct disorder are the primary reasons for referral to child and adolescent mental health services, and thus this is an important consideration. CD is a particularly troublesome condition, encompassing a range of socially unacceptable behaviours that have the potential to progress on to antisocial personality disorder (see Chapter 12) in many cases. CD has wide-reaching consequences that far exceed the impacts on the individual diagnosed and their family, and as such is considered to have significant social and community impacts that occur at great cost. Children and adolescents diagnosed with CD will often present with behaviours such as rule breaking, truancy from school, bullying behaviours towards others, property destruction, theft and aggression towards people and animals. These individuals are frequently seen in the criminal justice system.

Incidence and epidemiology

Conduct disorder rates of diagnosis range from around 2–10%, but the average is believed to be around 4%, and the condition is more likely to affect males than females (APA, 2013). CD in childhood is associated with higher rates of males being affected; however, when the condition's onset is during adolescence, the rates for males and females are similar (Erford et al., 2017).

Aetiology

The development of CD is a complex interplay between genetic predispositions, coupled with environmental vulnerability. This section will explore the aetiology and epidemiology of CD in more detail.

Genetic factors

CD is considered a moderately heritable condition. CD is more common in first-degree relatives with the condition, and in those who demonstrate highly heritable factors such as aggression and callous-unemotional traits (Blair, Leibenluft & Pine, 2014). CD is also more common in children whose parents have any of a range of serious mental health conditions such as schizophrenia or bipolar disorder, and substance use issues with alcohol (APA, 2013). It is likely that there are a number of genetic factors and when a vulnerable individual is exposed to an environment conducive to CD, the condition is more likely to occur (Salvatore & Dick, 2016). This means that in studies where genetics accounts for a moderate degree of CD presentations, shared environment consists of about 14% and is a substantial factor that needs to be considered (Salvatore & Dick, 2016).

Biological factors

Studies have suggested that individuals who have low levels of empathy also have higher levels of aggression (and vice versa), and this seems to be particularly evident in those with callous-unemotional traits such as those seen in CD (Blair, Leibenluft & Pine, 2014). It has also been suggested that those with reduced empathy levels have difficulty socialising with others. Principally, the amygdala is the area of the brain responsible for empathy, and dysfunction in this region may result in increased callous-unemotional traits and therefore CD and psychopathy (Blair, Leibenluft

& Pine, 2014). Interestingly, those who are impulsive or demonstrate poor judgement may also have a biological basis of origin with abnormalities within the prefrontal cortex of the brain. It has also been demonstrated that those with CD also have slower resting heart rates when compared with individuals who do not have this condition (APA, 2013).

Individual factors
Individuals diagnosed with CD will commonly present with similar personality traits, in particular the callous-unemotional trait that is highly affiliated with antisocial personality disorder and psychopathy. Callous-unemotional traits (or reduced prosocial behaviours) include reduced (or complete lack of) empathy and remorse, which makes it easy to victimise others or treat them poorly (Blair, Leibenluft & Pine, 2014). Other individual factors include lower intelligence quotient (IQ) test scores in those with CD (APA, 2013). Individuals with CD are also more likely to have had a mother who smoked during pregnancy and had a poor prenatal diet (Blair, Leibenluft & Pine, 2014).

Environmental factors
The majority of children who develop CD have come from a family environment that is dysfunctional and presents with many risk factors, such as violence and poverty. Higher incidence of punitive discipline from parents, abuse (physical, sexual, verbal, neglect) and disruptions and inconsistencies of care-giving are common (APA, 2013). Many of the consequences of childhood sexual abuse (such as self-harm/non-suicidal self-injury, suicide attempts, substance misuse, reduced social interactions and poor school achievement) are the same as those seen in CD (Maniglio, 2014). Maniglio (2014) explored the prevalence of sexual abuse in a multitude of individual research papers on conduct disorder and sexual abuse and found that 27% of those diagnosed with CD had been sexually abused. This is compared with 12% of females and 4.5% of males who report being sexually abused in Australia prior to the age of 15 (Australian Institute of Criminology, 2011). In addition, families are often larger than average and parents or caregivers may have a history of engaging in criminal activity and substance misuse (APA, 2013). There is often incidence of family violence, inadequate parental supervision and divorce or separation (Lewis et al., 2015).

Social environment also plays a part in the development of CD. Children with CD often come from communities where other 'delinquent' children or 'gangs' gravitate with like behaviours and the area may have a high crime rate and a low socioeconomic status (SES) (Erford et al., 2017) (see **Figure 19.1**).

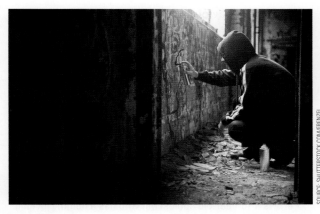

FIGURE 19.1
Children with CD will display early signs of antisocial behaviours, such as involvement in crime, and often draw the attention of law enforcement

Comorbidity
Children who have CD seem more prone to a number of other mental health conditions. Children with CD are at risk of an anxiety disorder at rates about three times higher than non-CD children and anxiety is more prevalent in females (Euler et al., 2015). Both attention deficit/hyperactivity disorder (ADHD) and oppositional defiant disorder (ODD) are commonly seen in young people with CD, in addition to learning disorders, substance use disorders and other serious mental health conditions (APA, 2013).

Clinical course
For many children with CD, behavioural issues emerge early in life and will usually be evident by the time the child begins school. Having said that, most children with CD will not be diagnosed until they are about 10 years of age, when they are more likely to demonstrate *enough* diagnostic requirements (Blair, Leibenluft & Pine, 2014). In the early presentation of the condition, children will usually demonstrate:

- impulsiveness
- early aggressiveness
- refusal to cooperate with others or with requirements.

In addition to these signs, possible signs of ADHD or ODD are often evident (APA, 2013; Blair, Leibenluft & Pine, 2014). ODD is often seen before CD emerges. While the course of CD may vary, for most the condition is well advanced by age 16, and it is unusual for it to emerge after this time (APA, 2013). As with many mental health conditions, the earlier that CD onsets, the poorer the outcomes, and this often paves the way for serious involvement in crime and increases the likelihood of imprisonment. In children who develop CD before age 10, the potential to develop antisocial personality disorder later in life is higher (Erford et al., 2017).

Adverse behaviours tend to change as the child ages and usually increase in seriousness and intensity; for example, sexual development may result in the adolescent raping someone; or with increasing physical strength, more serious altercations may occur where the injuries of victims increase in severity (APA, 2013). The individual with CD as a six-year-old-child may spend time annoying the family cat by pulling its tail, frightening or poking it. As the child grows older, behaviours tend to be more serious; for example, the same child at 12 years old may torture and kill the cat. It is important to note that CD is not diagnosed in individuals over the age of 18 years, and should such behaviours present in adulthood, a diagnosis of antisocial personality disorder may need to be explored further.

CASE **STUDY**

PERRY'S STORY

Perry is a 16-year-old adolescent who has a lengthy juvenile record. Perry dropped out of school completely when he was 15, but had very poor attendance, starting in high school, and has been expelled from three different public schools. Perry lives at home with his mother Karen and her partner Bill. His biological father Kevin lives in rural Queensland and he hasn't seen him for six years. Perry has five brothers and sisters, including an older brother who is in prison for armed robbery. Perry and his family live in public housing and often struggle to pay their bills. Karen works as an aged carer and Bill is an interstate truck driver. Many times, the police have been called to their home for domestic disputes stemming from alcohol misuse and violence. Perry himself has been in trouble with the police from a very young age. Over the years, he has been charged with theft, drug possession, graffiti and, more recently, assault. Perry has a tumultuous relationship with his mother and siblings and he dislikes Bill, who frequently uses physical violence as a means to manage his behaviours. His younger sister Tiarna is frightened of Perry. Karen is also afraid of Perry and he often uses his large physical presence to intimidate others. Last month, Perry killed a pregnant cat, dismembering it in the back shed 'to see what it looked like inside', and his increasingly aggressive behaviour is worrying his family. Karen is worried he will end up in prison like his brother, but concedes she doesn't know how to handle him any more.

Questions

1   Perry is demonstrating some worrying behaviours. Can you identify behaviours that are specific to CD in this case study?

2   What do you think the role of a social worker would be in Perry's case? How could the nurse and social worker collaborate to help his family?

Prognosis

For many children with CD, the outcomes are poor, particularly if they were diagnosed early and display behaviours that demonstrate a lack of empathy and remorse. Individuals who continue to display an antisocial trajectory of behaviour into adulthood will likely face a diagnosis of antisocial personality disorder and this occurs in up 50% of cases of CD (Blair, Leibenluft & Pine, 2014). Those adolescents who do not go on to develop antisocial personality disorder will often continue to experience significant mental health issues later in life.

Some of the more detrimental outcomes for CD include:

- a lack of education completion (exacerbated by truancy from school, a disregard for authority figures and low IQ)
- engagement in the criminal justice system through antisocial behaviours
- misuse of substances
- issues with employment
- issues with interpersonal relationships (Lewis et al., 2015).

Outcomes for females diagnosed with CD may include teen pregnancies, high incidence of domestic violence, depression, anxiety and borderline personality disorder (Lewis et al., 2015).

Prognosis is *improved* in individuals as adults who demonstrate the following:

- delayed onset of symptoms (preferably until adolescence)
- presence of prosocial behaviours (no callous-unemotional traits)
- presentation of less antisocial behaviours
- higher IQ
- lack of learning difficulties
- engaged in a healthy relationship with an adult (does not need to be a parent)
- peers who are not delinquent
- engaged in a hobby (such as music) or sport (such as football)
- no comorbid mental health conditions
- enrolled in school until at least 16 years of age (Andrews et al., 2013).

As can be seen, the presence of protective factors and positive social engagement and interactions is helpful in not only reducing the severity of CD, but in preventing the condition from progressing to antisocial personality disorder as well.

Conduct disorder and suicide

Wei and colleagues (2016) found in their study that individuals diagnosed with CD had higher rates of suicide attempts, and were also particularly troubled by comorbid mental health conditions that are more frequently associated with suicide attempts (such as depression and bipolar disorder).

Diagnostic criteria conduct disorder

The diagnostic criteria of CD are quite intricate and detailed as there are many diverse behaviours that must be present in order for an individual to be diagnosed with the condition. **Table 19.1** outlines the DSM-5 (APA, 2013) criteria in detail.

DIAGNOSTIC CRITERIA

Conduct disorder

TABLE 19.1
Diagnostic criteria conduct disorder

A. A repetitive and persistent pattern of behavior in which the basic rights of others or major age-appropriate societal norms or rules are violated, as manifested by the presence of at least three of the following 15 criteria in the past 12 months from any of the categories below, with at least one criterion in the past 6 months:

Aggression to people and animals
1. Often bullies, threatens, or intimidates others.
2. Often initiates physical fights.
3. Has used a weapon that can cause serious physical harm to others (e.g., a bat, brick, broken bottle, knife, gun).
4. Has been physically cruel to people.
5. Has been physically cruel to animals.
6. Has stolen while confronting a victim (e.g., mugging, purse snatching, extortion, armed robbery).
7. Has forced someone into sexual activity.

Destruction of property
8. Has deliberately engaged in fire setting with the intention of causing serious damage.
9. Has deliberately destroyed others' property (other than by fire setting).

Deceitfulness or theft
10. Has broken into someone else's house, building, or car.
11. Often lies to obtain goods or favors or to avoid obligations (i.e., "cons" others).
12. Has stolen items of nontrivial value without confronting a victim (e.g., shoplifting, but without breaking and entering; forgery).

Serious violations of rules
13. Often stays out at night despite parental prohibitions, beginning before age 13 years.
14. Has run away from home overnight at least twice living in the parental or parental surrogate home, or once without returning for a lengthy period.
15. Is often truant from school, beginning before age 13 years.

B. The disturbance in behavior causes clinically significant impairment in social, academic, or occupational functioning.

C. If the individual is age 18 years or older, criteria are not met for antisocial personality disorder.

Specify whether
- **Childhood-onset type:** Individuals show at least one symptom characteristic of conduct disorder prior to age 10 years.
- **Adolescent-onset type:** Individuals show no symptom characteristic of conduct disorder prior to age 10 years.
- **Unspecified onset:** Criteria for a diagnosis of conduct disorder are met, but there is not enough information available to determine whether the onset of the first symptom was before or after age 10 years.

Specify whether
- **Childhood-onset type:** Individuals show at least one symptom characteristic of conduct disorder prior to age 10 years.
- **Adolescent-onset type:** Individuals show no symptom characteristic of conduct disorder prior to age 10 years.
- **Unspecified onset:** Criteria for a diagnosis of conduct disorder are met, but there is not enough information available to determine whether the onset of the first symptom was before or after age 10 years.

Specify if:
- **With limited prosocial emotions:** To qualify for this specifier, an individual must have displayed at least two of the following characteristics persistently over at least 12 months and in multiple relationships and settings. These characteristics reflect the individual's typical pattern of interpersonal and emotional functioning over this period and not just occasional occurrences in some situations. Thus, to assess the criteria for the specifier, multiple information sources are necessary. In addition to the individual's self-report, it is necessary to consider reports by others who have known the individual for extended periods of time (e.g., parents, teachers, co-workers, extended family members, peers).
  - **Lack of remorse or guilt:** Does not feel bad or guilty when he or she does something wrong (exclude remorse when expressed only when caught and/or facing punishment). The individual shows a general lack of concern about the negative consequences of his or her actions. For example, the individual is not remorseful after hurting someone or does not care about the consequences of breaking rules.

TABLE 19.1
(Continued)

- **Callous—lack of empathy:** Disregards and is unconcerned about the feelings of others. The individual is described as cold and uncaring. The person appears more concerned about the effects of his or her actions on himself or herself, rather than their effects on others, even when they result in substantial harm to others.
- **Unconcerned about performance:** Does not show concern about poor/problematic performance at school, at work, or in other important activities. The individual does not put forth the effort necessary to perform well, even when expectations are clear, and typically blames others for his or her poor performance.
- **Shallow or deficient affect:** Does not express feelings or show emotions to others, except in ways that seem shallow, insincere, or superficial (e.g., actions contradict the emotion displayed; can turn emotions "on" or "off" quickly) or when emotional expressions are used for gain (e.g., emotions displayed to manipulate or intimidate others).

Specify current severity:
- **Mild:** Few if any conduct problems in excess of those required to make the diagnosis are present, and conduct problems cause relatively minor harm to others (e.g., lying, truancy, staying out after dark without permission, other rule breaking).
- **Moderate:** The number of conduct problems and the effect on others are intermediate between those specified in "mild" and those in "severe" (e.g., stealing without confronting a victim, vandalism).
- **Severe:** Many conduct problems in excess of those required to make the diagnosis are present, or conduct problems cause considerable harm to others (e.g., forced sex, physical cruelty, use of a weapon, stealing while confronting a victim, breaking and entering).

SOURCE: REPRINTED WITH PERMISSION FROM THE *DIAGNOSTIC AND STATISTICAL MANUAL OF MENTAL DISORDERS*, FIFTH EDITION, (COPYRIGHT ©2013). AMERICAN PSYCHIATRIC ASSOCIATION. ALL RIGHTS RESERVED.

Treatment of conduct disorder

Early intervention is key to addressing the behaviours and characteristics associated with CD. Given that for many children the development of CD stems from both familial *and* social origins, this is not an easy task and treatment is largely symptom management. It is also important to consider the impacts that family dysfunction have both in the inclination to seek help or treatment and the maintenance of treatment interventions. Some of the more common obstacles to treatment seeking include:

- reduced parental understanding of need for intervention
- logistics of keeping appointments
- socioeconomic factors
- educational level and health literacy
- social isolation
- embarrassment and fear of being labelled (Lewis et al., 2015).

Treatment for CD often focuses on the 'externalising behaviours' common to the condition.

Pharmacological

While there is no single medical treatment indicated for the treatment of CD, there are a couple of medications that have demonstrated some improvement in aggression and irritability. Aripiprazole and risperidone have both showed benefit (Blair, Leibenluft & Pine, 2014). It is important, however, to consider the risks of side effects in the use of antipsychotic medication and these must be weighed against any perceived benefits.

Stimulant medications such as those used to treat ADHD such as **methylphenidate** (e.g. Ritalin™) have also been used successfully to address aggression in individuals with CD (Blair, Leibenluft & Pine,

2014). While stimulants have fewer side effects than antipsychotics, they are not without risks, including increased anxiety, weight loss, dependence and insomnia.

Non-pharmacological

Parents of children with CD often require support and assistance in managing their child's behaviours, and their *responses* to these behaviours. After reading this section, it should be clear how much strain and difficulty caring for a child with CD would be experienced, and carers will often require mental health support too. Family-centred therapy has demonstrated effectiveness in the treatment of CD and involves the young person and their parents. In particular, efficacy has been demonstrated in assisting with improvements in parenting style, a reduction in offending and antisocial behaviours, a reduction in truancy from school, and improvements in social interactions with peers (Ronan et al., 2016). Other therapies that may be helpful include cognitive behavioural therapy (CBT) and behavioural modification strategies (Andrews et al., 2013). Where the child is still engaged in schooling, the classroom teacher should also be considered as an important contributor to the implementation of interventions and management strategies for the child.

Recovery

As mentioned previously, many children with CD will go on to develop antisocial personality disorder. Individuals who have CD *and* also demonstrate callous-unemotional traits present with poorer outcomes, and are less likely to experience recovery from or remission of the condition (Euler et al., 2015).

OPPOSITIONAL DEFIANT DISORDER

Like CD, **oppositional defiant disorder (ODD)** is a condition of disruption and impulsiveness and is characterised by angry or irritable and argumentative behaviours, and vindictiveness towards others. While it is common (indeed, normal) for children to test boundaries and develop an understanding of how far they can take something, children with ODD tend to take this behaviour to the next level. Children with ODD will also present as easily irritated and there are a number of adverse outcomes for children, adolescents and adults who are diagnosed with the condition.

Prevalence

Much like CD, ODD is fairly common in child and adolescent mental health settings and is seen in over 3% of the population, occurring slightly more often in males than females (APA, 2013). ODD is considered a relatively common condition and accounts for a large proportion of families accessing child and adolescent mental health services.

Aetiology and epidemiology

There are a number of mental health conditions that have had only limited research, and ODD and CD appear to be two of these conditions. When they are explored, they are often clustered together, making differentiating aetiology and epidemiology somewhat complicated. Nevertheless, this section aims to explore the causes and incidences of ODD.

Genetic factors and biological factors

Many of the studies on ODD are clustered with those around CD and differentiation between aetiology can be difficult. Many of the same identified genetic factors noted in CD are also possibly associated with ODD (e.g. brain abnormalities, reduced heart rate). Cortisol levels are also understood to play a role in the development of conditions where antisocial and aggressive behaviours are evident (Schoorl et al., 2016). Decreased levels of cortisol during times of stress may lead to fearlessness and reduced emotional capacity, which are traits commonly seen in externalising behavioural disorders.

Individual factors

Prenatal substance misuse (and *postnatal* substance misuse) has been identified as an aetiological factor in the development of ODD in some children (Russell et al.,2015). In particular, studies have linked in utero and childhood exposure to cocaine, alcohol and tobacco use as definitive factors associated with the development of ODD (Russell et al., 2015). Cocaine exposure has been linked to increases in aggression and other externalising behaviours (e.g. frustration, cheating, lying and property destruction) seen in ODD (and CD), and prenatal alcohol misuse highly correlates with ODD development in offspring (Russell et al., 2015). Childhood experiences of trauma have been associated with adverse and defiant behaviours.

Temperamental factors also play a role in the development of ODD development. Children who are reactive, have a reduced tolerance to frustration and are highly emotional are also considered suggestive to development of the condition (APA, 2013).

Children with ODD demonstrate challenging and disruptive behaviours that can result in parenting approaches that are punitive or harsh and do not actually address the issues; rather, these approaches exacerbate the challenging behaviours and cause family discord. Children with ODD may also reside in homes where there are inconsistencies with discipline, such as where a parent makes a threat of punishment, but fails to follow through with it (Tung & Lee, 2014). Children with ODD may also come from dysfunctional families where there is conflict and marital discord (Burke, Rowe & Boylan, 2014).

Environmental factors

Lower SES appears to be a factor for some children with ODD (Russell et al., 2015). In addition, being raised in a neighbourhood where there are higher rates of violence (including witnessing violence), crime, drug use and sales, lower rates of neighbourhood support and perceptions of danger demonstrate links to the development of ODD (Russell et al., 2015). Studies have also suggested that children who feel safe in the neighbourhood they live in are less likely to demonstrate problem behaviours and are more engaged within the community; in essence, this is social capital. Young minority groups, who feel disconnected from their neighbourhood, be it through racism, isolation or exclusion, also demonstrate higher rates of ODD (Russell et al., 2015).

Comorbidity

Studies have indicated that the comorbidity rates of ODD and other mental health conditions are as high as 92% (Pederson & Fite, 2014; Riley, Ahmed & Locke, 2016). Commonly, children with ODD have higher rates of progressing onto developing CD. The correlation between ADHD and ODD is also very high; children with either condition will meet criteria of the other condition in up to half of cases (Harvey, Breaux & Lugo-Candelas, 2016). Children with ODD demonstrate higher rates of development of both anxiety disorders and depression (APA, 2013).

Clinical course

With a likely onset in preschool-age children, ODD is rarely seen after early adolescence and for many children the condition is diagnosed before CD (APA, 2013). As the child progresses into adolescence and adulthood, behavioural issues may become more problematic and overt, and in adulthood can result in issues around employment, socialisation and interpersonal relationships.

Prognosis

Prognosis for ODD in children who demonstrate vindictiveness, rebelliousness and argumentativeness as major features of their condition have higher rates of progression on to CD and, as such, the outcomes are usually worse. In adults with ODD, there are a number of issues that can impact on many aspects of their life. Even in children who do not go on to develop CD, outcomes in adulthood can be challenging, with issues such as substance misuse, poor impulse control and antisocial behaviours making progression vocationally, socially and personally difficult. Children with ODD will often have to repeat schooling and so also may experience adverse peer relationships and rejection (Burke, Rowe & Boylan, 2014). Characteristics of ODD also seriously interfere with the child's ability to advance academically, and this has a flow-on effect into adolescence (Russell et al., 2015). ODD appears to also create impacts on employment opportunities (and retention of employment) and relationships with peers, family and the development of intimate relationships.

Oppositional defiant disorder and suicide

The potential for comorbidity with mood disorders such as major depressive disorder (see Chapter 10) and anxiety disorders (see Chapter 11) appears to make rates of suicide and attempted suicide in individuals with ODD higher, not necessarily the ODD *per se*. This seems heightened also in children who have comorbid ODD and ADHD, although there is conflicting research as to whether this occurs because of comorbidity (again with depression and anxiety) or as an independent factor associated with co-occurring ADHD and ODD (Dickerson Mayes et al., 2015). Regardless of the aetiology, the end result is evident; children with ODD have higher rates of both suicide attempts and deaths from suicide (Dickerson Mayes et al., 2015).

Diagnostic criteria for oppositional defiant disorder

Oppositional defiant disorder is characterised by the criteria listed in **Table 19.2**.

DIAGNOSTIC CRITERIA

Oppositional defiant disorder

TABLE 19.2
Diagnostic criteria oppositional defiant disorder

> **A.** A pattern of angry/irritable mood, argumentative/defiant behavior, or vindictiveness lasting at least 6 months as evidenced by at least four symptoms from any of the following categories, and exhibited during interaction with at least one individual who is not a sibling.
> **Angry/irritable mood**
> 1. Often loses temper.
> 2. Is often touchy or easily annoyed.
> 3. Is often angry and resentful.
> **Argumentative/defiant behavior**
> 4. Often argues with authority figures or, for children and adolescents, with adults.
> 5. Often actively defies or refuses to comply with requests from authority figures or with rules.
> 6. Often deliberately annoys others.
> 7. Often blames others for his or her mistakes or misbehaviour.
> **Vindictiveness**
> 8. Has been spiteful or vindictive at least twice within the past 6 months.
> **Note:** The persistence and frequency of these behaviors should be used to distinguish a behavior that is within normal limits from a behavior that is symptomatic. For children younger than 5 years, the behavior should occur on most days for a period of at least 6 months unless otherwise noted (Criterion A8). For individuals 5 years or older, the behavior should occur at least once per week for at least 6 months, unless otherwise noted (Criterion A8). While these frequency criteria provide guidance on a minimal level of frequency to define symptoms, other factors should also be considered, such as whether the frequency and intensity of the behaviors are outside a range that is normative for the individual's developmental level, gender, and culture.
>
> **B.** The disturbance in behavior is associated with distress in the individual or others in his or her immediate social context (e.g., family, peer group, work colleagues), or it impacts negatively on social, educational, occupational, or other important areas of functioning.
>
> **C.** The behaviors do not occur exclusively during the course of a psychotic, substance use, depressive, or bipolar disorder. Also, the criteria are not met for disruptive mood dysregulation disorder.
> *Specify* current severity:
> - **Mild:** symptoms are confined to only one setting (e.g. at home, at school, at work, with peers).
> - **Moderate:** Some symptoms are present in at least two settings.
> - **Severe:** Some symptoms are present in three or more settings.

Individuals with ODD will typically exert their frustration and hostility towards parents, teachers and other people of authority and this can cause significant issues for both the child and the people around them. Individuals with ODD are typically stubborn and prone to arguing with others and bear grudges of past feelings of injustices. Their anger and

TABLE 19.3
Pharmacologic treatments for ODD

MEDICATION	EFFECTIVENESS
Stimulants (Ritalin™ or Concerta™)	Studies have indicated a decline in oppositional behaviours in children with ODD and ADHD co-occurring.
Selective norepinephrine reuptake inhibitors (SNRIs)	Appropriate for children who cannot tolerate psychostimulants. Decline in oppositional behaviours in children with ODD and ADHD co-occurring.
Atypical antipsychotics (risperidone, aripiprazole, quetiapine)	In children with low IQ, a decline in aggressive and disruptive behaviours is seen. Decline in ODD in children with ADHD.
Mood stabilisers (lithium and carbamazepine)	Lithium has demonstrated efficacy in reducing aggressive behaviours. The effectiveness of carbamazepine is not clinically significant.

SOURCE: ADAPTED FROM HOOD, ELROD & DEWINE, 2015

frustration knows no bounds and they frequently find themselves frustrated with those around them, and with society in general.

There are issues with parenting styles at both ends of the spectrum in ODD; those parents who are controlling and restrictive, and those who are inconsistent, disordered or inadequate disciplinarians. Generally, children with ODD define their relationships with their parents as hostile and argumentative and these descriptors often translate to teachers and other authority figures also (Booker, Ollendick, Dunsmore & Greene, 2016).

Treatment of oppositional defiant disorder

Treatment of ODD is similar to that for CD and generally involves parenting style adjustments. As with CD, there is no medication clinically indicated for the treatment of ODD, and where medications are used, they should always be an adjunct to a psychological approach. Behavioural treatment approaches are one of the first-line approaches to the treatment of ODD, and the child's paediatrician or general practitioner may be one of the first individuals approached about behavioural concerns. Many advocates for childhood behavioural disorders suggest routine screening for externalising disorders such as ODD and CD, and more rapid preventative and responsive approaches to reducing the impacts later in life to the child, their family and society.

Non-pharmacological

Parent management training (PMT) is one approach that focuses on the interactions between the child and parents and utilises a reward-based approach to managing dysfunctional or challenging behaviours with good success (Hood, Elrod & DeWine, 2015). Other treatment approaches to ODD include collaborative problem solving (CPS), which is another intervention that seeks to address the child's emotional, frustration and problem-solving issues while heavily involving input from parents (Hood, Elrod & DeWine, 2015). While CBT is still used to treat ODD, its effectiveness is not as encouraging

as therapies that involve both the parents and the school.

Pharmacological treatments

Treatment of ODD with medication is not a first-line approach and there is currently no medication indicated for ODD. Pharmacological treatment when used will be similar to that used for CD (and ADHD), such as stimulants, and low dose antipsychotics like risperidone. While stimulants such as methylphenidate (Ritalin™ or Concerta™) have demonstrated efficacy in children with ODD, there are side effects such as insomnia and loss of appetite that necessitate serious considerations about their use. **Table 19.3** outlines pharmacological treatments for ODD and areas where efficacy has been demonstrated.

Recovery

Given research suggesting that over 90% of both children and adults with ODD will go on to develop a further mental health condition, there can be serious resulting issues even in the presence of appropriate and successful treatment of ODD. Nonetheless, in one study about 70% of individuals with ODD demonstrated recovery by age 18 (Riley, Ahmed & Locke, 2016). Outcomes for poor treatment responses and continuance of symptoms of ODD seem to be more likely where the individual is male and has an early onset of aggressive symptoms (Riley, Ahmed & Locke, 2016).

DISSOCIATIVE IDENTITY DISORDER

Imagine you have woken up to attend your mental health tutorial today; you begin to get dressed, take a shower, have breakfast and pack your bag with your laptop and books. Just before you leave, you remember you have forgotten your phone and go back into the kitchen to get it. When you enter the kitchen, you catch a glimpse of the shrubs outside the kitchen window. Suddenly, you are no longer Amy, a nursing student, but Ella, a frightened and scared 12-year-old girl who at one time hid in the backyard from her abusive father. This example reflects the life of someone with dissociative identity disorder (DID; formerly known as multiple personality disorder). The condition is associated with periods of memory loss and the experiencing of other personalities (which may be of different gender, age and nationality or life experiences).

Multiple personality disorder (MPD) is believed to have been studied in the late seventeenth century by a number of prominent names in the field of psychiatry (later including Sigmund Freud) who reported on hysteria and dissociation resulting from sexual abuse in a patient. Probably more noticeably, however, MPD became more prominent in the 1970s after the condition was featured in the award-winning movie *Sybil*, which explored the array of personalities within a young school teacher who was physically and sexually abused by her mother. In the text revision of the 1994 edition of the DSM, the condition was changed to DID to reflect the *division* of personality states rather than the evolution of separate individual states within the one person.

DID is a controversial disorder that has been refuted by many clinicians, and at times seen as being a condition that can be highly influenced upon suggestive consumers by curious practitioners. Despite its inclusion in the DSM, some clinicians and researchers are sceptical. One of the major factors for scepticism is whether the development of these distinct personalities is a result of trauma or abuse or it is a phenomenon influenced (or developed) by the clinician (Reed-Gavish, 2013).

In order to understand DID, it is important to identify the nature of **dissociation**. To dissociate is to experience a disruption in imperative psychological states of functioning such as cognition (our ability to understand), consciousness (our alertness), memory, identity and awareness of the environment (such as smell and sight). Some view the dissociative process as an involuntary progression of psychologically avoiding severely traumatic experiences, such as sexual abuse; simplistically, it is the psyche's way of protecting itself from the trauma being experienced. Many victims describe their abuse and subsequent dissociation as the only way they could cope with the horrific events happening to them. One such survivor described the need to escape the persistent sexual abuse after being abducted, 'There was a switch. I had to shut off… just went someplace else… you just do what you have to do to survive' (Middleton, 2013, p. 258).

Incidence and epidemiology

There is a lack of epidemiological research to identify the prevalence of DID in Australia and it would appear that it is quite rare. In the United States, prevalence rates are noted between 1.4% (females) to 1.6% (males) (APA, 2013).

While females are more likely to present as adults with DID in treatment settings, rates between males and females are generally consistent. Females more commonly display acute dissociative states (such as distressing flashbacks or hallucinations), while males are more likely to present as aggressive, violent or end up in the criminal justice system serving time for various offences. In males, the condition appears to be triggered by incarceration, further sexual abuse and warfare (APA, 2013).

CULTURAL CONSIDERATIONS

Possession, culture and DID

It is important to be mindful of the potential issues that culture may pose in the diagnosis of DID. In regions of the world where possession is not uncommon or is not considered a mental health issue (e.g. in some parts of South America and some African countries, or in those practising certain religions), it is important to be cognisant of this. The DSM-5 (APA, 2013, p. 295) differentiates actual DID from possession by the presence of '…conflict between the individual and his or her surrounding family, social, or work milieu; and is manifested at times and in places that violate the norms of the culture or religion'. It is also understood that DID is '…involuntary, distressing, uncontrollable and often recurrent or persistent…' (p. 295).

Differences in cultural beliefs can cause issues with treatment, and clinicians need to be sensitive and aware of the impacts of diverse cultural beliefs and how these may complicate treatment. Family and cultural beliefs play an important role in the treatment of mental health conditions and it would be remiss to assume these influences do not affect consumers. Similarly, it is important to acknowledge that belief in possession is not limited to particular countries, but also some religious practices, and therefore someone's beliefs or practices cannot be assumed merely from their cultural background. Practising in a culturally sensitive manner does not require the mental health nurse to agree with someone else's beliefs, but it is important to respect their right to this belief without dismissing it entirely.

Individual factors and environmental factors

DID is strongly associated with trauma. However, it is important to note that trauma is not strongly correlated to DID. This means that while the vast majority of people who have DID also have a history of traumatising experiences, most people who are traumatised do not have DID. Overwhelmingly, individuals with DID report strong histories of sexual abuse and neglect – in around 90% of cases (APA, 2013). High rates of other experiences that may be perceived as traumatising such as childhood illness and surgical procedures, experiences during war and prostitution have also been cited as possible causes of DID (APA, 2013). Childhood sexual abuse has been linked to a number of serious mental health issues such as self-harm behaviours, suicide and sexual aggression, and it is believed that the more serious the abuse, the more severe the dissociation (Yanartas et al., 2015).

Comorbidity

The most frequently seen comorbidity in DID is post-traumatic stress disorder (PTSD; see Chapter 18). Other comorbid mental health conditions include depression, anxiety, personality disorders, conversion disorder, other stress disorders, sleep disorders and substance-use disorders (APA, 2013).

REFLECT ON THIS

Trauma-informed practice

Being trauma-informed is a pertinent part of mental health care. There is a plethora of literature that tells us that trauma and mental illness are intimately related, and that many people living with a mental health condition have a past experience (or more) of trauma. Being a trauma-informed practitioner means being aware that the consumers in your care have most likely had a traumatic experience in their life and that this experience has impacted upon their mental health.

There are many things a mental health nurse can do when they practise in a trauma-informed manner. Some of these include:

- being trustworthy and honest
- resisting re-traumatisation
- collaborating, promoting, encouraging and facilitating choice.

Reflect upon five ways that you could be trauma-informed when working with a consumer who has a history of sexual assault. Ensure you are evidence-based in your responses.

Clinical course

Typically, DID manifests in childhood as a result of severe sexual and/or physical abuse or neglect, although it may present in older people who experience a trauma later in their life. The condition may be exacerbated by being removed from or leaving the location of abuse (often this is the home); when the individual's own children reach the same age that the abuse began for them; experiencing further trauma (minor or major); or the death or illness of the abuser (APA, 2013).

Prognosis

Outcomes for individuals with DID seem to be poorer for those who experienced long-term abuse, were delayed in receiving suitable treatment, have comorbid mental health conditions and were again traumatised in later life (APA, 2013).

Dissociative identity disorder and suicide

Suicide and self-harm/non-suicidal self-injury are very real concerns for individuals (and clinicians caring for someone with DID). More than 70% of individuals with DID have attempted to end their life through suicide (APA, 2013). It is important to consider that obtaining an accurate risk assessment of an individual with DID may be complicated, depending on the personality that is present during the assessment.

Diagnostic criteria for dissociative identity disorder

DID is characterised by the experience of more than two, distinct and separate personality states. For some cultures and individuals, this experience may be deemed 'possession'. As can be seen by criterion

A in **Table 19.4**, DID poses significant impacts on an individual's mental state, and as such can result in significant impacts towards social, occupational and interpersonal functioning.

DIAGNOSTIC CRITERIA

Dissociative identity disorder

TABLE 19.4
Diagnostic criteria dissociative identity disorder

A. Disruption of identity characterized by two or more distinct personality states, which may be described in some cultures as an experience of possession. The disruption in identity involves marked discontinuity in sense of self and sense of agency, accompanied by related alterations in affect, behavior, consciousness, memory, perception, cognition, and/or sensory-motor functioning. These signs and symptoms may be observed by others or reported by the individual.
B. Recurrent gaps in the recall of everyday events, important personal information, and/or traumatic events that are inconsistent with ordinary forgetting.
C. The symptoms cause clinically significant distress or impairment in social, occupational, or other important areas of functioning.
D. The disturbance is not a normal part of a broadly accepted cultural or religious practice. **Note:** In children the symptoms are not better explained by imaginary playmates or other fantasy play.
E. The symptoms are not attributable to the physiological effects of a substance (e.g., blackouts or chaotic behavior during alcohol intoxication) or another medical condition (e.g., complex partial seizures).

SOURCE: REPRINTED WITH PERMISSION FROM THE *DIAGNOSTIC AND STATISTICAL MANUAL OF MENTAL DISORDERS*, FIFTH EDITION, (COPYRIGHT ©2013). AMERICAN PSYCHIATRIC ASSOCIATION. ALL RIGHTS RESERVED.

Treatment of dissociative identity disorder

There is no specific treatment indicated for DID and practitioners rely on treating symptoms, comorbidities and impacts with a range of therapy-based and some pharmacological measures.

Non-pharmacological treatment

Talk-based therapies such as CBT, psychotherapy and therapies that involve creative avenues of expression (such as music or art therapy) are used in the treatment of DID. At times, family therapy may be useful; however, it is important to consider mandatory reporting laws in the event that the patient with DID is a victim of abuse, and that the choice to undergo family therapy may enable a perpetrator of abuse to remain in contact with the victim (see the 'Safety first' box). Hypnotherapy may also be used to treat DID.

Pharmacological treatment

Medications used to treat anxiety and depression, such as anxiolytics and selective serotonin reuptake inhibitors (SSRIs), may be used to manage the symptoms of DID. Pharmacological treatments such as antidepressants may also be used to manage comorbid depression or anxiety occurring in addition to DID.

GENDER DYSPHORIA

An ABS survey, *Same-sex Couples, Australian Social Trends,* showed in the previous five years a 32% increase in the number of Australians who identify as being in a same-sex relationship, perhaps indicating an increase in acceptance of sexuality differences in the community (ABS, 2013). Eleven per cent of Australians are of diverse sexual orientation (AHRC, 2014). **Gender dysphoria (GD)** is a condition experienced by individuals who feel their *natally* assigned gender differs from their gender identity. For example, a *natally* assigned male (an individual born as a male) feels that they are, in fact, a woman; that they identify as being female. **Dysphoria** is a feeling of unhappiness, anguish and distress. Gender dysphoria results in suffering and many individuals seek appropriate steps to change their gender, through surgery or hormonal treatment.

Terminology

It can be challenging to explore the different terminology used to define an individual's experience of their sexuality, or their desire to change it. **Table 19.5** explores the different terms used to define diversities of sexuality.

TABLE 19.5
Definition of terms related to sexuality

TERM	DEFINITION
Bisexual	A term used to describe someone who is sexually attracted to people, be that male or female.
Gay	A term used to describe a male or female (however, usually male) who identifies as homosexual.
Gender	Often considered socially constructed, gender is the cultural characteristic that constitutes a man or woman.
Gender assignment	The (natal) gender an individual is born with.
Gender-atypical or gender non-conformity	Behaviours or features that do not conform to the norm in society (e.g. a male dressing as a female).
Gender reassignment	Predominantly understood to be a legal term, which describes an individual who has changed their gender officially.
Gender identity	A personal feeling or understanding of one's own gender. This may include how a person may (or may) not align to traditional gender perceptions, e.g., masculine.
Gender dysphoria	Feelings of anguish or distress resulting from an individual's gender assignment (i.e., distress over the gender the individual has been born with).
LGBTQ(IA+)	An acronym used to indicate individulas who identify as lesbian, gay, bisexual, transgender, transsexual, queer, intersex, asexual and more.
Intersex	A term to describe individuals who are born with sexual anatomy that does not fit the norm or typical descriptions of male or female. Such individuals have been termed *ambiguous* by some within the medical profession.
Lesbian	A preferred term for a homosexual female.
Transgender	A general term used to describe individuals who transiently or frequently identify with a gender other than the one they were born with.
Transsexual	An antiquated term used to describe an individual who is attempting to undertake, or has undertaken, a social change from their birth (natal) gender, which often involves sex reassignment surgery and/or hormone therapy.
Queer or questioning	*Queer* is an umbrella term often used to describe all sexual identities and minorities mentioned in this table, such as those individuals who do not identify as heterosexual. *Questioning* is used to describe individuals who are yet to identify their sexual preference/identity/orientation, but who are exploring their feelings.

SOURCE: ADAPTED FROM THE UNIVERSITY OF WESTERN AUSTRALIA, 2015; REACHOUT AUSTRALIA, 2019

When engaging with any consumer, it is important to not make assumptions about their sexuality, assume they are in a heterosexual relationship or pass judgement. Consumers with GD may have a preferred name, and as such it is best to ask them what they would like to be known by.

Clinical presentation

Individuals will usually present with gender-preferred characteristics and patterns of speech, mannerisms and traits. When around people they are comfortable with, they may disclose experiencing distress at being 'trapped in the wrong body' and express feelings of being born with the wrong sexual organs. As an individual becomes more comfortable with expressing themselves as their preferred gender, they may change their name and live as someone of their preferred gender would.

CLINICAL **OBSERVATIONS**

Taking a sexual health history
Discussing a person's sexual preferences and behaviours can be difficult for any seasoned practitioner, but it is often noted as a particularly stressful experience for a student. It is, however, a very important part of the health history, and as such is something with which every nurse should be familiar. There are a number of links that can assist students on how to take a thorough sexual health history, including posing questions. The Australasian Sexual Health Alliance website provides some useful tips and assistance in taking a sexual health history: http://www.sti.guidelines.org.au/resources/how-to-take-a-sexual-history#how-to-take-a-sexual-history.

Prevalence

GD is a relatively rare condition and prevalence rates are somewhat difficult to obtain. Those who proceed with exploration of surgical and hormonal options are observed at rates of around 0.005–0.014% in males and 0.002–0.003% in females (APA, 2013). In Australia, it is estimated that about 1.7% of children born are **intersex** (AHRC, 2014). GD is understood to be higher in males; however, due to stigma it is likely to be underreported.

Aetiology and epidemiology

Understanding of GD continues to develop as more research is conducted in this area. This section explores the causes and prevalence of GD.

Individual and environmental factors

There appear to be some commonalities between parenting styles or issues in individuals who are later diagnosed with GD. In particular, parents who present as emotionally distant or unavailable and those who are overly controlling or excessively protective may be more likely to have children with GD (March & Schub, 2016). Children who have been rejected by their parents, and children who present with an 'atypical' temperament, may also be more inclined to GD (APA, 2013; March & Schub, 2016). Males who have GD are more likely to have older brothers, and older adolescents who develop GD also demonstrate higher rates of transvestism-fetish behaviours (e.g. requiring a thought of oneself as a woman in order to become sexually aroused) (APA, 2013).

Biological and genetic factors

It is believed that possible maternal imbalances in sex hormone levels may result in an increased chance of the resulting child developing GD (March & Schub, 2016). In addition, abnormalities in the size and shape of the hypothalamus may also be a contributing factor. Individuals with GD may have a family history of transsexualism in a relative (APA, 2013).

Comorbidity

Children with GD may demonstrate increased levels of behavioural and emotional problems, such as impulse-control issues, anxiety and depression (APA, 2013). In addition, autism spectrum disorders are more prevalent in individuals with GD (APA, 2013).

Clinical course

More often than not, individuals identify their sexuality as 'wrong' from a very early age and behaviours of cross-gender usually emerge in children around the ages of 2–4 years (APA, 2013). They may refuse gender-norm clothing or toys

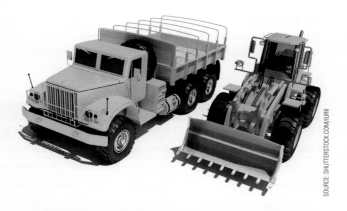

SOURCE: SHUTTERSTOCK.COM/IURII

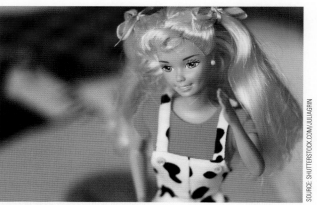

SOURCE: SHUTTERSTOCK.COM/JULIAGRIN

FIGURE 19.2
Toys are often marketed as toys for 'girls' or toys for 'boys'

(see **Figure 19.2**), instead opting to wear clothes in the gender they innately feel they are. **Natal-boys** may grow their hair long, shave their legs and prefer feminine games and toys. Natal-girls may cut their hair short, dress in boys' clothing and express a preference to grow up to be a man. Often, each will play with children of the desired gender. Boys with GD may refuse to stand to urinate, preferring to sit, and may express distress at having a penis and testes; in order to conceal erections, others will bind their genitals (APA, 2013). As the child ages and approaches puberty, they may become more distressed by the development of breast tissue, menstruation, hair and deepening of their voice. Adults with GD may hide their natal-gender from others, having chosen to dress and present as their preferred gender. Others may continue to struggle with society's perception of them.

Prognosis

In individuals who progress to gender-reassignment surgery (and where surgery is a success) prognosis is good. However, individuals with GD who are diagnosed later in life, are unemployed and have experienced loss of family demonstrate poorer outcomes (March & Schub, 2016). Individuals who have a poor surgical outcome and those who do not experience a positive engagement and attitude with health care providers also demonstrate poorer outcomes (March & Schub, 2016).

Gender dysphoria and suicide

Suicide rates in LGBTQ(IA+) individuals far exceed national averages for other Australians. Impacts of bullying, pressures to conform, stigma and intolerance of differences can add to the burden endured by many individuals who are exploring (or have confirmed) their sexuality. In addition to suicide, rates of self-harm are also high, and while highly distressing, self-penile castration has occurred in individuals with GD (March & Schub, 2016). For more information on suicide, and suicide among LGBTQ(IA+) individuals, see Chapter 20.

Diagnostic criteria

Because the characteristics and presentations of GD vary according to age, there are different classifications for different ages. This section lists the DSM-5 criteria for gender dysphoria in children (**Table 19.6**) and in adolescents and adults (**Table 19.7**).

DIAGNOSTIC CRITERIA

Gender dysphoria in children

TABLE 19.6
Diagnostic criteria gender dysphoria in children

A. A marked incongruence between one's experienced/expressed gender and assigned gender, of at least 6 months' duration, as manifested by at least six of the following (one of which must be Criterion A1):

1. A strong desire to be of the other gender or an insistence that one is the other gender (or some alternative gender different from one's assigned gender).
2. In boys (assigned gender), a strong preference for cross dressing or simulating female attire; or in girls (assigned gender), a strong preference for wearing only typical masculine clothing and a strong resistance to the wearing of typical feminine clothing.
3. A strong preference for cross-gender roles in make-believe play or fantasy play.
4. A strong preference for the toys, games, or activities stereotypically used or engaged in by the other gender.
5. In boys (assigned gender), a strong rejection of typically masculine toys, games and activities and a strong avoidance of rough-and-tumble play; or in girls (assigned gender), a strong rejection of typically feminine toys, games, and activities.
6. A strong dislike of one's sexual anatomy.
7. A strong desire for the primary and/or secondary sex characteristics that match one's experienced gender.

B. The condition is associated with clinically significant distress or impairment in social, school, or other important areas of functioning.

DIAGNOSTIC CRITERIA

Gender dysphoria in adolescents and adults

TABLE 19.7
Diagnostic criteria gender dysphoria in adolescents and adults

A. A marked incongruence between one's experienced/expressed gender and assigned gender, of at least 6 months' duration, as manifested by at least two of the following:

1. A marked incongruence between one's experienced/expressed gender and primary and/or secondary sex characteristics.
2. A strong desire to be rid of one's primary and/or secondary sex characteristics because of a marked incongruence with one's experienced/expressed gender (or in young adolescents, a desire to prevent the development of the anticipated secondary sex characteristics).
3. A strong desire for the primary and/or secondary sex characteristics of the other gender.
4. A strong desire to be of the other gender (or some alternative gender from one's assigned gender).
5. A strong desire to be treated as the other gender (or some alternative gender different from one's assigned gender).
6. A strong conviction that one has the typical feelings and reactions of the other gender (or some alternative gender different from one's assigned gender).

B. The condition is associated with clinically significant distress or impairment in social, occupational, or other important areas of functioning.

Specify if:
- **Posttransition:** The individual has transitioned to full-time living in the desired gender (with or without legalization of gender change) and has undergone (or is preparing to have) at least one cross-sex medical procedure or treatment regimen — namely, regular cross-sex hormone treatment or gender reassignment surgery confirming the desired gender (e.g., penectomy, vaginoplasty in a natal male; mastectomy or phalloplasty in a natal female).

Treatment

Prior to any surgical intervention, the consumer with GD will usually have to undergo rigorous psychological testing to ensure they are fully aware of the implications, longevity and risks associated with gender reassignment surgery. For many, surgery follows a period of hormonal treatment, psychotherapy and time (usually at least two years) living as one's preferred gender (Daly, 2016). Because of the high correlation between the experience of anxiety and depression in individuals with GD, anxiolytics and/or antidepressant medication may be indicated.

Hormonal

Hormonal treatment is often the first invasive step in gender reassignment and impacts the secondary sexual characteristics. Natal-males who are seeking feminine characteristics take oestrogen to:

- develop breast tissue
- develop feminine fat distribution (e.g. to hips)
- change hair patterns
- reduce muscle mass
- reduce penis, prostate, scrotum and testicle size
- reduce sex drive and spontaneous erections.

Natal-females who are seeking masculine characteristics take testosterone to:

- redistribute body fat
- cease menstruation
- increase muscle mass
- change sweat/odour (increases) and prominence of veins
- deepen the voice
- generate male growth of hair (on the face and body)
- shrink breasts.

It is important to consider that hormonal treatment comes with some potentially serious side effects (see **Table 19.8**).

TABLE 19.8
Risk factors for hormone treatment

TYPE OF TREATMENT	RISK FACTORS
Oestrogen treatment	Deep vein thrombosis (DVT) Embolism Stroke Changes in liver function
Testosterone treatment	Aggression Liver dysfunction Increases in red blood cells in blood (polycythaemia)

SOURCE: ADAPTED FROM MARCH & SCHUB, 2016

Surgical

Gender reassignment involves the removal of primary sexual characteristics and the surgical development of new sexual characteristics, such as the removal of the penis and testes, and the development of a vagina with muscle and tissue taken from the individual. Gender reassignment surgery usually involves multiple surgeries and involves:

- genital reconstruction surgery
- hysterectomy
- facial plastic surgery as necessary
- chest reconstruction or breast augmentation.

Satisfaction after gender reassignment surgery is high, with 97% of natal-female patients and 87% of natal-male patients happy with the results, although natal-females demonstrate higher levels of post-surgical functioning (March & Schub, 2016).

SAFETY FIRST

VIOLENCE AGAINST LGBTQ(IA+) INDIVIDUALS

While we are becoming more accepting and tolerant of diversity in Australia, there is still a way to go. The vast majority of individuals who identify as LGBTQ(IA+) report experiencing physical and/or verbal abuse because of their sexuality. Eighty per cent of this abuse occurs during school years, at imperative social times when many young people are exploring their sexuality and are greatly vulnerable to bullying. Experiences of abuse appear to increase significantly in male and female populations who identify as transsexual (AHRC, 2014).

According to the AHRC (2014), LGBTQ(IA+) individuals:

- are three times more likely to experience depression
- 26% of gay men and 23% of gay women have experienced verbal abuse because of their sexual orientation
- 47% of trans men and 37% of trans women have experienced verbal abuse because of their sexual orientation
- more than one-third of LGBTQ(IA+) individuals hide their sexual orientation or identify from others.

CONVERSION DISORDER

Conversion disorder is a condition classified as a somatic or symptom-related disorder and is sometimes also known as functional neurological symptom disorder. The individual with conversion disorder presents with various neurological symptoms suggestive of neurological impairment (e.g. Parkinson's disease), but upon further investigation, results are negative for such illnesses. Common presentations of conversion disorder include issues with speech, sudden paralysis or weakness to limbs, seizures or loss of sensory perceptions such as blindness (Yam et al., 2016). Diagnosis of conversion disorder can be exhaustive. Individuals usually present to their general practitioner or emergency department with symptoms that appear organic and may spend many months of invasive and costly testing in order to determine the causes of their condition. It is important to note that malingering or 'faking' their illness is not characteristic of conversion disorder, and in the event that this is suspected, a differential diagnosis of factitious disorder may be warranted (APA, 2013).

Prevalence

Conversion disorder is an uncommon condition affecting between 4–12 individuals in every 100 000 people (Merkler et al., 2016). Around 5% of individuals referred to neurology are understood to have conversion disorder (APA, 2013) and 1–3% of mental health outpatients have the condition (Erten, Yenilmez, Fistikci & Saatcioglu, 2013).

Aetiology and epidemiology

For most individuals, it would appear that conversion disorder is 'triggered' by a traumatic or stressful event, which may be a health condition, while for others it may stem from a psychological issue (APA, 2013); stress seems to play a role in up to 60% of diagnoses (Erten et al., 2013). While conversion disorder may affect an individual at any time of their life, it is most frequently seen in individuals between the ages of 15–35 years (Yayla et al., 2015). More commonly seen in females, conversion disorder appears to be more common in developing countries; in one study rates were more than three times greater than in developed regions of the world (Yayla et al., 2015).

Individual, genetic and environmental factors

Conversion disorder is more commonly seen in individuals who have a history of abuse and neglect stemming from childhood and temperamental traits which suggest poorly developed coping strategies (APA, 2013). More commonly seen in rural regions of developing nations with low SES, individuals with conversion disorder often present with low or poor health literacy (meaning they have poor knowledge of health conditions) and are often poorly educated (many not beyond primary school) (Erten et al., 2013; Yayla et al., 2015). The presence of a current neurological condition with a comparable symptom profile seems to result in a higher risk of conversion disorder (APA, 2013). For example, someone who already has epilepsy may present with psychogenic or non-epileptic seizures too.

Clinical course

Due to the varying nature and diversity of conditions present in conversion disorder, a clinical course is difficult to predict. Individuals who present with psychogenic seizures usually peak in their 30th year, while motor symptoms appear in the 40th year (APA, 2013). Symptoms, however, can be transient and recur. Erten and colleagues (2013) note that 48 months is the average period for which an individual has the condition.

Comorbidity

Comorbidity is commonly seen in those with conversion disorder and can further complicate treatment. Conditions seen more frequently in those with conversion disorder include anxiety disorders (namely, panic disorder), mood disorders, personality disorders, somatoform disorders and dissociative disorders (dissociation and derealisation are sometimes seen in conversion disorder) (APA, 2013; Yayla et al., 2015). One study indicated that the comorbidity of another mental health condition in

those with conversion disorder was over 83% (Yayla et al., 2015).

Diagnostic criteria

While the diagnostic criteria for conversion disorder are relatively simple and straightforward, there are a number of specifying types. **Table 19.9** explores the diagnostic criteria for conversion disorder.

DIAGNOSTIC CRITERIA

Conversion disorder (Functional neurological symptom disorder)

TABLE 19.9
Diagnostic criteria conversion disorder

A.	One or more symptoms of altered voluntary motor or sensory function.
B.	Clinical findings provide evidence of incompatibility between the symptom and recognized or medical conditions.
C.	The symptom or deficit is not better explained by another medical or mental disorder.
D.	The symptom causes clinically significant distress or impairment in social, occupational, or other important areas of functioning or warrants medical evaluation.

Specify symptom type:
- **With weakness or paralysis**
- **With abnormal movement** (e.g., tremor, dystonic movement, myoclonus, gait disorder)
- **With swallowing symptoms**
- **With speech symptoms** (e.g., dysphonia, slurred speech)
- **With attacks or seizures**
- **With anesthesia or sensory loss**
- **With special sensory symptom** (e.g., visual, olfactory, or hearing disturbance)
- **With mixed symptoms**

Specify if:
- **Acute episode:** Symptoms present for less than 6 months.
- **Persistent:** Symptoms present 6 months or more.

Specify if:
- **With psychological stressor** (*specify stressor*)
- **Without psychological stressor**

SOURCE: REPRINTED WITH PERMISSION FROM THE *DIAGNOSTIC AND STATISTICAL MANUAL OF MENTAL DISORDERS*, FIFTH EDITION, (COPYRIGHT ©2013). AMERICAN PSYCHIATRIC ASSOCIATION. ALL RIGHTS RESERVED.

Treatment

There is no specific treatment indicated for conversion disorder and much of the success of management of the condition lies in therapeutic treatment from a multidisciplinary perspective.

Pharmacological

There is no specific medication indicated for conversion disorder. It is important to ensure, however, that other comorbid mental health conditions are effectively treated and, as such, common medications include antidepressants and anxiolytics for symptoms of depression, anxiety and panic disorder.

Non-pharmacological

A number of talk therapies and interventions have been used successfully to treat conversion disorder. **Operant behavioural therapy** has been used successfully with an emphasis on the foundation that recovery will in fact occur (Yam et al., 2016). Operant behavioural therapy focuses on the premise that behaviours are learned responses and individuals can learn alternative behaviours that are more positive or productive than their present behaviours. Other treatments include hypnosis and CBT, and commonly the development of insight into the individual's condition, in addition to supportive rehabilitation as necessary, seems largely effective. Evidence suggests that rehabilitation that takes a multidisciplinary approach is most effective for conversion disorder, with the collaboration of psychiatry, psychology, physiotherapy, speech pathology, occupational therapy and other allied professionals within a recovery framework (Yam et al., 2016).

Conversion disorder and suicide

While there is little research into suicide in individuals with conversion disorder, the information that is available seems to suggest that rates are high. Suicide attempts in the order of 19–32% have been noted in individuals with conversion disorder (Güleç et al., 2014). It is believed that one of the contributing factors in suicide attempts and deaths from suicide is the period of lengthy diagnosis for conversion disorder, and the resulting distress that this causes. A presence of childhood adversity and trauma may also exacerbate suicidal tendencies (Güleç et al., 2014). Possible predictors of suicide in individuals with conversion disorder include:

- dissociative experiences
- alcohol abuse
- suicide attempts
- emotional neglect (Güleç et al., 2014).

Recovery

Individuals with conversion disorder may experience a rapid physical recovery from symptoms (Merkler et al., 2016). Results, however, vary widely. It is understood that at the first follow-up appointment, between 10–90% of individuals with motor symptoms are no longer experiencing such symptoms. Results for those with psychogenic (or non-epileptic) seizures are not as favourable, with response rates between 16–78% at follow-up (Merkler et al., 2016).

FACTITIOUS DISORDER

Factitious disorder is a somatic symptom condition perhaps best known for its notoriety in the media. You may have heard of the condition Munchausen by proxy (named after a fictitious character in a late-sixteenth-century book). This condition is now known as *factitious disorder imposed on another* and over the years has had a number of name changes. Individuals with factitious disorder imposed on another will purposefully hurt or make their victim ill (usually by poisoning them), seek frequent medical attention and often request a barrage of invasive, costly and painful tests. The perpetrator feels a sense of nurturing and enjoys the professional attention that medical staff provide. Some individuals have continued to poison their victim (who is often their child) while in hospital by putting toxic substances into food and even injecting faeces into intravenous lines to cause septicaemia. It is not uncommon for the victim to eventually die. This condition may also manifest in people where their pet (often a cat or dog) is the victim of their factitious disorder. When the condition is *imposed on self*, there have been two known reports of death from surgical complications (Baig et al., 2016).

Factitious disorder imposed on self results in feigning or falsification of symptoms, often in an attempt to receive sympathy, attention or nurturance from others. Individuals may interfere with medical testing, impersonate illness symptoms or self-injure (Yates & Feldman, 2016). Many individuals with this condition will have extensive medical histories, spanning large regions (including overseas), have an above-average understanding of medical processes and conditions, and demonstrate unreliable medical histories (Baig et al., 2016).

Generally, the symptoms individuals present with (be they *a proxy* or *imposed on self*) are:

- severe abdominal pain
- haemorrhage through self-venesection or misuse of anticoagulant medications
- impairment in neurological functioning
- major organ failure/damage
- self-ingestion of insulin
- self-venesection to demonstrate blood loss through anaemia
- cancer symptoms
- medical issues generated from misuse of anticoagulants and thyroid medications
- symptoms of AIDS (Baig et al., 2016).

It is thought that over the course of their medical career, doctors will encounter at least one individual with factitious disorder. Indeed, health practitioners working in emergency departments likely experience higher rates of interacting with someone with this condition. Yates and Feldman (2016) undertook an extensive literature review on factitious disorder and factitious disorder imposed on another and identified a number of key commonalities in case studies within the literature. These include similarities such as:

- Over 66% of individuals in their samples were female
- Average age mid-30s
- Presence of depression was common.

They also noted that for many individuals with either condition, illness was not so much *fabricated*, as it was *generated*. This includes injecting bacteria to create infection, and self-mutilating to induce dermatological conditions. Common medical specialities with high rates of the condition/s were noted in endocrinology, cardiology, dermatology, and neurology (Yates & Feldman, 2016).

Core features of factitious disorder and factitious disorder imposed by another, which support a diagnosis, include those listed in **Table 19.10**. These factors relate to both forms of the condition.

TABLE 19.10
Common behaviours seen in factitious disorder and factitious disorder imposed on another

ASPECTS OF CONDITION/S	COMMON FEATURES
Use of healthcare system	Extensive history of engagement in healthcare services
Patient provided information	Information may be difficult to corroborate; information is contrary, deceitful or deceptive presented in a dramatic manner
Presentation is atypical	Symptoms tend to be reported but not observed by medical staff (e.g., reports of seizures not witnessed); the condition does not follow a logical or expected sequence
Presentation is unable to be corroborated	Testing is unable to provide a definitive diagnosis, or is normal
There is evidence of deceit	Surveillance or observation of individual reveals tampering or fabrication of illness;
Behaviour of individual	Requesting invasive medical procedures; high knowledge of medical condition and/or terminology; argumentative with healthcare staff; non-adherence to treatment recommendations; refusal of psychiatry involvement
Further inspection suggests deceit	The individuals process of fabrication is revealed and etiology is able to be confirmed; this exploration reveals the individual's deceit conclusively
Treatment continues to fail	Origin of new symptoms or symptoms worsen despite treatment

SOURCE: ADAPTED FROM YATES & FELDMAN, 2016

It is important to note that individuals with factitious disorders are *not* motivated by monetary reward or benefits (such as compensatory claims for negligence or disability pensions); instead, their motivations are likely the care they receive when ill, feelings of control from deceiving medical personnel, euphoric feelings experienced after undergoing a procedure or often quite simply beyond the realm of our understanding (Yates & Feldman, 2016). One example of an individual with factitious disorder imposed on self underwent 42 surgical procedures, and was admitted to 650 hospitals on 850 occasions (Yates & Feldman, 2016). The cost to the health care system for unnecessary interventions for some individuals has exceeded millions of dollars.

Incidence and epidemiology

Because factitious disorders involve deception, they can be difficult to diagnose and so it is difficult to predict their occurrence. For the vast majority of medical practitioners, their patients are not attempting to deceive them, and as such they are usually not looking for symptoms to be fabricated. In hospital settings, it is believed that about 1% of individuals meet diagnostic criteria for factitious disorders (APA, 2013) and one study identified that 8% of individuals demonstrated behaviours consistent with illness deception (Bass & Halligan, 2014). Baig and colleagues (2016) note that diagnosis rates vary between 0.05–2.0%. The overwhelming majority of individuals with this condition are female and engage health care services as young adults (Yates & Feldman, 2016).

Aetiology

Individuals with factitious disorders often have a history of childhood abuse, neglect and separation from parents. Some may also have a past history of childhood medical conditions requiring hospital admissions, hypochondriasis, obsessions with their health and unstable interpersonal relationships (Baig et al., 2016). It is not uncommon for the adoption of the 'sick role' to be a past and present feature of the condition.

Individuals diagnosed with imposed on self factitious disorder are often themselves employed in the health care sector (Yates & Feldman, 2016). This may somewhat explain their desire for the 'adrenaline rush' of giving *or* receiving medical treatment. They may also be of higher intelligence.

Diagnostic criteria

Factitious disorders are conditions with brief diagnostic criteria that are easy to understand. The majority of individuals diagnosed with factitious disorders *induce* the illness or condition as opposed to *simulating* it or falsely reporting it. **Table 19.11** outlines the diagnostic criteria of these two conditions.

DIAGNOSTIC CRITERIA

Factitious disorder

TABLE 19.11
Diagnostic criteria factitious disorder

Factitious disorder imposed on self
A. Falsification of physical or psychological signs or symptoms, or induction of injury or disease, associated with identified deception.
B. The individual presents himself or herself to others as ill, impaired, or injured.
C. The deceptive behavior is evident even in the absence of obvious external rewards.
D. The behavior is not better explained by another mental disorder, such as delusional disorder or another psychotic disorder. **Note:** The perpetrator, not the victim, receives this diagnosis.

Factitious disorder imposed on another (previously factitious disorder by proxy)
A. Falsification of physical or psychological signs or symptoms, or induction of injury or disease, in another, associated with identified deception.
B. The individual presents another individual (victim) to others as ill, impaired or injured.
C. The deceptive behavior is evidence even in the absence of obvious external rewards.
D. The behavior is not better explained by another mental disorder, such as delusional disorder or another psychotic disorder. **Note:** The perpetrator, not the victim, receives this diagnosis. *Specify:* • **Single episode** • **Recurrent episode** (two or more events of falsification of illness and/or induction of injury).

SOURCE: REPRINTED WITH PERMISSION FROM THE *DIAGNOSTIC AND STATISTICAL MANUAL OF MENTAL DISORDERS*, FIFTH EDITION, (COPYRIGHT ©2013). AMERICAN PSYCHIATRIC ASSOCIATION. ALL RIGHTS RESERVED.

How are factitious disorders diagnosed?

Commonly factitious disorders are diagnosed upon presenting with unsubstantiated medical diagnosis (e.g. testing is contrary to reported symptoms) (Yates & Feldman, 2016). Other factors involved in diagnosis are information provided by other health care professionals that suggests fabrication, failure of treatment, behaviours evident, actual evidence of deception and, rarely, confession (Yates & Feldman, 2016). Some of the other potential warning signs of factitious disorders include:

- failure of illness symptoms to improve despite treatment
- severity or amount of symptoms surpass usual presentation for the same condition
- insisting to be admitted to hospital
- indication that some of the symptoms of the condition have been self-inflicted

- despite a barrage of tests and interventions, symptoms do not abate
- readiness to agree to interventions that may be high risk or painful
- disagreeing with results of tests that do not indicate illness
- prophesying further physical deterioration in condition
- multiple presentations to multiple different general practitioners, emergency departments and health clinics
- refusing to provide consent for medical practitioners to liaise with previous doctors (Feldman, 2013).

In cases of factitious disorder imposed by another, the perpetrator is often caught 'in the act' of poisoning or interfering with medical processes or equipment, sometimes on camera.

Comorbidity

Comorbid mental health conditions are commonly seen in factitious disorders; in particular, depression, personality disorders, substance misuse, anxiety disorders and eating disorders (Yates & Feldman, 2016).

Factitious disorders and self-harm/non-suicidal self-injury

The inclination to self-harm is high in individuals with this condition. For the majority, injury or illness is self-inflicted, and as such individuals with factitious disorders should be considered high risk of further self-harm. Close supervision is warranted around medical equipment and medications, and those with factitious disorder imposed on another are often found on camera in paediatric wards harming their child (Yates & Feldman, 2016). Over 10% of individuals with factitious disorder have attempted suicide.

Treatment

Harm reduction therapy is indicated in the treatment of factitious disorders; however, individuals with the condition are often very reluctant to seek treatment, and continue to perpetuate the belief that they are physically ill. Treatment of comorbid mental health conditions is important and may contribute to an improvement in functioning. Confrontation regarding the belief that the individual has a factitious disorder should be done in a calm and supportive manner because individuals with the condition respond better to, and are often looking for an empathic response. One study indicated that of the 75% of individuals confronted about their behaviours, only one in six admitted that they had deceived medical staff, and of them, only 12% consented to mental health treatment (Bass & Halligan, 2014). Where those identified with factitious disorder imposed on self eventually have children, there is increased risk of them imposing on their child.

Legal issues

Conservative estimates suggest that in the United States around 1200 cases of factitious disorder imposed on another occur annually (Feldman, 2013). When victims are removed from the presence of the perpetrator, symptoms abate and this is known as a *positive separation test*. The victim is usually an infant, unable to provide details of their suffering, and as such their carer does much of the 'talking' about the fabricated illness or condition for them (Feldman, 2013).

Presentation of perpetrators

As mentioned earlier, commonly the perpetrator of factitious disorder imposed on another is usually the child's mother. They tend not to stand out as different, and appear caring, concerned and upset by their child's condition. They may be assertive in their requests for invasive or painful tests and annoyed or angered when such tests return a negative result or are denied (Feldman, 2013). They will often insist on staying at the hospital with their ill child, only to return home fatigued, and often during this time the child improves suddenly and suspicion may be aroused in medical staff. The child may become ill again only upon the mother's return.

Recovery

There is a lack of research and evidence regarding the recovery potential and rates of those with factitious disorders; however, from the little that is available, recovery seems unlikely and rare. Individuals with factitious disorders are more likely to recover in environments where their need for nurturing is being addressed by compassionate people.

REFLECTION ON LEARNING FROM PRACTICE

Gender dysmorphia is a condition that can be difficult for people to understand due to the complexities involved in imagining that individuals could be born with a gender that does not reflect their sexual gender. GD is, however, increasingly becoming a topic of discussion in media and school alike, and requires a degree of sensitivity that comes with discussing such concepts. As demonstrated by the lived experience expert in this chapter, GD not only has implications for the individual who does not relate to their natal gender, but also for their parents, siblings and extended family.

Leigh's description of her experiences as a parent to a child with gender dysmorphia is powerful. As a health care clinician, what do you think you can do to ensure that you practise in a manner that does not contribute to the discrimination and judgement often experienced by Leigh, her son and their family?

CHAPTER RESOURCES

SUMMARY

- Conduct disorder is a serious condition affecting behaviour (e.g. school truancy, aggression, criminal activity, lack of remorse) that if left untreated may advance to antisocial personality disorder.
- Oppositional defiant disorder is a condition seen in childhood and can result in children who are resistive to direction from others.
- Dissociative identity disorder is a rare condition associated with the presentation of two or more distinct personality states, often in response to severe childhood sexual trauma.

- Gender dysphoria is a distressing condition resulting in a discord between one's natal gender and preferred gender.
- Conversion disorder is a somatic condition that mimics a range of neurological and sensory conditions often occurring in response to stress or trauma.
- Factitious disorders are conditions of illness fabrication where the individual either fabricates illness in themselves or in others.

REVIEW QUESTIONS

1 Conduct disorder may progress to antisocial personality disorder in individuals:
   a Over the age of 16
   b Who also present with callous unemotional traits
   c Over the age of 18
   d Who have been imprisoned
2 Conversion disorder is a somatic condition associated with the presentation of which type of symptoms?
   a Neurological
   b Cognitive
   c Pathological
   d Malingering
3 In dissociative identity disorder, reports of which of the following are higher?
   a Imprisonment
   b Trauma
   c Antisocial personality disorder
   d Delinquency
4 In gender dysphoria, what is the difference between natal-assigned gender and gender identity?
5 What are some of the fundamental differences between ODD and CD?

CRITICAL THINKING

1 What types of challenges may occur when engaging with a parent whose child has CD?
2 What possible consideration regarding your interviewing style may you need to make when interviewing a child with CD?
3 What feelings might be expressed by a consumer who believes they have multiple sclerosis but were instead diagnosed with conversion disorder?

USEFUL WEBSITES

- Child Mind Institute: https://childmind.org
- HEADSS – A Pyschosocial Interview for Adolescents: http://www.bcchildrens.ca/Youth-Health-Clinic-site/Documents/headss20assessment20guide1.pdf
- Safe Schools Coalition Australia: http://www.safeschoolscoalition.org.au
- Transcend: http://www.transcendsupport.com.au

REFLECT ON THIS

Interventions and resources

This chapter has covered a range of diverse and complex conditions that impact upon individuals, families and society as a collective. Conduct disorder and oppositional defiant disorder are good examples that present opportunities for early intervention to prevent future dysfunction and burden on the justice and healthcare systems, while dissociative identity disorder exemplifies the need for reporting and intervention for children who are in abusive situations. These conditions can all have long-lasting implications for mental health when intervention is not timely.

1 Choose one of the conditions in this chapter and consider how early intervention can prevent further harm to:
   • the individual
   • their family
   • society.
2 Now research what resources are available for early intervention in your area.

REFERENCES

American Psychiatric Association (APA). (2013). *Diagnostic and Statistical Manual of Mental Disorders (DSM-5)* (5th edn). Washington, DC: APA.

Andrews, G., Dean, K., Genderson, M., Hunt, C., Mitchell, P., Sachdev, P. & Trollor, J. (2013). *Management of Mental Disorders* (5th edn). Sydney: School of Psychiatry, University of NSW.

Australian Bureau of Statistics (ABS). (2013). *Same-sex Couples, Australian Social Trends, 4102.0*. Canberra: ABS. Retrieved from http://www.abs.gov.au/AUSSTATS/abs@.nsf/Lookup/4102.0Main+Features10July+2013.

Australian Human Rights Commission (AHRC). (2014). *Face the Facts: Lesbian, Gay, Bisexual, Trans and Intersex People 2014*. Canberra: AHRC. Retrieved from https://www.humanrights.gov.au/sites/default/files/FTFLGBTI.pdf.

Australian Institute of Criminology. (2011). Misconceptions about child sex offenders. *Trends & Issues in Crime & Criminal Justice*, 429. Canberra: Australian Government. Retrieved from http://aic.gov.au/media_library/publications/tandi_pdf/tandi429.pdf.

Australian Institute of Family Studies. (2016). *Mandatory Reporting of Child Abuse and Neglect*. Canberra: Australian Government. Retrieved from https://aifs.gov.au/cfca/publications/mandatory-reporting-child-abuse-and-neglect.

Baig, M.R., Levin, T.T., Lichtenthal, W.G., Boland, P.J. & Breitbart, W.S. (2016). Factitious disorder (Munchausen's syndrome) in oncology: Case report and literature review. *Psycho-Oncology*, 25, 707–11. doi:10.1002/pon.3906

Bass, C. & Halligan, P. (2014). Factitious disorders and malingering: Challenges for clinical assessment and management. *The Lancet*, 383, 1422–32.

Blair, J.R., Leibenluft, E. & Pine, D.S. (2014). Conduct disorder and callous-unemotional traits in youth. *New England Journal of Medicine*, 371(23), 2207–16. doi:10.1056/NEJMra1315612

Booker, J.A., Ollendick, T.H., Dunsmore, J.C. & Greene, R.W. (2016). Perceived parent–child relations, conduct problems, and clinical improvement following the treatment of oppositional defiant disorder. *Journal of Child & Family Studies*, 25, 1623–33. doi:10.1007/s10826-015-0323-3

Burke, J.D., Rowe, R. & Boylan, K. (2014). Functional outcomes of child and adolescent oppositional defiant disorder symptoms in young adult men. *Journal of Child Psychology and Psychiatry*, 55(3), 264–72. doi:10.1111/jcpp.12150

Daly, T.T.W. (2016). Gender dysphoria and the ethics of transsexual (i.e., gender reassignment) surgery. *Ethics & Medicine*, 31(1), 39–53.

Dickerson Mayes, S., Calhoun, S.L., Baweja, R., Feldman, L., Syed, E., Gorman, A.A., … Siddiqui, F. (2015). Suicide ideation and attempts are associated with co-occurring oppositional defiant disorder and sadness in children and adolescents with ADHD. *Journal of Psychopathological Behaviour and Assessment*, 37, 274–82. doi:10.1007/s10862-014-9451-0

Erford, B.T., Bardhoshi, G., Ross, M., Gunther, C. & Duncan, K. (2017). Meta-analysis of counseling outcomes for youth with conduct disorders. *Journal of Counseling & Development*, 95, 35–44.

Erten, E., Yenilmez, Y., Fistikci, N. & Saatcioglu, O. (2013). The relationship between temperament and character in conversion disorder and comorbid depression. *Comprehensive Psychiatry*, 54, 354–61.

Euler, F., Jenkel, N., Stadler, C., Schmeck, K., Fegert, J.M., Kölch, M. & Schmid, M. (2015). Variants of girls and boys with conduct disorder: Anxiety symptoms and callous-unemotional traits. *Journal of Abnormal Child Psychology*, 43, 773–85. doi:10.1007/s10802-014-9946-x

Feldman, M.D. (2013). *Playing Sick?.Untangling the Web of Munchausen Syndrome, Munchausen by Proxy, Malingering, and Factitious Disorder*. New York: Routledge.

Güleç, M.Y., Ýnanç, L., Yanartaþ, Ö., Üzer, A. & Güleç, H. (2014). Predictors of suicide in patients with conversion disorder. *Comprehensive Psychiatry*, 55, 457–62.

Harvey, E.A., Breaux, R.P. & Lugo-Candelas, C.I. (2016). Early development of comorbidity between symptoms of attention-deficit/hyperactivity disorder (ADHD) and oppositional defiant disorder (ODD). *Journal of Abnormal Psychology*, 125(2), 154–67. doi:org/10.1037/abn0000090

Hood, B.S., Elrod, M.G. & DeWine, D.B. (2015). Treatment of childhood oppositional defiant disorder. *Current Treatment Options for Paediatrics*, 1, 155–67. doi:10.1007/s40746-015-0015-7

Lewis, R.M., Petch, V., Wilson, N., Fox, S. & Craig, C.E. (2015). Understanding conduct disorder: The ways in which mothers attempt to make sense of their children's behaviour. *Clinical Child Psychology and Psychiatry*, 20(4), 570–84. doi:10.1177/1359104514538040.

Maniglio, R. (2014). Prevalence of sexual abuse among children with conduct disorder: A systematic review. *Clinical Childhood Family Psychological Review*, 17, 268–82. doi:10.1007/s10567-013-0161-z

March, P. & Schub, T. (2016). Gender dysphoria. *CINAHL Nursing Guide*. Ipswich, MA: EBSCO Publishing.

Merkler, A.E., Parikh, N.S., Chaundhry, S., Chait, A., Allen, N.C., Navi, B.B. & Kamel, H. (2016). Hospital revisit rate after diagnosis of conversion disorder. *Journal of Neurology, Neurosurgery and Neuropsychiatry*, 87, 363–6. doi:10.1136/jnnp-2014-310181

Middleton, W. (2013). Ongoing incestuous abuse during adulthood. *Journal of Trauma & Dissociation*, 14, 251–72. doi:10.1080/15299732.2012.736932

Pederson, C.A. & Fite, P.J. (2014). The impact of parenting on the associations between child aggression subtypes and oppositional defiant disorder symptoms. *Child Psychiatry & Human Development*, 45, 728–35. doi:10.1007/s10578-014-0441-y

ReachOut Australia (2019). *Gender and sexuality*, retrieved from https://schools.au.reachout.com/articles/gender-and-sexuality.

Reed-Gavish, M. (2013). Dissociation in abuse victims: Cognitive abuse within the incestuous family as a factor in the development of dissociative identity disorder. *Journal of Child Sexual Abuse*, 22, 444–61. doi:10.1080/10538712.2013.781093

Riley, M., Ahmed, S. & Locke, A. (2016). Common questions about oppositional defiant disorder. *American Family Physician*, 93(7), 586–91.

Ronan, K.R., Davies, G., Wikman, R., Canoy, D., Jarrett, M. & Evans, C. (2016). Family-centered, feedback-informed therapy for conduct disorder: Findings from an empirical case study. *Couple and Family Psychology: Research and Practice*, 5(3), 137–56.

Russell, A.A., Johnson, C.L., Hammad, A., Ristau, K.I., Zawadzki, S., Villar, L.D.A. & Coker, K.L. (2015). Prenatal and neighborhood correlates of oppositional defiant disorder (ODD). *Child Adolescent Social Work Journal*, 32, 375–81. doi:10.1007/s10560-015-0379-3

Salvatore, J.E. & Dick, D.M. (2016). Genetic influences on conduct disorder. *Neuroscience and Biobehavioral Reviews*, 91, 91–101. doi:org/10.1016/j.neubiorev.2016.06.034

Schoorl, J., van Rijn, S., de Wied, M., van Goozen, S. & Swaab, H. (2016). The role of anxiety in cortisol stress response and cortisol recovery in boys with oppositional defiant disorder/conduct disorder. *Psychoneuroendocrinology*, 73, 217–23. doi:org/10.1016/j.psyneuen.2016.08.0070

Tung, I. & Lee, S.S. (2014). Negative parenting behaviour and childhood oppositional defiant disorder: Differential moderation by positive and negative peer regard. *Aggressive Behaviour*, 40, 79–90.

University of Western Australia. (2015). *Sexuality and gender terms*, retrieved from http://www.student.uwa.edu.au/experience/health/fit/share/sexuality/definitions.

Wei, H.T., Lan, W.H., Hsu, J.W., Bai, Y.M., Huang, K.L., Su, T.P., Li, C.T., … Chen, M.H. (2016). Risk of suicide attempt among adolescents with conduct disorder: A longitudinal follow-up study. *Journal of Pediatrics*, 177, 292–6.

Yam, A., Rikards, T., Pawlowski, C.A., Harris, O., Karandikar, N. & Yutsis, M.V. (2016). Interdisciplinary rehabilitation approach for functional neurological symptom (conversion) disorder: A case study. *Rehabilitation Psychology*, 61(1), 102–11.

Yanartas, O., Ozmen, H.A., Citak, S., Zincir, S.B., Sunbul, E.A. & Kara, H. (2015). Childhood traumatic experiences and trauma related psychiatric comorbidities in dissociative disorders. *Bulletin of Clinical Psychopharmacology*, 25(4), 381–9. doi:10.5455/bcp.20140123030857

Yates, G.P. & Feldman, M.D. (2016). Factitious disorder: A systematic review of 455 cases in the professional literature. *General Hospital Psychiatry*, 41, 20–8. https://www.sciencedirect.com/science/article/pii/S016383431630072X

Yayla, S., Bakim, B., Tankaya, O., Ozer, O.A., Karamustafalioglu, O., Ertekin, H. & Tekin, A. (2015). Psychiatric comorbidity in patients with conversion disorder and prevalence of dissociative symptoms. *Journal of Trauma & Dissociation*, 16, 29–38. doi:10.1080/15299732.2014.938214

CONTEMPORARY ISSUES IN MENTAL HEALTH NURSING

Now that you have developed an understanding of the different mental health conditions, their treatments and their impacts on consumers, we will look at contemporary issues in mental health. While many of the concepts in this section have been discussed elsewhere in the book, they will be further expanded upon here; for example, suicide and non-suicidal self-injury are serious issues in mental health, and they will be explored in more detail in this section. With the importance of least-restricted environments, community mental health nursing is a pivotal part of the mental health care for many consumers and their families. This section also explores community mental health nursing, principles of recovery and carer and family involvement as well as issues of resilience, diversity and culture, and the role of the multidisciplinary team. Finally, mental health first aid is explored, to conclude this section.

CHAPTER 20

SUICIDE AND NON-SUICIDAL SELF-INJURY

Louise Alexander and Gylo (Julie) Hercelinskyj

LEARNING OUTCOMES

Upon completion of this chapter, you should be able to:

20.1 Explore the aetiology and epidemiology of suicide and explore suicide predictors in at-risk individuals as well as understanding protective factors

20.2 Develop an understanding of the theories of suicide

20.3 Understand cultural considerations and groups vulnerable to suicide

20.4 Understand the roles and responsibilities of the media in suicide

20.5 Understand how to assess the risk of suicide, including exploring strategies to initiate conversations with consumers about suicide

20.6 Understand non-suicidal self-injury and its aetiology and epidemiology

20.7 Explore assessment and collaborative care of consumers with non-suicidal self-injury behaviours

LEARNING FROM PRACTICE

The darkness was enveloping… there was no way I was going to make it out the other side. I couldn't bear to imagine that this life I was *enduring*, because that's essentially what it was… an endurance, a marathon of exhaustive proportions… was going to continue. I needed a way out. In the early days of this darkness, knowing that I had 'an out' was the only thing that actually kept me from ending it all then – the thought that I was in control of my destiny, that I *chose* to stay alive to fight another miserable day. But as my depression got worse (and it was unimaginable to me that it *could* get worse, but it did), this feeling of being in control wasn't enough. Nothing was enough. Everything was just too much. Intellectually, I knew I was depressed… intellectually, I knew there was probably some treatment out there, some magic pill, that could probably make me better, but I didn't feel worthy of it. These immense feelings of guilt were like a shroud over my very soul. I felt guilty for planning my death. What would become of my family?! How could I do this to them? But then I felt enormous guilt about being alive too…I was *such* a burden. Ending my life was the best thing that I could do for them. They would get over it eventually. Ah, the deals I made with my conscience. It was the ultimate no-win situation. There would be no winners in this

war. The breaking point, if you could call it that, came when I finally realised I had the courage to actually take the pills. I wasn't afraid of death…I was afraid of *living*. My sister found me, unconscious, and called an ambulance. It didn't work. I was so angry when I woke up and realised I wasn't dead… I couldn't even get that right! Two years, and two more serious suicide attempts later, I am still here. I am alive and I can honestly say it doesn't hurt any more. I see a psychologist regularly, and the medications I take for depression actually help. I have a purpose in life again and that purpose isn't to die any more. I've walked through the darkness and come out the other side. There is hope.

Cynthia, 59, suicide survivor

Cynthia has described her journey with depression and the feelings associated with her desire to die by suicide. Her narrative is strong and emotive, but a similar resonance is often shared by many people with a lived experience of suicidal ideation. How do you feel about working with consumers with suicidal ideation? How might these feelings influence your practice, both positively and negatively?

INTRODUCTION

The term 'suicide' originated from its parent term 'self-murder', probably in the mid-1500s, and through the ages there have been varied responses to suicide; some indifferent, some deeming it unlawful. Suicide is the deliberate act of ending one's life and is considered an intentional act. Suicide for many people is a means to an end. It is often not something they *want*, but they can see no other way out of their situation or their distress. For others, suicide is an impulsive, spontaneous reaction to a situation or stress and has perhaps not been 'thought out' or planned.

Almost one million people die from suicide worldwide every year, accounting for 1.4% of all deaths, and the majority of these individuals are from low- and middle-income countries (WHO, 2014). Suicide is the leading cause of death in Australians between the ages of 15–44 and comprises about 2.8% of all male and 0.9% of all female deaths (ABS, 2016a). While suicide rates in Australia have decreased over the past 10 years, deaths by suicide remain an important social consideration. Suicide is a preventable social health issue, and mental health nurses are in a prime position to help people at this most vulnerable time.

SAFETY FIRST ⚠

CONTENT WARNING – SUICIDE AND SELF-INJURY
This chapter explores both suicide and non-suicidal self-injury in detail. While these are both important concepts, and indeed social issues, for students to consider in their nursing practice, the authors acknowledge that this may be confronting for some readers. Lifeline is an Australian service that operates 24 hours a day, seven days per week and provides a free telephone service for people in crisis. The Australian Lifeline phone number is 13 11 14. In New Zealand, the phone number is 0800 543 354.

SUICIDE

While it may be tempting to assume that *all* suicide deaths are related to a mental health condition, this is not entirely the case. Overwhelmingly, the majority of people who take their own life *are* experiencing a mental health condition, in about 90% of cases (WHO, 2014). However, one cannot discount the role impulsivity to stressful situations plays in suicide. In addition, in low- and middle-income countries, where more impulsive methods of suicide are adopted (because they are available), this rate changes drastically to around 60% (in some studies from Asia, China and India). Later in the chapter, we look

at reducing access to means of suicide, resulting in reducing risk of death from suicide.

Terminology

You may wonder why we need to dedicate a section of this chapter to the way we phrase terminology when discussing terms such as suicide. However, when discussing suicide it is important to consider the language we use. It is no longer considered appropriate to use terms such as 'committed suicide', as this implies there is a criminal association, much the same as 'committing a murder' does. Some may argue that suicide is in fact illegal (and in some countries it *is* an offence); however, in Australia suicide is not an illegal act and therefore the language we use needs to reflect this. Other terms to be avoided include 'failed suicide attempt', as this implies the individual failed to achieve something that otherwise would have a desirable outcome such as 'failing an exam' or 'failing a driving test'. In addition, 'successful suicide' should be avoided as this suggests suicide is a favourable solution to a problem.

Appropriate terms and phrases to use when discussing suicide include the person:

- 'took their own life'
- 'died by suicide'
- was injured by a 'non-fatal suicide attempt'
- suicided (an acceptable term as the word is both a noun and verb).

Some other terms or terminology to consider when exploring suicide are:

- 'Suicide survivor' is a term used to describe the family and friends who have lost a loved one to suicide.
- **Suicidal ideation** refers to the thoughts associated with how to end one's life. This can vary from fleeting thoughts *to a detailed plan of suicide*.

Now that we understand the appropriate language to use when discussing suicide, we look at the *epidemiology of suicide*.

Incidence and epidemiology

Between 2010 and 2014, on average more than 2500 Australians took their lives annually and over 75% of those who died by suicide were males. The average age for someone to die by suicide is around 44 years for men and 42 years for women (Healey, 2014), and people in very remote locations rather than major cities are more likely to die (Parliament of Australia, 2011).

Aetiology

When looking at suicide, it is important to consider the areas of risk or those traits that are more commonly seen in people who die by suicide. **Table 20.1** explores some of the more common factors associated with increased risk of suicide.

TABLE 20.1

Risk factors – fatal-suicide attempt

Being of Aboriginal and/or Torres Strait Islander heritage
Experiencing a mental health condition such as psychosis, depression or an eating disorder
Alcohol or drug use (including those diagnosed with substance use disorder)
Being male
Being socially isolated
Social and/or geographical isolation
Bereaved by suicide (particularly if there is a recent family or friend loss)
Lesbian, gay, bisexual, transgender and intersex (LGBTQ(IA+)). This risk is even higher for LGBTQ(IA+) individuals who are also a: • migrant • refugee • Aboriginal or Torres Strait Islander
Voicing hopelessness about the future
Having a past non-fatal suicide attempt
Family violence or problems
Being recently discharged from a mental health hospital or receiving a reduction in treatment

While this list is not exhaustive, it does provide a unique picture of where the relative risks lie. When an individual presents with more than one of these risk factors, their individual risk may be much higher. For example, a young Aboriginal and Torres Strait Islander male living in remote rural Australia, who identifies as LGBTQ(IA+) and who has recently lost a friend to suicide, would present as a *significant* risk of death by suicide.

Socioeconomic status (SES) and suicide

Page et al. (2014) found in their study exploring links between suicide and socioeconomic status in Australians (18–34 years) that males in low SES were identified as a high risk of a fatal-suicide attempt, and that as SES increased, suicide risk decreased. The authors also suggest that SES plays a significant role in suicide, as does the presence of a mental health condition, and that there are benefits in targeting social deprivation as a means of promoting mental health *and* reducing suicide risk generally (Page et al., 2014).

Gender

Globally in high-income countries (such as Australia), men represent a significant proportion of the deaths resulting from suicide. However, in low- and middle-income countries, there is more parity between male and female deaths from suicide (WHO, 2014). In Australia, men die from suicide at a ratio of 4:1 compared with women and there are a number of possible reasons behind this. These include their chosen methods of taking their life (more lethal and more difficult to intervene or reverse), reduced ability to engage in help-seeking behaviours, and unwillingness to talk with others about their problems (AIHW, 2016).

In 2011–13, suicide was the leading cause of death in individuals aged 15–44 years and the fifth leading cause of death in those aged 45–64 years (AIHW, 2016). Men led death by suicide rates for all age levels in Australia, with particularly concerning high rates in the 85-plus age group (ABS, 2013). Hanging constitutes the most common method of suicide, followed by drug poisoning, use of firearms and other methods of poisoning such as carbon monoxide.

Suicide signs: predicting suicide

For the families left behind after a death by suicide, a myriad of questions are also likely left in their wake. Families and friends will ask: 'Why didn't they say something? How could I miss this? Why couldn't they ask for help?' Many people who make a non-fatal suicide attempt later describe feelings such as those mentioned by Cynthia in the opening vignette; overwhelming guilt about the burden their ongoing life places on others, and unworthiness of treatment. While it cannot be assumed that every person who dies by suicide had made their intentions evident to those around them, there are a number of factors or signs which *may* indicate a person is planning their own death. This leaves a potential opening for that individual to receive help. The act of choosing to die from suicide for many individuals is the culmination of a number of factors, and as such may be considered multifactorial. **Figure 20.1** indicates the various factors that may result in an increased chance of an individual dying by suicide, in addition to identifying those factors that may prevent this from occurring. As shown in the figure, it is a combination of these factors that changes an individual's 'risk profile' in relation to suicide; the more risks identified, the more significant the suicide risk. To counteract this, protective factors *significantly* aid in preventing death from suicide in much the same way that risk factors can cause suicide death. This means there is a checklist of possible indicators of suicide. This section explores the *possible* signs of impending suicide.

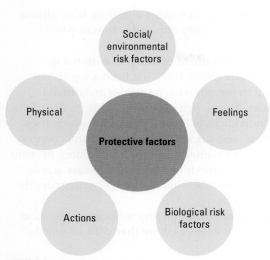

FIGURE 20.1
Suicide: risk and protective factors

Social/environmental risk factors

Living in a community where there has been an increase or spate of deaths by suicide poses a significant risk of others choosing to also engage in suicide behaviour. This is known as a *suicide cluster*. Individuals who are bereaved by suicide are more likely to engage in suicide behaviour themselves. Sometimes this occurs in schools and it has occurred in a number of Aboriginal communities. In Australia, the media has to be mindful of how it reports suicide and non-fatal suicide attempts due to this very reason; however, in countries where care in suicide reporting is not common practice, news-reported suicide methods have been 'copied', resulting in that particular method (no matter how bizarre) quickly becoming a top cause of suicide death (Chen et al., 2012). This same care must also be exercised when reporting celebrity deaths by suicide. In addition to suicide imitation, living in an environment where a person has access to the method of choice is an important consideration. In societies or communities where there is stigma regarding help-seeking behaviours, where there is poor mental health literacy and poor understanding of mental illness, the risk of suicide is higher (WHO, 2014).

Actions

An *invitation* in the context of suicide is a sign or possible suggestion made by a person who is considering their death by suicide. This includes things such as:

- giving away prized possessions
- finalising their will or final testimony or nominating a power of attorney
- uncharacteristic, or increases in, impulsive or reckless behaviour (such as drinking excessively, speeding)

- making broad emphatic statements such as, 'I won't be needing this any more'
- preoccupation with death (such as talking about death or researching it).

These factors may be worthy of further exploration, particularly in an individual with a history of a mental health condition and few protective factors.

Physical

It is quite common for people to experience physiological signs when distressed and the following signs *may* be evident in someone who is so distressed they no longer want to live:

- withdrawal
- difficulty sleeping
- reduced interest in personal appearance or grooming
- changes in appetite
- loss of libido
- self-injurious behaviours such as cutting or burning.

These physical signs make up a number of factors that may show an increased likelihood that an individual is contemplating ending their life.

Feelings

When talking with someone who is distressed or contemplating suicide, you may note a number of common themes. These common themes are often expressed by people who are planning suicide. Much like the physical manifestations of a possible suicide attempt, individuals who are contemplating their own death may experience or describe some of the following emotions:

- hopelessness
- helplessness
- guilt
- anger
- sadness
- worthlessness.

In addition to the individual overtly expressing these themes, you may also detect these elements within your conversation with them. For example, they may not openly say they feel guilty about something; rather they may appear to accept blame for things that are happening around them.

Risk factors

Along with social or environmental factors, there are a number of potential risk factors that are specific to the individual. These include their own personal risk factors, which may be influenced by things such as their mental health. The common individual risk factors are:

- experiencing a mental health condition
- a previous non-fatal suicide attempt or engaging in deliberate self-harm (DSH) (self-injuring) behaviours

- having experienced trauma, neglect or abuse
- having a chronic physical illness or experiencing chronic pain
- experiencing a triggering event such as a job loss, relationship breakdown or recent financial hardship.

Protective factors

As well as the many different risk factors associated with increased risk of death from suicide, there are **protective factors**. Protective factors are those that are seen to safeguard an individual from a mental health condition and/or suicide risk, and include the following:

- connection to family or friends with a stable and healthy relationship
- religion
- social support or engagement
- resilience (an individual's ability to manage and cope with stress and difficult circumstances)
- mental health literacy
- self-esteem.

Lethality and methods

The majority of people who take their own life are influenced by what is readily available in their immediate environment. This may be tall buildings (more common in countries such as Hong Kong and Singapore where falls/jumping account for large proportions of death from suicide), access to firearms (prevalent in the United States), proximity to train lines, in addition to 'iconic' suicide locations such as the Gap in Sydney, the Golden Gate Bridge in San Francisco or Aokigahara forest in Japan. Having access to the *means* of suicide increases the *risk* of suicide, particularly in individuals who are considering a poorly planned, impulsive suicide act (WHO, 2014).

While it may seem too simplistic that restricting access to an individual's desired method of completing suicide may prevent them from taking their own life, this is a relatively sound theory. The WHO (2014) notes that suicide bridge barriers, institution of firearm laws, restrictions in obtaining pesticides and modifying packaging guidelines on medicines have all had impacts on deaths from suicide globally. In particular, the ingestion of pesticides, which is attributed to around 30% of suicide deaths globally (mostly in Asian agricultural areas), is a method that can be potentially intercepted through access and packaging restrictions, as opposed to hanging, which

because of the ease of making a ligature from almost anything, is practically impossible to stall (WHO, 2014).

Since the enactment of uniform national gun laws in the late 1990s, there has been a significant reduction in firearm-related suicides in Australia (Chapman, Alpers, Agho & Jones, 2015). As mentioned earlier, individuals will use methods for which they have access, and suicide practices vary from country to country. For example, in the United States, firearms are common methods of suicide due to easy access. In Australia, the following methods of suicide are the most common:

- hanging, strangulation and suffocation, noted as the cause of death in more than 50% of suicide deaths
- drug poisoning (such as overdose) in around 14% of deaths
- other types of poisoning such as carbon monoxide poisoning (from car exhaust fumes) and alcohol in just under 7% of deaths
- drowning and jumping (among other means) account for the remaining methods (Healey, 2014).

REFLECT ON THIS

Suicide and the global pandemic

Suicide prevention is a priority area of health care for the Australian Government. Undoubtedly, people with mental health issues have experienced the effects of isolation and disruption during the COVID-19 pandemic. But how has the pandemic affected suicide rates in Australia? To date, the suicide rate does not appear to have increased due to COVID-19. Usually suicide rates tend to increase in times such as this because of unemployment. Moving forward, we might start to see suicide rates increase in countries where unemployment is high because of the pandemic and government support is low. Australians tend to unite in times of need, and the COVID-19 pandemic is a good example of this. Combined with general trust in government, this may have prevented an increase in suicide rates.

Question

Reflect upon the different social structures and financial interventions in Australia that may have had a positive impact on suicide rates during the pandemic. In particular, what role might government interventions such as JobKeeper and JobSeeker have played in preventing suicide among vulnerable people?

THEORIES OF SUICIDE

Given the heavy toll suicide has on communities, society and individuals alike, it is perhaps unsurprising that there are a number of theories regarding suicide, some of which are outlined in **Table 20.2**.

TABLE 20.2
Theories of suicide

THEORY OF SUICIDE	PRINCIPLES
Sociological theory (Durkheim, 1897)	Rationales for suicide in the sociological theory suggest four diverse motivators for suicide. 1 egoistic (based on loneliness) 2 altruistic (their death will benefit society; everyone is better off if they are dead) 3 anomic (socially detached) 4 fatalistic (socially burdened).
Hopelessness theory (Abramson, Metalsky & Alloy, 1989)	Overwhelming feelings of hopelessness are the driver for this theory of suicide. The individual does not feel there will be an end to their suffering and they feel that their life has no hope of improving.
Psychache theory (Shneidman, 1996)	Because of a failure to meet basic necessities of life, the individual experiences what is known as 'psychache' or severe psychological pain. The fewer healthy and positive options an individual has to alleviate their pain and suffering (if only for a short period), the more likely this will result in a lethal suicide attempt. The only way the individual can alleviate their suffering is to die.
Escape theory (Baumeister, 1990)	In escape theory the individual progresses through six stages resulting in eventual suicide: 1 Falling short of standards 2 Attributions to the self 3 High self-awareness 4 Negative affect 5 Cognitive deconstruction 6 Consequences of deconstruction (suicide).
Emotional dysregulation theory (Linehan, 1993)	This theory involves exposure to critical environments where emotional experiences are negative, ongoing and extreme in nature. Individuals experiencing dysregulation see suicide as a way of alleviating this distress.
Interpersonal-psychological theory (Joiner, 2005)	Three concepts are involved: 1 Feeling of disconnection with others (thwarted belongingness) 2 Feeling their ongoing existence is a burden to others (perceived burdensomeness) 3 Requires fearlessness regarding pain and thus death (acquired capacity). It is believed that once the individual has been through these three stages, their suicide is able to occur.

SOURCE: ADAPTED FROM NOCK, 2014

While this list is not exhaustive – for example, it fails to explore biological theories of suicide – it does give rise to the consideration of theoretical underpinnings and the role they may play in an individual's decision to end their life.

CULTURAL CONSIDERATIONS AND VULNERABLE GROUPS

While suicide is a global, social issue, there are a number of more vulnerable groups within Australian culture and society that are at greater risk of death from suicide. Factors in these groups include individual aspects such as culture or ethnicity, sexuality, age or occupation. This section explores these vulnerable and often minority groups in greater detail.

CULTURAL CONSIDERATIONS

Suicide and cultural factors
Within Australia, there are variations in the methods individuals use to die by suicide. While poisoning, carbon monoxide and hanging are the most frequent methods, there are variations between each state and territory (Too et al., 2017). In the Northern Territory, for example, hanging is most common, in Western Australia it is carbon monoxide, while Victoria has the highest proportion of suicide deaths by train. When researchers have investigated the reasons for this, many individuals who have had a non-fatal suicide attempt indicate that they knew of someone else who had used the method before (Too et al., 2017).

Other reasons for choosing a particular method include the ease of access, and how lethal, accessible and 'quick' the method is. For example, suicide death by jumping in front of a train is considered a widely accessible method that is perceived to be highly lethal, with minimal 'suffering'. In Victoria, survivors of suicide have indicated that these reasons were pivotal in their choice, but also more than half indicated they knew of someone who had died that way (Too et al., 2017).

It is important that clinicians acknowledge that particular locations, areas or means may be more romanticised in terms of suicide, and that this can increase the potential for continuing higher rates of a particular method and/or location. The research by Too and colleagues (2017) may suggest that this notion is widely distributed, even among cities.

Aboriginal and Torres Strait Islander peoples
Australian Aboriginal and Torres Strait Islanders have experienced notoriously poor health since British

settlement over 200 years ago. Prior to settlement, suicide was an unusual occurrence (Australian Government Department of Health and Ageing, 2013). While there have been movements to address the physical health issues of Aboriginal and Torres Strait Islander peoples, more recently there has been an urgent need to address their psychological needs. In Queensland, South Australia, Western Australia and the Northern Territory, Aboriginal and Torres Strait Islander people have suicide rates twice those of non-Indigenous Australians, and some extreme, remote regions have experienced substantial suicide clusters, including deaths of very young children (Australian Government Department of Health, 2013). It is believed that 95% of Aboriginal and Torres Strait Islander peoples have had a personal experience with suicide (Creative Spirits, 2013).

There are some specific risks or contributing factors to these high rates of deaths by suicide in the Aboriginal and Torres Strait Islander community, and **Table 20.3** explores these in more detail.

TABLE 20.3
Individual and community factors related to Aboriginal & Torres Strait Islander suicide rates

INDIVIDUAL FACTORS	Disadvantage and poverty Homelessness and/or dwelling overcrowding High unemployment Presence of both community and family suicide Alcohol and other drug use Lower levels of education (e.g. high school discontinuation rates) Neglect and family violence Incarceration
COMMUNITY FACTORS	Low social capital Low cultural capital High levels of community violence Low levels of youth engagement in community

SOURCE: ADAPTED FROM AUSTRALIAN GOVERNMENT DEPARTMENT OF HEALTH & AGEING, 2013

A number of measures are being taken to address the rates of suicide among Aboriginal and Torres Strait Islander peoples. Intervening and taking action in situations of children's exposure to domestic violence, neglect and substance misuse, while promoting positive social interactions and problem solving, are all strategies linked to reducing suicide within this population (Australian Government Department of Health & Ageing, 2013).

Other areas that may be addressed to reduce suicide include:

■ preventing access to alcohol (thus reducing alcohol-related violence and crime and psychosocial issues)

■ promoting schooling (thus improving self-esteem and problem-solving capabilities)

■ fostering healthy pregnancy (and thus foetal development and early life) through pregnancy and family violence education.

These are examples of long-term plans to address the growing problem of suicide among Aboriginal and Torres Strait Islander peoples through health promotion and illness prevention strategies. Other government strategies, which may be easier to implement, address issues such as access to after-hours mental health crisis services and counselling facilities.

Migrants

There are many challenges and benefits associated with migrating to a new country. In Australia, 28.2% of residents by mid-2015 were born overseas, the majority arriving from the United Kingdom, New Zealand, China and India (ABS, 2016b). Historically, suicide rates of individuals generally tend to correlate with those of the country from which they originated; for example, migrants from a country with a high suicide rate may have a higher rate of death from suicide in the country where they relocate. Similarly, it is important to explore the reasons why people choose to migrate. Recently, there have been increases in humanitarian reasons for people needing to leave their country of birth, including war, persecution and civil unrest. Chapter 18 explores trauma-related conditions such as post-traumatic stress disorder (a condition not uncommon in refugees) in greater depth. Some research has indicated that death from suicide in second-generation migrants is no greater than rates demonstrated in both local Australians and first-generation migrants (Law, Kõlves & De Leo, 2014). Others have suggested, however, that mortality rates with suicide as the cause of death have decreased among migrants from Western and Southern Europe and some parts of Asia, but there have been notable increases in suicide deaths from descendants of New Zealanders (Anikeeva et al., 2015). Despite reductions in suicide in most migrant populations, there is evidence of an *increase* in non-suicidal self-injury among this cohort. Improvements to migrant-specific community mental health services in regions with known elevated migrant populations and generalised acceptability of mental health diversity within communities, in addition to improved mental health literacy, are all factors expected to improve the rates of mental health, and by extension death from suicide, for Australian migrants.

Lesbian, gay, bisexual, transgender, queer, intersex, asexual or other (LGBTQ(IA+))

About 3.2% of Australians identify as lesbian, gay, bisexual, transgender, transexual, queer, intersex, asexual or other (LGBTQ(IA+)) (Wilson & Shalley, 2018). People who identify as LGBTQ(IA+) demonstrate rates of mental health conditions that are significantly higher than heterosexual individuals, and they are more likely to experience high or very high rates of psychological distress. Individuals who identify as LGBTQ(IA+) have non-fatal suicide attempts at rates that are 2–7 times higher than their heterosexual counterparts, and resulting higher rates of death by suicide; however, arguably this rate may be higher because sexual orientation is not determined simply from autopsy, or even readily identifiable by close family and friends (Meyer, Teylan & Schwartz, 2015). An inability to openly identify as LGBTQ(IA+) may be the very cause of a non-fatal suicide attempt or a suicide death. In the LGBTQ(IA+) population, non-fatal suicide attempt average age onset is 16 years, indicating the distress some youth feel when they are exploring and experimenting with their sexuality and the challenges associated with being 'different' (Rosenstreich, 2013). Some of the significant contributing factors to elevated rates of mental health conditions and suicide in LGBTQ(IA+) are their experiences of discrimination, prejudice and homophobia, in addition to confusion around their gender identity and distress related to sexuality acceptance. This is often further exacerbated in migrant LGBTQ(IA+) individuals who are also contending with potential cultural beliefs, stigma and misconceptions about homosexuality. LGBTQ(IA+) individuals have also been identified as a group more likely to be homeless or living in abject poverty, to drink alcohol at risky levels and/or misuse illicit drugs and leave school early (Rosenstreich, 2013). Many of these factors singularly are risk factors for mental health conditions, so LGBTQ(IA+) individuals are a cohort of particular concern with regard to mental health.

Older persons

When looking at mortality from suicide from a global perspective, older male adults consistently demonstrate rates significantly higher than others (WHO, 2014). Cobaugh, Miller, Pham and Krenselok (2015) note that in the United States older persons demonstrate higher rates of suicide and that restricting access to hazardous medicines (used in self-poisoning) and chemicals, and approaches that focus on prevention and medication education, may impact on this rate in the future. Wiktorsson et al. (2016) explored the rationale for suicide in older persons who had survived an attempt and found that physical illness and psychological anguish played significant roles in suicide motivations.

International research (Conwell, Van Orden & Caine, 2011; Koo, Kõlves & De Leo, 2017; Webb et al., 2018) has demonstrated that older individuals who die by suicide demonstrate characteristics such as being retired, living alone, having lower education levels, being widowed and having a diagnosis of depression, and studies in Australia

generally concur with these findings (Law, Kõlves & De Leo, 2015). Older persons are at risk of suicide if any of the following factors are present:

- high levels of emotional distress
- physical illness (such as cancer and lung illnesses)
- reduced capacity to undertake activities of daily living (such as toileting, showering, dressing)
- chronic pain
- presence of a mood disorder (Duberstein & Heisel, 2014).

While the aetiology of suicide in older persons may vary somewhat, thorough assessment and primary care providers who are able to appropriately assess and engage their patients are a vital factor in reducing suicide rates in this cohort. Depression is *not* a normal part of ageing and must be identified and treated accordingly.

'High-risk suicide' occupations

There are a number of occupations that have higher rates of suicide deaths than those experienced within the general population (see **Table 20.4**).

TABLE 20.4
Suicide rates by occupation in Australia

MALES	FEMALES
Construction work or labouring (there are likely links within this cohort including excessive alcohol consumption, lower SES, job insecurity, issues with relationships, predominantly male vocations and poor help-seeking behaviours)	Farming
Unskilled work	Clerical administration
Machine operating	Professionals
Farming	

SOURCE: ADAPTED FROM MILNER, NIVEN & LAMONTAGNE, 2014

Emergency workers such as paramedics and veterinarians also have elevated rates of suicide when compared with the general population (Milner, Niven & LaMontagne, 2014).

While this section has not been exhaustive in looking at all vulnerable groups, it discusses the more common groups who are at risk of death from suicide in Australia. It is also important to note that, globally, other factors such as incarceration (particularly detentions that breach humanitarian rights), persons who are seeking asylum, and persons living in countries with poor or no mental health care access are also more vulnerable to suicide (WHO, 2014).

THE ROLE OF THE MEDIA

The media has a powerful role to play in the prevention of suicide and education about mental health conditions. The WHO (2014) notes that in countries without media restrictions on reporting suicide deaths, the sensationalisation of suicide results in increases of the reported methods within the community. Social media also plays a serious role in the portrayal of suicide, including the numerous incidences where social media was a platform for provoking and assisting suicide in vulnerable people. There are a number of resources in Australia available to assist journalists in the reporting of suicide and mental illness in the media. *Mindframe* (Hunter Institute of Health, 2014) assists journalists to use appropriate language when discussing suicide, balancing stories on mental health conditions with positive aspects and refraining from providing information about suicide techniques. The media are also encouraged to provide crisis support contact details within their articles (both print and televised) for persons who are vulnerable. The WHO (2014) reports that suicide rates have decreased in regions where responsible media reporting has been enacted and that helpful social media reports about mental health have had a positive impact.

ASSESSING RISK OF SUICIDE

There are a number of techniques that the nurse can use when engaging with someone they feel may be at risk of suicide. There are also a number of strategies that can be helpful when having discussions around suicide and mental health. These can be challenging topics, which many students may be anxious about discussing. This section explores approaches to conversing with an individual about suicide.

Conversations

There are few conversations as feared or confronting as that of a discussion with someone who no longer wants to live. This is a time when the nurse will need to gently pack away any judgements or personal issues they may feel about suicide, and those who have died by suicide. These preconceived ideas are unlikely to benefit the conversation or the consumer. **Table 20.5** looks at some common thoughts around suicide from the perspective of the consumer and the student mental health nurse.

TABLE 20.5
Consumers' and student nurses' thoughts about suicide

CONSUMERS' CONCERNS	NURSES' CONCERNS
'They won't believe me, they'll think I am just looking for attention.'	'If I talk about suicide, I might put the idea in their mind and then it will be my fault.'
'I'm beyond help, I'm unworthy of their help.'	'I might say the wrong thing.'
'I don't think I can explain what I feel.'	'I don't know where to go with this discussion.'
'I'm so ashamed to talk about this.'	'What if they say "Yes", they do want to die…then what do I do?!'
'They'll try to stop me.'	'What if I can't help them?'

Things to say when discussing suicide

There are a number of things the nurse can do or say that can be helpful when conversing with someone who wants to die. While the following list is not exhaustive, it provides some ideas for how to talk about this difficult topic. Do:

- Take a deep breath…! Acknowledge that this is difficult for many experienced clinicians, too.
- Move to a safe, quiet area where privacy can be maintained and noise kept to a minimum.
- Slow the rate of your speech and lower your voice.
- Acknowledge how difficult this must be to discuss; for example, 'Thank you for confiding in me Cynthia, I can only imagine how difficult this must be for you.'
- Use therapeutic silence. When done correctly, this is a powerful communication skill that promotes elaboration, and values the peace that silence and simply 'being' with someone gives. It also allows an individual (particularly, if depressed) time to collect their thoughts and process their responses.
- Keep sentences short and clear. The individual may have difficulty concentrating on lengthy, verbose conversations.
- Be empathetic; this person is highly distressed, so your compassion and concern needs to be articulated.
- Use correct terms. It is okay to say the word 'suicide' or 'kill yourself' – these are explicit, overt terms and the meaning is obvious, as opposed to 'no longer be here', which could simply be interpreted as leaving the room or area, or going on a holiday.
- Consider asking the consumer what they think will happen when they die (without implying guilt); for example, 'Cynthia what do you think will happen if you die'?
- Ask open-ended questions.
- Take all threats and behaviours seriously.
- Debrief with a colleague and ensure you look after your own mental health.

Things not to say when discussing suicide

There are also a number of things that may make the situation worse when talking to someone who is contemplating suicide. Do not:

- panic; instead try to remain calm and take a few deep breaths
- compare other people's problems to try and minimise their problems
- tell them you know how they feel (even if you do)
- dismiss their concern by telling them not to worry about their problem/s
- argue with the individual about their reasons or rationales
- assure confidentiality; confidentiality is not absolute, and suicide is an example of when confidentiality *cannot* be guaranteed.

- try to fix their problem; it is important to listen, allow ventilation of feelings, frustration or anger, not to problem-solve
- start questions with 'You don't…
  - …want to die do you?'
  - …want to kill yourself do you?'
  - …think you'd be better off dead do you?'

Exercising care when discussing suicide

There are a few things that the mental health nurse should be considerate about when discussing suicide intention. Tread carefully with the following concepts:

- Reminding the person what they have to live for, as this can create increased feelings of guilt; asking, for example, 'What about your children?' Most certainly the person *has* thought about their children, and feels they are doing their best by them.
- Citing religious reasons for living.
- Stating that suicide is wrong. This may be *your* belief and you are entitled to that, but you need to refrain from statements that are judgemental.

Leading conversations

This section considers a range of ways to commence the conversation about suicide. Some examples of opening sentences are:

- 'Have you been having thoughts about suicide or killing yourself?'
- 'It sounds like things are really difficult for you at the moment. Sometimes when people are depressed they want to kill themselves. Is this something you can relate to?'
- 'You have mentioned many stressful events in your life at the moment. Have you considered killing yourself?'
- 'Aaron, have you ever felt like your life wasn't worth living any more'?
- 'Things sound difficult for you at the moment. What would you do if they got worse?'
- 'Cynthia, you sound like you are in a very dark place at the moment. Have you been thinking about ending your life?'

Plans

It is important to assess the individual's plan to establish how serious the risk is. Generally, the more 'thought out' a plan is, the more serious will be the attempt. For example, an individual who has decided on a *time* (when their family is at school/work), *method* (a firearm) and has *access* to the means which are lethal (they own a firearm) is at high risk of impending suicide. The following elements are important when assessing the individual's plan:

- When are they considering suicide (location)?
  - 'Have you thought about where you would kill yourself?'
  - 'Where do you think you will take the pills?'

- 'Has anything stopped you from carrying out your plan so far?'
- How are they going to take their own life (method/means)?
  - 'Have you considered how you plan to kill yourself?'
  - 'Sara, you mentioned that you know how many pills it would take. Could you tell me which pills you're considering taking?'
- Do they have access to the means?
  - 'You said that you were going to take an overdose of sleeping pills. Do you have any sleeping pills? How many? If not, how were you going to get them? When were you going to get them?' (Note, these questions should not be asked in quick succession; rather, await the response for each question, and then proceed).
  - 'What steps have you taken towards obtaining a firearm?'
- How lethal is the method?
  - Consider how lethal the proposed method is and how reversible it is, if at all. Firearms, jumping and hanging are quick methods of suicide that are highly lethal and difficult to reverse; while overdoses take longer and may be more easily intercepted and less lethal.

SAFETY FIRST

MURDER-SUICIDE

Individuals with a mental health condition are often incorrectly perceived as potentially violent. This is a damaging fallacy and, in fact, people with a mental health condition are more likely to be victims of crimes than perpetrators. It is important, however, to ensure when undertaking an interview with a consumer who presents with suicidal ideation that you explore the unlikely potential for risk to others, or risk of homicide. This may include a belief that their loved ones (such as children) would be better off dead with them. This is often a symptom of disturbed thinking associated with some mental health conditions. This may be more significant in individuals with dependants and little support, resulting in the notion that their dependants will be left alone when they die by suicide. Some potential questions to consider include:

- 'Dean, you've mentioned your family being better off without you. Have you thought about including them in your suicide plans?'
- 'Mohammed, sometimes when people are so distressed they think other people such as their children or partner would be better off dead too. Is this something you can relate to?'
- 'Have you thought about hurting anyone else when you think about suicide Tess?'

Suicide in inpatient settings

While suicide within the inpatient setting is a rare occurrence, it can and does happen, and nurses need to be vigilant. For example, in Victoria alone in 2014–15, there were seven suicide deaths within inpatient mental health units (Department of Health and Human Services, 2016). Inpatient setting suicides are particularly harrowing for staff, and even more importantly, for the consumer's loved ones. While their loved one is in hospital, it is likely that family and friends are feeling a sense of relief – that their family member is safe and protected – and the distress that a resulting suicide must cause is unimaginable. To prevent this tragedy occurring in an inpatient setting, there are a number of things the mental health nurse can do.

Vigilance

When preventing inpatient suicide and self-injury, it is most important to consider *access* to dangerous or potentially life-threatening objects. In particular, consider the following:

- adherence to prescribed medications (hoarding of medication for overdose) or a loved one unintentionally bringing in (even small) quantities of medicines such as paracetamol. Paracetamol can be lethal in overdose in as little as 10 g (20 tablets) and is both the leading cause of liver transplant and most commonly consumed drug in poisonings in Australia (Leang et al., 2014)
- access to ligatures (belts, ties, knitting wool, bras, shoe laces, drawstrings, power cords, etc.) and hanging points such as closet hooks, door jambs, roof fire sprinklers and bathroom areas
- access to sharp, cutting objects (e.g. razors, knives, scissors, mirrors, glass bottles/jars, cans, tins, etc.)
- access to chemicals (detergents, harmful soaps, floor cleaners, cleaning products, acetone, etc.)
- access to scalding/boiling hot water (ingestion of, or intentional scalding with)
- access to plastic bags
- access to lighters or matches.

Many of these items may be brought into the mental health unit in the consumer's own belongings, so searching and documenting belongings is usually mandated as hospital policy. Family and loved ones may also bring items in without considering the potential impact they may have. It is reasonable to think that many people would be unaware that one strip of paracetamol could be lethal.

It is important to also note that *absconding* (or leaving the hospital despite being a compulsory or involuntary consumer) is another cause for concern. Consumers who 'escape' the mental health unit have been known to take desperate measures to end their life (and succeeded in doing so), such as running in front of traffic or trains, and suicide is a leading reason for absconding.

By now it is probably apparent to you that the risk assessment with a consumer who has exhibited suicidal ideation or action is a vitally important role of the mental health nurse. Rapport development is vital when working with someone who is actively suicidal.

SAFETY FIRST

NO-SUICIDE CONTRACTS

At times, it may be necessary to obtain a verbal or written guarantee of safety (or a 'no-suicide' contract) from the consumer who is actively contemplating their suicide. While these contracts, from a research perspective, have demonstrated varied degrees of success, it is important to remember this strategy may be an option. No-suicide contracts require the individual to seek out staff (or an alternative coping strategy) when feeling unable to control their desire to make a suicide attempt. If anything, these contracts can generate a discussion about suicide and overtly demonstrate to the consumer that staff are available 24/7 to talk about their feelings. It is important to remember that a no-suicide contract does not replace adequate supervision, risk assessment and vigilance and must not be seen as a concrete guarantee of safety.

Observations

Each mental health unit will have its own policies for establishing, maintaining and terminating visual observations of a consumer who is at risk of suicide. Generally, visual observations may be:

- *15/60, 20/60, 30/60, etc.:* The consumer must be sighted in intervals *no greater* than 15/20/30 minutes. Generally, it will be required to detail what the consumer is doing during this time (see **Table 20.6**). Overnight, the observing nurse will likely need to demonstrate that respirations have been noted in the consumer.
- *1:1 special:* Consumers requiring this degree of observation are deemed a significant risk of suicide (perhaps they have made an attempt while an inpatient too) and must be in visual presence at all times. This usually includes during toileting and showering. Some policies may require the nurse supervising to be 'at arm's length' at all times. While seclusion and restraint rationales for most Australian states and territories include risk of self-injury, these methods are very restrictive and not conducive to maintaining therapeutic rapport. Consider the consumer who eventually confides their desire to die by suicide to the nurse who has been working with them extensively. Placing them in seclusion after declaring this would seem punitive and create a relationship where it may be considered best *not* to ventilate such feelings if the 'consequences' are so restrictive.

TABLE 20.6
Visual observations example

TIME	OBSERVATION	SIGNATURE	NAME AND DESIGNATION
1143 hrs	Lying on bed reading book; alert.	*Jenny Lewis*	Jenny Lewis (RPN)
1156 hrs	Lying on bed; respirations noted.	*P.Davis*	Peter Davis (RN)
1206 hrs	In kitchen, drinking water.	**AG Tran**	Alice Tran (RN)

PRN medication

In times of particular distress, as required (or PRN) medication may be useful. Anxiolytics such as diazepam may be prescribed for the short-term management of this distress, in addition to sedatives such as temazepam or zopiclone to help the consumer fall asleep. Chapter 11 explores the use of anxiolytics in more detail.

Impacts on carers and clinicians

The death of any loved one is a distressing and traumatic time for family and friends. It is normal for nurses to develop bonds and attachments to the patients under their care. A consumer suicide either under nursing care, or formally under the care of mental health services, can be a distressing time for staff. This section explores the different reactions and impacts of suicides on both carers and clinicians.

Carers

For many people, suicide remains a taboo subject; one that is not broached easily, even among close friends or family. Being a suicide survivor can be a lonely and difficult experience with many unanswered questions.

REFLECT ON THIS

Public awareness and suicide

One suicide death is one too many. There are a number of approaches we can take to address the suicide rate in Australia and make efforts to reduce it. These include targeting programs at the local community, state and national level. Public awareness campaigns that provide resources for Australians and guidelines for media are important in helping to reduce suicide deaths. Responsible media reporting of suicide and mental illness is particularly important when considering cluster suicides. We might consider what role the media plays in cluster suicide.

Reflect upon current public awareness campaigns. Compile a list of campaigns that you are familiar with and how you became aware of them. There is a method to how and why campaigns are targeted through certain platforms, and it is particularly dependent on the target audience or population. For example, domestic violence campaigns are often on the back of public toilet doors, where vulnerable women can access contact details in private, away from their abuser. Consider the appropriate platforms to target the following populations about suicide. You will need to take into consideration the manner in which the targeted population group engage with media, technology and information:

- adolescents
- young mothers
- older mothers
- young men

- older men
- retirees
- non-English-speaking people
- Indigenous people
- LGBTQ(IA+) people.

An important role of government is ensuring people who come into contact with individuals experiencing suicidality are adequately trained and supported. In communities that are bereaved by suicide, postvention services are important considerations in preventing future suicide. People who are bereaved by suicide are particularly vulnerable themselves to suicide, so it is important to ensure that these people are targeted. How is this issue addressed among Aboriginal and Torres Strait Islander peoples, where suicide rates in small communities are high?

Fostering social capital where community engagement and inclusion are cultivated is helpful in capacity-building in communities where suicide rates are higher, such as Aboriginal and Torres Strait Islander communities. Consider your local community.

1. How are social capital and community engagement fostered?
2. Reflecting on your understanding of causes of suicide (such as isolation, mental illness, unemployment, alcohol and drug use, etc.), what types of community engagement programs or activities are available in your area that may indirectly prevent suicide?

While every individual grieves in their own way, there are a number of commonalities seen among survivors of suicide, and these include:

- Guilt at 'not seeing it coming' or 'not taking threats seriously'. This guilt may also be experienced due to a feeling of 'relief' that their loved one's mental anguish and suffering is over.
- Anger with the individual: 'Their suffering is over but ours has only just begun.' In the event the individual was under the care of mental health services, this anger may also be directed at such services for failing to prevent the death. This anger may also be projected onto other people perceived to be contributors to the suicide, perhaps a bully or an ex-partner.
- Embarrassment or shame that their loved one died from suicide, and subsequent failure to identify suicide as the cause of death when discussing it for fear of stigmatisation or lack of understanding or empathy from others. This can also be experienced as awkward or uncomfortable silences when they *do* tell someone their loved one died by suicide, because people often don't know how to react.

It is important to offer counselling to families or carers affected by suicide. In addition, there are a number of organisations dedicated to helping suicide survivors, and people affected by suicide may benefit from joining these groups.

Clinicians

Clinicians caring for a consumer who dies by suicide will also experience a range of feelings, even though these are certainly not the same experiences as those of loved ones. The following are possible responses to suicide:

- anger and a feeling of failure; in particular due to all the progress you may have thought you had made
- grief
- concern, particularly if the consumer was under the care of mental health services and their death results in a coronial investigation
- wondering, 'Is there anything else I could have done?'
- feeling despondent or that there are few rewards in your role as a mental health nurse.

As an active member of the interdisciplinary team, it is important that the nurse takes opportunities to discuss their own feelings and concerns. This may include attending clinical supervision sessions or mandatory critical incident debriefing sessions, which are both excellent opportunities to explore feelings about suicide. Mental health nursing is often an emotionally taxing or draining profession and it is important for the mental health nurse to take care of their own mental health so that they are able to balance the demands of the job, with a need for appropriate relaxation and 'down time'. The following are good ways to de-stress:

- exercising
- speaking to an external counsellor (they will be able to provide the objectivity that someone within the unit cannot)
- catching up with friends
- laughing – an excellent de-stress activity and is great for cardiac health
- taking time off work, or requesting a unit change if things become too difficult.

SELF-HARM/INJURY (NON-SUICIDAL SELF-INJURY)

The reasons why a person might take their life by suicide have been explored in depth in the preceding sections. This section looks at the issue of non-suicidal self-injury. Non-suicidal self-injury has been referred to at other points in the text (e.g. see Chapters 8, 9 and 19) as self-harm or deliberate self-harm (DSH). The definition of non-suicidal **self-injury** used here is the act of behaving in a way that intentionally causes harm or injury to oneself with a non-fatal outcome (Madge at al., 2008; NICE, 2012). In this chapter, we will use the term 'non-suicidal self-injury', keeping in mind that this injuring behaviour, while intentional, has a non-fatal outcome. At times you will see this term shortened to 'self-injure' or 'self-injury' as this language is also used to describe non-suicidal self-injury. This injury can be through a variety of means, which are explored later in the chapter.

A person who engages in non-suicidal self-injury is just attention seeking right?

The movie *The Da Vinci Code* (Brown et al., 2006) contains a scene where a character is flogging himself. The character did not display this behaviour in public. He wore clothes that hid the physical results of his behaviour. He did not draw attention to himself. Yet he felt compelled to injure himself repeatedly, seemed to go into an almost trance-like state as he prepared himself and was relieved when he reached the conclusion. This self-injuring behaviour was not attention seeking. And when we think of non-suicidal self-injuring behaviour in the context of mental health, the first crucial point we must remember is such behaviour is not attention seeking. It is most often the result of a person in great distress being unable to communicate this distress in a less physically damaging way or who has tried to talk but not been heard by others. Other myths surrounding self-injury include:

- *Non-suicidal self-injury is a suicide attempt:* Self-injury is usually used as a coping mechanism – it is not a suicide attempt. However, one unintended consequence may be death if the individual injury sustained is more critical than intended.

- *A person who engages in non-suicidal self-injury is mentally unwell:* Self-injury is not a diagnosed mental health condition and it is not listed in DSM-5 (APA, 2013). While some people who engage in self-injuring actions will have an underlying mental health issue, it is not appropriate to say that every person who self-injures will also have a mental health condition.
- *A person who engages in non-suicidal self-injury has borderline personality disorder (BPD):* In order for a person to receive a diagnosis of BPD, they must demonstrate a range of clinical features, which may include self-injury. However, it should never be assumed that a person who self-injures has BPD.
- *Only young people engage in non-suicidal self-injuring behaviour:* While non-suicidal self-injury is more commonly noted in younger people, it is incorrect to assume that adults do not self-injure (Scanlan & Purcell, 2010).

It is important to remember that myths such as these perpetuate negative stereotypes and maintain a stigmatised view of self-injury.

Defining non-suicidal self-injury

The term 'self-harm (injury)' is a broad one and there have been many attempts to define it. The WHO defined deliberate self-harm as behaviour that was intended to inflict self-harm (injury), but without suicidal intent (Platt et al., 1992). Work by Madge et al. (2008, p. 670) defined self-harm as being an 'act with a non-fatal outcome…'; that is, harm that involves a self-injurious behaviour, ingestion of a prescribed substance, recreational substance use or ingestions of a non-digestible substance or object.

You will often hear and read the terms 'self-harm', 'self-injury', 'deliberate self-harm', 'self-mutilation' and 'parasuicide' used interchangeably. The language we use to describe this behaviour will have an impact on how people view this issue and the judgements they make about people who engage in self-harming behaviour. Using terms such as 'deliberate' can imply a conscious or intentional choice that could have been avoided. Parasuicide is used to convey the idea that a person has inflicted injury on themselves without the actual intent of suiciding. Using these terms in contemporary mental health practice is now viewed as stigmatising and derogatory (Long, Manktelow & Tracey, 2013).

Epidemiology

Rates of non-suicidal self-injuring behaviour are difficult to estimate accurately. For every person who presents for assessment and treatment following a non-suicidal self-injury episode, there will many more who do not. It is estimated that less than 13% of young people who engage in non-suicidal self-injuring behaviour will present for hospital treatment (Rowe et al., 2014). Non-suicidal self-injury is seen to be an issue that is especially prevalent among adolescents, and more commonly seen as a behaviour that females engage in, with a large number of young women requiring hospital admission and treatment (AIHW, 2014; Madge et al., 2008). Evidence suggests 1 in 10 young people in Australia have self-injured without suicidal intent (Lawrence et al., 2015). Lifetime prevalence rates are higher, with 17% of Australian females and 12% of males aged 15–19 years, and 24% of females and 18% of males aged 20–24 years reporting non-suicidal self-injury at some point in their life (Martin et al., 2010). Self-injurious behaviour is also thought by some researchers to be a risk factor for later suicide. Mars et al. (2014) argue that suicide and self-injury with suicidal intent are in fact overlapping behaviours distinguished by a number of distinct characteristics. Self-injury tends to decline with age (Rowe et al., 2014).

Methods of non-suicidal self-injury include:

- self-cutting
- self-battery (banging one's head or limbs)
- jumping from heights
- burning oneself
- overdosing
- ingesting toxic substances.

Aetiology

While non-suicidal self-injury is not a mental illness and is not classified as a mental health condition in the DSM-5 (APA, 2013), it is listed as one of the diagnostic criteria for BPD (see Chapter 12).

There are a number of underlying reasons for non-suicidal self-injury. These include self-injuring as a response to stress, the means of communicating distress, difficulty in dealing with problems in life or a non-fatal suicide attempt. As with suicide, it is important to look at the risk factors associated with non-suicidal self-injury, as shown in **Table 20.7**.

TABLE 20.7
Risk factors for non-suicidal self-injury

POTENTIAL SELF-INJURY RISK FACTORS
Socioeconomic disadvantage
Family factors (loss, separation, divorce, interpersonal conflict)
Trauma (physical/sexual)
Mental health conditions (depression and anxiety disorders)
Heavy alcohol consumption (at levels of misuse/dependence)
Bullying
Female gender
Antisocial behaviour

SOURCE: ADAPTED FROM HEERDE ET AL., 2015; MARS ET AL., 2014; MOLLER, TAIT & BYRNE, 2013

Cultural considerations and vulnerable groups

Because non-suicidal self-injury is such a broad term, it is important to remember that behaviours that are culturally unacceptable in one culture may be acceptable in other cultures, even if the impact of the behaviour results in self-inflicted physical or psychological damage. For example, in Australia the rates of people smoking have decreased dramatically in recent decades as people recognise the short- and long-term health impacts of this behaviour. This is in contrast to alcohol consumption, which many people would argue is an intrinsic part of Australian culture. Also, non-suicidal self-injury can occur as a part of religious practices, such as self-flagellation, or as a form of political or social protest, such as fasting. While a great deal of research looks at non-suicidal self-injury as a particular concern for young people, people of any age can self-injure. However, there are specific groups of younger people who are thought to have a higher risk of engaging in non-suicidal self-injuring behaviour. These include:

- females
- people with a diagnosis of a mental health condition
- Aboriginal or Torres Strait Islander people
- people in immigration or youth detention
- people from rural and remote areas
- lesbian, gay, bisexual, transgender, queer and intersex (LGBTQ(IA+)) people (Robinson, McCutchen, Browne & Witt, 2016).

While it is often quite easy to think about the various risk factors associated with non-suicidal self-injuring behaviour, it is also necessary to identify what protective factors might reduce the risk of a person engaging in non-suicidal self-injuring behaviour. **Tables 20.1**, **20.3** and **20.7** list risk factors for suicide, and these help in identifying some possible protective factors. For instance, a young person who has a positive relationship with their parents which involves open communication may find this a protective factor. Developing a range of coping skills can also be a protective factor. Other protective factors such as experiencing a sense of belonging to various groups as well as developing social networks can also be a protective factor.

Why does a person engage in non-suicidal self-injuring behaviour?

There are a variety of reasons why a person may engage in non-suicidal self-injuring behaviour, including:

- feeling disconnected
- a need for control
- feeling numb
- expression of feelings
- as a coping mechanism
- isolation
- punishment
- addictive behaviour

- identity
- emotions
- issues with peers/family/work
- bullying
- low self-esteem
- alcohol and other drugs issues
- physical health problems
- sexual problems
- difficulties with their partner.

ASSESSMENT AND COLLABORATIVE CARE FOR CONSUMERS WHO EXPERIENCE SELF-INJURING BEHAVIOURS

Living with persistent and/or an acute episode(s) of non-suicidal self-injuring thoughts or behaviour requires a collaborative approach to working with consumers and their families/carers. A person who self-injures may not be experiencing suicidal thoughts, but the behaviour is a means of communicating their distress or regulating their emotions. However, the potential for unintended suicide must also be assessed for and incorporated in the care process with consumers and their families. The assessment and care planning processes can be divided into short- and long-term management. There are a number of key actions that should be followed in caring for a person who has self-injured.

These key actions relate to knowledge, attitudes, values and behaviours:

- A person who has self-injured must be treated with the same respect and unconditional positive regard as any other person for whom care is provided. This includes respecting privacy, maintaining confidentiality and recognising that the experience of non-suicidal self-injury is a distressing one for the consumer.
- It is essential that a person who has self-injured is kept informed and involved in all aspects of care and management to the degree that they are able to participate in the acute management stage.
- Recovery-oriented practice with a person who has self-injured must include appropriate education and training for staff, working with people who have self-injured as part of the learning process and ongoing review and updating of their knowledge and skills. This includes knowledge and understanding of legal and ethical considerations such as mental capacity and consent and relevant mental health legislation.

These key actions relate to assessment of needs, and risk and acute management:

- Acute general hospital management involves treating the effects of the injury through coordinated multidisciplinary care. First responders such as paramedics as well as ED staff should always have activated charcoal on hand in the event that the person has self-injured through ingesting a toxic substance. The earlier (within one hour of ingestion) this can be taken, the higher the chance that absorption of the ingested substance can be reduced or even prevented (NICE, 2012).

- Treatment of any physical consequences of the self-injury must be dealt with immediately. This includes adequate pain relief/analgesia for any medical procedures. This does not mean that any psychosocial/mental health/risk assessment must not be commenced, but it will be prioritised in relation to physical health in the emergency phase; for example, treatment of a paracetamol overdose. You will also see samples for analysis such as urine samples, blood samples and/or samples of vomit.

- Once stabilised, the person must have a comprehensive psychosocial and mental health assessment done as soon as possible and this would normally be undertaken by a member of the mental health team assigned to the ED. This assessment must include the reasons underlying the current episode of self-injury, assessment of suicidal thoughts and intent, depression and/or feelings of hopelessness, any risk factors associated with self-injury and a social history. Refer to Chapter 7 for more information on assessment.

Longer-term management

As with short-term assessment and management, long-term management for people who have self-injured must be a collaborative process based on ongoing assessment of needs. **Table 20.8** outlines the elements of specialist mental health assessment of needs and risk.

TABLE 20.8
Assessment of needs and risks

ASSESSMENT OF NEEDS	
	• Strengths/skills/coping strategies
	• Mental health problems/illness (e.g. depression in older people)
	• Physical health/illness (comorbidities)
	• Social circumstances and problems
	• Psychosocial and occupational functioning, and vulnerabilities, recent and current life difficulties (e.g. personal, family and financial problems)
	• Psychological signs of possible self-injury
	• Assessment of need for different types of interventions (e.g. psychological, substance use rehabilitation, physical treatment)
	• Treatment for any associated conditions
ASSESSMENT OF RISK	• Methods and frequency of current and past self-injury
	• Current and past suicidal intent depressive symptoms and their relationship to self-injury
	• Mental health issues and their connection to self-injury
	• Personal and social situations preceding self-injury, such as specific heightened periods of emotions and changes in relationships
	• Specific risk factors and protective factors that may increase or decrease the risks associated with self-injury
	• Significant mood changes, changes in sleeping and eating patterns, social withdrawal, hiding or washing their own clothes to avoid any blood resulting from cutting being seen by others, avoiding events where their arms or legs are exposed (e.g. swimming)
	• Unexplained injuries/physical complaints (e.g. abdominal pains), dressing inappropriately for the climate in order to avoid signs of non-suicidal self-injury
	• Coping strategies and relationships that the person has used to either successfully limit or avoid self-injury or to contain the impact of self-injury to themselves
	• Relationships that may increase the risk of self-injury

SOURCE: ADAPTED FROM HEADSPACE, 2018; NICE, 2011

Care planning

Care planning is based on consistent assessment and plans for both the ongoing health and well-being of the person as well as managing future risk. Plans must include strategies related to how to prevent escalation of non-suicidal self-injury, reduce harm arising from non-suicidal self-injury or reduce or stop non-suicidal self-injury, reduce or stop other risk-related behaviour, improve social or occupational functioning, improve quality of life, and improve any associated mental health conditions. Care plans are developed collaboratively with the person and other members of the multidisciplinary team and should be focused on developing achievable short- and longer-term goals that are success focused, including steps to help people move towards meeting their goals, together with the supports the person needs to help them on their journey and the roles of different team members who may be involved (NICE, 2011).

A risk management plan should be a clear component of the care plan. Specific risk factors that increase the potential for a person to self-injure should be identified and listed in collaboration with the person. A crisis plan should clearly state the self-management strategies a person can use and also how to access services during a crisis should self-management strategies fail (NICE, 2011). Examples of self-management strategies that a person can use when experiencing the need to self-injure are:

- wearing an elastic band around their wrist and snapping it when they have an urge to self-injure
- drawing red lines on their body where they usually cut or hurt themselves
- holding ice cubes in their hands, or in the areas they usually self-injure
- punching a bed, pillow or punching bag or participating in vigorous exercise
- scratching a picture on a piece of wood
- breaking the object they would usually hurt themselves with
- running their hands under freezing water
- clapping until their hands sting
- massaging where they want to hurt themselves
- writing down thoughts when they become stressed.

Together with the strategies outlined above, there are a number of psychological interventions that focus on helping people who self-injure that aim to increase coping resources, problem-solving and interpersonal communication skills. These interventions include dialectical behaviour therapy, psychodynamic therapy and brief interpersonal therapies. These have been identified as useful in working with people with a diagnosis of BPD (RANZCP, 2004). There will also be a need to manage any concurrent mental health issue the person is experiencing such as depression, schizophrenia or borderline personality disorder (NICE, 2011). The care planning process is explored in Chapter 12. Psychological interventions focus broadly on helping the consumer to identify triggers and stress responses, and identifying new ways of managing these distressing thoughts and the resulting stress.

The person's experience of non-suicidal self-injury

Given its emotive nature, it is essential that mental health nurses think about the impact of non-suicidal self-injury on people who experience this behaviour. Important questions to consider are:

- What drives a person to self-injure?
- How easy is it for a person to seek help?
- What is their experience of seeking help like?

Evidence shows that people who self-injure experience stigma, negative interactions with health care professionals, and do not feel respected and/or treated with dignity (Long, Manktelow & Tracey, 2012; Youd, 2013). People can be made to feel they are seeking attention inappropriately, wasting health care resources and/or that they are being ridiculed (SBU, 2015). This results in people being less likely to seek help from formal health services.

The experience of carers and clinicians

Working with people who self-injure can be emotionally demanding. Best practice requires mental health nurses, as part of the multidisciplinary team, to have a high level of communication skills and self-awareness. This is because their knowledge and attitudes will be reflected in their clinical practice and will impact on the experience of the person who self-injures and the likelihood that they access services for treatment in the future if needed. Mental health nurses working with people who self-injure need to have access to regular clinical supervision where they can discuss and develop an understanding of any emotional impact experienced and self-care strategies they can implement.

CASE **STUDY**

MARIE: ONE EXPERIENCE OF SELF-INJURY

Marie is studying Year 12 at high school and is hoping to study social work at university. She has presented at the GP clinic and is seeing the mental health nurse practitioner, following her stepfather's discovery of her numerous cuts and small circular scabs on her forearms and legs.

Marie is the oldest of three children. Her two brothers are significantly younger than her as they are the children of her mother's second marriage. Her mother is an academic and her father works as a computer analyst. She recalls growing up in a very competitive household, with both her parents constantly challenging her to work harder and do better than them at school. She did not have an extensive friendship network as she was repeatedly told she had to focus on 'being the best'. Any outside activities were chosen

for her. At the same time, her parents were frequently absent due to their own professional commitments. Marie grew up feeling alone and isolated from other people.

Marie's parents separated when she was 11 years old, leaving Marie feeling confused but unable to speak about her feelings as both parents did not want to talk about the reasons for their separation. Marie started cutting herself at the age of 13. Marie felt increasingly isolated and angry, but felt she had no one to speak to about her feelings.

'I was constantly told to focus on my studies, feelings were seen as useless. I felt like I was exploding inside and no one could see. Cutting and burning myself was something I was in control of, something I chose to do and it was so superficial I could hide it easily,' she tells the practice nurse.

With her mother's remarriage and subsequent arrival of her brothers, Marie's cutting increased in frequency and intensity. 'I feel…no I find I need to cut myself every day now and I have gone to cutting myself on my arms and legs – but no one was supposed to know. But I started burning myself as well to get the release when the cutting stopped doing it for me. If my stepfather hadn't got suspicious and started questioning me I wouldn't be here.'

Questions

1 What risk factors do you assess as contributing to Marie's current self-injuring behaviour?
2 What protective factors are evident in Marie's story?
3 Based on Marie's story, what strategies could Marie and the mental health nurse develop for Marie to use when she feels the need to self-injure?
4 Describe the roles and responsibilities of the various members of the multidisciplinary team working with Marie and her family.

REFLECTION ON LEARNING FROM PRACTICE

Consumers with suicidal thoughts will often experience feelings such as those described by Cynthia. Feelings of worthlessness, guilt at being alive but also feeling guilty for wanting to die are constant themes that mental health nurses will hear consumers speak about. Consumers will speak of not necessarily wanting to die, but having a stronger desire to not live.

These conversations can be challenging and uncomfortable for mental health nurses, who either may have had little experience with suicide and/or are students who have previous professional experience of suicide, or personal experience through family or friends. Part of a student's professional learning and development is to see how the mental health nurse creates space through therapeutic engagement based on respect for the person and a non-judgemental attitude to facilitate a conversation whereby consumers such as Cynthia can be open about their feelings and the mental health nurse works with them as they move forward. The key is having hope for the future and helping Cynthia to entrust others to hold this hope with and for her during those times when she is unable to do so for herself.

CHAPTER RESOURCES

SUMMARY

- Suicide is a complex phenomenon that can occur in the presence or absence of a mental health condition, and is understood to result from a number of factors.
- There are a number of diverse theories around suicide and these can help us understand an individual's motivations.
- Suicide rates differ according to culture and location, and some groups are more prone to suicide (e.g. Indigenous Australians).
- The media has an important role in informing Australians about current news events, underpinned by particular responsibilities in reporting sensitive topics such as suicide.

- Professional nursing practice requires nurses to engage with consumers who are experiencing suicidal ideation. This requires a degree of sensitivity to ensure that conversations with consumers about suicide are safe.
- Self-injury differs from suicide by intent, and while there is some overlap between the two, they are separate phenomena.
- Assessment of self-injury involves addressing acute episodes, long-term management strategies that focus on safety, identifying risk factors, developing alternative coping strategies, reducing risk and addressing underlying issues related to self-injuring behaviour.

REVIEW QUESTIONS

1 Vulnerable groups identified as being at a higher risk of experiencing self-injury are:
   a Young women
   b Young people in immigration youth detention centres
   c Consumers experiencing psychosis
   d All of these options
2 You are working on a unit where Amy who has a history of self-injury has just been admitted. You overhear two registered nurses talking, when one says, 'You know she's just an attention-seeking brat.' Based on your understanding of self-injury, this statement reflects:
   a A common misconception people hold about self-injury
   b The years of experience the registered nurse has working with consumers who self-injure
   c The stigma associated with self-injury
   d a and c

3 Evan discloses suicidal thoughts to the mental health nurse during a mental health assessment. What would be the most appropriate intervention that the mental health nurse should implement?

   a Document the conversation and repeat the mental health assessment as soon as possible

   b Close supervision as per the organisation's policy and encourage Evan to speak with clinical staff

   c Report the conversation to the senior nurse and ask them to follow up

   d Place Evan in seclusion for his own safety

4 What are the aspects of the acute management of a consumer who has self-injured?

5 What are the overall goals of psychological interventions utilised in working with consumers who self-injure?

CRITICAL THINKING

1 Consider your own feelings and thoughts on suicide and self-injury. What personal traits and/or beliefs do you think you possess which will make working with someone who is suicidal difficult? How do you think you are able to help?

2 A young consumer's parent asks you about the difference between self-injury and suicide. How would you explain the difference to them?

3 How effective are non-suicide contracts, according to the current evidence?

USEFUL WEBSITES

- Headspace: https://headspace.org.au
- Lifeline: http://www.lifeline.org.au
- Reach Out: http://www.au.reachout.com
- Suicide Prevention Australia: https://www.suicidepreventionaust.org

REFLECT ON THIS

Vicarious trauma and self-care

Suicide and self-harm are sensitive issues that can be emotionally taxing for people who work in health care. Vicarious trauma (VT; or as it is sometimes known, compassion fatigue) is a concept that is gathering momentum with regard to its effects on the mental health workforce. Vicarious trauma is essentially the impact of listening to other people's traumatic experiences, such as abuse and victimisation. Vicarious trauma builds over time and can result in some of the following symptoms:

- feeling angry on behalf of consumers who have been victimised

- insomnia and rumination
- issues maintaining professional boundaries
- feeling cynical and pessimistic.

To protect yourself from VT and burnout, it is important that you take care of your own mental health as you embark on your journey as a nurse. Consider what self-care strategies you will employ when you begin your nursing career. Ideally, you should consider implementing them now so that you have good coping strategies when you graduate.

REFERENCES

Abramson, L.Y., Metalsky, G.I. & Alloy, L.B. (1989). Hopelessness depression: A theory-based subtype of depression. *Psychological Review*, 96, 358–72. doi:10.1037/0033-295X.96.2.358

American Psychiatric Association (APA). (2013). *Diagnostic and Statistical Manual of Mental Disorders (DSM-5)* (5th edn). Washington, DC: APA.

Anikeeva, O., Bi, P., Hiller, J.E., Ryan, P., Roder, D. & Han, G.S. (2015). Trends in migration mortality rates in Australia 1981–2007: A focus on the National Health Priority Areas other than cancer. *Ethnicity & Health*, 20(1), 29–48. doi:10.1080/13557858.2014.883368

Australian Bureau of Statistics (ABS). (2013). *Causes of Death, Australia, 2011*. Cat. no. 3303.0. Canberra: Commonwealth of Australia. Retrieved from http://www.abs.gov.au/ausstats/abs@.nsf/Lookup/3303.0Chapter222011.

Australian Bureau of Statistics (ABS). (2016a). *Causes of Death, Australia 2014. Cat. No. 3303.0*. Canberra: Commonwealth of Australia. Retrieved from http://www.abs.gov.au/AUSSTATS/abs@.nsf/allprimarymainfeatures/47E19CA15036B04BCA2577570014668B?opendocument.

Australian Bureau of Statistics (ABS). (2016b). *Migration, Australia. Cat. No. 3412.0*. Canberra: Commonwealth of Australia. Retrieved from http://www.abs.gov.au/ausstats/abs@.nsf/mf/3412.0.

Australian Government Department of Health. (2013). *Aboriginal and Torres Strait Islander Suicide: Origins, Trends and Incidence*. Retrieved from http://www.health.gov.au/internet/publications/publishing.nsf/Content/mental-natsisps-strat-toc~mental-natsisps-strat-1~mental-natsisps-strat-1-ab.

Australian Government Department of Health and Ageing. (2013). *National Aboriginal and Torres Strait Islander Suicide Prevention Strategy.* © Commonwealth of Australia. Retrieved from http://www.health.gov.au/internet/main/publishing.nsf/Content/1CE7187EC4965005CA25802800127B49/$File/Indigenous%20Strategy.pdf.

Australian Institute of Health and Welfare (AIHW). (2016). *Leading Causes of Death.* Canberra: AIHW. Retrieved from http://www.aihw.gov.au/deaths/leading-causes-of-death.

Baumeister, R.F. (1990). Suicide as escape from self. *Psychological Review*, 97, 90–113.

Brown, D., Calley, J., Grazer, B., Hallowell, T., Howard, R., McGill, K. & Velis, L. (Producer) & Howard, R. (Director). (2006). *The Da Vinci Code.* [Motion Picture]. Culver City, CA: Columbia Pictures.

Chapman, S., Alpers, P., Agho, K. & Jones. M. (2015). Australia's 1996 gun law reforms: Faster falls in firearm deaths, firearm suicides, and a decade without mass shootings. *Injury Prevention*, 21, 355–62. doi:10.1136/ip.2006.013714rep

Chen, Y.Y., Liao, S.F., Teng, P.R., Tsai, C.W., Fan, H.F., Lee, W.C. & Cheng, A.T.A. (2012). The impact of media reporting of the suicide of a singer on suicide rates in Taiwan. *Social Psychiatry and Psychiatric Epidemiology*, 47, 215–21. doi:10.1007/s00127-010-0331-y

Cobaugh, D.J., Miller, M.J., Pham, T.T. & Krenselok, E.P. (2015). Risk of major morbidity and death in older adults with suicidal intent: A cross-sectional analysis from the National Poison Data System, 2000–2009. *American Geriatric Society*, 63(3), 501–7. doi:10.1111/jgs.13323

Conwell, Y., Van Orden, K. & Caine, E.D. (2011). Suicide in older adults. *Psychiatric Clinics of North America*, 34(2), 451–68. doi:10.1016/j.psc.2011.02.002

Creative Spirits. (n.d.). Aboriginal culture. People: Aboriginal suicide rates. Retrieved from http://www.creativespirits.info.

Department of Health and Human Services. (2016). *Chief Psychiatrist's Annual Report 2014–2015.* Melbourne: State of Victoria.

Department of Parliamentary Services. (2011). *Suicide in Australia.* Canberra: Parliament of Australia. Retrieved from http://www.aph.gov.au/About_Parliament/Parliamentary_Departments/Parliamentary_Library/pubs/BN/2011-2012/Suicide.

Duberstein, P.R. & Heisel, M.J. (2014). Person-centred prevention of suicide among older adults. In M.K. Nock (ed.), *The Oxford Handbook of Suicide and Self-injury.* Oxford Handbooks Online. doi:10.1093/oxfordhb/9780195388565.013.0009

Durkheim, E. (1897). *Suicide.* New York: Free Press.

Healey, J. (2014). *Suicide Prevention.* Thirroul, NSW: Spinney Press.

Heerde, J.A., Toumbourou, J.W., Hemphill, S.A., Herrenkohl, T.I., Patton, G.C. & Catalano, R.F. (2015). Incidence and course of adolescent deliberate self-harm in Victoria, Australia, and Washington State. *Journal of Adolescent Health*, 57(5), 537–44. doi:http://dx.doi.org/10.1016/j.jadohealth.2015.07.017

Hunter Institute of Health. (2014). *Reporting and Portrayal of Suicide.* Canberra: Australian Government Department of Health. Retrieved from http://www.mindframe-media.info/for-media/reporting-suicide#cc.

Joiner, T.E. (2005). *Why People Die By Suicide.* Cambridge, MA: Harvard University Press.

Koo, Y.W., Kõlves, K. & De Leo, D. (2017). Suicide in older adults: Differences between the young-old, middle-old, and oldest old. *International Psychogeriatrics*, 29(8), 1297–1306. doi:10.1017/S1041610217000618

Law, C.K., Kõlves, K. & De Leo, D. (2014). Suicide mortality in second-generation migrants, Australia, 2001–2008. *Social Psychiatry and Psychiatric Epidemiology*, 49(4), 601–8. doi:10.1007/s00127-013-0769-9

Law, C.K., Kõlves, K. & De Leo, D. (2015). Influences of population-level factors on suicide in older adults: A national ecological study from Australia. *International Journal of Geriatric Psychiatry*, 31, 388–95. doi:10.1002/gps.4343

Lawrence, D., Johnson, S., Hafekost, J., Boterhoven De Haan, K., Sawyer, M., Ainley, J. & Zubrick, S.R. (2015). *The Mental Health of Children and Adolescents. Report on the Second Australian Child and Adolescent Survey of Mental Health and Wellbeing.* Canberra: Department of Health. Retrieved from https://www.health.gov.au/internet/main/publishing.nsf/Content/9DA8CA21306FE6EDCA257E2700016945/%24File/child2.pdf.

Leang, Y., Taylor, D.M., Dargan, P.I., Wood, D.M. & Greene, S.L. (2014). Reported ingested dose of paracetamol as a predictor of risk following paracetamol overdose. *European Journal of Clinical Pharmacology*, 70, 1513–18. doi:10.1007/s00228-014-1756-0

Linehan, M.M. (1993). *Cognitive-behavioral Treatment of Borderline Personality Disorder.* New York: Guilford Press.

Long, M., Manktelow, R. & Tracey, A. (2013). We are all in this together: Working towards a holistic understanding of self-harm. *Journal of Psychiatric and Mental Health Nursing*, 20(2), 105–13. doi:10.1111/j.1365-2850.2012.01893.x

Madge, N., Hewitt, A., Hawton, K., Wilde, E.J.D., Corcoran, P., Fekete, S., … Ystgaard, M. (2008). Deliberate self-harm within an international community sample of young people: Comparative findings from the Child & Adolescent Self-harm in Europe (CASE) Study. *Journal of Child Psychology and Psychiatry*, 49(6), 667–77. doi:10.1111/j.1469-7610.2008.01879.x

Mars, B., Heron, J., Crane, C., Hawton, K., Lewis, G., Macleod, J., Tilling, K. & Gunnell, D. (2014). Clinical and social outcomes of adolescent self harm: Population based birth cohort study. *British Medical Journal*, 3(49). doi:10.1136/bmj.g5954

Martin, G., Swannell, S.V., Hazell, P.L., Harrison, J.E. & Taylor, A.W. (2010). Self-injury in Australia: A community survey. *Medical Journal of Australia*, 193(9), 506–10.

Meyer, I.H., Teylan, M. & Schwartz, S. (2015). The role of help-seeking in preventing suicide attempts among lesbians, gay men, and bisexuals. *American Journal of Suicidology*, 45(1), 25–36. doi:10.1111/sltb.12104

Milner, A., Niven, H. & LaMontagne, A. (2014). Suicide by occupational skill level in the Australian construction industry: Data from 2001 to 2010. *Australian and New Zealand Journal of Public Health*, 38(3), 281–5. doi:10.1111/1753-6405.12205

Moller, C.I., Tait, R.J. & Byrne, D.G. (2013). Self-harm, substance use and psychological distress in the Australian general population. *Addiction*, 108(1), 211–20.

National Institute for Health and Care Excellence (NICE). (2011). *Self-harm in over 8s: Long-term management.* Retrieved from https://www.nice.org.uk/guidance/CG133.

National Institute for Health and Care Excellence (NICE). (2012). *Self-harm: Longer-term management.* London: NICE.

Nock, M.K. (2014). *The Oxford Handbook of Suicide and Self-Injury.* Oxford: Oxford University Press.

Page, A., Morrell, S., Hobbs, C., Carter, G., Dudley, M., Duflou, J. & Taylor, R. (2014). Suicide in young adults: Psychiatric and socio-economic factors from a case-control study. *BMC Psychiatry*, 14, 68. doi:10.1186/1471-244X-14-68

Platt, S., Bille-Brahe, U., Kerkhof, A., Schmidtke, A., Bjerke, T., Crepet, P., … Faria, J.S. (1992). Parasuicide in Europe: The WHO/EURO multicentre study on parasuicide. I. Introduction and preliminary analysis for 1989. *Acta Psychiatrica Scandinavica*, 85(2), 97–104. doi:10.1111/j.1600-0447.1992.tb01451.x

Robinson, J., McCutcheon, L., Browne, V. & Witt, K. (2016). *Looking the Other Way: Young People and Self-harm*. Melbourne: Orygen, The National Centre for Excellence in Youth Mental Health.

Rosenstreich, G. (2013). *LGBTI People Mental Health and Suicide* (revised 2nd edn). Sydney: National LGBTI Health Alliance.

Rowe, S.L., French, R.S., Henderson, C., Ougrin, D., Slade, M. & Moran, P. (2014). Help-seeking behaviour and adolescent self-harm: A systematic review. *Australian & New Zealand Journal of Psychiatry*, 48, 1083–95. doi:10.1177/0004867414555718

Royal Australian and New Zealand College of Psychiatrists (RANZCP) Clinical Practice Guidelines Team for Deliberate Self-harm. (2004). Australian and New Zealand clinical practice guidelines for the management of adult deliberate self-harm. *Australian and New Zealand Journal of Psychiatry*, 38, pp. 868–84.

SBU. (2015). Self-harm: Patients' experiences and perceptions of professional care and support. SBU alert report. Retrieved from http://www.sbu.se/contentassets/4b3a210e262742c9aede925a23889cb5/self_harm_patients_experiences_perceptions_professional_care_support_201504.pdf.

Scanlan, F. & Purcell, R. (2010). *Mythbuster: Sorting Fact from Fiction on Self-harm* (pp. 1–6). Melbourne: Headspace National Youth Mental Health Foundation. Retrieved from https://headspace.org.au/assets/Uploads/Resource-library/Health-professionals/self-harm-mythbuster.pdf.

Shneidman, E.S. (1996). *The Suicidal Mind*. New York: Oxford University Press.

Too, L.S., Bugeja, L., Milner, A., McClure, R. & Spittal, M.J. (2017). Predictors of using trains as a suicide method: Findings from Victoria, Australia. *Psychiatry Research*, 253, 233–9.

Webb, C.A., Cui, R., Titus, C., Fiske, A. & Nardoff, M.R. (2018). Sleep disturbance, activities of daily living, and depressive symptoms among older adults. *Clinical Gerontologist*, 41(2), 172–80. doi:10.1080/07317115.2017.1408733

Wilson, T. & Shalley, F. (2018). *What is the size of Australia's non-heterosexual population?* Retrieved from https://blog.ukdataservice.ac.uk/australias-non-heterosexual-population/

Wiktorsson, S., Berg, A.I., Wilhelmson, K., Fässberg, M.M., Van Orden, K., Duberstein, P. & Waern, M. (2016). Assessing the role of physical illness in young old and older old suicide attempters. *International Journal of Geriatric Psychiatry*, 31, 771–4.

World Health Organization (WHO). (2014). *Preventing Suicide: A Global Imperative*. Luxembourg: WHO Press.

Youd, J. (2013). Clinical update: Self-harm, expert opinion. *Nursing Standard*, 28, 16.

CHAPTER 21

RECOVERY AND RESILIENCE IN MENTAL HEALTH

Peri O'Shea

LEARNING OUTCOMES

Upon completion of this chapter, you should be able to:

21.1 Understand the concept of recovery and recovery-oriented mental health

21.2 Explore why nurses need to be trauma-informed and the features, principles and focus of trauma-informed and recovery-oriented practice

21.3 Demonstrate how to work with, support and learn from peer workers

21.4 Understand how to support the changes in service provisions occurring due to the increasing awareness and understanding of recovery orientation and trauma-informed practice

21.5 Understand how to reflect and support each other as a team

21.6 Understand how to reflect on recovery ethics and the impact your own history can have on your practice and understand how to manage risk without risking recovery

---

LEARNING FROM PRACTICE

You can hear Evie coming down the corridor outside even before she arrives. The abuse and vitriol, currently being directed at security and the staff member who are escorting her, is loud, spiteful, full of strongly offensive language and threats. You are feeling, angry, stressed, frustrated and a little bit frightened because you know that you will be the target of her tirade the minute she comes through that door. You are near the end of a long and exhausting shift. You know Evie well, she has been here many times before and it has never been easy, but lately she has been even less cooperative, more violent and it seems that she is being readmitted and then sectioned more often. You knew she was coming up but you hoped that maybe they'd keep her in ED a little longer so she'd arrive after you'd left for the day. Just your luck the wheels of the hospital turned a bit faster than they usually do and you're stuck with her. The door is opening.

What you do next has the potential to significantly change Evie life forever.

The thoughts and feelings expressed by the mental health nurse will impact on how she greets and responds to Evie's needs. What does the nurse need to understand about Evie and her possible feelings regarding this admission? How should this underpin her approach to welcoming Evie onto the unit?

INTRODUCTION

As described in Chapter 1, the history of mental health represents a variety of ways in which consumers have been viewed and the treatment options available and offered to them. In recent years, there has been a strong commitment to mental health reform to ensure that good mental health and well-being is the core business of service development, delivery and evaluation. This reform has led to a commitment to supporting people with a lived experience of a mental health condition in their recovery journey and also supporting their families and other important people in their lives. In this chapter, we explore the central ideas of recovery, resilience and trauma-informed practice.

RECOVERY AND RECOVERY-ORIENTED PRACTICE

Recovery refers to 'recovery of life'. Recovery is about a person being able to live their life the way they would like to live it; making choices and working towards life goals with or without ongoing symptoms of illness. For many people with a lived experience of a mental health condition, recovery means a return to a meaningful life that is not dominated or dictated by a mental health condition.

The Australian Government, through the National Framework of Recovery Oriented Mental Services (AHMAC, 2013a, p. 2), defines recovery as 'being able to create and live a meaningful and contributing life in a community of choice with or without the presence of mental health issues'.

Recovery is very personal and different for every person. Individual recovery is defined by the person who has the mental health condition based on what is meaningful to them. The focus of recovery is on the person, with the person's hopes and aspirations at the fore. Each person's recovery goals are personalised or unique, and they cannot be set or evaluated by others. Slade and Longden (2015, p. 10) emphasise the personal quality of recovery, asserting that: 'Recovery is best judged by the person living with the experience'.

This understanding of recovery is significantly different compared with more traditional ways of working with people with a mental health condition, which are now often referred to as 'medical models', 'clinical recovery' or 'biomedical approaches' (Slade et al., 2014). Traditionally, the focus of mental health treatment tended to be on diagnosis and recovery from, or control of, symptoms. Recovery in the personal sense, as outlined in this chapter, is different from the medical conception of a 'cure' or a condition being cured or controlled. Recovery is defined by a person's ability to live a life that is meaningful to them, a life that is no longer defined by illness.

The relationship between recovery and treatment

While recovery represents a significant shift in the way we view mental illness and treatment, it does not exclude people from seeking treatment if they require or choose it. Many people seek clinical treatment and continue to use medication as part of their recovery. Recovery, however, shifts power to the person with a mental health condition to explore their own mental health and symptoms and to make choices about how best to alleviate and/or live with symptoms. With the increased emphasis on individual choice and control, many people have found non-medical ways of alleviating their symptoms. Some common examples are physical exercise, meditation, yoga or mindfulness and healthy diets. These approaches are strongly supported by studies that show a strong correlation between physical health and mental health and well-being and the positive impact that diet and exercise can have on a person's mental health (Colton & Manderscheid, 2006; Curtis, Newall & Samaras, 2012; NMHC, 2016). Other non-medical ways or 'personal medicines', as consumer advocate Patricia Deegan (2005) has called them, include: being involved in the arts, working or playing with children, and engaging in intellectual pursuits like maths (Deegan, 2005).

The shift of control from the health system to the consumer has also assisted many people who have experienced trauma. Trauma in large part is an experience of being unable to control or stop something extremely bad from happening. Trauma experience involves a loss of power or being overpowered by other(s) in some way (Clark, Classen, Fourt & Shetty, 2014; Kezelman & Stavropoulos, 2012). For individuals experiencing trauma, the ability to make choices and take control of their own recovery is itself a process of healing and can result in significant improvement in their mental health (Browne & Hemsley, 2008; O'Brien & Golding, 2003; Deegan, 2005; Mead & Copeland, 2000). With recovery-oriented practice and the shift of control from medical interventions to personal choice, there has also been a shift in the way that many people view their symptoms. Many people who 'hear voices', for example, might continue to hear them but, rather than deny them or try to be rid of them, they have decided to 'take ownership' of 'their voices' – deciding when they will listen to them and when they will ignore them (adapted from Hearing Voices, n.d.).

The recovery process and journey

Recovery is often referred to as a '*journey*'. For many people with a mental health condition, it is the '*process*' of recovery that is key. For many who have experienced mental health challenges, the *recovery journey* is not necessarily a straightforward and predictable, time-limited path, as might be the case with healing a broken bone, for example (see **Figure 21.1**). Recovery is often a journey of growth and learning: trialling new ways of living and being, celebrating when things work well and learning from what does not work so well. Recovery is a continuous process of learning, exploration, discovery and relearning – of finding new meaning and purpose.

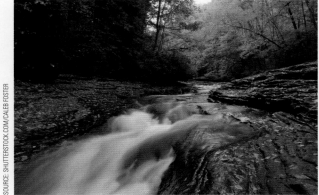

SOURCE: SHUTTERSTOCK.COM/CALEB FOSTER

FIGURE 21.1
Ralph Waldo Emerson famously quoted that life is a journey, not a destination

An early and widely used definition of recovery from Anthony (1993, cited in Slade, 2009, p. 4) encapsulates this in the following description:

> [Recovery is] a deeply personal, unique process of changing one's attitudes, values, feelings, goals, skills, and/or roles. It is a way of living a satisfying, hopeful, and contributing life even within the limitations caused by illness. Recovery involves the development of new meaning and purpose beyond the effects of mental illness.

CULTURAL CONSIDERATIONS

Recovery within cultural traditions
Recovery is about individual choice and power, so differences are already considered as part of the approach. There are, however, cultural considerations regarding how recovery is approached. Some cultures, such as those of Aboriginal and Torres Strait Islander peoples, for example, tend to have stronger connections to family and community than non-Indigenous Australians. This might mean there is more involvement by the family and/or community in a person's recovery journey, and if these ties have been broken, supporting the person to mend these connections might be of vital importance. Spirituality also differs and has different emphases dependent on a person's culture. Cultures also view mental health conditions in varying ways, with some people experiencing significant discrimination, stigma or misunderstanding within their community.

Recognition of recovery as a framework
Recovery is recognised and supported internationally (Deegan, 2005; Jacob, Munro & Taylor, 2015; Slade, 2009). In Australia, the National Mental Health Commission worked with consumers, carers, service providers and other stakeholders to develop a 'contributing life framework' (NMHC, 2013). This framework encapsulates common recovery goals, as depicted in **Figure 21.2**.

A national framework for recovery-oriented mental health
The federal government has also provided a policy platform to support recovery-oriented service provision

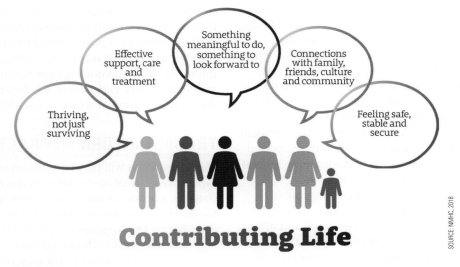

SOURCE: NMHC, 2018

FIGURE 21.2
A contributing life framework

TABLE 21.1
The domains of recovery-oriented practice

DOMAIN	DOMAIN NAME	DOMAIN DESCRIPTION
Domain 1	Promoting a culture and language of hope and optimism	A service culture and language that makes a person feel valued, important, welcome and safe, communicates positive expectations and promotes hope and optimism – central to recovery-oriented practice and service delivery
Domain 2	Person first and holistic	Putting people who experience mental health issues first and at the centre of practice and service delivery; viewing a person's life situation holistically
Domain 3	Supporting personal recovery	Personally defined and led recovery at the heart of practice rather than an additional task
Domain 4	Organisational commitment and workforce development	Service and work environments and an organisational culture that are conducive to recovery and to building a workforce that is appropriately skilled, equipped, supported and resourced for recovery-oriented practice
Domain 5	Action on social inclusion and the social determinants of health, mental health and well-being.	Upholding the human rights of people experiencing mental health issues and challenging stigma and discrimination; advocating to address the poor and unequal living circumstances that adversely impact on recovery.

SOURCE: AHMAC, 2013B

through its *National Framework for Recovery-oriented Mental Health Services: Policy and Theory* (AHMAC, 2013a). The principles of recovery are outlined in the *National Framework for Recovery Oriented Practice: Guide for Practitioners and Providers* (AHMAC, 2013b).

The domains of recovery-oriented practice and service delivery as outlined in this framework are listed and described in **Table 21.1**.

Understanding the domains of recovery-oriented practice

These five domains help nurses to ensure their practice is recovery-oriented by giving guidance on what both the nurse and the mental health service should be doing in this area, providing a useful framework for monitoring and evaluating both professional practice and the practices and culture of the service.

The first domain is about promoting a culture of hope and optimism. This is about believing all people have the capacity to recover and holding this hope for people until they can hold it for themselves. It is about believing in the person's capacity to recover, communicating with them and working with them in hopeful ways that ensure they know the nurse has faith in their capacity.

The second domain is a reminder that mental health nurses (and all members of the multidisciplinary team) are working with whole people, not just a diagnosis or symptoms. While this may appear evident, in clinical settings it is easy to lose sight of the person when care, clinical treatment and maintaining general order can often eclipse personal service.

The third domain is about supporting people to make choices and set goals for their own recovery. It also is a reminder that recovery is personal and unique to each person. While recovery is not necessarily about recovering from symptoms, it is important to note that neither is it the polar opposite to clinical practice or treatment, which can be an important part of somebody's recovery goals.

The fourth domain is focused on changing and adapting workplace cultures and ensuring that staff are trained and resourced to work in recovery-oriented ways. This textbook is an example of this domain in operation. Recovery is not just about how the nurse as an individual works with people, but how the whole mental health team works with people. While many of the concepts of recovery may seem obvious, as they are about basic human decency and respect, moving towards truly recovery-oriented services requires significant cultural change.

The fifth domain is important in creating cultural and social change in and beyond mental health services. It acknowledges that the principles of recovery extend beyond individual service delivery. Recovery is everyone's business, so everyone has a responsibility to take action, of being part of the action to ensure social inclusion and that the social determinants of health promote recovery-oriented practice.

Later in this chapter we explore in more detail how to work with people to support their recovery using these domains and other common features of effective recovery-oriented services. First, however, we examine the effects of trauma on recovery. Being trauma informed – that is, knowing how best to work with people who have experienced significant trauma – is an essential feature of recovery-oriented practice.

TRAUMA-INFORMED PRACTICE

Many consumers will present to health services with an experience of significant trauma. As described in earlier chapters, a history of trauma is a common feature of the development of many mental health conditions (see Chapter 18). For many people, the trauma is long-standing, such as childhood trauma, and their experience of trauma may be the reason or catalyst for their current symptoms of a mental health condition (Clark et al., 2014; Kezelman & Stavropoulos, 2012).

There is also significant trauma experienced in having a mental health condition due to discrimination, relationship breakdown and social and economic marginalisation and disadvantage. The social and life circumstances of many people with mental health challenges are likely to include situations and events that are potentially traumatising. Stigma, poverty, poor or severed family relationships, social exclusion, perpetuating traumatic relationships, homelessness or inappropriate housing can all lead to significant experiences of trauma. People with a mental health condition are also more likely than the general population to be in jail (Ackland, 2011), be the victim of domestic violence or other violent crimes (Clark et al., 2014), or have their children removed from their care (Sheehan & Levine, 2005) – all of which can be traumatic.

There is also significant trauma experienced by consumers within mental health services from the workers purportedly there to help and support them (Clark et al., 2014; LeBel, Huckshorn & Caldwell, 2010). Previous experiences of trauma within health services and with other official establishments, such as criminal justice systems or education institutions, can make it difficult for people to trust others, especially people in positions of authority (Clark et al., 2014).

The recollections of 'Sandra', cited in Thornicroft, Rose and Kassam (2007, p. 114), illustrate how traumatic an incident of restraint and enforced medication can be:

> There were between six and eight staff members, I'm not sure, I can't remember too much. I didn't have a very clear vision. I saw people surrounding me, holding me by the hand, holding me by the legs. I don't think it was something they had to do. There was no talking. They would have helped better if they had more understanding and more talking... more respect. I felt really bad. While I was in hospital I tried to complain but I don't know if anybody was listening. It was a nightmare.

Understanding the potential for trauma and re-traumatisation

People who have been traumatised are at significant risk of being re-traumatised in situations where they feel unsafe. This can also be triggered by situations that remind people of previous trauma. This can happen in mental health services where punitive or coercive practices are used or when the person feels they are being controlled or dominated in some way by others (Clark et al., 2014; Kezelman & Stavropoulos, 2012). When people access the health service, and have experienced trauma in services and other establishments in the past, they may view the practitioner as a threat, as they are seen as a person in authority or part of the establishment. Hence, when people first access the service, the nurse could initially be seen as someone to be feared rather than supportive. How to build a person's trust and alleviate fear are important features of trauma-informed practice and are discussed in more detail in the next sections.

Staff are also at risk of experiencing trauma or being re-traumatised when working in mental health services. With one in five people in the general community affected by a mental health condition at any one time (ABS, 2007), at least this proportion of people working in mental health services may have experienced a mental health condition and many of these will have an experience of significant trauma. In services where staff are fearful of violence or reprisal, or feel they have to act in aggressive or harmful ways to maintain control and safety, staff experience high levels of vicarious trauma (Clark et al., 2014; LeBel, Huckshorn & Caldwell, 2010). The term 'vicarious' means to observe or hear about another person's experience, which can result in the generation of similar 'feelings'. Therefore, vicarious trauma is trauma experienced from hearing a story, or witnessing something traumatic. Trauma-informed services are places where people who have previous experiences of trauma can feel safe from persecution and re-traumatisation. Trauma-informed services are safer for everyone, (Clark et al., 2014; Kezelman & Stavropoulos 2012), as trauma-informed practice reduces the risk of traumatisation, re-traumatisation and vicarious trauma for both consumers and staff.

The first and foremost consideration when working with people who have experienced trauma is to take care not to perpetuate or add to their traumatic experiences (Clark et al., 2014; Kezelman & Stavropoulos, 2012). When working with someone who has experienced or is experiencing trauma, it is important to help them to feel safe. Mental health nurses can help consumers feel safe by asking them what would make them feel most safe, right now, in this place. Because all people are different, have had different experiences and also have different things that help them feel safe, assumptions should never be made about what will make someone feel safe – always ask. For some people, for example, a human touch is reassuring, for others any touch at all would be re-traumatising; and while some people prefer company, others need alone time.

The term trauma-informed practice

We have established that most consumers within clinical mental health settings are likely to have experienced some traumatic events and may be suffering from trauma at the point of entry to the service. In addition to making sure that their current experience is not made more traumatic, there are a number of ways the mental health nurse can work with consumers to help them recover life after trauma. This is called **trauma-informed care/practice**.

The word *practice* is used in this chapter because the concept of care does not fit with the recovery model. While most nurses working in the mental health field do so because they care *about* people, it is important, in shifting power to self-determination, that we move away from caring *for* people, and instead *support people to care for themselves* to their capacity.

Features of trauma-informed practice

Trauma-informed practice has the following features:
- recognition that most service users and many staff members may have experienced significant trauma
- conscious and active design of practices and environments aimed at ensuring that people feel safe and are not traumatised or re-traumatised
- respectful acknowledgement and interest in the role that trauma may have played in a person's life experience and possibly their experience of mental health challenges
- strengths-based practice – honouring the person's resilience and survival in the face of trauma
- recovery-oriented – choice, and control in particular, are important features when working with people who have experienced significant loss of choice and control.

Creating trust and safety on arrival

Many people enter mental health services in traumatic circumstances; for example, the experience of being restrained and brought into an emergency department by armed police would be traumatic for most people. When people arrive in the service, staff need to consider what their last 12 to 24 hours may have been like.

Part of the job of the mental health nurse is to help people to feel welcome and safe upon point of entry. Unfortunately, history and the environment are often working against the mental health nurse in achieving this. The person might have been at this or similar services before when they did not feel safe, heard or respected, and felt and were hurt. Furthermore, the closing of the locked doors, an over-lit clinical setting and the glass 'fishbowl' of the staff station, can all project feelings of fear and hurt.

The most important thing you can do at the point of entry is to make the person feel welcome and safe. Some things that you can do to help people to feel welcome and safe are:
- come out to meet them, making an effort to ensure they are feeling welcomed, safe and comfortable
- greeting them with a mindset of being pleased they are there and hopeful that they can be supported to recover
- asking them what would make them feel safer
- taking an interest in them

- orienting them to the environment (e.g., location of room, toilet, telephone, communal areas etc.).

Once you know something about them, there are a number of things you can do to help them settle in depending on their preferences. These include:
- giving them some space or solitude, if this is what they ask for (assessments can wait until a little later)
- providing some physical comfort – a quiet room, warm socks, headphones, weighted blanket (see more on sensory tools and environments below)
- introducing them to other people living at the service. This should be done as soon as the person is ready – it can be daunting to suddenly be living with strangers
- giving them something to do – a useful task or activity
- giving them more information about the service and their rights and responsibilities.

Focusing on strengths and resilience

Being trauma informed is not necessarily about knowing all the details of someone's trauma. Retelling trauma details can be re-traumatising and knowing the details of someone's trauma is not usually necessary to work with them to support their recovery. If a person trusts the mental health nurse and feels ready to tell them details of their experiences, however, this can be a great step in developing an empathetic relationship.

When people tell their story, keep in mind the following:
- Be careful not to judge – you have not lived their life (see **Figure 21.3**).
- Show interest without pushing for more details than they are ready to share.
- Share something of yourself to ensure the exchange is reciprocal and more balanced (see Chapter 5 on self disclosure).
- Acknowledge the enormity (for them) of what they have experienced, but do not dwell on it.
- Take your lead from the person as to how dreadful or shocking their story is. Be careful not to overdramatise based on your own experiences – this will feel like judgement.

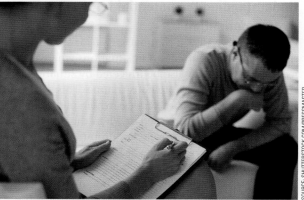

SOURCE: SHUTTERSTOCK.COM/PRESSMASTER

FIGURE 21.3
When people tell their story, it is important not to judge them

- Thank them for trusting you and honouring you to hear their story.
- Comment on or ask questions that highlight where they drew on their own strengths and resilience.
- Remind them of any obligations you might have to share certain details of their story with others and the reason for doing this (do this before they share any details with you and also advise them during and afterwards of any details you will need to pass on to other members of the multidisciplinary team).

Trauma-informed for all

Trauma-informed practice benefits everyone: people who have experienced trauma, other service users and staff, whether they know about the consumer's story or not. Trauma-informed practice will minimise or eliminate the possibility of people experiencing further trauma within the health service. Furthermore, integrating trauma-informed practice within a recovery-oriented service provision opens up

opportunities for people to obtain tools, support and personal insight into their own strengths, resilience and power. All of these can help them to overcome the negative effects of previous trauma and help them to armour themselves against the negative effects of future traumatic events (Deegan, 2005; Mead & Copeland, 2000). People usually will not want to tell a nurse about their trauma until they trust them. It is important not to insist or push someone for information they are unable or unwilling to share at this time.

Consumers can still be supported in trauma-informed ways without having revealed the details of their experiences. Trauma-informed practice involves working with everyone on the basis they may have experienced trauma – it is about creating safer environments, finding out what makes people feel safe, developing trusting relationships and supporting people in their recovery.

EVIDENCE-BASED PRACTICE

Increasing understanding of trauma-informed care

Title of study

Safe and collaborative communication skills: A step towards mental health nurses implementing trauma-informed care

Authors

Sophie Isobel and Cynthia Delgado

Background

The authors of this paper identify that a challenge in implementing trauma-informed care (TIC) relates to the lack of clarity in translating the philosophy of TIC into practice. The authors argue that while successful implementation of TIC requires changes at all levels of mental health service delivery, mental health nurses through their use of therapeutic use of self and the nurse–consumer/carer relationship are in a pivotal position to use principles of TIC in their daily interactions and collaboration with consumers. The authors describe the delivery and evaluation of a trauma-informed communication workshop, which focused on an increased understanding of the possible impact to consumers because of trauma and developing communication strategies that would be implemented as part of their daily interactions with consumers.

Design and participants

Seventy-three registered nurses working in acute inpatient mental health were invited to attend 10 one-day workshops over a two-year period. The workshop included establishing the use of practical strength-based and communication exercises, discussion of the neurobiological and psychological impacts of trauma and the use of two role

play scenarios based on clinical experience of the workshop developers with a simulated consumer (paid actor). In these scenarios, staff interacted with the actor using a trauma-informed approach. The workshop concluded with a discussion on the use of peer support and clinical supervision in sustaining reflective practice.

A 5-point Likert scale questionnaire was used to capture workshop participants' thoughts about the benefits of the workshop and to assist in ongoing development of future workshops.

Results

The authors report that while participants were initially concerned about and resistant to the use of role play, their feedback indicated they found the process enlightening in terms of their own practice and that of their colleagues.

Conclusion

While peer feedback and reflection was at times uncomfortable, it was seen as very useful. The questionnaire responses showed that participants had limited self-reported knowledge of TIC prior to the workshop. The workshop experience improved this understanding, particularly in relation to how to incorporate TIC into their daily practice.

Implications

Clinicians such as mental health nurses need to understand and recognise the possible impacts of trauma on consumers and develop communication approaches to implement trauma-informed care into their practice.

SOURCE: ISOBEL, S. & DELGADO, C. (2018). SAFE AND COLLABORATIVE COMMUNICATION SKILLS: A STEP TOWARDS MENTAL HEALTH NURSES IMPLEMENTING TRAUMA INFORMED CARE. *ARCHIVES OF PSYCHIATRIC NURSING*, 32(2), 291–6. DOI:HTTPS://DOI.ORG/10.1016/J.APNU.2017.11.017

WORKING WITH PEOPLE

While recovery is a personal and consumer-directed journey, it is often a journey that is shared. Many people need or appreciate help and support to recover, and the nurse plays a vital role in this. The key things the practitioner can do to support a person's recovery are to:

- believe in their ability and capacity to recover and hold hope for the person
- work with the person, not on symptoms
- take a holistic approach to the person's health
- support choice
- encourage and facilitate participation
- take the time to build trust.

These and some other strategies are expanded on below.

Be hopeful

First and foremost, recovery is about hope. In working in a recovery-oriented way, it is important that for the nurse to believe, and be seen to believe, in the recovery of the people they work with. No matter how unwell a person is, there are always things to be hopeful about, at that particular moment and into the future.

Often people have lost hope through life experiences, where they may have been judged by themselves and others as failing in some way. Many people with a mental health condition have also been given a diagnosis accompanied by a damning prognosis that appeared to banish any hope of living a meaningful life (Mead & Copeland, 2000). We now know that people with a mental health condition can and do recover (Deegan, 2005). If the nurse can effectively show someone that they believe in them and their recovery, holding their hope for them until they can believe in themselves, this is a wonderful gift from which they can build their recovery (Russinova, 1999). Weick and Chamberlain (2000) have observed: 'Professionals communicating their belief in the inner strength and resourcefulness of a person, family, or community becomes the beginning step in restoring people's faith in themselves and in their capacity to influence the shape of their lives.'

Communicating hope

When holding hope for someone it is important to be aware of, acknowledge and communicate hope in ways that are congruent with the individual's life experiences and perception of reality. People who have suffered severe trauma can have difficulty being hopeful about what might be seen to them as hopeless (Coulter, 2014). As Coulter (2014, p. 55) observes:

> Trauma has the potential to lead to major psychological pathology and one must be particularly aware of avoiding adopting an inappropriately 'sunny' or overoptimistic disposition when engaging victims/survivors in a therapeutic process, as this would probably be received by the client as disrespectful or minimising of their experience.

A focus on hope may also lose relevance in different cultural contexts or when working with people who belong to or identify with communities where people have experienced significant marginalisation or adversity. Saunders, Sherwood and Usher (2015), for example, found that for Indigenous Australians living in communities where disadvantage is high, hope is difficult to envisage. Berry et al. (2011, p. 125S) also found that for many people who live in rural and remote communities, declining economic conditions and extreme climatic conditions can 'lead to an experience of hopelessness at a community level… undermined cohesion in many communities, and just living in a declining area is detrimental to mental health'.

Nevertheless, being hopeful and holding hope for others not only assists people in their recovery but is also a much healthier way for the mental health nurse to work. Mental health services can be very difficult places to work in. Having hope and faith in the people they are working with and, perhaps more importantly, faith in one's capacity to support people to recover, results in higher work satisfaction and safer workplaces for all, both physically and emotionally. In contrast, despair, hopelessness and a lack of faith in the effectiveness of the nurse's work can lead to burnout and physical and mental health issues (Delaney, 2006). A workplace where people feel hopeless or ineffective can also lead to a culture of fear where there is increased use of draconian, punitive practices as a way of attempting to regain control (Brophy et al., 2016). Fearful, unhopeful workplaces where draconian measures are adopted to keep order instigate and perpetuate trauma for service users and staff (Clark et al., 2014; Delaney, 2006).

Work with the person, not on symptoms or diagnosis

Recovery relates to the person and their life, not their mental health condition. Recovery-oriented service is about working *with* people, not *on* people or even *for* people. When we work with people we find out what works best for them, what motivates them, what makes them laugh and what upsets them. We also share some of ourselves and find out new things about ourselves as working with people is a reciprocal activity, not a one-way street. People are much more than their mental health condition, and taking the time to find out who they are is always worthwhile. Do they have any children, pets, other relatives, carers? What do they want from life? What do they want from you? How can you support them to 'meet the challenges' to achieve their aspirations?

People want to recover and engage and contribute to society. Prominent survivor advocate Patricia Deegan (n.d., para 3) articulates the aspirations of people with mental health challenges: 'The need is to meet the challenge of the disability and to re-establish a new and valued sense of integrity and purpose within and beyond the limits of the disability; the aspiration is to live, work and love in a community in which one makes a significant contribution'.

Recovery is also about the whole of life – not just about today, but about yesterday and tomorrow. Mental health recovery works for all ages. Everyone from the youngest to oldest person has the capacity to recover.

Take a holistic approach to the person's health

Working with people holistically to support their recovery includes considering a person's physical health. Physical and mental health are closely aligned. People with a mental health condition have a higher mortality rate than the general population (Ahire et al., 2013; Lambert et al., 2017). Many people with a mental health condition die earlier, with estimates being 14–23 years earlier than the average mortality age of the general population (NMHC, 2016).

Furthermore, most die from diseases and conditions that are not directly related to their mental health condition (Ahire et al., 2013; NMHC, 2016). Social and economic disadvantage, discrimination and side effects of medication are the main reasons people with a mental health condition are more likely to die up to 17 years earlier than the general population. They also are more likely to have diabetes, to smoke, have poor dental health, and experience side effects from medications, including significant and rapid weight gain and poor circulation, increasing risk of metabolic syndrome which can lead to heart disease and stroke (Colton & Manderscheid, 2006; Curtis et al., 2012; Lambert et al., 2017; NMHC, 2016).

The NMHC has launched an awareness campaign called 'Equally-Well: Quality of Life – Equality in Life' aimed at improving the physical health of people living with a mental health condition in Australia. **Figure 21.4** demonstrates this need for a more holistic approach to health for people who have a mental health condition.

Discrimination, which can lead to inadequate and inappropriate physical health interventions for people with a mental health condition, occurs within health services (Coffey, 2009). Many people have had experiences of being denied proper treatment for physical illness or injury due to a focus on their mental health history that has led to discrimination or mistreatment (Happell et al., 2016; Thornicroft, Rose & Kassam, 2007). This includes: people being triaged into mental health facilities when they have broken bones or other obvious physical injuries or medical conditions; people known to have a mental health condition being denied an ambulance without a police escort when there are no symptoms of a mental health condition; and physical health issues not being noticed or overlooked due to the focus on the mental health issues (Coffey, 2009; Happell, Platania-Phung & Scott, 2013; Thornicroft, Rose & Kassam, 2007).

People with severe mental illness are particularly at risk. They are:

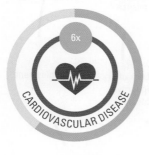

Six times more likely to die from cardiovascular disease.

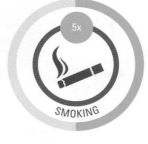

Five times more likely to smoke.

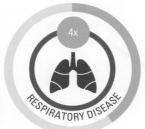

Four times more likely to die from respiratory disease.

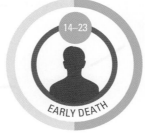

Likely to die between 14 and 23 years earlier than the general population.

SOURCE: NMHC, 2016, P. 10

FIGURE 21.4
The need for a more holistic approach to health

The recovery-oriented mental health practitioner should be interested in and mindful of people's physical health needs as well as their mental health needs. Supporting a person to visit the dentist, change their diet and exercise regimen or talk to the doctor about changing their medication (if the side effects are of concern to them) can significantly contribute to their mental recovery and well-being as well as improving their physical health (Curtis, Newell & Samaras, 2012; Lambert et al., 2017; NMHC, 2016). The need to care for all aspects of a person's well-being is also specified in the standards of practice for mental health nurses, which state: 'The mental health nurse collaboratively plans and provides ethically based care consistent with the mental, physical, spiritual, emotional, social and cultural needs of the individual' (ACMHN, 2010, p. 6).

When working with people holistically, it is important to consider the many different factors that may have contributed to their current mental and physical health challenges. The well-being consensus showing many of the factors that can contribute to both poor physical and mental health is depicted in **Figure 21.5**.

Support and facilitate choice

Often in traditional practice, people who have difficulties accessing and retaining information would be seen as lacking 'capacity' and have choices made for them (Browne & Hemsley, 2008). In a recovery-oriented service, staff work with the person to establish the best ways to present information to them at the time and to adapt the delivery of information to ensure the person can both access and process it. No matter how unwell a person is, they usually have capacity to make some choices. The health worker's role is to work with them to establish the level of choices that they are comfortable with making at the time. Mental health legislation can limit some of the choices people can make when they are unwell (see Chapter 3). It is important that nurses are clear about exactly what choices people can make and those they are not able to make and to communicate this clearly to them. It is also important that legislation is not

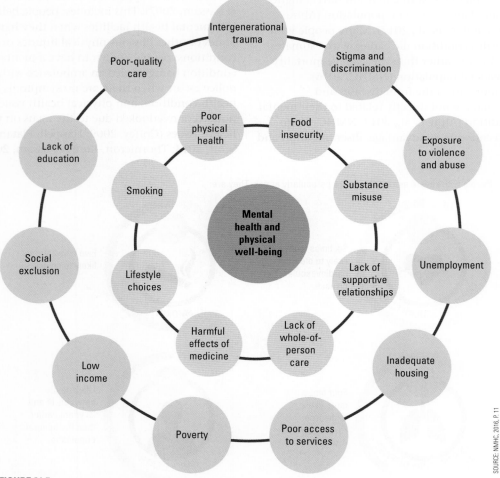

SOURCE: NMHC, 2016, P. 11

FIGURE 21.5
The many factors that can contribute to poor physical and mental health

used to prevent the person from making choices that are not prohibited by that legislation. No matter how unwell a person appears to be, they should always be asked if they would like to choose if they are able to, and be well informed about what has been decided on their behalf and why, when they do not have a choice. When people are engaged in these ways, they usually have a much greater capacity to make informed choices than their current behaviour or level of symptoms may indicate.

Choices and limitations

When we are discussing choice, it is important to acknowledge that the mental health nurse also has a number of limitations on the choices that they can make within the workplace. In mental health settings, nurses will be working under legislation, policy and guidelines that limit their choices about how to work with consumers. It is important not to give people the impression they have choices when the choice is unfair or not really a choice at all. When supporting people to make their own choices, nurses must ensure that the choices communicated are realistic and fit within the choices that are able to be made. An example of this might be where the person chooses, as part of their recovery goals, not to take medication, but they are under a legal directive that includes they must take medication. They may have choices, however, about which medication they take, how they take it and how long they take it for. In discussing choice in this situation, it would be important to be realistic about the limitations of the person's choices and to help them to make choices within these limitations. The nurse might also be able to support them to set goals for working towards a reduction in medication or a lifting of legislative requirements with improved self-regulation. Even in this example, the consumer still has a choice to not take their medication willingly. The nurse's role in this case would be to ensure that the person fully understands the likely outcomes of this choice. To maintain a relationship of trust and respect, the nurse should also consider discussing with them what their own limited choices would be in such a scenario and what they would be required to do as part of their job in complying with the legal requirements of the person's treatment if they did not themselves comply. To be able to do this effectively, the nurse also needs to know the limits and consequences of their choices when working with people in their particular workplace.

Supporting and facilitating participation

The participation of people who have a mental health condition is a very important feature of recovery-oriented service delivery. It is important that people with a mental health condition (and people more generally) are able to participate in all decisions that affect them (Browne & Hemsley, 2009). The adage 'Nothing about us without us' is just as relevant in the mental health sector as it is in the rest of the disability sector (Deegan, 2005).

Participation of mental health consumers should occur at all levels, from individual case planning; to service delivery and service quality improvement processes; to service advisory and governance processes; and also at state and national policy levels. Participation is a fundamental human right as enshrined in Article 25 of the International Covenant of Civil and Political Rights (United Nations, 1976).

Consumer and carer participation is also mandated in many government policies, including in the National Standards for Mental Health Services (Department of Health and Ageing, 2010): 'Standard 3. Consumer and carer participation' where mental health services are directed to ensure that: 'Consumers and carers are actively involved in the development, planning, delivery and evaluation of services'.

The benefits of participation

Participation results in better services, policies, guidelines, laws and practices, and also facilitates individual recovery (Browne & Hemsley, 2009). Ensuring the people you work with are supported to participate in their own recovery, and the running and improvement of your services, is not only the right thing to do, it is the best thing to do. Participation of people in their own treatment and recovery is a crucial element of recovery. We know that coercion hinders and stalls recovery (Brophy et al., 2016), and we also know that people do not recover just because other people would like them to. Recovery from a mental health condition is a personal journey (Slade, 2009). No matter how hard others work to assist a person to recover, they cannot make them recover. Recovery can only occur once the person owns and drives their own recovery.

Roles when participating

If there is a team of people working with a person, the consumer should be the team leader of their own recovery. As outlined earlier in this chapter, recovery is about personal choice and personal direction; it is not about what clinicians, psychiatrists, nurses, social workers or even family believe is the best thing for the person. While all of these people can make important and useful contributions to people's recovery, ultimately, the only person who can actually enact and drive their recovery is the person themselves (Deegan, 2005; Mead & Copeland, 2000).

The mental health practitioner has an important role in supporting and facilitating people to lead their own recovery. The mental health nurse is an important member of the 'recovery support team', as they hold specific expertise and experience that the service user and other members of the team may not have. A good team has members with a diversity of expertise and experience on which to draw. All other members of the team also hold specific expertise and experience that they can contribute. The consumer, and often their families and significant others, will also have particular knowledge, expertise and experience that no one else can know (Jacob, Munro & Taylor, 2015).

Focus on people's strengths and resilience

Recovery is a strengths-based practice. With the focus on what people can do rather than on what they cannot do, recovery allows people to take control of their life and shift their focus from their illness to their future. Traditional approaches tend to be deficit focused, which means they focus on symptoms and behaviours seen to be inappropriate. When the focus is on deficits, the person often feels helpless, hopeless and often identifies as a victim. In the deficit model of practice, the person is more likely to stay reliant and dependent on a system that is keeping them unwell (Deegan, 2005; Mead & Copeland, 2000). On the other hand, a focus on a person's strengths and resilience can shift their view of themselves from *victim* to *survivor*. It is important to work from a framework that acknowledges that everyone has strengths from which they can draw. The mental health nurse's job is to help people identify and recognise their strengths and to draw on them in their recovery journey. As Deegan observes: '…we learn that even when people present with obvious vulnerabilities they also have strengths. Their strengths are in their passions, in their skills, in their interests, in their relationships and in their environments. If mental health practitioners look for strengths they will find them' (cited in Rapp & Goscha, 2011).

When you work with people that have experienced significant trauma it is very helpful to identify and focus on the person's strengths, and recognise and acknowledge their resilience and the strategies they have used to survive (Coulter, 2014). Resilience indicates a capacity to resist stress and cope with adverse conditions. It derives from the Latin word '*resilio*', meaning to adapt and bounce back from a disruptive event (Coulter, 2014).

The capacity for resilience is the reason people can and do recover from a mental health condition. It is this confidence in people's resilience that allows us to hold hope for people. People who have experienced significant adversity have demonstrated the capacity '…to adapt, cope, rebound, withstand, grow, survive,

and define a new sense of self' (Ridgway, 2004, cited in Deegan, 2005, p. 29).

People with a mental health condition demonstrate a great capacity for resilience. In every traumatic situation people express or enact some level of resilience even if they are not consciously aware of it. People with a mental health condition are often seen and spoken about as being 'out of control', 'lacking insight' or 'self-destructive', when the reverse is often the case. Symptoms of a mental health condition or behaviours labelled as inappropriate might be very appropriate within the context of the person's experience. Mental illness itself is often the body and mind's way of surviving significant trauma (Kezelman & Stavropoulos, 2012). When working with people who have experienced significant trauma, the best questions to ask them are ones like: 'How did you survive? How is it you are still here to talk with me today?'

When people with a mental health condition tell their story, the nurse should focus their questions and comments on the strengths they demonstrated and their resilience in the face of adversity. The details of the trauma will largely include actions and situations over which the person may have felt they had little or no control and retelling the details can remind them of their powerlessness and feelings of fear and failure. Conversely, when they are helped to consider where they demonstrated strength and resilience in their life story, the focus can be brought to where they held power and made positive decisions. This can help the consumer to reframe their story, providing space and opportunity for healing. As Coulter (2014) has observed: 'Glimmers of hope and optimism can arise through the interviewing process itself, even following extreme trauma. A first step is to encourage clients to move from a relatively helpless victim position to that of a survivor, when a more active role becomes possible' (Coulter, 2014, p. 55).

Bannink (2008, p. 220, cited in Coulter, 2014, p. 55) suggests some key questions to assist people to reframe their experience from being a *victim* to being a *survivor*. These are:

- What helped in the past, even if only marginally?
- How do you succeed in getting from one moment to the next?
- Could it be worse than it is? Why is it not worse?

Support access to treatment and care when required

Recovery is not the polar opposite of clinical approaches. Most consumers with a serious mental health condition find some clinical treatment and medications complementary or enabling in their recovery. Many people are interested in alleviating the symptoms of their illness that might hinder their recovery. The emphasis or focus of recovery, however, is inverse. Traditional medical and clinical approaches focus on and work *on* the illness, and recovery from this viewpoint would be an absence or alleviation of symptoms. The recovery approach, conversely, focuses on and works *with* the person, and any medical or clinical treatment would be part of the recovery plan guided by the person rather than being the main focus.

It is important to acknowledge that when recovery was first introduced, the comparison with clinical approaches was much more polarised. In early evolutions of the recovery model there were often tables that outlined the differences between clinical and personal recovery. Recovery is part of a social movement aimed at addressing social inequalities, breaches of human rights and a reclaiming of power (Deegan, 2005). The word itself is reclaiming a known word that clinically, and perhaps even colloquially, has a 'recovery from symptoms' meaning. People who had been hurt and disempowered by impersonal, punitive treatments saw recovery as a way of reclaiming lost power, so it is not surprising that earlier proponents of the recovery approach were against traditional approaches; a prominent section of the movement of this time was called 'anti-psychiatry' (Murray, 2014).

As recovery is about choice and recovering life, however, an individual's recovery can include traditional, clinical treatment. Many people will choose to seek treatment and/or take medication as part of their recovery. This is where the expertise and support of the mental health nurse will often be sought, as part of the role to support and assist the consumer's recovery, keeping in mind that, historically, mental health treatments disempowered and severely hurt people.

Build trust and rapport

As noted, recovery is about building trust and rapport with the consumer. Building trust is not the same as making friends, although trust is an important part of friendship. An essential part of building trust is being truthful and authentic. As discussed above, there will be boundaries within the mental health service workplace that will limit choices. In a truthful, authentic relationship, it is important to be clear about these boundaries and rules. Also important in building trust is being clear about the nature of the relationship within the mental health service, and how rules, boundaries and roles can affect the power within the relationship. In almost all cases, the nurse will have more power in this relationship than the consumer. To build and maintain trust, it is important to acknowledge this.

Rapport requires reciprocation, with people being prepared to share something of themselves, show their humanity and show vulnerabilities. Well-known mental health 'survivors' Shery Mead and Mary Ellen Copeland (2000, p. 320) discuss the importance and power of reciprocation:

> Health care professionals need to relate to us that they have their own struggles and own that change is hard for all. They need to look at our willingness to 'recover' and not perpetuate the myth that there is a big difference between themselves and people they work with.

Trust is not something that can be demanded from another person. It has to be earned. It is also something that often takes time to build, especially when working with people who have been hurt or betrayed by others they have trusted in the past, perhaps even with mental health services. Hence, as Rapp (1998) points out, finding ways to meaningfully engage with people is an important first step in building trust: 'Given the importance of the relationship as the bedrock of work, and the painful histories of professional and interpersonal relationships experienced by people with a severe mental health condition, engagement is viewed as the indispensable and critical first step'.

Once the nurse has earned the consumer's trust, the nurse has a responsibility to esteem and respect that trust. It is important to always remember that it can be more disempowering and harmful for a person to feel betrayed by someone whom they trusted than by someone they did not trust. Nevertheless, building trust is a very important step in building an effective relationship with another person and effectively supporting the consumer in their recovery.

Use respectful, recovery-oriented language

Communication is key, but the type of communication is also extremely important. You may have noticed that we have underlined subtle differences in phrases such as 'working *with* people, not *on* them', which demonstrate how changing one word in a sentence can change the meaning.

Language is an important factor in mental health recovery. The way we use and interpret language can empower or disempower. We can discriminate, stigmatise and exclude people through words, even inadvertently. The Devon Partnership Trust and Torbay Care Trust (2008, p. 2, cited in MHCC NSW, 2013, p. 1) emphasises: 'Words are important. The language we use and the stories we tell have great significance to all involved. They carry a sense of hope and possibility or can be associated with a sense of pessimism and low expectations, both of which can influence personal outcomes.'

To support people through recovery it is important that we use language that promotes and supports recovery. To ensure recovery-oriented language is used, talk to people as people, taking care not to reduce people to symptoms, behaviours or diagnosis in the words used directly to them or when talking to others about them – including when writing in their file.

To avoid discriminatory language and remain focused on a person as a whole, it is important to use person first language (as you would also do with someone with a disability); for example, phrases such as a 'person with mental health challenges' as opposed to a 'mentally ill person'.

When talking about a person's behaviour it is important to accurately describe the behaviour rather than label it. Many of the labels commonly used in mental health settings are derogatory and unhelpful and often block our ability to see what is really going on for the person; for example, a label of 'manic' in a file or handover instead of a description that a person was 'having difficulty sleeping' could mean the reasons why the person was not sleeping and how they could best be helped are not explored. Disrespectful language and derogatory labels can also perpetuate power imbalances within mental health services, further disempowering consumers. Derogatory comments about mental illness or about people who have mental health challenges can make the workplace unsafe for colleagues who may also have an experience of mental health challenges.

Create and support environments that aid recovery

Recovery occurs in environments that are supportive of recovery. This is not just about the culture of the service or style of working with people, but the working environment. Environments that support recovery are environments where people feel safe, comfortable, respected and important as human beings.

Often mental services are designed to control and regulate service users, rather than work with them. They often have locked doors and safe areas such as glass lockable offices from where staff can observe consumers. On the other hand, there is often no corresponding safe area for consumers or places where they can go to be alone, be unobserved or have a quiet conversation. Many mental health services have features that perpetuate coercive measures such as seclusion rooms while having few or no environmental features that encourage or facilitate self-regulation or support de-escalation such as sensory rooms (Brophy et al., 2016).

While the justification for mental health services to be designed in these ways is, ironically, to ensure safety, environments where people feel unsafe, disrespected or disregarded make people fearful and/or resentful and increase the risk of violence within the service (Brophy et al., 2016; O'Brien & Golding, 2003). This is beginning to be recognised and the physical design of services is slowly changing, corresponding with the nation-wide quest to reduce the incidence of seclusion and restraint within public mental health services (Brophy

et al., 2016; NMHCCF, 2009). There also has been a corresponding development in what practitioners can do as alternatives to restraining or secluding people. One set of tools that is being recognised and used more in mental health settings is sensory modulation approaches. These might include further use of occupational therapy focusing on sensory modulation and setting up environments and using tools (or 'toys') that support sensory modulation (Champagne & Koomar, 2012) – see **Figures 21.6** and **21.7**.

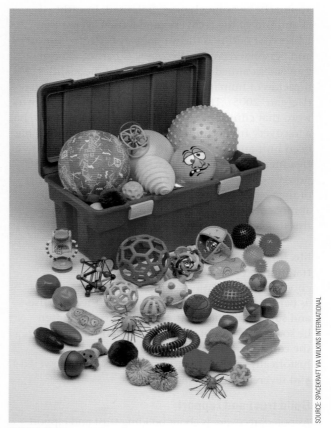

SOURCE: SPACEKRAFT VIA WILKINS INTERNATIONAL

FIGURE 21.6
A sensory toolkit

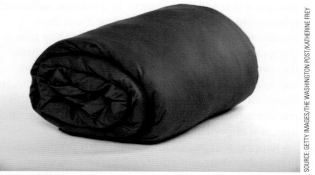

SOURCE: GETTY IMAGES/THE WASHINGTON POST/KATHERINE FREY

FIGURE 21.7
Weighted blankets can have an immediate calming effect

The mental health practitioner has many options to make the physical environment within the service more recovery oriented. These include:

- using soft furnishings – cushions and soft toys
- turning the seclusion room into a self-opted time-out room with sensory 'toys', weighted blankets, socks, soft music (and headphones), soft comforting furniture and lighting that can be dimmed
- painting walls softer colours, with furnishings in good condition and as welcoming and homely as possible
- not putting cages around the television or other items of value – this not only affects the quality of picture/sound but clearly says, 'We don't trust you' or 'We think you will break this'; some people may perceive that there are violent people around and the space is not safe. If items are in good condition and work properly, most people will respect them
- coming out as often as possible from the glass office and talking to people, and never using the glass as a barrier to ignore people or keep them waiting. Some services now have windows that are kept open to lessen the barrier.

BE AN 'AGENT OF CHANGE' FOR RECOVERY-ORIENTED AND TRAUMA-INFORMED PRACTICES

Although both recovery-oriented and trauma-informed practice are well supported in theory and policy, there is still some way to go before these approaches are fully embedded at the frontline within mental health services. Practices in many services are still dominated by traditional medical and clinical approaches that emphasis diagnosis, control and cure (Deegan, 2005; Mead & Copeland, 2000). Interventions, such as seclusion and restraint, are still widely used in residential mental health services (Brophy et al., 2016) and Mental Health Acts in all states and territories in Australia continue to legalise and condone enforced treatments, which are contrary to recovery principles and human rights (Brophy et al., 2016).

Graham Thornicroft, in his book *Shunned* (2006, cited in Coffey, 2009), found that professional workers specifically trained and educated to work with people with a mental health condition are seen by those in receipt of services as some of the most pessimistic and negative towards mental illness. Furthermore, Thornicroft found that those receiving care see that the therapeutic relationship, '(blending care, concern and threat) is at best a mixed blessing, and at worst a dishonest amalgam of both help and control' (Thornicroft, 2006, p. 153, cited in Coffey, 2009).

Service provision is changing as awareness and understanding of recovery-oriented and trauma-informed practice increases. However, it is difficult for many people who have been working in a particular way for many years to change how they work (Glisson & Williams, 2015; Mead & Copeland, 2000; Newman, O'Reilly, Lee & Kennedy, 2015) and there is pushback from some clinicians who believe that their current practice does not need changing (Lauritzen, Reedtz, Van Doesum & Martinussen, 2014) and/or are concerned about relinquishing power and control related to existing hierarchies (LeBel, 2006; Park et al., 2014). Hence, culture change takes time and can be very challenging to achieve where the existing culture is strong and resistant to change (Glisson & Williams, 2015). Culture change to ensure recovery-oriented service provision depends on current nurses being open to new learning and innovation and new nurses coming into the service with new knowledge (Lauritzen et al., 2014; Park et al., 2014) in addition to **peer workers** being embedded in services in advisory and peer support roles (Gillard & Holley, 2014; NMHC, n.d.).

As outlined in **Table 21.1**, Domain 5 in the *National Framework for Recovery-oriented Mental Health Services* is 'Organisational commitment and workforce development' (AHMAC, 2013b). The practitioner who understands the benefits of recovery-oriented and trauma-informed practice, and the disadvantages and dangers of more traditional approaches, has a responsibility to ensure their practice is recovery-oriented and trauma-informed, and has a role to play in assisting their service and team members to also understand and work in recovery-oriented and trauma-informed ways. This can be achieved by demonstrating recovery-oriented and trauma-informed practice; respectfully questioning unhelpful or harmful language or practices; mentoring other staff; and supporting and advocating for peer workers in the service and engaging in regular personal and team reflection of practice (discussed below).

THE PEER WORKFORCE AND RECOVERY

Another important element of recovery support is the role that peer workers play. Peer supporters or workers are people who have a lived experience of mental health challenges who work or volunteer in roles where they draw on their own lived experience to support other consumers and/or the consumer movement more broadly.

A peer support relationship is equal and mutual, with an emphasis on learning together. In the intentional peer support model, people learn how to respectfully challenge each other to move out of the passive 'patient role' and start moving on with the rest of their lives. It is described as: 'People with lived experience have unique expertise that can be transformative for people who access services, their families, carers and for mental health services and systems' (Mental Health Commission of NSW, 2016, p. 1).

Peer workers are experts by experience. Employing peer workers has a positive impact on the quality of services and client outcomes. Consumers can more readily relate to and trust other people who have experience of a mental health condition or mental health challenges and, by the fact that they are now employed and are seen by service users to be functioning professionally and socially at a high level, they provide evidence of recovery and engender hope. As Julie Repper, Associate Professor of Recovery, University of Nottingham (cited in Mental Health Commission of NSW, 2016, p. 3) points out: 'Peer workers stand as a living testimony to the potential of everyone with mental health problems to recover.' Fay Jackson, Deputy Commissioner Mental Health Commission of NSW (2014, cited in Mental Health Commission of NSW, 2016, p. 4) supports this with the observation that: 'Peer workers model recovery and resilience to the people they support, other staff, partners, families, other services and the community at large'.

Services also often find that peer workers are an invaluable source of information and advice on how best to work with people in recovery-oriented approaches. As people with an experience of mental illness, many peer workers have experienced significant trauma (Rossiter et al., 2015), including within mental health services (Bonner, Lowe, Rawcliffe & Wellman, 2002). Peer workers are also often supportive in shifting the culture of the service to more recovery-oriented and trauma-informed in their approaches.

The benefits of peer support work are well recognised in Australian policy and guidelines. The Summary of Actions within the Australian Government Response to Recommendations to the National Mental Health Commission's review of Mental Health Programmes and Services (2014), for example, states:

> The Commonwealth… recognises the value of a mental health peer workforce…. The National Mental Health Commission has also progressed important work in this area and will be looked to in building upon existing work and further promoting the mental health peer workforce as an important component of quality, recovery-focused mental health services.

In 2013, the NMHC funded the development of training resources for a nationally recognised qualification for peer workers, the Certificate IV in Mental Health Peer Work, in recognition of this growing workforce and the value that peer workers provide for consumers and services (NMHC, n.d.).

Learning from peer workers

Peer workers have unique qualities and expertise that cannot be emulated, and there is much that other non-peer workers can learn from them. Peer workers tend to be better at building trust and rapport with service users than non-peer staff. While this is largely due to the recognition of shared experiences and understandings, it is also because peer workers tend to be less judgemental and less restricted by real, or imagined, culture-driven assumptions, boundaries and hierarchies that can prevent clinical and other staff within mental health services from developing real rapport with service users. 'Peer support holds minimal assumptions about people's capabilities and limits. It avoids categories and hierarchical roles' (Mead & Copeland, 2000, p. 319).

Peer workers are more able to develop and support reciprocal relationships where they also share something of themselves with service users so that their engagements tend to entail some level of mutual support. According to Mead and Copeland (2000, p. 319), 'mutual support is a process in which the people in the relationship strive to use the relationship to become fuller, richer humans'. Newman et al. (2015, p. 172) found that building relationships was a key element of good recovery-oriented service delivery and that 'there is a need for a fundamental shift in the context of the provider–service user relationship to fully facilitate service users' engagement in their care' to facilitate and support recovery. Clinicians and other practitioners often cite or use current boundaries and professional guidelines as reasons not to engage in authentic reciprocal relationships. This merely upholds unhelpful and unnecessary power imbalances that can re-traumatise and disempower people. This is rarely done deliberately. Perhaps the biggest block for mental health clinicians in building rapport with and having mutual support-type engagements with consumers is the idea of 'caring' *for* people. Caring for people can be the antithesis of recovery – caring keeps people dependent, perpetuates power imbalances and focuses on deficits rather than strengths. As Mead and Copeland (2000, p. 319) assert: 'Though clinical relationships may never truly be mutual or without some assumptions, we can all work to change our roles with each other in order to discard the kinds of paternalistic relationships some of us have experienced in the past'. This can be a challenging dichotomy for the nurse, whose traditional roles are primarily seen as caring and support.

RECOVERY ETHICS AND REFLECTION

Our worldview, or how we view the world based on our experiences of it, affects how we make choices. We all have different life experiences and hence different worldviews. The mental health nurse will work with a diversity of people from different backgrounds and different life experiences; they might question the life choices of others. When we work with people and find ourselves feeling uncomfortable or judging them or their decisions, it is usually because their worldview is different to our own.

Know your worldview

When we work with people, it is important to ask ourselves, 'How is my worldview influencing what I am currently thinking, saying or doing?' The exciting thing is that by opening ourselves up to other worldviews, our worldview can grow and change. When the choices of others are difficult to understand or accept, we can ask ourselves, 'How could I reframe this differently?' Mead and Copeland (2000, p. 320) assert that 'health care professionals need to continue to examine their own roadblocks to change, understand where they get "stuck" and dependent, and look at their own less-than-healthy ways of coping'.

Mead and Copeland (2000) suggest considering the following questions when reflecting on our thoughts, actions and practices:

- How much of our own discomfort are we willing to sit with while someone is trying out new choices?
- How are our boundaries continuously being redefined as we struggle to deepen each individual relationship?
- What are the assumptions we have about this person, by virtue of his/her diagnosis, history and lifestyle?
- How can we put aside our assumptions and predictions in order to be fully present to the situation and open to the possibility for the other person to do the same?
- What are the barriers that might prevent both of us from stretching and growing (Mead & Copeland, 2000, pp. 319–20)?

Hard choices and 'dirty hands'

Michael Waltzer (1973) explores how difficult decisions can leave us with what he calls 'dirty hands', meaning that there is (or appears to be) no clean or perfect solution or decision that can be made at the time. This will be the day-to-day reality in many mental health services. Mental health legislation endorses coercive practices, including individuals being detained and medicated against their will. Many services are busy and at times hectic, and the overall ambience may not be conducive to building supportive relationships and facilitating environments where people feel safe. Hence, we are all human and sometimes we will do things or act in ways that we do not feel okay about. This is when we should acknowledge what Waltzer calls a 'dirty hands' decision. The issue, however, is not so much that we made this decision or acted in a certain way, but that the dominant culture of many services ignores or justifies difficult 'dirty hands' decisions as something that had to be done, without engaging in reflective practice (Brophy et al., 2016). This can result in unquestioned draconian, coercive practices that traumatise both consumers and staff (Brophy et al., 2016).

Reflecting on a 'dirty hands' decision

It is important to recognise and acknowledge 'dirty hands' decisions so as to reflect upon them. The mental health nurse should reflect upon these decisions individually, with their team and also with consumers where the decision affected them. Reflection should include what could have been done differently, what processes might need to change to allow a different outcome next time, and what would have been done the same and why. On reflection, it might be decided that, given all the circumstances and the limitations the nurse was working within, that they made the best decision they could at the time. The difference is that, with reflection, the nurse can move on without further feelings of discomfort.

Don't risk recovery

We live in a risk averse society and mental health services often have many rules and functions designed to mitigate risk. Slade, Adams and O'Hagan (2012, p. 2) highlight the discordance between recovery and risk aversion, asking the question; 'Is a recovery-orientated mental health system compatible with sociopolitical expectations that a mental health system will manage risk and provide social control?'. Focus on risk and control can hinder recovery (Newman et al., 2015; Slade, Adams & O'Hagan, 2012). For example, a person might be refused leave from an inpatient service to socialise or gain some independence due to a concern about the risk of them absconding. While the nurse has a duty of care to consumers and must follow rules and regulations to ensure safety, they should be careful not to over-limit a person's choices and freedoms under the guise of protecting them. When thinking about risk there are two things to consider:

1   People may make choices different from the choices we would make, but that does not make them wrong.
2   We all learn through trial and error and our best learning occurs when things are not quite working out the way we hoped or envisaged (Davidson et al., 2006; Mead & Copeland, 2001).

As outlined earlier, the recovery journey is a journey of discovery. People grow and learn 'through taking positive risks' (Mead & Copeland, 2001, p. 319). According to Mead and Copeland (2001), some ways to assist people in taking positive risks are to encourage and support them to:

- make life and treatment choices for themselves
- build their own crisis and treatment plans
- choose their own relationships and spiritual practices
- create the life of their choice.

Davidson et al. (2006) assert that rather than see everyone and every situation as high risk, services should appropriate risk assessment and management systems to identify circumstances where there might be a significant risk. 'Within the context of a recovery-oriented system of care, the competent conduct of risk assessments will be needed precisely in order to identify the rare circumstances in which people cannot be allowed to act in ways that put others or themselves at risk' (p. 644). Davidson et al. (2006) also make the point that most people with mental health challenges do not pose a significant risk to themselves or others and that making across-the-board assumptions about risk is not best practice.

When thinking about risk, we can ask ourselves: 'What is the risk of not supporting people to recovery and being trauma informed?'

REFLECTION ON LEARNING FROM PRACTICE

What should we do, then, as Evie is walking through the door? We want Evie to feel welcomed and that we are glad that she is here so we can work with her and support her recovery. To do this, we need to reflect on how we are thinking about Evie and how much of this is influenced by our own perceptions and circumstances. How could we reframe, or rethink about, Evie's behaviour? How much of our own behaviour has or could potentially influence Evie? We need to also have faith in our ability to assist Evie.

If we are thinking of Evie as a troublemaker, timewaster, nuisance and/or frightening, or as someone we cannot help, then we cannot authentically welcome her. People are very perceptive if we are thinking, 'I wish she wasn't here' or 'I wish I wasn't here', it would not be surprising if Evie did not want to be there either.

An authentic welcome might go some way to de-escalating Evie's behaviour. However, if the behavioural roles are entrenched over many instances, Evie might not have quite caught up with your reframing and might still need to do more before her behaviour calms. Having worked with her before, you might already know some of her preferences and what helps her to feel calm and safe – whether she might like to go directly to her room and have some quiet time or a sleep, go directly to the shared space and catch up with other consumers, or sit with you or another worker for a while and have a chat. If you are not sure, ask her what she would like to do. This might require some flexibility in admission or assessment procedures, but is worthwhile so as to have a positive admission and instead

of having to restrain or seclude Evie – and the delay in completing assessment would be the same.

Moving forward, you might introduce Evie to the peer workers for support, and also sit with her and chat about what's happening in her life. Check with her that she feels safe and comfortable in the service and what you might be able to do to assist her to be and feel safer. Take an interest in Evie as a person – not her symptoms or even her mental health specifically. Ask her what she would like to achieve while she is here and when she leaves, and how you and others in the service can help her. This might be a number of conversations over a period of days or even weeks while your relationship strengthens and trust builds. It is important that these are discussions – not you asking questions and Evie responding, but a genuine exchange. Go in to bat for Evie help her to identify and meet her goals, and address any risk-aversive practices or decisions that are holding her back unnecessarily. Use respectful and affirming language and question the language of other staff if it is not strengths-based and respectful.

By the time Evie leaves, you will be pleased for her and how well she is going. You are going to miss her. But this is what you work towards, seeing consumers move forward with their lives. Your role is to facilitate that process and work with Evie. You also know that just down the corridor is someone else with whom you will strive to develop that same therapeutic connection and travel with on this part of their journey in all its richness and complexity.

CHAPTER RESOURCES

SUMMARY

- Recovery refers to recovery of life with or without ongoing symptoms of a mental health condition. Recovery-oriented service delivery is practice that supports and facilitates people to recover to live a life that is meaningful to them. When working within a recovery framework, it is important to build relationships of trust and rapport with service users.

- Many people who have a mental health condition also have experienced significant trauma. It is important to acknowledge people's trauma and ensure that your practice and the service culture and environment do not perpetuate or trigger previous trauma. You should work with people in a strengths-based way, helping them to identify and focus on their strengths and resilience, assisting them to reframe their perception of themselves from that of a victim to a survivor.

- It is important to understand and acknowledge how our worldview is affecting our judgement and to properly reflect on decisions or actions that might have left us feeling uncomfortable.

- Working with and learning from consumers, carers and peer support workers, as well as actively reflecting on our practice, is essential for team members to understand and learn from the impact of care decisions made and how to continue to improve our practice.

- Peer workers play an important part in the recovery team due to their unique expertise and experience, the shared understanding and experience they have with service users and the hope they engender by being there.

- We should ensure people have the freedom and control to take risks in their recovery, acknowledging that we all learn through trial and error. While we have a duty of care, we are risking hurting rather than helping people if we deny them the freedom to recover on their terms.

REVIEW QUESTIONS

(Note: More than one answer can apply to some questions)

1 When working with a person to support their recovery, what should you do?
   a Be hopeful that they can recover and that you can support them in their recovery
   b Ensure they have the correct medication
   c Focus on their mental health condition and help them to become symptom free
   d Be careful not to share any of your life or story with them

2 When you work with people with a mental health condition, you should be aware they are most likely to have an experience of:
   a Attempted suicide
   b Trauma
   c Divorce
   d Behaving violently towards others

3 When working with people who have experienced trauma, it is most important for you to:
   a Find out all about it
   b Help them to feel safe
   c Focus on their resilience
   d Tell them that they don't need to worry any more and just look to the future

4 When things don't go according to plan and you feel uncomfortable or unsure of how you responded, you should:
   a Rationalise that this is the way things are done here or you didn't really have a choice
   b Acknowledge that it was a hard decision and think about what you might do the same or differently next time
   c Critically reflect on the incident with other team members
   d Remember that no one is perfect

5 When you are working and a consumer asks for leave to smoke off the hospital grounds, you should:
   a Say no, as they might not come back
   b Say yes, even though you have some reservations about their safety
   c Conduct a risk assessment
   d Tell them that they shouldn't smoke

CRITICAL THINKING

1 In order to implement recovery-oriented principles in practice and for them to be of benefit to consumers, it is essential that we understand what these principles mean. Consider the following principles: self-determination; hope; personal growth.

   a What do these terms mean for the person with a lived experience of a mental health condition?
   b What do these terms mean for mental health nurses when working with the individual?

2   How is resilience important to a person's mental health? What behaviours build resilience?

3   A student peer asks you to explain trauma-informed practice to them. How would you do this?

4   The balance between 'caring' and 'doing' can be difficult for nurses working in mental health to achieve, particularly those new to this specialty. How do you think you will balance the need for fostering autonomy in consumers with your caring role?

5   Why is reflection so important in the context of reviewing 'dirty hands' decisions that are sometimes made by clinicians in mental health settings?

USEFUL WEBSITES

- Australian Government. Principles of Recovery Oriented Practice: http://www.health.gov.au/internet/publications/publishing.nsf/Content/mental-pubs-i-nongov-toc~mental-pubs-i-nongov-pri
- NEAMI International: http://www.neaminational.org.au

- Patricia Deegan: https://www.patdeegan.com/pat-deegan
- Recovery is: excerpt of a public lecture given by Dr Larry Davidson in Sydney in 2013 that identifies developments in the way in which recovery is now understood: https://www.youtube.com/watch?v=8p5l36yNPnY

REFLECT ON THIS

Trauma-informed practice

Understanding and practising in a recovery-oriented and trauma-informed way is the cornerstone of contemporary mental health service delivery for all members of the multidisciplinary team. However, as you have seen, it is not always easily incorporated into practice. In this chapter, you have read about a number of ideas that will be the basis of your own journey in embedding these approaches in your own practice. Reflect on the following questions in relation to your discipline.

1   How have these ideas been explored in your own learning? What concepts did you find challenging to understand?

2   In what ways does your current worldview influence or impact on your own developing practice?

3   How do you 'work with the person, not on symptoms or diagnosis' as stated in the chapter?

4   Work through the questions posed by Mead and Copeland (2000) presented in this chapter. Which questions were more challenging to reflect on? Why do you think this was the case (dig deeper!)? What strategies could you use to further understand and 'know' your worldview?

5   How has working on clinical placement in your discipline with people who have a mental health condition helped you widen your worldview? What will you incorporate into your ongoing learning and practice in mental health and other clinical areas?

REFERENCES

Ackland, R. (2011). Modern prescription for mental illness: Go directly to jail. *Sydney Morning Herald*, 29 July, p. 15.

Ahire, M., Sheridan, J., Regbetz, S., Stacey, P. & Scott, J. (2013). Back to basics: Informing the public of co-morbid physical health problems in those with mental illness. *Australian and New Zealand Journal of Psychiatry*, 47(2), 177–84.

Australian Bureau of Statistics (ABS). (2007). *National Survey of Mental Health and Wellbeing: Summary of Results*. Canberra: ABS. Retrieved from http://www.abs.gov.au/ausstats/abs@.nsf/7d12b0f6763c78caca257061001cc588/3f8a5dfcbecad9c0ca2568a900139380!OpenDocument.

Australian College of Mental Health Nurses (ACMHN). (2010). *Standards of Practice for Australian Mental Health Nurses 2010*. Canberra: ACMHN.

Australian Government, National Mental Health Commission. (2014). 2014 Contributing Lives Review. http://www.mentalhealthcommission.gov.au/our-reports/our-national-report-cards/2014-contributing-lives-review.aspx

Australian Health Ministers' Advisory Council (AHMAC). (2013a). *A National Framework for Recovery-oriented Mental Health Services: Guide for Practitioners and Providers*. Canberra: Commonwealth of Australia. Retrieved from http://www.health.gov.au/internet/main/publishing.nsf/content/67d17065514cf8e8ca257c1d00017a90/$file/recovgde.pdf.

Australian Health Ministers' Advisory Council (AHMAC). (2013b). *A National Framework for Recovery-oriented Mental Health Services: Policy and Theory*. Canberra: Commonwealth of Australia. Retrieved from http://www.mhima.org.au/pdfs/Recovery%20Framework%202013_Policy_theory.pdf.

Berry, H., Hogan, A., Owen, J., Rickwood, D. & Fragar, L. (2011). Climate change and farmers' mental health: Risks and responses.

Asia-Pacific Journal of Public Health, 23(2_suppl), 119S–132S. doi:10.1177/1010539510392556

Bonner, G., Lowe, T., Rawcliffe, D. & Wellman, N. (2002). Trauma for all: A pilot study of the subjective experience of physical restraint for mental health inpatients and staff in the UK. *Journal of Psychiatric and Mental Health Nursing*, 9, 465–73. doi:10.1046/j.1365-2850.2002.00504.xhttp://onlinelibrary.wiley.com/wol1/doi/10.1046/j.1365-2850.2002.00504.x/full

Brophy, L.M., Roper, C.E., Hamilton, B.E., Tellez, J.J. & McSherry, B.M. (2016). Consumers and their supporters' perspectives on barriers and strategies to reducing seclusion and restraint in mental health settings. *Australian Health Review*, 40(6), 599–604.

Browne, G. & Hemsley, M. (2008). Consumer participation in mental health in Australia: What progress is being made? *Australasian Psychiatry*, 16(6), 446–9.

Byrne, L., Happell, B., Welch, T. & Moxham, L.J. (2013). 'Things you can't learn from books': Teaching recovery from a lived experience perspective. *International Journal of Mental Health Nursing*, 22, 195–204.

Champagne, T. & Koomar, J. (2012). Evaluating sensory processing in mental health occupational therapy practice. *OT Practice*, 17(5), CE1–CE8.

Clark, C., Classen, C., Fourt, A. & Shetty, M. (2014). *Treating the Trauma Survivor: An Essential Guide to Trauma-Informed Care*. Florence: Taylor and Francis.

Coffey, M. (2009). Shunned: Discrimination against people with mental illness. *Journal of Psychiatric and Mental Health Nursing*, 16(1), 108.

Colton, C. & Manderscheid, R. (2006). Congruencies in increased mortality rates, years of potential life lost, and causes of death among public mental health clients in eight states. *Preventing Chronic Disease*, 3(2), A42.

Coulter, S. (2014). The applicability of two strengths-based systemic psychotherapy models for young people following type 1 trauma. *Child Care in Practice*, 20(1), 48–63.

Curtis, J., Newall, H. & Samaras, K. (2012). The heart of the matter: Cardiometabolic care in youth with psychosis. *Early Intervention in Psychiatry*, 6(3), 347–53.

Davidson, L., O'Connell, M., Tondora, J., Styron, T. & Kangas, K. (2006). The top ten concerns about recovery encountered in mental health system transformation. *Psychiatric Services*, 57(5), 640–5.

Deegan, P. (2005). The importance of personal medicine: A qualitative study of resilience in people with psychiatric disabilities. *Scandinavian Journal of Public Health*, 33(66 suppl.), 29–35.

Delaney, K. (2006). Evidence base for practice: Reduction of restraint and seclusion use during child and adolescent psychiatric inpatient treatment. *Worldviews on Evidence-based Nursing*, 3(1), 19–30.

Department of Health and Ageing. (2010). *National Standards for Mental Health Services*. Canberra: Commonwealth of Australia. Retrieved from http://www.health.gov.au/internet/main/publishing.nsf/Content/mental-pubs-n-servst10.

Gillard, S. & Holley, J. (2014). Peer workers in mental health services: Literature overview. *Advances in Psychiatric Treatment*, 20(4), 286–92. doi:10.1192/apt.bp.113.011940

Glisson, C. & Williams, N.(2015). Assessing and changing organizational social contexts for effective mental health services. *Annual Review of Public Health*, 36, 507–23. https://doi.org/10.1146/annurev-publhealth-031914-122435

Gray, S., Ferris, L., White, L.E., Duncan, G. & Baumle, W. (2019). *Foundations of Nursing: Enrolled Nurses* (2nd edn). South Melbourne: Cengage.

Happell, B. (2014). Consumer participation in the education and training of mental health nurses: Issues paper. Published by the Queensland Mental Health Commission.

Happell, B., Ewart, S., Bocking, J., Platania-Phung, C. & Stanton, R. (2016). 'That red flag on your file': Misinterpreting physical symptoms as mental illness. *Journal of Clinical Nursing*, 25(19–20), 2933–42.

Happell, B., Platania-Phung, C. & Scott, D. (2013). Mental Health Nurse Incentive Program: Facilitating physical health care for people with mental illness? *International Journal of Mental Health Nursing*, 22(5), 399–408.

Hearing Voices Network. (n.d.). *Hearing Voices Coping Strategies*. Retrieved from http://www.hearing-voices.org/wp-content/uploads/2012/05/Hearing_Voices_Coping_Strategies_web.pdf.

Isobel, S. & Delgado, C. (2018). *Safe and collaborative communication skills: A step towards mental health nurses implementing trauma informed care*. Archives of Psychiatric Nursing, 32(2), 291–6. doi:https://doi.org/10.1016/j.apnu.2017.11.017.

Jacob, S., Munro, I. & Taylor, B. (2015). Mental health recovery: Lived experience of consumers, carers and nurses. *Contemporary Nurse*, 1–13.

Kezelman, C. & Stavropoulos, P. (2012). *The Last Frontier: Practice Guidelines For Treatment of Complex Trauma and Trauma Informed Care and Service Delivery*. A Blue Knot Foundation (formerly Adults Surviving Child Abuse).

Lambert, T.J.R., Reavley, N.J., Jorm, A.F. & Oakley Browne, M.A. (2017) Royal Australian and New Zealand College of Psychiatrists expert consensus statement for the treatment, management and monitoring of the physical health of people with an enduring psychotic illness. *Australian and New Zealand Journal of Psychiatry*, 51(4) 322–37. doi:10.1177/0004867416686693

Lauritzen, C., Reedtz, C., Van Doesum, K. & Martinussen, M. (2014). Implementing new routines in adult mental health care to identify and support children of mentally ill parents. *BMC Health Services Research*, 14, 58.

LeBel, J., Huckshorn, K.A. & Caldwell, B. (2010). Restraint use in residential programs: Why are best practices ignored? *Child Welfare*, 89(2), 169–87.

Mead, S. & Copeland, M. (2000). What recovery means to us: Consumers' perspectives. *Community Mental Health Journal*, 36(3), 315–28.

Mental Health Commission of NSW. (2016). *Employer's Guide for Implementing a Peer Workforce*. Sydney: Mental Health Commission of NSW. Retrieved from http://peerworkhub.com.au/wp-content/uploads/2016/05/Business-Case.pdf.

Mental Health Coordinating Council (MHCC) NSW. (2013). *Recovery Oriented Language Guide*. Sydney: MHCC. Retrieved from http://www.mhcc.org.au/wp-content/uploads/2018/05/Recovery-Oriented-Language-Guide_2018ed_v3_201800418-FINAL.pdf.

Murray, H. (2014). 'My place was set at the terrible feast': The meanings of the 'anti-psychiatry' movement and responses in the United States, 1970s–1990s. *Journal of American Culture*, 37(1), 37–51.

National Advisory Council on Mental Health (NACMH). (2009). *Fourth National Mental Health Plan: An Agenda for Collaborative Government Action in Mental Health*. Canberra: Commonwealth of Australia. Retrieved from https://www.health.gov.au/internet/main/publishing.nsf/content/9A5A0E8BDFC55D3BCA257BF0001C1B1C/$File/plan09v2.pdf.

National Mental Health Commission (NMHC). (n.d). *Mental Health Peer Work Development and Promotion*. Retrieved from http://www.mentalhealthcommission.gov.au/peerwork.

National Mental Health Commission (NMHC). (2013). *A Contributing Life: The 2013 National Report Card on Mental Health and Suicide Prevention*. Sydney: NHMC. Retrieved from http://www.mentalhealthcommission.gov.au/media/94321/Report_Card_2013_full.pdf.

National Mental Health Commission (NHMC). (2014). *The National Review of Mental Health Programmes and Services*. Sydney: NMHC. Released under CC BY 3.0. Link to license: https://creativecommons.org/licenses/by/3.0/au/.

National Mental Health Commission (NMHC). (2016). *Equally Well Consensus Statement: Improving the Physical Health and Wellbeing of People Living with Mental Illness in Australia*. Sydney: NMHC. Retrieved from https://mentalhealthcarerstas.org.au/wp-content/uploads/2017/07/Equally-Well-booklet.pdf.

National Mental Health Commission (NMHC). (2018). *Monitoring Mental Health and Suicide Prevention Reform: National Report 2018*. Sydney: MHMC. Retrieved from: http://www.mentalhealthcommission.gov.au/media/245211/Monitoring%20Mental%20Health%20and%20Suicide%20Prevention%20Reform%20National%20Report%202018.pdf.

National Mental Health Consumer and Carer Forum (NMHCCF). (2009). *Ending Seclusion and Restraint in Australian Mental Health Services*. Retrieved from https://nmhccf.org.au/sites/default/files/docs/seclusion_restraint.pdf.

Newman, D., O'Reilly, P., Lee, S.H. & Kennedy, C. (2015). Mental health service users' experiences of mental health care: An integrative literature review. *Journal of Psychiatric and Mental Health Nursing*, 22, 171–82.

O'Brien, A. & Golding, C. (2003). Coercion in mental healthcare: The principle of least coercive care. *Journal of Psychiatric and Mental Health Nursing*, 10(2), 167–73.

Park, M., Zafran, H., Stewart, J., Salsberg, J., Ells, C., Rouleau, S., Estein, O. & Valente, T. (2014). Transforming mental health services: A participatory mixed methods study to promote and evaluate the implementation of recovery-oriented services. *Implementation Science*, 9, 119. https://doi.org/10.1186/s13012-014-0119-7

Ramon, S., Healy, B. & Renouf, N. (2007). Recovery from mental illness as an emergent concept and practice in Australia and the UK. *International Journal of Social Psychiatry*. Sage Publications, 53(2).

Rapp, C. (1998). *The Strengths Model: Case Management with People Suffering from Severe and Persistent Mental Illness*. New York: Oxford University Press.

Rapp, C. & Goscha. R. (2011). *The Strengths Model*. New York: Oxford University Press.

Rossiter, A., Byrne, F., Wota, A., Nisar, Z., Ofuafor, T,. Murray, I., Byrne, C. & Hallahan, B. (2015). Childhood trauma levels in individuals attending adult mental health services: An evaluation of clinical records and structured measurement of childhood trauma. *Child Abuse & Neglect*, 44, 36–45. https://doi.org/10.1016/j.chiabu.2015.01.001

Russinova, Z. (1999). Providers' hope-inspiring competence as a factor optimizing psychiatric rehabilitation outcomes. *Journal of Rehabilitation*, 65(4), 50–7.

Saunders, V., Sherwood, J. & Usher, K. (2015). If you knew the end of the story, would you still want to hear it?: The importance of narrative time for mental health care. *The Qualitative Report*, 20(10), 1594–608. Retrieved from https://nsuworks.nova.edu/tqr/vol20/iss10/4.

Sheehan, R. & Levine, G. (2005). Parents with mental illness: Decision-making in Australian Children's Court cases involving parents with mental health problems. *Journal of Social Welfare and Family Law*, 27(1), 17-30.

Slade, M. (2009). *100 Ways to Support Recovery. A Guide for Mental Health Professionals. Rethink Recovery Series, Volume 1*. Retrieved from https://recoverylibrary.unimelb.edu.au/__data/assets/pdf_file/0005/1391270/100_ways_to_support_recovery.pdf.

Slade, M. (2010). Mental illness and well-being: The central importance of positive psychology and recovery approaches. *BMC Health Services Research*, 10, 26.

Slade M., Adams N. & O'Hagan M. (2012). Recovery: past progress and future challenges. *International Review of Psychiatry*, 24, 1–4.

Slade, M., Amering, M., Farkas, M., Hamilton, B., O'Hagan, M., Panther, G., … Whitley, R. (2014). Uses and abuses of recovery: Implementing recovery-oriented practices in mental health systems. *World Psychiatry*, 13, 12–20. doi:10.1002/wps.20084

Slade, M. & Longden, E. (2015). The empirical evidence about mental health recovery: How likely, how long, what helps. *BMC Psychiatry*, 15(285).

Stacey, G. & Stickley, T. (2012). Recovery as a threshold concept in mental health nurse education. *Nurse Education Today*, 32, 534–9.

Thornicroft, G. (2006). *Shunned. Discrimination against People with Mental Illness*. New York: Oxford University Press.

Thornicroft, G., Rose, D. & Kassam, A. (2007). Discrimination in health care against people with mental illness. *International Review of Psychiatry*, 19(2), 113–22.

United Nations. (1976). *International Covenant on Civil and Political Rights*. Geneva: UN Human Rights Office of High Commissioner. Retrieved from http://www.ohchr.org/EN/ProfessionalInterest/Pages/CCPR.aspx

Waltzer, M. (1973). Political action: The problem of dirty hands. *Philosophy and Public Affairs*, 2(2), pp. 160–80.

Weick, A. & Chamberlain, R. (2000). Putting problems in their place: Further explorations in the strengths perspective. In D. Saleebey (ed.), *The Strengths Perspective in Social Work Practice* (2nd edn, pp. 39–48). New York: Longman.

Wynaden, D. (2010). There is no health without mental health: Are we educating Australian nurses to care for the health consumer of the 21st century?. *International Journal of Mental Health Nursing*, 19, 203–9. doi:10.1111/j.1447-0349.2010.00671.x http://onlinelibrary.wiley.com/doi/10.1111/j.1447-0349.2010.00671.x/abstract

THE FAMILY'S ROLE IN CONTEMPORARY MENTAL HEALTH SERVICE DELIVERY

Gylo (Julie) Hercelinskyj

LEARNING OUTCOMES

Upon completion of this chapter, you should be able to:

22.1 Consider the various ways in which families are defined

22.2 Describe theories related to family structure and function

22.3 Explore the factors influencing the family's experience of care-giving

22.4 Apply the concept of resilience to the family's experience of care-giving

22.5 Understand that mental health nurses work with families

22.6 Identify the mental health nurse's role in assessing and working with families

22.7 Review strategies for increasing family resilience

22.8 Explore the consumer's view of family care-giving

LEARNING FROM PRACTICE

As an academic, I taught the concept of family for a number of years. I gave various definitions of families for students to reflect on. I taught students about primary and secondary families, blended, step and merged families; resilient, meshed and dysfunctional families.

My brother Tom was born into a family. He had two parents and two sisters. I remember how close he and our sister were. They laughed and fought, then cried and finally laughed again. They did those things that younger siblings do that would drive me, their big sister crazy.

Tom went to school and was a happy gregarious person who had lots of friends. Mum and Dad had the same hopes for Tom as they did for my sister and me. Go to school, have a career and find someone special. Nothing earth-shattering; just the things that any parent wants for their child.

However, things didn't go the way Mum and Dad hoped. And it's a moot point as to what came first, the drugs or the mental health issues. Did Tom self-medicate with drugs to try and control his symptoms? Or did the symptoms start as a result of Tom's drug use, with Tom then using drugs to try and deal with his symptoms? It was the early 1980s and Tom was part of a new wave of young people presenting with issues that we now recognise and cleverly label as dual diagnosis.

So what happened to our family? Like so many others in those days, we all floundered. It didn't matter that as a mental health nurse I understood the psychopathology of Tom's diagnosis and could explain the symptoms and medications. My brother was unwell, he did not want to take his medication and his relationships with us were at times what could only be described as fractious. During those early years, I often felt as if I was standing on a precipice. I was a mental health nurse for goodness sake; I should have been able to recognise the slow insidious onslaught of symptoms that Tom was experiencing. The increasing withdrawal from family, the signs of drug use and the questions Tom would ask that didn't seem quite logical to my parents, but which they would try their best to answer. But I was also his sister and by the time Tom's symptoms became increasingly evident I had been away from home for some years and so had missed the opportunity to ask my parents for more specific information. Those years were characterised by uncertainty, feelings of failure, times where we had no contact with Tom for perhaps several months, and a sense of grief at what we saw as the loss of the gorgeous young man we once knew.

We lost Tom in 2011, and while we did not have regular contact with him for a number of years, we grieved for our loss. We still do.

Jo, nurse academic

INTRODUCTION

In 2015, the Australian Bureau of Statistics (2013) estimated that there were 2.7 million unpaid carers in Australia, providing savings of just over $60 billion to the Australian Government (Deloitte Access Economics, 2015). There has been a steady move over the last 30 or so years to promote families assuming responsibility for care-giving. These changes occurred at the same time that moves were made to implement deinstitutionalisation within Australian mental health service delivery. The increasing contribution of families to the management and support of consumers living with a mental health condition has become a central guiding feature in health policy and delivery of social services to people living with a diagnosis of a chronic illness, as noted as early as 1982 (Walker, 1982). The concept of community care was described by Walker (1982, p. 5) as 'help and support given to individuals including children... in non-institutional settings... provided by informal, quasi-formal or formal helpers... or a combination of all three'. Barbarin, Hughes and Chesler (1985) believed that families respond to stressors such as chronic illness as an interactive group rather than isolated individuals. This idea of the family as an interactive group suggests that while families are comprised of distinct people, the way in which they understand and respond to circumstances such as caring for a family member with a diagnosis of a mental health condition will also be as a group.

Therefore, in this chapter we consider how families are conceptualised as both a collection of unique individuals as well as a group who are interrelated in terms of function, roles and responsibilities. In this chapter, we also consider how the consumer's experience of a mental health condition can impact on the family and all members.

WHAT IS A FAMILY?

As suggested in the 'Learning from practice' reflection at the beginning of this chapter, there are different ways of understanding what constitutes a family. In Australia, many forms of family exist; authors such as Carter and McGoldrick (2005) considered that family was a group of people connected by blood and/or emotional bonds, and who have developed patterns of interacting with each other and forming relationships within the family unit. Family members have both a shared history and a shared future. Systems theory also provides a definition of family. As a system, families are seen to be a self-organising group forming a whole, which is greater than the sum of each individual part. This system will be based on a set of rules; for example, rules about child, sibling and parental roles and identities. Other theories about families suggest that families go through specific stages or life cycles, while more contemporary ideas describe the way in which individual, interpersonal, group and wider societal factors impact on the individual's and the family's development and experiences.

The Australian Bureau of Statistics (2013) also defines the family in the Australian context as consisting of two or more persons, one of whom is at least 15 years of age, who are related by blood, marriage (registered or de facto), adoption, step or fostering, and who usually reside in the same household. In Jo's experience, family was not restricted necessarily to blood ties or formalised relationships as defined by legislation or social or cultural norms. For her, a person creates a family of people who care for and about each other. This view of family reflects the idea that family refers to the significant people in a person's life. This is not limited to biological relatives but also friends, carers and the broader community (Young, O'Hanlon & Weir, 2016).

We now consider these theoretical ideas and why it is important for mental health nurses to have an understanding of them.

THEORIES REGARDING FAMILY STRUCTURE AND FUNCTIONING

There are three major groups of theories regarding family structure and functioning. These are family systems theory, family life cycle theory and ecological theory.

Family systems theory

Using ideas from work in cybernetics (McLeod, 2013), family systems theory views the family as a system that is comprised of interrelated components (the family members). The connection between family members is shared and repetitive, as the 'system' (family) works to maintain equilibrium or homeostasis. It is like a heating system. This system is made of interrelated parts. The overall goal is to reach a predetermined temperature and keep people warm and comfortable. If there is a change in one component of the heating system, there will be a change in how the system operates.

Therefore, in terms of the idea of a family *system*, changes to one part of the 'system' (a family member) will impact on the other components, both at the individual level and the system (family) as a whole. This is because a system (family) operates according to a set of rules. Each part of the system (family) has a particular set of role(s) and/or responsibilities. When all components are able to fulfil these roles and responsibilities, the system (family) is stable. However, if one component (family member) cannot complete/meet their roles and responsibilities, there will be a subsequent impact on the whole system (family).Therefore, when one member of a family receives a diagnosis of a mental health condition (e.g. depression), this event will reverberate through the entire household. There will be changes to the usual roles and responsibilities of family members, and adjustments will be more or less successfully made. Understanding this enables mental health nurses to provide appropriate information, support and assistance to family members as they adjust to a new life, both individually and as a family.

Development and family life cycle theory

This theoretical perspective provides a framework to understand the expected changes or stages a family is said to go through over the lifetime of its members. The key elements of this theory are:

- families develop and evolve over time in terms of membership, roles and responsibilities
- family members are considered in the context of their individual development as well as the development of the family unit
- there are specific stages of the family life cycle. Duvall (1977) proposed the following eight stages in the family life cycle:

1 Newly married couple with no children
2 Childbearing family (newborn infants until approximately three years of age)
3 Family with young children (children three to six years of age)
4 Family with school-age children (up to the age of 12 years)
5 Family with adolescents (children from 13 to 20 years of age)
6 Launching grown children (from first child leaving home to the last child)
7 Family without children (empty nesters and retirement)
8 Family in later life (retirement to death)

Again, think of the potential repercussions to families when a member (e.g. a parent) receives a diagnosis of a mental health condition. What are the possible consequences of this in relation to the children's emotional, physical and social well-being? What are the social and economic implications for the family as whole? What impact might this event have on parental roles and responsibilities?

Bronfenbrenner's bioecological systems theory

This theory identifies five environmental systems that impact on a person's development from childhood because of their interactions with their environment. Various contexts such as work, family and education influence the child's development over the course of their lifespan. Importantly, the relationship between the person and their environment is a reciprocal one. Bronfenbrenner conceptualised his theory as a process–person–context–time model (Tudge, Mokrova, Hatfield & Karnik, 2009). Because this theory looks at lifetime development, it highlights how these external systems affect families and each individual within in it (Bronfenbrenner, 1986), as well as the importance of socialisation and culture to an individual's development. Bronfenbrenner's ideas looked at how biology and environment shaped a person's development, hence the name. The five structures of a person's environment as identified by Bronfenbrenner are identified in **Table 22.1**.

TABLE 22.1
The five systems of Bronfenbrenner's bioecological systems theory

STRUCTURE	CHARACTERISTICS
1 The microsystem	The physical and social environment a person interacts with. Examples include community resources (e.g. parks/play areas), family, school, peers and church. The individual's interactions will impact on them as well as influence the particular environmental source; e.g. the interaction between a newborn infant and their primary carer will impact on the infant's attachment to the primary carer as well as on the primary carer's feelings of confidence in their role.
2 The mesosystem	Relationships/links between two or more microsystems. For example, an adult who is experiencing difficulties at work may find they are still in a bad mood when they get home, resulting in increased arguments.
3 The exosystem	Settings that an individual may not have direct contact with but which can still have an influence on their development. This includes the media, health and social services, and governments. For example, repeated media coverage of negative events can impact on an individual's views of and interactions with people who have a particular medical condition or who are homeless.

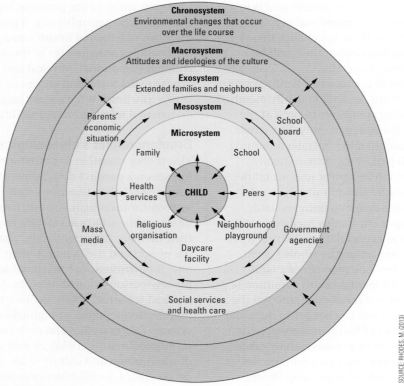

FIGURE 22.1
Bronfenbrenner's ecological system

STRUCTURE	CHARACTERISTICS
4 The macrosystem	The larger cultural context in which the micro, meso and exosystems are set. Culture includes beliefs, attitudes, customs and laws.
5 The chronosystem	The system in which the other systems are located. It refers to the personal, social, political and historical events and changes that occur during an individual's life.

SOURCE: ADAPTED FROM SIGELMAN, WALKER & GEORGE-WALKER, 2016

Figure 22.1 illustrates these systems, their main features and their relationships to each other.

If there are disruptions to a child's immediate environment (microsystem) through events such as one parent receiving a diagnosis of a mental health condition, the child may or may not have access to the necessary support, education and nutrition to foster optimal physical, emotional and social development.

THE FAMILY'S EXPERIENCE OF CARING FOR A LOVED ONE WITH A MENTAL HEALTH CHALLENGE

The relationship between family members involves the expenditure of emotional energy and practical resources by all family members. This is particularly evident in the context of the caring role that families have in relation to a loved one with a mental health issue.

Caring for someone living with a mental health condition can have significant physical, emotional and social impacts on the family's well-being. The impact of caring not only affects individuals within the family but the family unit as a whole. Families can experience a sense of constant anxiety, which also takes a toll on their emotional and physical well-being, both personally and in their wider social relationships.

Events such as involuntary admission (also referred to as compulsory treatment in some jurisdictions), multiple admissions of a family member, behaviour and choices by consumers that seem to be in opposition to recommended management strategies can increase the experience of burden for family members (Hallam, 2007). Lack of knowledge and understanding regarding mental health conditions from a personal perspective, as well as a lack of understanding from extended family and social networks, can increase confusion and a sense of isolation, leading to fewer opportunities for social interaction and support (Cohen et al., 2011).

Table 22.2 outlines a number of impacts that families can experience as a result of caring for a family member who has a mental health issue.

Importantly, however, families can also experience what Rugkåsa (2015, pp. 66–7) describes as 'personal growth'. Whether it is learning new skills to assist them in caring for a family member, or developing

TABLE 22.2
Impacts of caring on families

TYPE OF IMPACT	CONSEQUENCES
Emotional	• Anxiety • Worry • Guilt • Increased risk of personal mental health issues such as depression • Feeling shut out of the consumer's life • Grief and sense of loss for previous relationship
Social	• Isolation • Reduced income/employment difficulties • Disruptions in education (particularly for children) • Impaired family communication and relationships • Role reversal (e.g. children taking on parental roles for younger siblings or parents)
Physical	• Tiredness/exhaustion • Sleep disturbances • Exacerbation of pre-existing physical conditions (e.g. hypertension)

SOURCE: ADAPTED FROM ENNIS & BUNTING, 2013; RUGKÅSA, 2015

personal resources and independence in coping with events and situations, the family can continue to learn and grow along with their loved one. It is as if they have a lived journey that is complementary to that of the consumer. These ideas are explored later in the chapter when we consider resilience and families. The following sections outline some factors that influence the family's experience of caring for a loved one with a mental health issue.

Cultural factors

While Rugkåsa (2015) argues that it is important not to limit our understanding of a family's experience of caring to only their cultural identity, cultural norms and values impact significantly on the expectations, roles and experiences of family members as they experience their loved one's mental health journey.

The responsibility for family care-giving inevitably falls to a close family member. Hernandez, Barrio and Yamada (2013) note the figures indicate that the cultural norms regarding this caring impact on the extent to which different cultural groups will have the family member diagnosed with a mental health condition residing at home with them. Culture will also have a significant impact on the extent to which families provide support. The presence of family support can be seen as a protective factor for consumers and has been shown to be associated with higher levels of psychosocial functioning (Guada, Brekke, Floyd & Barbour, 2009). Some authors also argue that cultures where family connection and support are highly valued and provided are associated

with lower levels of negative physical, social and emotional burden for carers (Suro & Weisman de Mamani, 2013).

Gender

Women are more likely than men to be caregivers of relatives (Cançado Monteiro Savassi & Modena, 2013; Stewart et al., 1994). In this care-giving role, women assume what Strauss (1984, p. 99) describes as 'types of work'. They bear the primary responsibility for the care of their family member (Lubkin, 1990). This care-giving role is not without its costs. While referring to 'the family', given that it is the female member who usually assumes this role, the cost of care-giving would be expected to impact on that person.

CASE **STUDY**

THE FAMILY'S BURDEN OF CARE

Scott is 77 and was recently assessed by the aged psychiatry assessment and treatment team (APATT) and diagnosed with dementia. His family have avoided seeking help as there has been disagreement between members as to whether Scott's increasing confusion and memory problems were a sign of something significant or just a case of 'dad getting older'.

Over the next 12 months, a range of additional supports were introduced to assist Scott to remain in his home. This included daily visits by district nurses to assist Scott with his personal hygiene and medication administration as well as Meals on Wheels. However, Scott has been having increasing periods of confusion and was found by police wandering around his local shopping centre after closing. Scott was disoriented and agitated, hitting out at the police. Following this incident, the family decided that Claire, the youngest daughter, should quit her job as a teacher's aide to care for their father. This change in role has been very challenging for Claire and she is both physically and mentally exhausted by the end of the day. Recently, Scott has become incontinent, he is having increasing difficulty communicating verbally and his condition has deteriorated rapidly. Claire is considering placing her father into full-time care, but feels guilty. She says, 'He took care of me when I was young, I feel bad palming him off.'

Questions

1   What physical, emotional, social and/or economic impacts could Claire be at risk of experiencing as a carer for her father?

2   What resources and supports are available for family members/carers in your jurisdiction?

3   What are the benefits and challenges of implementing family-inclusive recovery-oriented practice for consumers, families and clinicians?

Role changes, overload and strain, changing expectations, financial burdens, emotional strain, anxiety and fatigue are all possible consequences of the care-giving role (Lubkin, 1990; O'Neill & Ross, 1991). A person's individual experience of the care-giving role needs to be explored and validated.

FAMILIES AND RESILIENCE

There are many definitions of resilience, but all share certain characteristics. One definition of resilience indicates a relationship between vulnerability, risk and coping. Thinking about resilience has also developed to consider who is likely to be a more resilient person. Early ideas of resilience focused on resilient people being those who possessed innate or biological characteristics that led them to be more resilient, while more contemporary definitions define resilience in terms of behaviours/skills that people can *learn* and *develop* because psychological and environmental factors have an impact on the extent to which a person can learn resilient behaviours. Definitions of resilience are also invariably related to the individual, not the family. In the context of this chapter, Walsh (2016) describes family resilience as the way in which the family positively withstands and rebounds from adversity.

Understanding resilience is important in the context of the family's experience of supporting a family member diagnosed with a mental health condition, as it is rare for anyone (individual or groups) to never confront a challenging situation during their lives. The concept of self-efficacy (Bandura, 1977) is linked to the idea of resilience. Families in which individual members experience a higher sense or degree of self-efficacy can contribute more effectively to both their own resilience, as well as to family resilience. This would involve the capacity to implement coping strategies, experience higher levels of competence and confidence, as well as having a sense of making a positive contribution to their individual and family's sense of well-being; all of these factors contribute to resilience.

Zauszniewski, Bekhet and Suresky (2009) identify a range of what they refer to as indicators of family resilience. These indicators are:

- *acceptance:* understanding of the circumstances that exist and the impact of this
- *hardiness:* the capacity to be flexible in the face of adversity, maintain a positive outlook, seek support as needed and use effective coping skills in the care-giving role
- *mastery:* the degree to which family members/ caregivers feel they have control regarding what happens to them
- *hope:* the ability to find meaning in changing circumstances, and use memories and strengths

of relationship to develop a sense of purpose moving forward into the future. This is integral to a family's capacity to cope with a diagnosis of a mental health condition for a family member
- *self-efficacy:* the belief that a person can cope with challenging situations/achieve goals. It is linked with confidence
- *sense of coherence:* the belief that family members can make sense of the world around them, manage events and relationships, be able to access the necessary supports when needed and live a meaningful life as a family
- *resourcefulness:* cognitive and behavioural skills that family members use to prevent potentially negative thinking and feeling impacting on daily life as well as the capacity to use external supports when able to be independent (adapted from Zauszniewski, Bekhet & Suresky, 2010).

Hernandez, Barrio and Yamada's 2013 study on hope and burden among Latin American families of adults with schizophrenia also explored the question of whether hope was a factor associated with a decrease in negative outcomes such as burden. The results of their study demonstrated that when a family member had increased hope for the consumer's future, there was a decrease in the experience of family burden. The 'Evidence-based practice' box further explores this study.

Principles of family resilience

Walsh (2016) identifies a number of principles related to family resilience. Three of those principles that are particularly relevant to an understanding of family resilience in the context of mental health are:

1. Crisis and ongoing stressors can affect the whole family, posing risks not only for individual dysfunction but also for relational conflict in family breakdown.
2. Individual resilience is best understood and fostered in the context of the family and larger social world. Individuals and families interact with each other and with broader sociocultural influences, including organisations and institutions involved in the delivery of mental health.
3. Considering resilience more broadly than simply a set of innate traits promotes a strengths-based view of individuals and families that mental health nurses can use to promote an increased sense of resilience for family members. This involves facilitating and fostering connectedness and mutual support, promoting connections with extended family, providing clear information and working collaboratively and proactively with families to identify issues impacting on them and interventions to address these issues (Walsh, 2016).

EVIDENCE-BASED PRACTICE

The significance of hope for resilience

Title of study

Hope and burden among Latino families of adults with schizophrenia

Authors

Mercedes Hernandez, Concepcion Barrio and Anne-Marie Yamada

Background

This 2013 study tested the hypothesis that if a family experienced high levels of hope for the consumer's future, they would experience lower levels of burden.

Participants

Researchers recruited outpatient adults who had a diagnosis of schizophrenia and asked each consumer to invite a family member they considered to be most involved in their care, who they relied on for support and with whom they had at least weekly contact. Participants were recruited from two community-based mental health programs in an urban area of Los Angeles which had an ethnically diverse population.

Method

This was a quantitative study that used a number of surveys to measure the following variables: family burden, hope, consumer symptoms, consumer length of illness and acculturation. The sample consisted of 54 families. Participants were adults diagnosed with schizophrenia.

Results

The research team found strong support for their hypothesis that increased hope for the future was negatively correlated with family burden. That is, if a family member experienced high levels of hope they would be likely to experience less feeling of burden. Hope was associated with a number of areas of family burden, including family interaction and the physical and emotional impact on family members, but not financial burden. That is, even though family members may experience financial strain, this did not negatively influence their feelings of hope. Cultural factors and the impact these had on family expectations of care-giving were part of the role that was also noted and the recommendation for further research into this area was made.

Conclusions

An interesting point made by the authors related to the need to explore the possibility of a two-way connection between hope and family burden. While this study explored hope as an indicator of burden, there is a need to investigate the extent to which burden may influence feelings of hope.

Implications

The authors believe this study highlights the need for clinicians to consider the role of hope in working with Latin American families.

SOURCE: HERNANDEZ, M., BARRIO, C. & YAMADA, A.-M. (2013). HOPE AND BURDEN AMONG LATINO FAMILIES OF ADULTS WITH SCHIZOPHRENIA. *FAMILY PROCESS*, 52(4), 697–708. DOI:10.1111/FAMP.12042

MENTAL HEALTH NURSES WORK WITH FAMILIES

In order for nurses to address the needs of consumers and families, there is an implicit assumption that each individual experiences their own reality and that nurses must learn to hear the voices of the consumers and families with whom they work. In working effectively with consumers' mental health, nurses must understand the experiences and meaning that chronic illness has for the family as well as the individual (Anderson & Bury, 1988, p. 1). Contemporary mental health services policy identifies the centrality of families to the ongoing support and care for people living with a mental health condition, but what is the impact of this role on families?

It is now recognised that mental health service delivery must be responsive to families as well as the individual consumer so that families are able to support their family member (Health.Vic, 2011). Family-inclusive recovery-oriented practice recognises the pivotal role that families play in supporting people who have a lived experience of a mental health condition. Family-inclusive practice also recognises that families will have experiences with mental health services; they will have an experience of how their family member has been treated; and they will have their own experiences of interacting with clinicians, which may or may not be positive. Family-inclusive practice requires that clinicians are respectful of and towards families and carers, recognising the role they play in the consumer's life and providing support and interventions that are tailored to meet their needs and support their family member. It also recognises that family members have needs as well and provides support and access to resources that may be required (Young, O'Hanlon & Weir, 2016).

ASSESSING FAMILY STRUCTURE, FUNCTION AND DYNAMICS

In working collaboratively with consumers, it is essential that mental health nurses understand the individual in the broader context of their immediate and extended family network. One of the key ways to do this is through the use of assessment tools, which present important information regarding family structure and dynamics. Assessment is vital in understanding the impact of factors on the family's well-being at both an individual and group level in order to collaboratively plan and implement appropriate intervention strategies.

Genograms

Genograms were first developed in the mid 1980s (McGoldrick, Gerson & Petry 2008). A genogram is a like a family tree. It visually records family members and their relations over a minimum of three generations (McGoldrick, Gerson & Petry, 2008). Besides recording the specific members of a family, the genogram also represents the nature of the relationships between family members and types of issues or patterns across generations, which is why it is essential that at least three generations are depicted. Importantly, contemporary genograms not only identify biological family relationships but, in keeping with more current understandings of family, identify all relationships considered under the term of family by the person. The genogram also provides important health history. Key health history information found in a genogram includes physical and mental health, family violence/abuse, the quality of relationships between family members such as conflicted relationships, and physical and mental health issues. There are a number of software applications that can be used to generate a genogram, although in clinical practice genograms are also drawn by hand. Specific symbols are used to construct a genogram. These symbols will present features such as gender, age, date of birth and death, relationship status and the quality of relationships between different

family members; and while each organisation and/or software application will have individual differences in the symbols it uses to represent certain aspects of a genogram, there are a number of universal symbols that are used. At the beginning of this chapter, Jo reflected on her family's experience of their loved one Tom's life. **Figure 22.2** illustrates some key features of a genogram for Tom and his family.

Tom's genogram identifies that his family has been under considerable stress in recent years. Since 1991, there have been a number of deaths in Tom's family. These were the death of his father, grandparents and older sister. These losses in a relatively condensed period of time had a profound impact on Tom, particularly his grandparents passing, as he was very close to them.

Ecomaps

Ecomaps are another useful assessment tool that nurses can use. An ecomap visually represents the social and personal relationships between individuals within a family and their environment. The ecomap uses the same symbols as a genogram, which makes it easier to use both resources together to build a more holistic understanding of a family. Some of the key features that an ecomap identifies include:

- the connection of individual family members to their community
- the strength and quality of connections between individuals and community support networks/ institutions
- awareness of the significant connections a family has with external people and organisations/

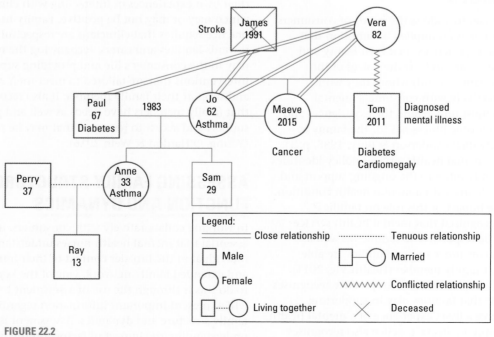

FIGURE 22.2
Tom's genogram

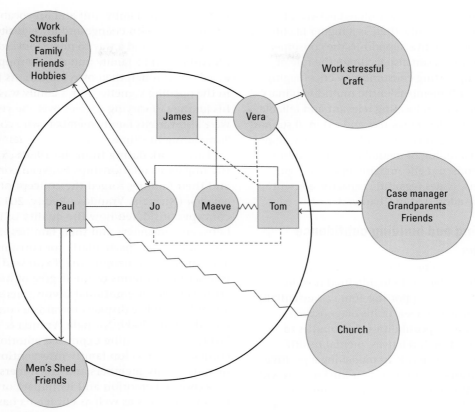

FIGURE 22.3
Sample ecomap of Tom's family (prior to 2011)

institutions and the extent to which these connections are supportive or unsupportive

- the impact of the connection between the individual and the environment through the use of an arrow to indicate whether resources and energy are flowing from an individual or to them
- connections that are stressful, usually represented by a jagged line
- an avenue for family discussion
- an objective and consistent picture of family connections to the external environment
- like the genogram, captures often complex information in a clear visual way.

Figure 22.3 illustrates a sample ecomap for a segment of Tom's family. This ecomap would have been constructed prior to Tom's death.

STRATEGIES FOR PROMOTING FAMILY RESILIENCE

Previously in this chapter, we considered the concept of resilience as it applies to families who live with and care for a consumer with a lived experience of a mental health condition. However, knowing how the concept is relevant to understanding a family's experience is only half of the equation. Effective mental health nursing practice is also based

on implementing collaborative, evidence-based interventions. In this section, we explore some strategies that mental health nurses can implement to promote family resilience.

Communication

In order to promote confidence in their capacity to support their loved one and each other, mental health nurses must facilitate transparent and respectful communication. This requires the development of rapport and trust so that family members are more likely to engage in the important conversations regarding supporting their loved one. Chapter 5 outlines the processes involved in the communication; refer to this chapter to review these ideas.

Education

If families are to effectively support their loved ones living with a mental health condition, it is essential that they have a clear understanding of the consumer's situation, and this requires clear, open communication between the multidisciplinary team, the consumer and the family. Yet it is clear in the relevant privacy legislation that the consumer's right to privacy is of prime importance; the degree to which one or more family members may be involved in supporting a consumer must rest with that person. However, where communication can be fostered between the consumer and their family, there is a higher likelihood that they can be an active support to the consumer. Mental health nurses can also facilitate the role of the family in supporting consumers by encouraging them to work with members of the multidisciplinary team, who can assist in locating relevant and reliable resources such as internet sources and external support groups. In particular, mental health nurses can support ongoing understanding of mental health conditions, treatment options and encouraging open dialogue with consumers. Issues regarding capacity, consent and privacy are addressed in Chapter 3.

Understanding and building confidence and strengths

In the 'Learning from practice' vignette at the beginning of this chapter, Jo highlighted how her family's experience of supporting Tom was essentially grounded in a negative view of his diagnosis, treatment and future possibilities. For families to effectively support their relatives, mental health nurses have an essential role in modelling a positive **strengths-based** approach in their interactions with the consumer. It is also about helping family members recognise that they can contribute in a positive way to the consumer's personal recovery journey. What this means is that families learn to view health as something to be achieved daily as opposed to health being simply the absence of illness. Strategies such as praising efforts and achievements, and **reframing** perceived problems into opportunities for growth and change, are just as important as recognising a person's limitations.

Strengthening family supports

When family members feel supported both within the immediate family context and broadly through extended family and friends, their resilience strengthens. Having access to extended family, social and community networks, and civic participation in cultural and faith-based organisations, provides not only social but practical and emotional support to families.

CONSUMERS' VIEWS OF THE FAMILY IN SUPPORTING THEM THROUGH THEIR JOURNEY

The diagnosis of a mental health condition does not affect isolated individuals; its impact strikes at the very core of the family unit and irrevocably stamps a family's life with change and uncertainty as well as the need to find a way to move forward, both as individuals and a family unit as they support their loved one through their own journey. As Jo explains in the opening vignette, Tom's family was involved in his journey to varying degrees over the years. There were also various family members who connected with Tom during this time.

Early work dating from the 1960s exploring the impact of relationships between consumers and their families forged the concept of *expressed emotion* (Nirmala, Vranda & Reddy, 2011). This concept considered how the quality of interactions between consumers and their families impacted on relapse rates, particularly for consumers with a diagnosis of schizophrenia. Expressed emotion is described in terms of the degree of hostility, criticism and/or emotional involvement that a family member displays towards a consumer (Guada et al., 2009; Nirmala, Vranda & Reddy, 2011). Understanding expressed emotion enables clinicians to develop family interventions that include family members and consumers. Research on expressed emotion and its impact on consumers, family members as well as clinicians has continued (Guada et al., 2009; Mubarak & Barber, 2003; Scazufca & Kuipers, 2001).

However, much of the work around expressed emotion has focused on the family's experience of caring for a family member diagnosed with a mental health condition and the consumer's view of their relationships with family members and the extent to which families play a role in their journey has only been explored more intensely in recent years. The degree to which families are involved in the lives of consumers living with mental health challenges varies due to the unique characteristics of each family. Research by Cohen et al. (2013) suggests that consumers want family involvement, but also worry about the impact of any involvement on both themselves and family members. Being supportive is viewed as important by consumers and involves values, qualities and actions such as being patient, tolerant, understanding and encouraging (McCann, Lubman & Clark, 2012). Alternatively, family conflict and lack of support compromises the recovery journey (McCann, Lubman & Clark, 2012). The 'Evidence-based practice' box highlights some of the factors influencing family involvement in the care of consumers living with a diagnosed mental health condition.

EVIDENCE-BASED PRACTICE

Family involvement in care

Title of study

Preferences for family involvement in care among consumers with serious mental illness

Authors

Amy N. Cohen, Amy L. Drapalski, Shirley M. Glynn, Deborah Medoff, Li Juan Fang and Lisa B. Dixon

Background

Understanding the preferences of consumers regarding family involvement in their lives and experiences of mental health and mental illness is essential in order for mental health nurses to offer holistic person- and family-centred care. Research by Cohen et al. (2013), explored this important issue. Arguing that there was a mismatch between the preferences of consumers and families and the actual services available, this project explored the preferences for family involvement by consumers.

Participants

232 consumers in the United States of America recruited from two veteran service networks; all participants were over the age of 18 years, had a formal diagnosis of schizophrenia, schizoaffective disorder, bipolar disorder, major depression with psychotic features or psychotic disorder not otherwise specified; and had had at least two outpatient mental health visits and contact with a family member or caregiver in the past six months.

Results

Results from this project showed that consumers believed that family involvement would be beneficial in helping them manage their illness and would contribute to lower stress for family members. Consumers also noted that family involvement could lead to less personal privacy and lack of time for family members to meet other responsibilities. The importance of a shared decision-making process was noted by the authors as being essential to addressing these concerns.

Conclusion

An important finding was that the extent to which the consumer believed that family involvement would be beneficial predicated the degree of desired family involvement and reflected the important hope that families can be a supportive pathway to improvement.

Implications

In discussing the implications of this study, the authors noted the extent to which consumers believed that family involvement was beneficial as well as noting concerns about personal privacy and the capacity for family members to meet other responsibilities. The authors also identified the importance of shared decision-making.

Questions

1   What does the term 'shared decision-making' mean to you?
2   Based on your understanding of this chapter, who is or should be involved in the process of shared decision-making? As well as nurses, what role do various members of the multidisciplinary potentially have? Think about health professional groups such as pharmacists, midwives (particularly in perinatal mental health) and social or welfare workers.

SOURCE: COHEN, A.N., DRAPALSKI, A.L., GLYNN, S.M., MEDOFF, D., FANG, L.J. & DIXON, L.B. (2013). PREFERENCES FOR FAMILY INVOLVEMENT IN CARE AMONG CONSUMERS WITH SERIOUS MENTAL ILLNESS. *PSYCHIATRIC SERVICES*, 64(3), 257–63. DOI:10.1176/APPI.PS.201200176

CULTURAL CONSIDERATIONS

Respecting differences: culture and care-giving

While culture is seen to have an impact on the way in which families will understand and take on care-giving roles, it is important not to generalise. Each family is ultimately unique and will have a range of factors influencing their care-giving activities. Culture adds dimension and depth to how a family understands the care-giving role as well as their experience of caring, but it does not solely define it. The 'Evidence-based practice' box earlier in this chapter explored a study by Hernandez et al. (2013) that highlights how culture can influence the care-giving role.

REFLECTION ON LEARNING FROM PRACTICE

At the beginning of this chapter, Jo described the impact of her brother Tom's diagnosis on their family. The idea of recovery and its importance to Tom's personal journey with his mental health condition was not understood in the 1980s when he was first diagnosed. The understanding of Tom's experience was grounded in symptom control and what he had lost in terms of his future. Yet Jo now knows that in the midst of all of this, Tom was still her brother – changed, but still Tom. And as the years went by Tom's disconnection and isolation from his family started to decrease. He loved his grandmother and would go there for coffee. When Jo spoke with her grandmother, she would say, 'Tom came for coffee', and Tom's grandfather would make sure that he left with a clean pair of socks and shoes. Their grandmother spoiled him, hugged him and laughed with him. His relationship with their mother became less strained as they both sought and began to find a common space to communicate. He lived in supported accommodation and undertook adult education and work experience opportunities. He had family around him whom he felt comfortable with and the rest of the family knew where he was, knew he was safe and that he was engaging with others. He had dinner each week with his cousin and aunt. But the years took their toll physically, and Tom had a number of physical health issues to contend with. As a nurse, Jo knew the incidence of mental health problems and co-occurring physical health problems was high and she worried about his health. Tom was diagnosed with diabetes and chronic respiratory problems, issues clearly attributable to his long-term poor diet, lack of exercise and long history of heavy smoking.

Tom passed away in 2011 when he was just 47 years old. In the last couple of years of his life, Jo believes Tom finally found a sense of being settled and content.

So, what is a family? For Jo, family is the group of people you collect around you as you go through life, people who care about what happens to you even though they may not see you often. They are the people in the background who just want you to be safe and happy, they are the people who buy your favourite food to cook when you go for dinner. They go shopping with you and when they have to they make difficult decisions with you and sometimes for you. Family are the people who matter in your life and you matter in theirs. Tom had family and Tom mattered.

The experience of caring of Jo's family highlights the number of complex issues involved in a family's experience of living and caring for a consumer diagnosed with a mental health condition. Over the years, Jo and her family experienced a range of sometimes conflicting emotions. They felt love, compassion and a sense of duty to Tom, but also frustration. In the early years there was a sense of isolation from extended family as well as anxiety and constant worry when Tom would disappear. In Jo's view it is essential that the multidisciplinary team, including mental health nurses, promote increased family understanding of the consumer's experience through education and support, and encourage the family's capacity to support their family member living with a mental health condition.

CHAPTER RESOURCES

SUMMARY

- We are all born into a family and we will spend our lives with families in various shapes and forms. Families provide the foundation for developing our understanding of the world around us and interacting with other people. Families provide the context for our ongoing growth and development.
- Family care-giving is seen as integral to supporting consumers on their personal recovery journey.
- Families can experience a range of impacts as a consequence of the care-giving role. While in many instances these impacts can be negative, it is also important to recognise that families can experience personal growth as well.

- While resilience is often described in terms of the individual, the concept is equally as important for families.
- Mental health nurses have an important role in assessing family strengths and challenges as part of their role in working with consumers and families.
- As part of the multidisciplinary team, mental health nurses can assist families to develop resilience in a number of ways. This includes encouraging open communication, education, building confidence and increasing family supports.
- Research indicates that consumers value the support and input from family members and the degree to which family members are involved will be a reflection of the unique characteristics of each family.

REVIEW QUESTIONS

1   Eric says that in spite of the challenges of his recent diagnosis, he and his family are working on a plan to help him recognise when he is starting to experience signs of a relapse and feeling hopeful for the future. The term that best describes this is:

a   Relieved
b   Coping
c   Adapting
d   Resilience

2 Family has been defined as:
   a A group of people who live together and may or may not be biologically related
   b A system where the whole is greater than the sum of its parts
   c A personal construct for each individual
   d All of the above
3 A family genogram is:
   a A visual representation that illustrates support systems and stressors in the external environment of the immediate family
   b An assessment tool that reports on the individual's perception of their family's relationships
   c A specialised form of a family tree that records information about family members and their relationships and health history over at least three generations
   d An assessment of a family's capacity to respond to a crisis
4 A family ecomap is:
   a A visual representation that illustrates support systems and stressors in the external environment of the immediate family

b An assessment tool that reports on the individual's perception of their family's relationships
   c A specialised form of a family tree that records information about family members and their relationships and health history over at least three generations
   d An assessment of a family's capacity to respond to crisis
5 Theories are useful to the extent they help us explain a series of facts or a phenomenon. What do you think are the benefits and limitations of the family life cycle, ecological systems and family systems theories?
6 In the 'Learning from practice' vignette, Jo reflects on how mental health nurses need to be more actively involved in assessment and support. How could the mental health nurse use the assessment tools described to gather important information about Jo's family?
7 What factors impact on the extent to which consumers may feel supported and welcome family support as part of their recovery journey?

CRITICAL THINKING

1 Select one of the theories regarding family structure and function in this chapter. Think of a family you know and consider to what extent they reflect the key features of the theory you selected. In what ways does this family differ from the theory you selected?
2 Consider the following scenario: Ramandeep has been admitted to the acute mental health inpatient unit. He is 23 years old. His parents request information on his progress and how they can assist. How would you need to respond to this request?

3 Families often provide a significant care-giving and support role for the consumer living with a diagnosis of a mental health condition. This can impact on the emotional, social and physical health of family members. What resources exist in the community to support families in your region or state/territory?
4 Read the article 'Family burden, family health and personal mental health' (Ennis & Bunting, 2013). What issues are important in understanding and recognising the impact of family burden on family caregivers? What role can nurses play in supporting family caregivers?

USEFUL WEBSITES

- Children of Parents with a Mental Illness: http://www.copmi.net.au
- Family Mental Health Support Services (FMHSS): https://www.dss.gov.au/our-responsibilities/mental-health/
programmes-services/family-mental-health-support-service-fmhss#family
- SANE Australia: https://www.sane.org/mental-health-and-illness/facts-and-guides/292-families-friends-carers

REFLECT ON THIS

Resilience and families
Resilience from a personal perspective is addressed in Chapter 21. This chapter has introduced you to how the concept of resilience is important to a family's journey of living with a loved one experiencing a mental health condition. Consider how resilience is important to families and families' experiences of a crisis such as the COVID-19 pandemic.

REFERENCES

Anderson, R. & Bury, M. (1988). *Living with Chronic Illness: The Experience of Patients and Their Families*. London: Allen and Unwin.

Australian Bureau of Statistics (ABS). (2013). *What Is a Family? 6224.0.55.001 – Labour Force, Australia: Labour Force Status and Other Characteristics of Families. June 2012*. Retrieved from http://www.abs.gov.au/ausstats/abs@.nsf/Products/6224.0.55.001~Jun%202012~Chapter~What%20is%20a%20Family%3F.

Bandura, A. (1977). Self-efficacy: Towards a unifying theory of behaviour change. *Psychological Review*, 84, 191–215. doi:http://dx.doi.org.ezproxy2.acu.edu.au/10.1037/0033-295X.84.2.191

Barbarin, O.A., Hughes, D. & Chesler, M.A. (1985). Stress, coping and marital functioning among parents of children with cancer. *Journal of Marriage and the Family*, 47(2), May, 473–80.

Bronfenbrenner, U. (1979). *The Ecology of Human Development*. Cambridge, MA: Harvard University Press.

Bronfenbrenner, U. (1986). Ecology of the family as a context for human development: Research perspectives. *Developmental Psychology*, 22(6), 723–42. doi:10.1037/0012-1649.22.6.723

Cançado Monteiro Savassi, L. & Modena, C.M. (2013). The different facets of the suffering of the person who gives care: A review about the caregiver. *Revista de Atencao Primaria a Saude*, 16(3), 313–19.

Carter, B. & McGoldrick, M. (2005). *The Expanded Family Life Cycle: Individual, Family and Social Perspectives* (classic edn). Boston, MA: Allyn & Bacon.

Cohen, A.N., Drapalski, A.L., Glynn, S.M., Medoff, D., Fang, L.J. & Dixon, L.B. (2013). Preferences for family involvement in care among consumers with serious mental illness. *Psychiatric Services*, 64(3), 257–63. doi:10.1176/appi.ps.201200176

Cohen, L., Ferguson, C., Harms, C., Pooley, J.A. & Tomlinson, S. (2011). Family systems and mental health issues: A resilience approach. *Journal of Social Work Practice*, 25(1), 109–25. doi:10.1080/02650533.2010.533754

Deloitte Access Economics. (2015). *The Economic Value of Informal Care in Australia in 2015*. Carers Australia. Retrieved from https://www2.deloitte.com/au/en/pages/economics/articles/economic-value-informal-care-Australia-2015.html.

Duvall, E.M. (1977). *Marriage and Family Development* (5th edn). Philadelphia, PA: J.B. Lippincott.

Ennis, E. & Bunting, B.P. (2013). Family burden, family health and personal mental health. *BMC Public Health*, 13, 255. doi:10.1186/1471-2458-13-255

Guada, J., Brekke, J.S., Floyd, R. & Barbour, J. (2009). The relationships among perceived criticism, family contact, and consumer clinical and psychosocial functioning for African-American consumers with schizophrenia. *Community Mental Health Journal*, 45(2), 106–16. doi:10.1007/s10597-008-9165-4

Hallam, L. (2007). How involuntary commitment impacts on the burden of care of the family. *International Journal of Mental Health Nursing*, 16(4), 247–56.

Health.Vic. (2011). *Framework for Recovery-oriented Practice*. Melbourne: Department of Health and Human Services. Retrieved from https://www2.health.vic.gov.au/about/publications/policiesandguidelines/Framework-for-Recovery-oriented-Practice.

Hernandez, M., Barrio, C. & Yamada, A.-M. (2013). Hope and burden among Latino families of adults with schizophrenia. *Family Process*, 52(4), 697–708. doi:10.1111/famp.12042

Lubkin, I.M. (1990). *Chronic Illness: Impact and Interventions* (2nd edn). Boston, MA: Jones and Bartlett Publishers.

McCann, T.V., Lubman, D.I. & Clark, E. (2012). Views of young people with depression about family and significant other support: Interpretative phenomenological analysis study. *International Journal of Mental Health Nursing*, 21(5), 453–61. doi:10.1111/j.1447-0349.2012.00812.x

McGoldrick, M., Gerson, R. & Petry, S. (2008). *Genograms: Assessment and Intervention* (3rd edn). New York: W.W. Norton & Company.

McLeod, J. (2013). *An Introduction to Counselling*. Maidenhead, Berkshire: Open University Press.

Mubarak, A.R. & Barber, J.G. (2003). Emotional expressiveness and the quality of life of patients with schizophrenia. *Social Psychiatry and Psychiatric Epidemiology*, 38(7), 380–4. doi:10.1007/s00127-003-0645-0. Retrieved from https://link-springer-com.ezproxy2.acu.edu.au/content/pdf/10.1007%2Fs00127-003-0645-0.pdf.

Nirmala, B., Vranda, M. & Reddy, S. (2011). Expressed emotion and caregiver burden in patients with schizophrenia. *Indian Journal of Psychological Medicine*, 33(2), 119–22. doi:http://dx.doi.org.ezproxy1.acu.edu.au/10.4103/0253-7176.92052

O'Neill, G. & Ross, M.M. (1991). Burden of care: An important concept for nurses. *Health Care for Women International*, 12, 111–21.

Rhodes, M. (2013). *How Two Intuitive Theories Shape the Development of Social Categorization*. Child Dev Perspect, 7: 12–16. doi:10.1111/cdep.12007.

Rugkåsa, J. (2015). *Care and Culture: Care Relations from the Perspectives of Mental Health Caregivers in Ethnic Minority Families*. Cambridge: Cambridge Scholars Publishing.

Scazufca, M. & Kuipers, E. (2001). Perception of negative emotions in close relatives by patients with schizophrenia. *British Journal of Clinical Psychology*, 40, 167–75.

Sigelman, C., Rider, E. & De George-Walker, L. (2016). *Life Span Human Development* (2nd Australian and New Zealand edn). South Melbourne: Cengage Learning Australia.

Stewart, M.J., Ritchie, J.A., McGrath, P., Thompson, D. & Bruce, B. (1994). Mothers of children with chronic conditions: Supportive and stressful interactions with partners and professionals regarding caregiving burdens. *Canadian Journal of Nursing Research*, 26(4), 61–82.

Strauss, A. (1986). Chronic illness. In P. Conrad & R. Kern (eds), *The Sociology of Health and Illness: Critical Perspectives* (2nd edn). New York: St Martin's Press.

Suro, G. & Weisman De Mamani, A.G. (2013). Burden, interdependence, ethnicity, and mental health in caregivers of patients with schizophrenia. *Family Process*, 52(2), 299–311. doi:10.1111/famp.12002

Tudge, J.R.H., Mokrova, I., Hatfield, B.E. & Karnik, R.B. (2009). Uses and misuses of Bronfenbrenner's bioecological theory of human development. *Journal of Family Theory & Review*, 1(4), 198–210. doi:10.1111/j.1756-2589.2009.00026.x

Walker, A. (1982). *Community Care, the Family, the State and Social Policy*. Oxford: Basil Blackwell Publications and Martin Robertson and Company.

Walsh, F. (2016). *Strengthening Family Resilience* (3rd edn). New York: Guilford Press.

Young, J., O'Hanlon, B. & Weir, S. (2016). *From Individual to Families: A Client-centred Framework for Involving Families*. Melbourne: The Bouverie Centre. https://www.bouverie.org.au/images/uploads/Bouverie_Centre_Framework.pdf.

Zauszniewski, J.A., Bekhet, A.K. & Suresky, M.J. (2009). Effects on resilience of women family caregivers of adults with serious mental illness: The role of positive cognitions. *Archives of Psychiatric Nursing*, 23(4), 412–22.

Zauszniewski, J.A., Bekhet, A.K. & Suresky, M.J. (2010). Resilience in family members of persons with serious mental illness. *Nursing Clinics of North America*, 45(4), 613–26. doi:https://doi.org/10.1016/j.cnur.2010.06.007

CHAPTER 23

THE MULTIDISCIPLINARY TEAM

Gylo (Julie) Hercelinskyj

LEARNING FROM PRACTICE

Students often worry about going on placement in mental health. Their questions centre on concerns about what to say, and being afraid they will 'say the wrong thing'. The other major concern is what the mental health nurse does – what is their role exactly? What is the multidisciplinary team? How do they prepare for clinical placement in mental health? There doesn't seem to be a clear vision or understanding of the role of the mental health nurse. Students will ask what the routine on an inpatient unit is, who are the other disciplines they will meet and how will they know if they are 'doing the right thing'. They struggle with the language of mental health, the idea of recovery as it applies to mental health practice and service delivery, and even how this knowledge is transferable to other clinical contexts. There is often an academic or intellectual interest in the subject but the reality of working with consumers and clinicians can be a worrying matter. As an educator, this is the challenge I face every time I work with a new group of students. In my experience, the more preparation a

student has the more they will achieve during their clinical placement. The key is to help them move past their own preconceptions, lack of knowledge prior to their studies or their own experiences with mental health services either personally or through family or friends. This could lead to an internal struggle as they try to resolve this tension, or come to the realisation that the role of the mental health nurse is actually broad and complex. A student once said that prior to studying mental health and clinical placement, they did not know that mental health nurses did anything other than administer medications.

Nurse educator, 20 years' experience

A student's experience in mental health is shaped by a number of factors, as the nurse educator in this excerpt has identified. In this chapter, you will explore how the multidisciplinary team is essential to mental health care, and to your learning, and reflect on the role of consumers and carers as members of this team.

INTRODUCTION

The multidisciplinary team can be defined as a group of health care professionals who contribute to the planning and management of an individual's health care needs through their different areas of expertise. In contemporary mental health service delivery, care is delivered by this type of team. In mental health, it is thought that care delivered by a multidisciplinary team is more effective and leads to better health outcomes because of the often complex and varied set of issues a consumer living with a mental health condition can experience (Bowen, 2014). As the comment made by the student nurse in the opening vignette suggests, sometimes it can be difficult to know exactly who each member of the team is and what their specific role entails. In 2001, the World Health Organization (WHO) stated that nurses, as part of the multidisciplinary team, are especially relevant in the management of mental health conditions.

A significant part of your professional development as a nurse will be understanding the concepts underpinning the role of the multidisciplinary team and experiencing this in the clinical environment. Therefore, in this chapter we review a number of important considerations related to the multidisciplinary team, teamwork and its place within current mental health care planning and delivery.

THE MULTIDISCIPLINARY TEAM

The nurse contributes to a range of activities as part of the team. A team in general terms is a group of people who work together to achieve a goal or complete a task. We now look at the multidisciplinary team in more detail.

Early ideas regarding the multidisciplinary team

Renouf and Meadows (2012, p. 325) state 'much mental health work is organised as teamwork, and the mental health team is one of the main vehicles of collaborative work'. This statement puts the mental health team at the centre of mental health care delivery. It is directly oppositional to the idea that it is an end product of different occupational groups occupying a shared space and working with the same group of consumers.

Multidisciplinary approaches to health are an integral part of mental health care service delivery. Policy directives regarding primary care increasingly call for teamwork and cooperation in multidisciplinary group practice (Belanger & Rodriguez, 2008). Dennis (2006) believes that interdisciplinary work in its most positive sense provides the opportunity for consumers to receive care influenced by a range of professional understandings that should improve the quality and diversity of care options offered.

Exploring the idea of the 'team'

Typically, teams are considered relatively stable structures that are task oriented and have a shared purpose and goal (Renouf & Meadows, 2012). So effective multidisciplinary teamwork really boils down to working successfully as a group member. So what is a group? There is no single definition, but some common themes emerge in the literature. These include the idea that groups are goal directed, governed by expectations or rules and involve different members who have different roles. If we consider these ideas, we can identify that most people already spend a great deal of time working and socialising in groups. The multidisciplinary team is another group, of which the nurse will be part.

In clinical practice, the term used most commonly is the **multidisciplinary team**. However, some authors believe that most teams in mental health are either multidisciplinary or transdisciplinary in composition and purpose, with mental health nurses making up the bulk of team membership (Ndoro, 2014; Renouf & Meadows, 2012).

Table 23.1 presents a summary of the various types of teams employed within the health care context.

TABLE 23.1

Different types of health teams

Interdisciplinary team (IDT)	Used in the 1970s when research suggested that lives were saved by better coordination and collaboration in health services. Interdisciplinary teams are understood to build upon the expertise of each other's disciplines.
Multidisciplinary team (MDT)	Members from a range of disciplines who work in parallel. There is coordination, collaboration and conferring. In contrast to the interdisciplinary team, the multidisciplinary team tends to work in silos, around each other.
Transdisciplinary team (TDT)	Teams where there is professional boundary overlap
Interprofessional collaborative team (IPCT)	A range of disciplines collaborating in mutually supportive teams, optimising the skills and knowledge of each individual to the fullest extent
Multi-professional team (MPT)	Professional practitioners who work in parallel. There are clear role definitions, specified tasks, hierarchical lines of authority and high levels of professional autonomy

SOURCE: ADAPTED FROM BENNETTS ET AL., 2012; STONE, 2010

Renouf and Meadows (2012, p. 228) define the multidisciplinary team as comprising 'members from a range of disciplines working in parallel, coordinating, cooperating and conferring'. This is contrasted with the characteristics of the interdisciplinary team, which 'has all the features of multidisciplinary teams and in addition requires a system of collaboration, which brings joint activity and some degree of shared responsibility' (p. 229). Different again, transdisciplinary teams 'comprise a range of professions, place little emphasis on individual team members' different disciplinary backgrounds, but use a common set of axioms and integrated methods and concepts' (p. 229). It becomes apparent from this table that while the literature refers overwhelmingly to the multidisciplinary team and this is the term commonly used in clinical service delivery, the definitions provided by Renouf and Meadows would suggest the use of the term 'multidisciplinary' is somewhat ambiguous. This ambiguity may well contribute to role ambiguity and role strain.

Roles in the multidisciplinary team

Who are the members of the multidisciplinary team, and what do they do? Put simply, the people who make up any team are those individuals who have the range of knowledge and skills to contribute towards achieving the team's goals. In the case of the mental health multidisciplinary team, this means that health professionals from a range of disciplines can be members of the team. **Table 23.2** outlines some of the key members of the mental health multidisciplinary team.

Renouf and Meadows (2012) say that the multidisciplinary team has specialist roles and responsibilities as well as shared ones. All members of the multidisciplinary team will be responsible for establishing and maintaining a professional therapeutic relationship with consumers and carers. All team members will also contribute to the assessment process. However, different team members will focus on different aspects during the assessment process, as well as undertake different interventions that relate to the specific expertise of their discipline;

TABLE 23.2
Roles in the multidisciplinary team

STAFF	ROLE
Registered nurse	A registered nurse who, after completing a postgraduate specialist qualification in mental health, works in partnership with the consumer, carers and the other members of the multidisciplinary team to meet the holistic health care needs of consumers Roles include: assessment, planning and evaluation care within a recovery-oriented model of care, education, mental health promotion, advocacy in partnership with consumers, acute practice, community practice, psychotherapy, advanced practice and mental health nurse practitioner. All these roles include case management
Psychiatrist	A registered medical practitioner with specialist qualifications in psychiatry. Responsible for physical and psychiatric assessment, confirming the diagnosis of a mental health condition, prescribing medications and authorising treatment options
Psychologist	Holds specialist qualifications in clinical psychology and conducts assessments (such as IQ testing), psychological screening, interpreting results as well as practising specific therapies such as cognitive behavioural therapy and talking therapies
Social worker	Assesses the individual, family and community support systems that a consumer can access and use in the process of their recovery journey Places emphasis on the strengths of consumers and their families in the assessment of a person's needs
Occupational therapist	Works with consumers and carers to maximise occupational, social and daily living skills Provides specialised assessment of functioning in areas such as social skills or ability to perform activities of daily living such as shopping, cooking and mobility
Mental health consumer worker	Participates in activities such as mental health service planning, mental health service evaluation and peer support roles
Other personal care staff	Include personal services officers and personal care attendants who assist consumers with specific needs such as activities of daily living
Registrar	A registered doctor who is completing specialist training through a medical college
Pharmacist	A health professional who dispenses prescriptions, and provides education and information regarding drugs to consumers, carers and other health professionals
Enrolled nurse	In Australia, anyone who completes a Diploma in Nursing can work in a variety of clinical areas including mental health
Clinical nurse specialist	A registered nurse who is a senior member of staff in a practice area such as mental health Often practises in the acute mental health care setting and will have completed postgraduate education in mental health
Mental health nurse practitioner	A registered nurse who has advanced nursing practice in a clinical leadership role in a specific clinical area for at least five years. Also has demonstrated research, education and management skills and has completed a Master's level qualification as a nurse practitioner Must be authorised to practise in this role by the relevant nursing and midwifery registration body. Can work in public or private health networks in rural, remote and primary health care settings If eligible, can access the Medicare Benefits Schedule (MBS) and the Pharmaceutical Benefits Scheme (PBS) in Australia

EVIDENCE-BASED PRACTICE

How different disciplines understand and conduct mental health assessments

Title of study

Perspectives of a nurse, a social worker, and a psychiatrist regarding patient assessment in acute inpatient psychiatry settings: A case study approach

Authors

Bridget Hamilton, Elizabeth Manias, Phil Maude, Timothy Marjoribanks and K. Cook

Background

This study provides a useful way in which to understand the different perspectives that health disciplines bring to their role using the example of the assessment process.

Participants

The participants comprised a nurse, social worker and psychiatrist who were employed in separate inpatient units.

Methods

The authors used a descriptive case study method to explore health professionals' perspectives on patient assessment in the mental health setting.

Results

Two of the major themes from this study related to the distinctive way in which each clinician undertook assessment and the place they gave to patient involvement in the assessment process. Nursing assessment differed from other disciplines in its focus on the consumer's behaviour and interactions in the immediate environment of the inpatient unit. There was less consideration of the

broader social or personal context of the consumer. The nursing assessment was often framed in medical terms. The assessment of the social worker indicated a focus on the consumer's usual community context and information was often sourced from other family members who were also included in the social worker's assessment. A medical diagnosis was central to the social worker's understanding of the consumer prior to meeting with them. For the psychiatrist, diagnosis was integral to any assessment they engaged in. Relevant information about social factors contributed to the diagnostic process.

Implications

This study demonstrates that each discipline is to some degree using a medical framework of understanding to collect and describe information, interpret and understand that information from within their disciplinary lens. Each discipline has also mapped the boundaries in their practice through the role they enact in the assessment process. Within the context of this study each discipline appears to give priority to some elements of the assessment over others, notably the degree to which they used the social context of consumers to inform the assessment. Also of importance is the degree to which all three disciplines used a medical lens to frame their understanding and description of the assessment and subsequent rationale for the choice of interventions. However, this study was conducted in an inpatient environment and cannot be generalised to the broader context of the community setting.

SOURCE: HAMILTON, B., MANIAS, E., MAUDE, P., MARJORIBANKS, T. & COOK, K. (2004). PERSPECTIVES OF A NURSE, A SOCIAL WORKER, AND A PSYCHIATRIST REGARDING PATIENT ASSESSMENT IN ACUTE INPATIENT PSYCHIATRY SETTINGS: A CASE STUDY APPROACH. *JOURNAL OF PSYCHIATRIC AND MENTAL HEALTH NURSING*, 11, 683–9.

for example, a psychiatrist will prescribe medications, a social worker will consider the community supports a consumer may wish to access, and a registered nurse can provide psychoeducation on a particular medication that the consumer has been prescribed. Renouf and Meadows (2012) also argue that the different roles undertaken will also be dependent on the clinical context in which a team member is working.

CHARACTERISTICS OF EFFECTIVE TEAMWORK

For the multidisciplinary team to work effectively, all members must have a clear sense of what their role is and how this contributes to effective teamwork. Some of the benefits of a team approach to mental health service delivery include:

- increased productivity and role sharing; for example, case management and psychoeducation
- team-based problem identification and decision making, which promotes ethical practice.

Each member of the multidisciplinary team has knowledge and skills that are considered to be discipline specific to their approach to their work. But they also bring a shared set of knowledge and skills to working with consumers and carers. This combination promotes a broader, shared understanding of the health and recovery approaches to working with consumers and carers.

Multidisciplinary teams also provide the opportunity for new and innovative ways of thinking about and addressing consumer recovery goals.

There are several factors that constitute effective teamwork generally and in the mental health multidisciplinary team context specifically. These include:

- respect and trust
- accountability
- clear and complementary roles
- ability to recognise and work through conflict
- being goal directed.

We now consider each of these factors in more detail.

Respect and trust

A team comprises individuals who each has a unique disciplinary focus or lens through which they assess, understand and plan interventions in partnership with consumers. For a team to work effectively, mutual respect and trust are essential. This enables team members to feel that their distinct disciplinary/lived experience contribution is valued and integrates with the overall goals and work of the team. This trust and respect is demonstrated through clear, open communication, addressing issues respectfully and being accountable.

Accountability

While clinicians bring their individual expertise to a team, all team members share accountability for the decisions made by the team. When accountability is shared, people are more highly motivated and able to work effectively together as a group.

Clear and complementary professional roles and group behaviours

In this section we look at the professional roles people have as part of the multidisciplinary team, and the related aspect of the role behaviours that people can engage in to help the team achieve its goal(s).

Professional roles

When a person is asked, 'What do you do for a living?', it is common to hear them refer to their position title; for example, 'I am a nurse' or 'I am a teacher'. Explaining what a nurse does is usually described in terms of their place of employment, specific tasks or functions, who they work with and perhaps examples of their work. What is being described is the nurse's role. If there is confusion, lack of clarity or misunderstanding in these descriptions, other people may wonder exactly what it is that the person does.

Professional roles are best understood by considering role theory. According to Conway (1988, p. 63), role theory is concerned with and predicts 'how people will perform in a given role or the circumstances under which certain behaviours would be expected'.

Roles have recognisable patterns of behaviours and expected behaviours assigned to them. Role expectations refer to the position-specific demands made of, or obligations felt by, the person occupying that role (Hardy & Hardy, 1988). There are also expectations regarding the behaviour of the individual or group with whom the different professionals interact. Furthermore, to make the complex nature of roles even more apparent, each of these individuals will have a set of role expectations they are required to meet. In professional relationships, colleagues and

peers all have their own role in relation to the context of the others (Kahn et al., 1964); that is, each member of the team will come from a discipline with their own occupational understanding, knowledge and skills (MacAteer, Manktelow & Fitzsimons, 2016). Each individual health professional (such as the mental health nurse) is required to understand and meet the expected requirements of their role. These individual roles that each person performs within the scope of practice will also be combined to reach group decisions. Where the expected professional and organisational requirement of each person's role matches those of the individual or group, there is role congruence. However, where there is incongruence between the professional and organisational expectations of a mental health nurses role and that of the mental health nurse themselves, there is role conflict.

Role conflict is viewed by Kahn et al. (1964) as either the discrepancy between the role expectations within various roles or when individuals have differing perceptions of how a role should be performed. In other words, conflict occurs when an individual experiences stress from a difference or contradiction in one work role compared with another (Wickham & Parker, 2007). Role conflict can also take place when there are varying expectations by others towards the person occupying a particular role (Kahn et al., 1964). The key feature of this conflict is a breakdown in communication in role expectations between two or more people. We discuss conflict in more detail below.

Role behaviours

Not only does effective multidisciplinary teamwork mean that each member must have a clear sense of what unique functions they bring to the team and what characteristics they share, but they must understand the various behaviours that can be seen in the team. By understanding this, it is possible to build on the strengths of various members at different points in the team's work. Some roles are related to the functions and tasks of the group. These are referred to as **task behaviours**, which are the behaviours that are helpful in getting the task completed. Other roles are related to maintaining relationships and communication between group members to assist in achieving the goal of the group. These are referred to as **maintenance behaviours** and are aimed at maintaining a climate for group activities, to reduce conflict and to encourage contributions from all team members. The original authors of this work on role behaviours, Benne and Sheats (1948, 2007), also identified a number of roles that individual group members may adopt to satisfy individual goals or needs. **Table 23.3** identifies a number of task and *maintenance functions* – those behaviours that relate to maintaining social relationships.

TABLE 23.3
Task and maintenance behaviours

TYPE OF BEHAVIOUR	BEHAVIOUR	EXAMPLE
Task behaviours	Initiating	Defining the issue or task the group must complete, providing ideas about how to proceed or giving directions
	Seeking information/opinions	Asking for information or asking for clarification
	Giving information/opinions	Providing information that is factual rather than relying on opinions
	Clarifying and elaborating	Reducing/eliminating confusion/ambiguity by giving examples, defining key terms or ideas, or explaining
	Summarising	Communicating the main ideas discussed/developed by a group in a clear concise manner that captures the key points, identifying discrepancies/common themes, etc.
	Consensus testing	Establishing whether the group is satisfied as a whole with the outcome of the task and final decision
Maintenance behaviours	Harmonising	Acting as a mediator, promoting behaviours aimed at reducing tension between group members
	Encouraging	Recognising the contributions of group members, providing encouragement, being friendly
	Gatekeeping	Enabling contributions from everyone, keeping communication flowing between all group members
	Trust building	Communicating openly and being non-judgemental helps to establish trust
	Compromising	Offering or accepting compromises, someone acknowledging when they are incorrect in order to achieve group goals and maintain group cohesion
	Standard setting	Considering whether the group is satisfied with how it will go about addressing the task, looking at the factors it needs to consider and possibly resolve before they can complete the group activity Deciding how to identify/address disputes

SOURCE: ADAPTED FROM PORTEUS, N.D.

Recognising and addressing conflict

One of the key features of effective group work is the capacity to recognise and address conflict. Before considering how groups can address conflict, it is important to consider what conflict is and why it arises.

Within the context of the multidisciplinary team, conflict can occur when there is disagreement between various team members regarding matters such as identification of consumer issues, management options and/or values and interests of different group members (Balzer Riley, 2017). This conflict occurs at an interpersonal level, between members of the group. Unresolved conflict within the multidisciplinary team leads to ineffective outcomes for consumers and carers, as well as professional dissatisfaction and role conflict for mental health professionals such as nurses (MacAteer, Manktelow & Fitzsimons, 2016; Ndoro, 2014).

DeVito (2016) identifies that conflict within a group can occur because of context differences; for example, when there are perceived differences in how the group should actually go about achieving a particular task and/or conflict between people in the group. Kindler (1996) highlights four principles that are essential for effectively addressing conflict:

1 ensuring dignity and respect of all members of the group
2 empathic listening
3 recognising and working to achieve common goals between people and in groups
4 valuing diversity and distinctiveness.

Often, conflict is considered something that should be avoided at all costs, and if conflict occurs in a group situation such as the multidisciplinary team it is regarded as demonstrating poor working relationships between team members. However, while the experience of conflict can be stressful, it has both positive and negative aspects (DeVito, 2016). The reason conflict can be positive is that team members have the opportunity and are professionally required to explore the particular, contentious issue and work towards a potential solution or resolution. Underpinning this strategy is the need to communicate assertively. Assertive communication is addressed later in the chapter.

Horizontal violence

One significant form of conflict that can occur between clinicians is **horizontal violence**. Also referred to as **bullying**, horizontal violence is acknowledged as a significant workplace issue for all health clinicians including mental health nurses. It was estimated that in Australia in 2010 the total cost of workplace bullying was between $6–36 billion annually (Victorian Auditor-General's Report, 2016), with this figure most likely including the impact of horizontal violence.

Horizontal violence in the mental health setting is characterised by behaviour (verbal and/or physical) that is abusive or hostile, occurs over a period of time and involves a range of behaviours that publicly or privately humiliate, intimidate or threaten a nurse. Behaviours that constitute horizontal violence include criticising, undermining efforts of the individual, name calling, isolating a person, ignoring them, eye rolling, public humiliation, refusing to provide assistance and assigning unreasonable tasks (Becher & Visovsky, 2012). Clear, assertive communication, self-care, speaking with a trusted friend or colleague, reporting horizontal violence through the appropriate organisational processes, seeking support through counselling and learning to say no are all important skills for nurses to develop.

Addressing conflict in the multidisciplinary team

The key to addressing conflict in the multidisciplinary team relates to building effective communication between team members. If conflict is not resolved, there are implications for the working relationship between team members and the extent to which the team effectively achieves its goals. Each team member has responsibilities and is accountable for their own practice and the successful completion of group tasks.

In terms of the multidisciplinary context and conflict between team members, the first point to remember is: who is at the centre of the team? That is, why is the team in place to begin with? The multidisciplinary team exists to work collaboratively with consumers and carers in identifying the consumer's health-related needs, managing any challenges in meeting those needs and facilitating the consumer's recovery journey. Therefore, it is clear that the consumer is at the centre of the multidisciplinary team, not any one health professional. Recognising this is the first way in which the team can begin to address any potential conflict. When the multidisciplinary team is clear about the reason for the existence and the centrality of the consumer's place within the team, moving forward to resolve any potential conflict becomes possible.

Assertive communication is viewed as a crucial way in which conflict can first be recognised and then addressed. Assertive communication provides the opportunity to identify and address problems between people. Assertiveness is the capacity to stand up for one's rights by expressing thoughts and feelings in a direct and transparent manner. The key to being

assertive is ensuring that this communication does not violate the rights of the person to whom the communication is directed (Eunson, 1994, 2016). Assertive communication within the multidisciplinary team is an essential skill for all team members. Importantly, it is a skill that can be learned, and improved with practice (Balzer Riley, 2012).

There are some strategies that contribute to communicating assertively. When a person communicates assertively, they use language that demonstrates three things:

1   Self-awareness of how they react to certain events, their understanding of these reactions and how they influence their thoughts and emotions. This self-awareness will be reflected in their communication and behaviour towards other people.

2   Being aware of the other person and how one's own style communication can impact on them.

3   Effective listening; speaking openly and honestly about the situation they are in, what they think about it and how it makes them feel. Communicating assertively requires us to recognise our emotions, the emotions of others, and to manage them.

There are other ways of communicating. There are times when we may wish to avoid potential conflict, or may not have the confidence to speak up assertively and so we communicate **non-assertively**; that is, in a way that aims to reduce conflict by appeasing the other person, perhaps being overly apologetic or acting in a subservient manner. Alternatively, we may find it difficult to manage our emotions in a situation in an assertive manner. We may believe we are right about a matter and behave and communicate in a way that belittles the other person as we seek to demonstrate that we are 'right'. This is referred to as **aggressive communication**.

There are a number of characteristic behaviours and ways of communicating that demonstrate an assertive nurse. An assertive nurse:

- is confident
- listens and checks their understanding of the situation by asking questions
- has assessed the situation and gathered the information they need to address the issue and communicates this clearly and concisely
- is congruent in their verbal and non-verbal communication (Lampert & Youl, 2016).

Balzer Riley (2017) provides a succinct and useful pro forma that can be used to help nurses to communicate assertively. Called the DESC process, it enables the mental health nurse to work their way through a conflict situation. The process is:

- **D**escribe the situation
- **E**xpress what you think and feel

TABLE 23.4
Communicating assertively

PROCESS STEP	EXAMPLE	RATIONALE
Describe the situation	When you insult me during handover, like today….	Be specific about the behaviour/event and state the facts.
Express what you think and feel	I am confused as to what has happened to cause this.	Using the identifier 'I' shows that you own your response. The aim is to reduce the chance of the other person becoming defensive.
Specify your request	If there is an issue with my work, could you please speak with me individually.	Specific what you would prefer. In this example, you are not refusing to have the conversation, but stating there is an alternative way to go about it.
outline the **C**onsequences of your request being met	We can then both talk in an uninterrupted manner.	This shows that there are positive outcomes for both parties.

- **S**pecify your request
- outline the **C**onsequences of your request being met.

  Table 23.4 illustrates the DESC process in action.

Being goal directed

An effective team will be clear about the goals it is seeking to achieve. In the context of the mental health multidisciplinary team, this means co-creating with consumers and carers a plan within a recovery-oriented framework. It is essential that all team members share this goal. If there are other issues or **hidden agendas** that team members bring to their practice, this creates the potential for conflict (as discussed above). Generally, when all members of a team share the same goals they are more likely to be involved and have a sense of commitment to achieving those goals.

BECOMING A MEMBER OF THE MULTIDISCIPLINARY TEAM: INTEGRATING INTO THE TEAM AS A STUDENT NURSE

As a student completing a course in nursing, a critical component will involve clinical learning placements. Clinical learning placements are an essential part of the educational journey. They provide the opportunity for the student to integrate theory into practice. Part of this clinical learning experience will involve working with the multidisciplinary team in a variety of clinical settings. Joining a multidisciplinary team will be an integral component of the student nurse's socialisation into nursing practice, as they learn about the roles and responsibilities of a nurse generally, as well as within the multidisciplinary team. The amount of time the student nurse spends on clinical placement in a mental health setting will vary between universities. Therefore, it is essential to make the best use of this time. Research shows that positive

clinical placements are associated with increased interest in working in particular areas. Students rank mental health nursing low as a preferred career choice, but supportive, positive clinical learning experiences can contribute to a change in perception and increase interest in mental health nursing (Happell, 2008; Muldoon & Riley, 2003; Rushworth & Happell, 2000; Wells, McElwee & Ryan, 2000). Feeling welcome rather than being seen as a burden to staff was viewed positively by student nurse respondents in nursing research. The following statements reflect some of the experiences that contribute to a positive experience within the mental health multidisciplinary team:

> The staff were really friendly. They joked a lot and said it's okay if you don't know what you're doing just yet, it's your first day and they were very together as a group of people (SN1).

> (I was made to feel) very, very welcome. Everyone was really nice and willing to answer questions, willing to give information even without being asked a question (SN7).

> They didn't expect me to be perfect (SN1).

> They let you sit in on one on one interviews that they (nurse) did and said if you had any questions just ask them and if you weren't sure about anything and kept telling us to ask the patient how, rather than going through them because they will tell you, most of them. Pretty much just giving you the chance (SN2).

Source: Hercelinskyj, 2010

The student's role is a complex one. The student nurse is designated as supernumerary, and enters the field for a limited amount of time. Yet they are expected within this short time frame to integrate into the mental health multidisciplinary team and demonstrate the requisite degree of competency against practice standards for registered nurses (NMBA, 2016).

Charleston and Happell's (2005) study on **preceptorship** acknowledged the connection between students and preceptor as crucial to a positive clinical experience in mental health. Being encouraging, integrating students into their practice and demonstrating good practice were considered active ways in which mental health nurses encourage learning.

Therefore, it is clear that thinking about and exploring strategies to maximise the benefits of the clinical placement are essential. This is relevant to not only meeting, interacting and collaborating with consumers and carers, but also in increasing the student mental health nurse's understanding and confidence in working as part of the mental health multidisciplinary team.

Preparing for clinical placement

A clinical placement in mental health is an exciting time during nursing studies, but it can also be stressful. The following points may be of use in preparing for a clinical placement in mental health:

1   Be prepared. This may sound obvious, but sometimes the obvious is overlooked! Because you will be notified of the type of venue you will be attending, it is always useful to do some research on that venue, looking for information such as the services the venue provides and the type of staff working there. This strategy will give you a beginning understanding of the specific context you will be going into. This can help you feel more confident in those first few days on clinical placement.

2   Think about your own learning objectives for your clinical placement. When you start to think about the questions you have in relation to a mental health placement it is more likely that you will be able to identify questions and learning objectives related to clinical practice; for example, learning about different medications, attending interviews with consumers and observing electroconvulsive therapy. However, it can be a little more challenging to think about questions or objectives related to working within and understanding the multidisciplinary team. Here are some possible questions to consider:

   – Who are the members of the multidisciplinary team in the particular context that I will be working in?

   – How do members of the multidisciplinary team communicate with each other?

   – What is the distinction between the generic and discipline-specific roles of different team members?

   – How are consumers and/or carers integrated into the multidisciplinary team?

   – Are regular team meetings held? How are information and decisions communicated and documented? How often are these decisions reviewed, and who does these reviews?

3   Review your clinical learning objectives and clinical assessment tool prior to commencing placement. You should clearly see within any tool that you use where you are required to focus on your role within the multidisciplinary team. For example, the clinical assessment tool that you use may have an objective related to demonstrating that you collaborate with the multidisciplinary health care team to provide comprehensive nursing care (Australian Catholic University, 2016).

During clinical placement

In order to get the most out of the clinical learning placement and begin to understand the role of the multidisciplinary team, the following strategies are recommended:

1   Ask questions. If you want to understand how the multidisciplinary team works, then being involved in discussions is essential. The more questions you ask, the more information you gain and this will help in developing your understanding of how the multidisciplinary team works within the mental health context.

2   Be proactive. Talk to people and find out what your buddy nurse or preceptor is doing and ask them how you can assist. Staff notice when you are interested and they invariably reciprocate. This helps you to develop a deeper understanding of how specific health professionals work individually and as team members.

3   Keep in touch with your university lecturer as well as your buddy nurse during your placement. If you encounter or find yourself involved in potential conflict within the team, it is important to have someone to talk to about your concerns.

4   As with any aspect of clinical placement, do not undertake any activity unless you have had the relevant learning at university prior and you feel comfortable with taking it on. Always ask for help and have someone work through a particular activity with you first so that you can observe and ask questions. Remember, the importance of assertive communication, understanding and accepting that learning is lifelong – not just something you engage in as a student – is essential. It is essential to always work within your scope of practice.

SAFETY FIRST

SCOPE OF PRACTICE

Scope of practice refers to those practices, procedures and activities that a health professional such as a nurse can perform that is in keeping with their professional registration. Scope of practice is determined by the education, knowledge, qualifications, competency and experience of the clinician and the legislated authority (NMBA, 2018). This is because the nurse is in the process of learning through education, development of psychomotor skills, clinical learning experiences, assessment, feedback and evaluation on their practice, responsibilities and accountability to the registered nurse. When applied to the role of a student, scope of practice means the student nurse can perform care; that they have the learned theory; they have been shown how to carry out that care and/or task; and they have practised under supervision within a Bachelor of Nursing program. The student nurse must be fully aware of what their scope of practice is at all times and never undertake any care or task that does not sit within this scope of practice. When in doubt, they refer to the clinical educator and buddy nurse/preceptor for clarification before undertaking any clinical activity. They must also be familiar with the professional conduct guidelines of their nursing registration body.

RESEARCH ON CONSUMERS' VIEWS ON THE ROLE OF THE MENTAL HEALTH NURSE AS A MEMBER OF THE MULTIDISCIPLINARY TEAM

It is essential to remember that consumers are the integral member of the multidisciplinary team. This is clearly because it is their health needs and goals that fundamentally direct the activities of the whole team. Therefore, it is a collaborative process. Without the consumer, there would be no multidisciplinary team. It is important to consider the experience of consumers in working with the multidisciplinary team and how they describe the role of the mental health nurse and their experience of receiving care.

Important factors identified by consumers include:

- behaviours such as having sufficient time for the development of a therapeutic relationship
- developing a shared understanding of the issues encountered by the consumer
- the capacity of clinicians such as mental health nurses to be open in the relationship without relying on preconceived ideas or understandings regarding mental health conditions and their clinical presentation.

REFLECT ON THIS

Learning about the multidisciplinary team

Read the article 'A mulitidisciplianry learning experience contributing to mental health rehabilitation' by Moxham and colleagues (2017). This paper explored participants' experiences of engaging with people experiencing a mental health condition. The project, which was called the 'Recovery Camp', provided multidisciplinary health education to healthcare students by providing opportunities for them to engage with people experiencing mental health conditions, and to become more confident in their communication with each other and actively participate in collaborative work. Participants were invited to reflect on their experiences and explore what they had learned during the camp. Participants spoke about developing an increased understanding of people's lived experience with mental illness and, importantly, recognising their contribution as active members of the multidisciplinary team.

Questions

After reading the article, reflect on the following questions:

1 How important is it for people experiencing a mental health condition to be a contributing member of the multidisciplinary team? Why?
2 Reflect on the concepts explored in Chapter 21 to help you consider the following questions:
   a How confident do you currently feel in interacting with people experiencing mental illness? Why?
   b What knowledge, skills, support and learning opportunities would help you to build your confidence?

CASE **STUDY**

ROLES WITHIN THE MULTIDISCIPLINARY TEAM

Chen is a 33-year-old woman who has been receiving treatment for a recent episode of depression. Chen was diagnosed with bipolar affective disorder following the birth of her first child 13 years ago and has had several admissions when she has experienced symptoms of depression and mania. Prior to this admission, Chen had been living in a women's refuge with her youngest child for five weeks. Chen's older children are in the care of her parents, with whom she has little contact. Chen also has limited contact with her two siblings.

Chen had left her current partner following several episodes of domestic violence. She was referred to the refuge after presenting at the emergency department with her child in a distressed state and showing physical signs of injury. Over the course of her stay at the refuge, Chen became increasingly withdrawn and isolated herself from others, experienced sleep and appetite disturbances and expressed her distress about where she would go after she left the refuge as she did not have the money to pay rent and had to take unpaid leave from her job as a sales assistant.

Staff became concerned when she started expressing thoughts of suicide. At this time, her daughter was placed in the care of welfare officers and Chen was admitted to the acute inpatient mental health facility.

Chen's depression has improved enough that she can leave and be cared for under the community team. Chen meets with the multidisciplinary team. Chen informs the team that she has been discussing returning to her abusive partner because she feels at least she will have a roof over her head and it may help her get her youngest child back.

Questions

1 What mental health clinicians would be likely to be involved in the team meeting regarding Chen's discharge and ongoing management?
2 What potential issues might the multidisciplinary team identify?
3 What would be the various roles of the team members you have identified in question 1?
4 What role would Chen take in this meeting?

Features like clear, open communication, being non-judgemental and not patronising are important characteristics of positive interactions with mental health nurses identified by consumers. Trust is essential, as this is linked to feelings of safety (Gilburt, Rose & Slade, 2008; Johansson & Eklund, 2003). Conversely, organisational systems that do not support teamwork, are overly formalised with little opportunity for informal discussions, and do not integrate specialist services as required, can precipitate less successful teamwork activity (Kutash et al., 2014).

Emotional labour and mental health nursing

Student nurses learn that the core of mental health nursing practice is the therapeutic relationship established with the consumer. From clinical experience, students will also discover that mental health nurses work as members of the multidisciplinary team in complex environments that can be both challenging and rewarding. Implementing a therapeutic relationship requires the mental health nurse to use themselves therapeutically, implement and maintain professional boundaries, demonstrate self-awareness of the impact of their practice and interactions with consumers, families, carers and colleagues, utilise specific skills, and practise within their scope of practice and legislative requirements as well as organisational policies and procedures. The reality of practice is that the emotional (as well as physical) work involved in mental health nursing is often not recognised or acknowledged.

Emotional labour is described as the effort required to suppress one's own emotions in order to effectively care for others and also care for oneself (Edward, Hercelinskyj & Giandinoto, 2017). Emotional labour has been linked with burnout and attrition. It is also thought to provide opportunities for developing (Edward, Hercelinskyj & Giandinoto, 2017) **emotional intelligence** and resilience. The key is how the mental health nurse is able to address and work through clinical practice issues in a positive way. This is an important concept in mental health nursing, because of the complex lived experience of consumers and their families as well as the issues surrounding practice. The need for self-care is essential. Practices such as supervision, reflective practice, caring for oneself physically, supportive management and team environments are essential.

REFLECTION ON LEARNING FROM PRACTICE

Having worked with students over a number of years, I am always struck by the sense of anticipation and trepidation that many students simultaneously experience before they undertake a clinical learning placement in mental health. Yet many students return from clinical placement with stories to tell. Often these stories centre on the consumers they meet and their deepening understanding of a consumer's lived experience. What is also clear is their understanding of the role of the mental health nurse as a member of the multidisciplinary team. Students will use phrases such as, 'They worked really well together', 'Everyone was equal on the team' or 'They welcomed and encouraged me'. Other

students speak about the experience of being part of the multidisciplinary team and how they share this knowledge with them. Students will have often been able to see how their studies had prepared them, making statements such as, 'I got the theory when I was there – it made sense'.

Reflections such as these highlight the need for successful preparation not only about the theory of mental health, but the practice and role of the mental health nurse as part of the multidisciplinary team. The more prepared students are before they attend clinical placement, the more likely they are to find the experience a positive one.

CHAPTER RESOURCES

SUMMARY

- The multidisciplinary team is a specialised type of group with members from different disciplines. The membership may change as the specific needs and requirements of the group change. However, a range of discipline-specific professionals can be involved and at all times the consumer and carer should be integral parts of the multidisciplinary team.
- Team structures have distinctive features but also share overlapping characteristics. Within any group there are a number of roles that a person may assume. The purpose of these roles is to facilitate the team in meeting its goals or tasks.

- This chapter has looked at the experience of the student nurse as part of the multidisciplinary team. The importance of understanding the student nurse's role within the multidisciplinary team has been highlighted in some strategies on making best use of the clinical placement in relation to becoming a member of the multidisciplinary team.
- The consumer is an integral member of the multidisciplinary team. Research clearly shows that consumers value being active members of the team. They have a clear idea about how mental health nurses, in particular, can contribute in a positive way to care planning and management. They also highlight the importance of being listened to and being actively involved in their own care.

REVIEW QUESTIONS

1 Assertive communication is characterised by the following behaviours:
   a Confidence
   b Listening and understanding the issue
   c Respect for the other person's point of view
   d All of the above
2 Which of the following is not a feature of effective teamwork?
   a Open, clear communication between team members
   b The pursuit by individual team members of their own goals
   c Ability to recognise and work through conflict
   d All team members share accountability for the decisions made by the team
3 What does teamwork mean to you? Reflect on your experience of working in a multidisciplinary team. Does your experience match your personal definition? What were the positive aspects and challenges of working in a multidisciplinary team?

4 List three learning objectives you would like to achieve when you undertake a clinical learning experience in mental health. What strategies and/or resources could you implement to help you achieve these objectives?
5 How would you respond to the following situation? You are working with Flora, a 27-year-old female diagnosed with borderline personality disorder. Flora confides in you that she has razors hidden in her room that she plans to use to self-harm. Feeling that this is outside your scope of practice, you approach a senior nurse, Richard, and explain the conversation you just had with Flora. Richard rolls his eyes and says, 'Just another PD, she's found a new target in you. She does this all the time. You students are so gullible.'
6 John and his family are taking part in a family meeting with the multidisciplinary team. What factors will influence John's feelings regarding the efficacy of the team meeting and his involvement in the meeting?

CRITICAL THINKING

1   Reflect on a previous clinical experience. How were you made to feel welcome in the multidisciplinary team? What roles did team members take on? How were decisions made?

2   What are the advantages and challenges of communicating assertively within a multidisciplinary team?

3   What skills do you believe are important for working effectively in a team?

USEFUL WEBSITES

- ANMF Clinical Placement tips: https://otr.anmfvic.asn.au/articles/clinical-placement-tips
- RCNi: https://journals.rcni.com/nursing-standard/effective-communication-and-teamwork-promotes-patient-safety-ns.29.49.50.e10042

- Who Safety Curriculum: https://www.who.int/patientsafety/education/curriculum/who_mc_topic-4.pdf

REFLECT ON THIS

Role of the paramedic in the MDT
In Table 23.2, the registered paramedic was not listed as a member of the multidisciplinary team in the context of acute and community-based mental health service delivery. Yet, as McCann and colleagues (2018) point out, paramedics are frequently the first responders to people experiencing mental health and/or substance use issues. Read their article and reflect on the following questions:

1   What major themes arose out of this research?

2   In what contexts might mental health nurses and paramedics work together? What might be the advantages and challenges of such an approach?

Alharbi, Jackson and Usher (2020) consider the impact of the COVID-19 pandemic on the experience of compassion fatigue.

3   How can you apply their ideas to nurses working in mental health?

4   Why is it important to understand this and what strategies might be useful in addressing compassion fatigue?

REFERENCES

Alharbi, J., Jackson, D. & Usher, K. (2020). The potential for COVID-19 to contribute to compassion fatigue in critical care nurses. *Journal of Clinical Nursing*, 29(15–16), 2762–64.

Australian Catholic University. (2016). *Faculty of Health Sciences. National Competency Assessment Schedule*. Retrieved from https://leo.acu.edu.au/pluginfile.php/1616380/mod_resource/content/1/NRSG%20262%20Nursing%20Competency%20Assessment%20Schedule%202016.pdf.

Balzer Riley, J. (2017). *Communication in Nursing* (8th edn). London: Elsevier Health Sciences.

Becher, J. & Visovsky, C. (2012). Horizontal violence in nursing. *MEDSURG Nursing*, 21(4), 210–13.

Belanger, E. & Rodriguez, C. (2008). More than the sum of its parts? A qualitative research synthesis on multi-disciplinary primary health care teams. *Journal of Interprofessional Care*, 22(6), 587–97.

Benne, K.D. & Sheats, P. (1948). Functional roles of group members. *Journal of Social Issues*, 4(2), 41–9. doi:10.1111/j.1540-4560.1948.tb01783.x

Benne, K.D. & Sheats, P. (2007). Functional roles of group members. *Group Facilitation*, 8, 30–5.

Bennetts, W., Callander, R., Cavill, M., Fossey, E., Meadows, G., Naughtin, G. & Renouf, N. (2012). Working collaboratively. In G.

Meadows, J. Farhall, E. Fossey, M. Grigg, F. McDermott & B. Singh (eds), *Mental Health in Australia. Collaborative Community Practice* (3rd edn). South Melbourne: Oxford University Press.

Bowen, L. (2014). The multidisciplinary team in palliative care: A case reflection. *Indian Journal of Palliative Care*, 20(2), 142–5. doi:10.4103/0973-1075.132637

Charleston, R. & Happell, B. (2005). Attempting to accomplish connectedness within the preceptorship experience: The perception of mental health nurses. *International Journal of Mental Health Nursing*, 14(1), 54–61.

Conway, M.E. (1988). Organisations, professional autonomy, and roles. In M.E. Hardy & M.F. Conway (eds), *Role Theory. Perspectives for Health Professionals*. Stamford, CT: Appleton and Lange.

Dennis, S. (2006). The tip of the iceberg. In C. Gamble & G. Brennan (eds), *Working with Serious Mental Illness. A Manual for Clinical Practice* (vol. 2). Edinburgh: Elsevier.

DeVito, J.A. (2016). *The interpersonal communication book* (14th edn). Boston, MA: Pearson.

Edward, K.-L., Hercelinskyj, G. & Giandinoto, J.-A. (2017). Emotional labour in mental health nursing: An integrative systematic review.

International Journal of Mental Health Nursing, 26(3), 215–25. doi:https://doi.org/10.1111/inm.12330

Eunson, B. (1994). *Communicating for Teambuilding: The Communication Skills Series*. Milton: John Wiley & Sons.

Eunson, B. (2016). *C21. Communicating in the 21st Century* (4th edn). Milton: John Wiley & Sons.

Gilburt, H., Rose, D. & Slade, M. (2008). The importance of relationships in mental health care. A qualitative study of service users' experiences of psychiatric hospital admission in the UK. *BMC Health Services Research*, 8(92). Retrieved from http://www.biomedcentral.com/1472-6963/8/92.

Hamilton, B., Manias, E., Maude, P., Marjoribanks, T. & Cook, K. (2004). Perspectives of a nurse, a social worker, and a psychiatrist regarding patient assessment in acute inpatient psychiatry settings: A case study approach. *Journal of Psychiatric and Mental Health Nursing*, 11, 683–9.

Happell, B. (2008). The importance of clinical experience for mental health nursing – Part 1: Undergraduate nursing students' attitudes, preparedness and satisfaction. *International Journal of Mental Health Nursing*, 17(5), 326–32.

Hardy, M.E. & Hardy, W.L. (1988). Role stress and role strain. In M.E. Hardy & M.E. Conway (eds), *Role Theory. Perspectives for Health Professionals* (vol. 2).Upper Saddle River, NJ: Prentice Hall.

Hercelinskyj, G. (2010). Perceptions of professional identity in mental health nursing and the implications for recruitment and retention. (Doctor of Philosophy), Charles Darwin University, Darwin.

Johansson, H. & Eklund, M. (2003). Patients' opinion on what constitutes good psychiatric care. *Scandinavian Journal of Caring Sciences*, 17, 339–46. Retrieved from https://www.ncbi.nlm.nih.gov/pubmed/14629636.

Kahn, R.L., Wolfe, D.M., Quinn, R.P., Snoek, J.D. & Rosenthal, R.A. (1964). *Organisational Stress. Studies in Role Conflict and Ambiguity*. New York: John Wiley & Sons.

Kindler, H.S. (1996). *Managing Disagreement Constructively: Conflict Management in Organizations* (rev. edn). Menlo Park, CA: Crisp Publications.

Kutash, K., Acri, M., Pollock, M., Armusewicz, K., Serene Olin, S.-C. & Hoagwood, K. E. (2014). Quality indicators for multidisciplinary team functioning in community-based children's mental health services. *Administration and Policy in Mental Health and Mental Health Services Research*, 41(1), 55–68. doi:10.1007/s10488-013-0508-2

Lampert, L. & Youl, Z. (2016). Nurse Life. How to be assertive. Retrieved from https://www.ausmed.com/articles/how-to-be-assertive.

MacAteer, A., Manktelow, R. & Fitzsimons, L. (2016). Mental health workers' perception of role self-efficacy and the organisational climate regarding the ethos of recovery. *British Journal of Social Work*, 46(3), 737.

McCann, T.V., Slavic, M., Ferguson, N., Bosley, E., Smith, K., Roberts, L., … Lubman, D.I. (2018). Paramedics' perceptions of their scope of practice in caring for patients with non-medical emergency-related mental health and/or alcohol and other drug problems: A qualitative study. *PLoS One*, 13(12). doi:http://dx.doi.org/10.1371/journal.pone.0208391

Moxham, L., Patterson, C., Taylor, E., Perlman, D., Sumskis, S. & Brighton, R. (2017). A multidisciplinary learning experience contributing to mental health rehabilitation. *Disability and Rehabilitation*, 39(1), 98–103. doi:10.3109/09638288.2016.1146358

Muldoon, O.T. & Reilly, J. (2003). Career choice in nursing students: Gendered constructs as psychological barriers. *Journal of Advanced Nursing*, 43(1), 93–100.

Ndoro, S. (2014). Effective multidisciplinary working: The key to high-quality care. *British Journal of Nursing*, 23(13), 274–7.

Nursing and Midwifery Board of Australia (NMBA). (2016). *Registered Nurse Standards for Practice*. Melbourne: NMBA.

Nursing and Midwifery Board of Australia (NMBA). (2018). *Code of Conduct for Nurses*. Melbourne: NMBA. Retrieved from https://www.nursingmidwiferyboard.gov.au/Codes-Guidelines-Statements/Professional-standards.aspx.

Porteus, A. (n.d.). Roles people play in groups. Retrieved from https://web.stanford.edu/group/resed/resed/staffresources/RM/training/grouproles.html#hinder.

Renouf, N. & Meadows, G. (2012). Working collaboratively. In G. Meadows, B. Singh & M. Grigg (eds), *Mental Health in Australia. Collaborative Community Practice* (vol. 2). South Melbourne: Oxford University Press.

Rushworth, L. & Happell, B. (2000). 'Psychiatric nursing was great, but I want to be a "real" nurse': Is psychiatric nursing a realistic choice for nursing students? *Australian and New Zealand Journal of Mental Health Nursing*, 9(3), 128–37.

Stone, J. (2010). Attempting to speak the same language: Interprofessional collaborative practice (ICP) – definitions and terminology. *Nursing Review*, 10–11.

Victorian Auditor-General's Report. (2016). *Bullying and Harassment in the Health Sector. PP No 148, Session 2014–16*. Melbourne: Victorian Government Printer. Retrieved from http://www.audit.vic.gov.au/publications/20160323.Bullying/20160323.Bullying.pdf.

Wells, J.S., McElwee, C.N. & Ryan, D. (2000). 'I don't want to be a psychiatric nurse': An exploration of factors inhibiting recruitment to psychiatric nursing in Ireland. *Journal of Psychiatric and Mental Health Nursing*, 7, 79–87.

Wickham, M. & Parker, M. (2007). Reconceptualising organisational role theory for contemporary organisational contexts. *Journal of Managerial Psychology*, 22(5), 440–64.

World Health Organization (WHO). (2001). *The World Health Report 2001: Mental Health – New Understanding, New Hope*. Geneva: WHO. Retrieved from https://www.who.int/whr/2001/en/whr01_en.pdf?ua=1.

COMMUNITY MENTAL HEALTH CONTEXT

Karen Hall

LEARNING FROM PRACTICE

My life had been difficult at times as my mother suffered from bipolar I disorder and I would often have to take care of the family during the times she was in hospital or when she was so sick she couldn't get out of bed. When I was 18, I got a job as a receptionist for a large trucking company and worked in this position for 18 months. Just before my 20th birthday, things started to change.

I found I couldn't go to work and after several weeks of not answering phone calls from work, they terminated my employment. I became increasingly concerned that my family were poisoning my food and that the water in our house was contaminated with a deadly virus. I ceased eating with the family and would eat canned food in my room, and came out of my room only after my family had gone to bed. My family had changed and my mother had become possessed by the devil. My brother no longer acted like my real brother and I began to believe he was an impostor. I could only trust my father and he worked long hours, so I rarely spoke with him. There were times when the demon that possessed my mother would talk to me, telling me evil and frightening things and I would run out of the house down the road screaming for it to leave me alone. I would often hear my mother on the phone ringing mental health triage and her own case manager requesting they come to see me.

At my father's request, I spoke to the lady at triage and she asked me to go for an assessment in the local mental health clinic, but I decided not to go, as I did not need any assistance, and told them it was my mother who should be attending. The next week the clinic staff attended my house and after they asked me several questions, they rang for an ambulance and I was admitted to the inpatient unit with what they called a 'first episode psychosis'. Discharged after 10 days, I was placed on a community treatment order and forced to attend the local mental health clinic weekly. I was started on olanzapine but didn't take the medication. They then forced me to have a risperidone injection every two weeks. After several weeks, I found I was no longer scared at home and my mother was more like my old mother. I began to eat with the family again and was now showering every day. I had previously gone up to four months without showering. Six months later, I managed to get a job with a call centre and still work there. The community team discharged me after nine months and I no longer need medication. Although angry at the time, I am now grateful to the community team who spent many hours trying to assist me.

Jodie, 22, a consumer

INTRODUCTION

This chapter discusses the significant historical factors that have shaped what is known today as community mental health. It explores the social aspects that affect the mental health of communities and the government initiatives that have been established to address these issues. It defines the many different clinical community teams and their roles and identifies their functions. As many mental health issues require specialist treatment, this chapter also explores the functions and achievements of specialist services.

HISTORICAL FACTORS OF COMMUNITY MENTAL HEALTH CARE

Historically, it was common for people with severe mental health issues to be treated in large psychiatric institutions, isolated and independent of general community areas. The *patients* (now referred to as consumers) would live, work and play at the institution and many of them had no contact with people outside of the institution. Hospital stays were lengthy, and some patients remained in these large institutions for decades. Community treatment was reserved only for those with less severe mental health conditions and was delivered by general practitioners and psychiatrists (Bedell, Hunter & Corrigan,1997).

Deinstitutionalisation

The development of new pharmacological interventions in the 1950s along with the strengthening civil rights movement led to better mental health outcomes and the community recognition that, ethically, people with mental health issues had the right to live freely in the community (Hungerford et al., 2015).This in turn started a process known as *deinstitutionalisation*, which occurred in many developed countries through the 1960s to 1990s. *Patients* (the use of this term would continue for some time) were transferred into the community and a large number of psychiatric institutions closed their doors. The process of deinstitutionalisation led to the establishment of community-based care and the relocation of inpatient beds from psychiatric institutions to general hospitals. Despite the movement of people diagnosed with various mental health conditions into the community, mental health resources and funding did not follow. In New South Wales in 1994, for example, 90% of people with severe mental health issues were living in the community, yet approximately 90% of the funding for mental health was still given to the hospital system. The large demand for a small number of services saw many consumers slip through the system, which led them to living in disadvantaged conditions in poor-quality accommodation, prisons or homelessness (Rosen, 2006; Saugeres, 2011); this in turn, increased the stigma associated with mental health issues (Holmes & Jacob, 2014). While there is little doubt that poor planning for deinstitutionalisation of mental health consumers led to these issues, it is important to also consider other factors that were involved. The development of the nuclear family as the dominant family structure, changes to the legal system, increased demand on housing markets and budget cuts may have contributed to the increasing numbers of mental health consumers being incarcerated or homeless (Winkler et al., 2016).

SOCIAL DETERMINANTS OF MENTAL HEALTH

The World Health Organization's Ottawa Charter (WHO, 1986) first identified the **social determinants of health** as peace, shelter, education, food, income, a stable eco-system, sustainable resources, social justice, and equity (WHO, 2016).

In 2014 the **social determinants of mental health** were selected in order to improve mental health and reduce inequities (WHO & Calouste Gulbenkian Foundation, 2014). These determinants are the economic and social conditions that influence individual and group mental health status and they are the same as the social determinants of health (refer to **Figure 24.1**). Mental health issues are more likely to emerge in social conditions of 'discrimination and social exclusion; adverse early life experiences; poor education; unemployment, underemployment, and job insecurity; income inequality, poverty, and neighbourhood deprivation; poor access to sufficient healthy food; poor housing quality and housing instability; adverse features of the built environment; poor access to health care' (Compton & Shim, 2015, p. 4).

Strategies to address these issues were established by the WHO Mental Health Action Plan 2013–2020, in which services and initiatives were developed to span across an individual's life span and be life stage appropriate (WHO, 2012). The strategy aims to ensure quality perinatal care, childhood, adolescent and family, older age and gender support. It includes ensuring the individual's access to income, food, nutrition, water, sanitation, housing and employment. On a community level, it aims to establish trust and safety, reduce violence and crimes, ensure adequate health services, consumer rights and education, and reduce discrimination and inequality (WHO, 2013).

The Mental Health Action Plan 2013–2020 (WHO, 2013, p. 1; see also **Table 24.1**) envisaged:

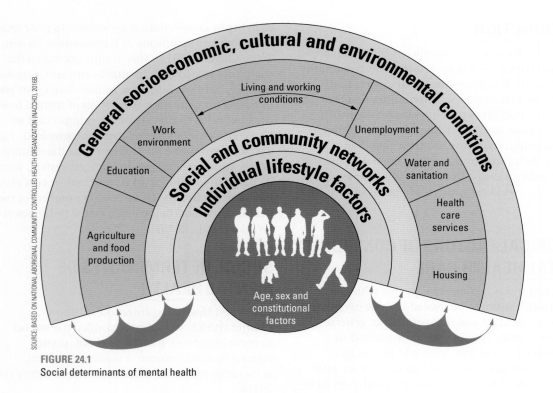

SOURCE: BASED ON NATIONAL ABORIGINAL COMMUNITY CONTROLLED HEALTH ORGANIZATION (NACCHO), 2016B.

FIGURE 24.1
Social determinants of mental health

TABLE 24.1
Principles of the WHO Mental Health Action Plan 2013–2020

UNIVERSAL HEALTH COVERAGE	UNIVERSAL RIGHTS	EVIDENCE-BASED PRACTICE	LIFE COURSE APPROACH	MULTI-SECTOR APPROACH	EMPOWERMENT OF PERSONS WITH MENTAL DISORDERS AND PSYCHOSOCIAL DISABILITIES
Persons with mental health issues should be able to access essential health and social services that enable them to achieve recovery and the highest attainable standard of health.	Mental health strategies, actions and interventions for treatment, prevention and promotion must be compliant with the Convention on the Rights of Persons with Disabilities and other international and regional human rights instruments.	Mental health strategies and interventions for treatment, prevention and promotion need to be based on scientific evidence and/ or best practice, taking cultural considerations into account.	Policies, plans and services for mental health need to take account of health and social needs at all stages of the life course, including infancy, childhood, adolescence, adulthood and older age.	A comprehensive and coordinated response for mental health requires partnership with multiple public sectors such as health, education, employment, judicial, housing, social and other relevant sectors as well as the private sector, as appropriate to the country situation.	Persons with mental disorders and psychosocial disabilities should be empowered and involved in mental health advocacy, policy, planning, legislation, service provision, monitoring, research and evaluation.

SOURCE: WORLD HEALTH ORGANISATION (WHO), 2013

a world in which mental health is valued, promoted, and protected, mental disorders are prevented and persons affected by these disorders are able to exercise the full range of human rights and access high-quality, culturally appropriate health and social care in a timely way to promote recovery all in order to attain the highest possible level of health and participate fully in society and at work free from stigmatization and discrimination.

PRIMARY MENTAL HEALTH CARE

Primary mental health care aims to improve the mental health of those living in the community, with its focus being on prevention rather than cure (Hungerford et al., 2015). Primary mental health care recognises that mental health is best achieved by engaging people in the community, being socially inclusive, where people are free from discrimination and violence and have access to appropriate resources (Shim & Rust, 2013). It involves promoting positive mental health, nurturing resilience and addressing consumers' mental health needs in the community setting. Primary mental health care also is often the consumer's first point of engagement with health professionals and services. If the contact is well managed, it can promote mental well-being, achieve early identification of mental health needs and prevent future episodes (WHO & Calouste Gulbenkian Foundation, 2014). Primary mental health care is in keeping with the Australian state and territory Mental Health Acts, which mandate a person be treated in the least restrictive environment, ideally the community, close to where they live and work. Primary mental health has three broad aims. These are to:

1 achieve inclusion and reduce social disparities in health
2 offer services that meet community needs and expectations
3 integrate health and wellness education into all sectors (WHO & Calouste Gulbenkian Foundation, 2014).

For more information, see Chapter 21, which discusses resilience and recovery in depth.

Primary health services and initiatives

Primary health services are generally the first point of contact the consumer has with a health service and this precedes any hospital admissions. The Australian Government has developed a number of initiatives to address health issues in the community setting.

General practitioners

In Australia, general practitioners (GPs) are the first and main point of entry into the health care system. They coordinate care, advise, refer and offer treatment to patients and this may continue over a person's lifetime. As a primary health service, GPs are the most frequently consulted professionals for mental health reasons (Dezetter et al., 2013).

The National Survey of Mental Health and Wellbeing (2007) used an interview-based household survey that measured the prevalence of mental health issues in people living in the community. It found that 45% of Australians aged 16–85 years had at some point in their lifetime experienced a mental health condition and in the period from 2006–07 the most frequently consulted professional for the mental health condition was their GP (25%), followed by seeing a psychologist (13%) (Australian Bureau of Statistics [ABS], 2007).

The Mental Health Nurse Incentive Program

In July 2001, the Australian Government introduced the Mental Health Nurse Incentive Program (MHNIP). This program aimed at increasing the accessibility of mental health care for consumers with severe mental distress in the primary health setting. It funds community-based general practices, private psychiatric practices and other organisations to enable them to employ mental health nurses within coordinated clinical care for people with severe mental health conditions (Department of Health, 2016). In 2015, in response to the National Mental Health Commission's Review of Mental Health Programmes and Services, the Australian Government made reforms to this program. These reforms saw the movement of primary mental health programs, such as the MHNIP, from Medicare Locals to Primary Health Networks (PHNs) in July 2016 to increase accessibility and to establish a more streamlined mental health response. Admission into the program is determined by GPs and psychiatrists, and consumers must meet specific eligibility criteria (see **Table 24.2**).

The mental health nurse role may include, but is not limited to, establishing a therapeutic relationship with the consumer, liaising with family, carers and stakeholders as appropriate, review of and response to the consumer's mental state, monitoring and administration of medication and encouraging

TABLE 24.2
Eligibility criteria for MHNIP

CONSUMER ELIGIBILITY CRITERIA FOR MHNIP
The consumer has been diagnosed with a mental disorder according to the criteria defined in the ICD-10 *Classification of Mental and Behavioural Disorders Diagnostic Criteria for Research* (WHO, 1993) or the *Diagnostic and Statistical Manual of Mental Health Disorders* (DSM-5; APA, 2013).
The disorder is significantly impacting their social, personal and work life.
The consumer has had at least one hospital admission for their mental disorder or they are at risk of needing hospitalisation in the future if appropriate treatment and care is not provided.
The consumer is expected to need ongoing treatment and management of their mental disorder over the next two years.
The GP or psychiatrist employed to treat the patient by the organisation participating in the MHNIP will be the main person responsible for the patient's clinical mental health care.
The consumer has given permission to receive treatment from a mental health nurse.
Eligible organisations must engage the services of a mental health nurse credentialled with the Australian College of Mental Health Nurses.

SOURCE: ADAPTED FROM DEPARTMENT OF HEALTH, 2016

adherence, coordinating services and supporting the consumer in their recovery.

Access to Allied Psychological Services (ATAPS)

Another primary mental health initiative by the Australian Government is Access to Allied Psychological Services (ATAPS). This program allows consumers in a 12-month period to access up to a maximum of 12 and under exceptional circumstances, 18 individual and 12 group sessions with mental health professionals. Consumers can attend psychologists, social workers, mental health nurses, occupational therapists and Aboriginal and Torres Strait Islander health workers with specific mental health qualifications (Department of Health, 2014b).

Better Access to Psychiatrists, Psychologists and General Practitioners through the MBS (Better Access) initiative

In 2006, the Australian Government introduced the Better Access to Psychiatrists, Psychologists and General Practitioners through the Medicare Benefits Schedule (Better Access) initiative. Under this initiative, Medicare rebates are available to consumers for selected mental health services provided by GPs, psychiatrists, psychologists, social workers and occupational therapists with the aim to improve outcomes and easy access for people with a clinically diagnosed mental disorder (Department of Health, 2015a).

Mental Health First Aid Training

Mental Health First Aid Training is another government initiative, established for frontline community workers, financial and legal workers, relationship counsellors, and education and health care workers. The training is designed to help these workers better identify and appropriately respond to the needs of people at risk of suicide or who have attempted suicide and keep them safe until clinical services are involved (Department of Health, 2014d). Refer to Chapter 26 for further discussion.

Mental Health Services in Rural and Remote Areas (MHSRRA)

The Mental Health Services in Rural and Remote Areas (MHSRRA) program provides rural and remote areas with allied health and nursing professionals, including social workers, psychologists, occupational therapists, mental health nurses, Aboriginal health workers and Aboriginal mental health workers (NTPHN, 2016). MHSRRA provides for the provision of mental health services in rural and remote communities where, traditionally, people do not have access to services or previously had little or no access to mental health services, especially the remote areas of the Top End of Australia (Department of Health, 2015b). It

also provides funding to non-government health organisations such as Northern Territory Aboriginal Medical Services and the Royal Flying Doctor Service to provide services for Aboriginal and Torres Strait Islander peoples.

THE ROLES OF THE MENTAL HEALTH NURSE

Community mental health nurses care for people experiencing mental distress in a community setting. Their primary role is to work alongside people and their carers to assist in the consumer's personal recovery. In the community setting, they work within a multidisciplinary team that may include psychiatrists, social workers, psychologists, occupational therapists and GPs. Often, all staff perform the same role and discipline-specific skills are employed when they can be of benefit to the consumer.

Mental health clinical community teams

Community mental health teams follow up with new and existing consumers at clinics, in their own homes or in a designated place of mutual convenience. Most mental health teams use an **assertive outreach** approach to follow up with consumers that results in either staff being involved with consumers for extended periods of time or providing more episodic or crisis care. Clinicians employed in these roles are frequently involved in **clinical review**, monitoring the consumer's mental state, promoting medication adherence and safety, as well as liaising with and referring to more generalist services, including GPs, for ongoing support. In the case of a consumer known to a mental health service, the team offers ongoing support and case management and may be involved in early transition from inpatient admissions to community-based mental health care.

Acute Community Intervention Services (ACIS)

Acute Community Intervention Services (ACIS) provide a timely response to a person's acute mental health distress and aim to minimise the impact on and increase safety of consumers, carers and the community. ACIS offer comprehensive, evidence-based assessment and short-term treatment in the community. They are also involved in facilitating acute inpatient admissions and early discharge management (EDM). ACIS provide a 'three-pronged approach to front-end mental health care: 1. Telephone triage; 2. Emergency department assessment and care; 3. Acute assertive community outreach' (Department of Health, 2014a, p. 1).

SAFETY FIRST

HOME VISITS

It is essential that the nurse explores possible dangers and risks before home visiting and conducts a risk assessment. Potential considerations for a risk analysis may include:

- checking if the person has access to weapons
- ensuring there are no impediments to access to the house/unit (exits are identified, stairs and pathways are cleared)
- identifying whether the person keeps any dogs or other animals
- checking whether the person has a history of violence (consumer, family or otherwise)
- familiarising themselves with the neighbourhood (e.g. whether it is considered a safe area, and whether the time for the visit is a safe time)
- checking that the home has sufficient lighting
- considering whether the person is a new assessment, and if so, whether the visit should be conducted as a pair
- ensuring they have mobile phone access and reception
- ensuring they do not park in any area where their exit could be blocked, such as single-lane driveways
- ensuring someone knows where they are at all times.

See also the sample risk assessment at http://staging.mhcc.org.au/media/5856/check-sheet-6-assessments.pdf.

Mental health triage

In Australia, emergency response teams or mental health triage teams offer the clinical entry point to mental health support and treatment for consumers, carers and primary health services (Department of Health, 2010). Mental health triage teams provide timely support, assessment, response, referral and coordination over the telephone or in the hospital's emergency department. These highly skilled clinicians determine and initiate the type and urgency of response required based on their assessment of distress, risk, dysfunction and disability. After a thorough biopsychosocial assessment and documentation, the clinician decides if there is a need, or potential need, for further intervention by the mental health service, or whether referral to another service should be considered. Consideration is given to symptoms of acute psychosis, suicidal behaviour or thought, and risk of harm to self and others, including children and pregnancies (Ministry of Health, NSW, 2012). Where a mental health triage assessment indicates that specialist mental health services are required (or possibly required), a more comprehensive assessment is provided through the intake assessment to specific community teams or inpatient units. Mental health triage is essentially responsible for the:

- management of inpatient beds
- assessment and referral and service coordination of public mental health.

Crises and assessment teams

Crises and assessment services are known by different names across Australia; for example, psychiatric crisis intervention services (PCIS), intensive treatment teams (ITT), community assessment and treatment (CAT) services, and crisis assessment and treatment teams (CATTs). CATTs are mobile, multidisciplinary teams designed to assess and treat consumers during acute episodes of mental health distress offering support 24 hours, seven days a week. They provide care in the community and without this crisis intervention, the consumer would be at risk of admission to a psychiatric inpatient service. CATT teams also function to facilitate and support the consumer's early discharge from hospital by offering intensive support seven days a week in the community. This in turn results in a reduction of admissions and a decrease in duration of hospital stay (Kim et al., 2015; Udechuku et al., 2005). Qualitative studies have shown that consumers and other stakeholders value the accessibility, the time given for them to tell their stories, continuity of care, practical help, ability to be treated at home, access to a psychiatrist and 24-hour access that these teams provide (Wheeler et al., 2015).

Police, ambulance and clinical early response teams (PACER)

PACER teams have been implemented in a small numbers of countries, including the United States, Canada and Australia, and the first Australian team was piloted in Melbourne's south-eastern suburbs in 2007. PACER teams provide a quick crisis community response to people experiencing mental health crises or causing behavioural disturbances. This involves police and senior mental health clinicians working together effectively to provide support, assessment and intervention that can prevent the need for the unnecessary hospitalisation of the consumer. It is often police officers who are the first responders to consumers experiencing a mental health crisis and, with minimal training in mental health and the responsibility for the consumer's safety, police often resort to transporting the consumer to hospital. The establishment of PACER teams has allowed for the person to receive a more immediate assessment and treatment in the community. The frequency of this is supported by a study assessing all presentations to a Sydney emergency department (ED) found that 2334 presentations (4% of all presentations) were for mental health issues and 20% of the mental health presentations to the ED arrived with police (Lee et al., 2008). Allen Consulting Group (2012) evaluated the outcomes of time to access assessment, proportion of consumers requiring transportation to hospital ED, and the cost-effectiveness of this initiative (the first Victorian PACER team) over a 16-month period. PACER was found to be less costly, reducing the time to assessment and resulted in fewer consumers being transported to hospital ED for care; 19% of cases with PACER were transported to hospital as compared with 82% of cases with police response (Allen Consulting Group, 2012). The PACER teams were also found to be responsible for a diverse array of non-hospital psychosocial referrals for consumers to housing, welfare and addiction services. This highlights the importance of considering the cause of the presenting crisis and how to best address this can have a significant input in reducing attendance at EDs. PACER was also found to enhance collaboration and communication between police and mental health services (Allen Consulting Group, 2012; Lee et al., 2015).

Specific criteria exist for requesting PACER assistance, and these include:

- Clinical assessment of a person's mental state is required.
- Advice is required on appropriate mental health referrals.
- Advice is required on appropriate consumer transport options in regard to sedation and restraint.
- Advice is required on appropriate de-escalation techniques.
- Intervention strategies are required to reduce the frequent use of emergency services (Evangelista et al., 2016).

Community care teams (CCTs)

Community care teams (CCTs) vary in their response times from short-term case management for acute psychiatric presentations to longer-term case management and recovery for more residual mental health presentations. The most common diagnosis for people receiving support from a CCT is schizophrenia, followed by depression, bipolar disorder and schizoaffective disorder (AIHW, 2015a). CCTs are multidisciplinary teams comprising mental health nurses, occupational therapists, social workers, psychologists, medical officers and psychiatrists, carers and **consumer consultant** (also known as a peer worker – see Chapter 21). Most consumers attend clinics or engage with community staff voluntarily and a few consumers may be required to attend as compulsory consumers, having been placed on a community treatment order (CTO). The multidisciplinary team provides primary education, liaising with GPs and other service providers, relapse prevention, medication management, recovery planning and support, skills training and service

referral. Different disciplines perform the primary role of case management and may also engage in discipline-specific interventions.

Case management

Case management remains the most common form of mental health service delivery in the community, being utilised mainly by consumers with severe, persistent mental health conditions or high impact mental distress. Case managers coordinate consumer care, navigating through an often confusing array of fragmented services. Initially, case management was introduced to reduce hospital presentations, but the role has expanded to include assessment, linking, monitoring and evaluation services, supporting consumers' recovery, monitoring medication adherence and promoting autonomy and empowerment (Palmer, 2013). In Australia, supporting the recovery of the consumer through recovery-oriented practice has seen a shift from medical models to strengths-based recovery approaches. The adoption of the strengths-based model has led to reported outcomes of increased numbers of individuals living independently, increased numbers of consumers being competitively employed or involved in tertiary education, and decreased hospital admissions (Petrakis, Wilson & Hamilton, 2013). The strengths-based model suggests that people can recover, reclaim and transform their lives; that all people have unique strengths, talents and skills; and that community provides a key to helping people achieve well-being (Rapp & Goscha, 2006). Refer to Chapter 21 for discussion of the strengths-based model.

Eventual discharge from compulsory treatment

Non-clinical social support programs

The Mental Health Community Support Services (MHCSS) program (formerly Psychiatric Disability Rehabilitation and Support Services) is a type of social and welfare support initiative provided by state and territory governments to assist people living with mental distress (AIHW, 2015a). One program that is part of this group of services is the Personal Helpers and Mentors (PHaMs) program, an Australian Government initiative to improve recovery outcomes for people who have a lived experience of mental health issues, to help consumers to better manage their activities of daily living and reconnect to their community. PHaMs services provide biopsychosocial support and assist consumers by establishing links between consumers and services. PHaMs also ensures services accessed by participants are coordinated, integrated and complementary with other services

CASE **STUDY**

CTOs AND MANAGING INDEPENDENCE

Adam is a 37-year-old male who resides in a 30-bed special residential service (SRS). He has a long history of schizoaffective disorder that was diagnosed at age 25 years. His father misused alcohol and was often violent towards Adam, so he left home at 15 years of age and lived on the streets until age 17 when he had his first inpatient admission to the child and adolescent mental health services (CAMHS) ward. Adam's father is now deceased. Adam's mother lives in a social housing unit and Adam has contact with her occasionally. She often requests that Adam move in with her, but each time he has done so Adam becomes both physically and mentally unwell. Social workers at the mental health service have recorded that his mother takes away his pension and neglects Adam. Adam also wants to live with his mother.

Adam is currently on a CTO and is required to attend his local community treatment clinic once a fortnight; each time he receives Risperidol Consta 50 mg IM to treat his delusional symptoms. At times, Adam smokes marijuana, when he becomes mentally unwell and often fails to attend the clinic to receive his medication. When he becomes unwell he tends to run away from the SRS and live rough on the streets. Although Adam is street smart and knows where to find food and bedding, he has been attacked and stabbed in the past and fails to attend to his hygiene, which has resulted in serious skin conditions.

Adam has a financial administrator – the State Trustees – who ensure his accommodation is paid and he does not spend all his money on drugs. Adam hates this restriction. He has only one close friend at the SRS and spends most of his days in his room. He refuses to attend any of the activities provided by the accommodation.

Questions

1 Adam is on a treatment order managed in the community. What are the legal requirements of a CTO? What are the legal implications for Adam of not attending the clinic?
2 Should Adam be allowed to move in with his mother?
3 Should Adam be allowed to manage his own finances? How could you assist this to happen responsibly?
4 Utilising a biophyschosocial model, what interventions, referrals or services could the case manager initiate that may be helpful to Adam's recovery.

in the community. It is estimated that consumer involvement is increasing by an annual average rate of 15% (AIHW, 2015a). The service has also been embraced by Aboriginal and Torres Strait Islander peoples, who represent 3% of the Australian population (ABS, 2013), making up approximately 13% of PHaMs participants (AIHW, 2015a).

SPECIALISED COMMUNITY SERVICES

Specialised community services are comprised of highly experienced mental health clinicians with detailed and expert knowledge in their field. Some of the areas of specialisation are described in this section.

Perinatal mental health services

Perinatal mental health issues can affect the person before, during or after the birth of a child. The most common presentations are depression and anxiety, with 1 in 10 women and 1 in 20 men experiencing perinatal depression (AIHW, 2012; Panda, 2016). A less common but higher risk presentation is puerperal psychosis, which poses a greater risk to mother and baby. Most women and men initially seek assistance from their GP but may at times require referral to specialist perinatal mental health services. These services offer timely support, treatment and management for mothers and families experiencing mental health issues before, during or after the birth of a child. They are comprised of midwives, maternity and child health nurses, mental health nurses, psychologists, GPs and psychiatrists all working together to get the best outcomes for the family. NICE guidelines (2014) recommend early assessment and treatment for the best outcomes and suggest the person be assessed by competent practitioners within two weeks and receive professional referral and psychological intervention within one month.

CLINICAL **OBSERVATIONS**

Health care professionals caring for women in the perinatal period who are at risk of developing or have mental health issues should monitor the mother regularly for symptoms throughout pregnancy and the postnatal period, particularly in the first few weeks after childbirth.

To reduce postpartum psychosis, better identification and a greater understanding of prophylactic and acute treatment would have a significant impact on maternal and child welfare, and service costs.

SOURCE: NICE, 2014

Older persons' mental health services

Older persons' mental health services are specialist mental health services for people aged 65 years and over. These services are commonly known as aged persons mental health (APMH) and are available to consumers with mental health issues or severe **behavioural difficulties** associated with organic disorders such as dementia. This age group requires specialised services due to the high incidence and need to manage comorbid mental health and chronic health issues (see **Figure 24.2**). APMH services include community-based APMH teams, intensive community

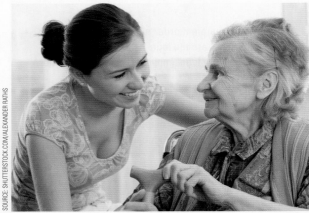

SOURCE: SHUTTERSTOCK.COM/ALEXANDER RATHS

FIGURE 24.2
Older persons require specialised services due to the high incidence of comorbid mental health and chronic health issues

treatment programs and access to residential care. The primary care APMH team can offer early identification and treatment of dementia and, in turn, better outcomes and a slower progression of cognitive deficits.

Despite increasing interest in the early diagnosis of dementia, it still remains underdiagnosed and undertreated. To increase the incidence of diagnosis and combat the issue of time constraints in primary care, new brief screening tests have been developed and found to be as clinically robust as the more time-consuming mini mental state examination (MMSE). These tests include the General Practitioner Assessment of Cognition (GP-COG), the Mini-Cog Assessment Instrument, the Memory Impairment Screen (MIS) and the six-item Cognitive Impairment Test (CIT). The Memory Alteration Test (MAT) tests verbal, episodic and semantic memory (De Mendonça Lima, 2015). Although older persons have a lower prevalence of severe mental health disorders than younger age groups (ABS, 2007), they are at greater risk of developing anxiety and depression (10–15%), social isolation and suicidal ideation (Haralambous et al., 2009). Certain sub-groups, in particular permanent aged care residents, are at an even higher risk of developing depression, with 52% of residents having either mild, moderate or major symptoms of depression (AIHW, 2013).

Homelessness

Mental health issues are often a causal factor of housing instability, which includes living in

CASE **STUDY**

THE ROLE OF THE AGED PSYCHIATRIC ASSESSMENT AND TREATMENT TEAM

Sophie is a 75-year-old lady experiencing an episode of major depression. She lives alone but has regular contact with her two daughters. Most of Sophie's friends have died or are in aged care accommodation, and her husband passed away six years ago. This has left her isolated and now, with her depression, she stays at home sleeping most of the day and hoping to die.

Sophie has many comorbid physical issues as she has severe chronic obstructive pulmonary disease (COPD) which has resulted in significantly reduced lung function and difficulty walking more than 50 metres. She rarely seeks assistance or attends doctor's appointments as she feels everything is hopeless and nothing will improve. She does not have a regular GP.

Sophie receives house cleaning support from the local council and has a community worker from a local agency (funded by the Commonwealth carers service) who takes her to the local shopping centre once a week. For the past four weeks, Sophie has refused to go with the carer, stating she is too unwell.

Sophie has lost a significant amount of weight over the past year and now weighs only 42 kg. She is no longer able to open jars or bottles in the house and finds her walker is too heavy to lift. She smokes 10 cigarettes a day and drinks three to four glasses of wine at night. Her drinking has increased from only two to three glasses a week four months ago.

After a fall last week, Sophie had an admission to the short stay unit and was seen by client liaison, who referred her to the aged psychiatric assessment and treatment team (APATT), and she was started on citalopram 20 mg for her depression.

Questions

1   What are the symptoms that suggest Sophie may be suffering from depression?
2   How would you establish a therapeutic relationship with Sophie?
3   Utilising a biopsychosocial model, what interventions, referrals or services could the APATT initiate that may be helpful to Sophie?
4   What is the specific role for the APATT clinician in Sophie's case?

marginalised housing and homelessness; and, conversely, being homeless tends to be a major factor in the development of mental health issues such as anxiety and depression (Johnson & Chamberlain, 2011). This is supported by ABS (2014) research that found people who had experienced mental health issues in the previous 12 months were four times more likely to have a history of homelessness than people without these disorders; and 13% of those who had experienced a psychotic disorder reported at least one period of homelessness in the preceding 12 months (Harvey, Killackey, Groves & Herrman, 2012). Specialist homelessness services (SHS) are community services funded by the Australian Government to provide support to clients who are homeless or at risk of homelessness. One in four persons who accessed these services in 2013–14 experienced current mental distress and required assistance as a result of housing crises or domestic violence. This compares with those people not experiencing mental distress, who stated the main reason for accessing the services was domestic violence (AIHW, 2015b). It is estimated that the demand for homelessness services by people with mental health issues is increasing by 12% per annum (AIHW, 2015b). In 2017–18, the number of consumers with a current lived experience of mental distress supported by the SHS exceeded 81 000 clients, which was a 4% increase from the preceding 12-month period (AIHW, 2018). These services assist in finding housing and shelter, and identifying and treating the mental distress of what is often a transient population. Many areas have specialised outreach teams that provide assistance to those who are homeless or at risk of homelessness through assertive outreach, providing comprehensive assessment, case management, allied health care and clinical care. These teams often work alongside other community services and are referred to as Homeless Outreach Program (HOP), Homeless Outreach Psychiatric Service (HOPS) or Homeless Health Outreach teams (HHOTs).

Aboriginal and Torres Strait Islander mental health services

The Aboriginal and Torres Strait Islander population is at increased risk of experiencing poor social and emotional well-being. This is often attributed to the harsh colonisation of Australia and the *Aborigines Act 1905*, which led to what is known today as the stolen generation. The removal of children from their families and cultural background led to issues around unresolved grief, loss, trauma, a sense of alienation from cultural ties and destruction of traditional lifestyles. This in turn led to greater poverty, chronic illnesses, high levels of psychological stress and higher unemployment, resulting in poor-quality

health and reduced life expectancy compared with non-Indigenous Australians (DHHS, 2015; Dudgeon, Milroy & Walker, 2014). Despite the reports of high psychological distress, fewer Indigenous Australians attend government-provided psychological or psychiatric services than do non-Indigenous Australians, and this is further reduced for Indigenous Australians living in remote areas (AIHW, 2014). The hospitalisation rate for mental health-related conditions for Indigenous Australians was 1.9 times the rate for non-Indigenous Australians (28 per 1000 compared with 15 per 1000), with the rate for Indigenous men 2.3 times the rate for non-Indigenous men, and for Indigenous women 1.7 times the rate for non-Indigenous women (AIHW, 2014).

The National Aboriginal and Torres Strait Islander Health Plan (2013–2023) provides an 'evidence-based policy framework as part of the overarching COAG approach to Closing the Gap in Indigenous disadvantage' (Commonwealth of Australia, 2015, p. 18). The goal of this health plan is the establishment of a healthy, empowered life connected to culture and country for Aboriginal and Torres Strait Islander peoples. This is achieved through addressing the underlying social determinants that lead to poor health (Commonwealth of Australia, 2015). The health plan suggests a multidisciplinary primary intervention approach that offers screening and early intervention, and social and welfare support including access to employment, education and housing, counselling and pharmacotherapy. Also recommended in the plan are case coordination, 24-hour access to the advice of a specialist mental health clinician, community education programs, mental health literacy, mental health first aid and early childhood programs; along with well-supported Aboriginal Mental Health Workers and a strong emphasis on cultural safety and the inclusion of people with mental health issues in community engagement processes (Tilton &Thomas, 2011).

CULTURAL CONSIDERATIONS

Considering the meaning of health

Depending on a person's cultural background, health may not simply mean the physical well-being of an individual as promoted by allopathic medical practice, but may also refer to the social, emotional and cultural well-being of the whole community. For Aboriginal and Torres Strait Islander peoples, health is seen in terms of the whole-of-life view incorporating the cyclical concept of life–death and relationship to the land.

SOURCE: NACCHO, 2016A

Forensic mental health services

Forensic mental health services are specialist services for people who are at risk or involved in the criminal legal system (Hungerford et al., 2015). The rates of mental health disorders are up to six times higher in forensic populations than in the broader community (AIHW, 2011) and studies of Australian court defendants also show high rates of mental health conditions (Elsayed, Al-Zahrani & Rashad, 2010). The Australian Institute of Health and Welfare (AIHW) reported that during a two-week census period in 2010, 31% of prison entrants across most Australian states and territories, with the exclusion of New South Wales and Victoria, reported some history of mental health issue, with only 16% taking medication for a mental health condition (AIHW, 2011). Forensic mental health professionals provide assessments, advice and reports for the courts and prisons, manage treatment and recovery of the consumer, and coordinate care across all settings including pre-release planning and linking with mainstream community mental health services. They are often employed to provide court assessment or liaison, assist the courts, or provide support and advocate for those attending court who have mental health issues. In addition, forensic mental health services offer specialised community support for both clinicians and offenders.

Specialty areas of interest may include offences such as arson and working with perpetrators of sexual assault, and forensic services run programs tailored to prevent individuals with serious mental health issues reoffending while addressing the intricate needs of the mental health condition. By streamlining forensic mental health services and supporting clinicians in treating offenders with mental health conditions, outcomes such as recidivism and higher concordance to treatment plans can be achieved. Health care professionals within the forensic setting also have a role in research, education and training (Martin et al., 2012).

Child and adolescent mental health services

Child and adolescent mental health services (CAMHS) provide specialist mental health services up until 18 years of age and youth services (CYMHS) provide specialist services to young adults from 18–25 years. Mental health issues affect around 15% of children under 18 years of age and the emergence of behavioural disorders such as oppositional defiant and conduct disorders is seen in young children. The onset of high-prevalence disorders such as anxiety, mood and substance use as well as psychotic disorders like schizophrenia also occurs in adolescence and young adults (McGorry, Purcell, Goldstone & Amminge, 2011). The onset of mental health issues in this period of emotional growth, changing roles and increasing

independence requires a specialist response capable of consumer and family support in order to ensure a better prognosis and reduce social isolation. It is evident that 'early age of onset has been shown to be associated with a longer duration of untreated illness and poorer clinical and functional outcomes' (McGorry et al., 2011, p. 301). The most common presenting mental health issues in this age group are impulsive behaviours/self-harming/non-suicidal self-injuring behaviours (12%), drug and alcohol use, depression and anxiety (Headspace National Youth Mental Health Foundation, 2016). It is also estimated that approximately 30% of adolescents aged 12–20 have thought about suicide at some point in their lives, with around 20% reporting having had such thoughts in the previous year (Orygen, 2015). Eating disorders are another mental health issue that emerges in this age group and they are associated with a high mortality rate. Research suggests that health promotion and prevention, enhancing protective factors and/or reducing early warning signs, and media literacy lead to a reduction in the incidence of this disease (NEDC, 2010). With all this in mind, CAMHS and CYMHS services have a distinct ability to reduce the national burden of disease; and strategically targeted specialty services that engage the individual and the family and offer acute crisis care, intensive follow-up both pre- and post-inpatient admission, case management and linking to other services are essential components for these services.

Refugee and culturally and linguistically diverse (CALD) communities

Cultural and linguistic diversity is a core feature of the Australian population, with Victoria alone being home to over 200 different nationalities. This diversity challenges services to be culturally inclusive and competent and respond to the differing needs of immigrants, refugees and asylum seekers (Minas et al., 2013).

> Several factors have been found to be associated with increased risk of mental disorder among immigrants. They include limited English proficiency, separation from cultural identity, loss of close family ties, lack of opportunity to make effective use of occupational skills, trauma exposure prior to migration, and the many stresses associated with migration and adjustment to a new country (Minas et al., 2013, p. 14).

Due to migrant and refugee underutilisation of mental health services and language difficulties, clear figures on the incidence of mental health issues in these populations are unavailable, but evidence suggests that mental distress in immigrant communities is similar to that in host populations (Minas et al., 2013).

Refugees and asylum seekers, however, are at greater risk of developing mental health issues or suicidal ideation than the general population as a result of prolonged detention, exposure to trauma and violence and loss of cultural identity (Minas et al., 2013). Specialist community CALD programs for mental health include the Mental Health in Multicultural Australia (MHiMA) project, which provides advice and support to providers and governments on mental health and suicide prevention for people from CALD backgrounds (Mental health in Multicultural Australia, 2011). Access to Allied Psychological Services (ATAPS) also provides specific targeted services to people from CALD communities. The Programme of Assistance for Survivors of Torture and Trauma (PASTT) delivers mental health and other support to permanently resettled humanitarian entrants, those on temporary visas, and people have experienced torture and trauma, as well as capacity building for health professionals assisting this group of individuals. The Department of Health funds a number of projects under the National Suicide Prevention Programme (NSPP), which include a focus on CALD communities, such as the Queensland Programme of Assistance to Survivors of Torture and Trauma NEXUS project. The Migrant Resource Centre's Phoenix Centre Suicide Prevention project aims to build partnerships with and provide support for key organisations that provide services to CALD groups and includes planning and training for professionals to respond to those at risk of suicide (Department of Health, 2014c).

Individual recovery plans

In the community setting, nursing care plans are called individual recovery plans (IRP). The purpose of these plans is to support the individual in identifying meaningful goals to support their recovery journey. The consumer guides and takes responsibility for the process.

The following nursing care plan explores how consumers and mental health nurses work together in developing recovery-focused goals that are consumer-focused and driven.

NURSING CARE PLAN

Context

Tom is a 45-year-old man with a long history of schizophrenia. He lives in a supported accommodation service (SRS) with 45 other residents. Tom has experienced hearing derogatory voices since the age of 16 and despite having been prescribed many different medications, he has never really had a lot of relief from them. Tom has no friends, keeps to himself and sees his family only once every two years. Tom believes that one of the other residents is a demon that wants to control his body and often feels very afraid, packs up all his belongings and runs away from the SRS and sleeps rough. During these times, he also fails to adhere to his medication and his voices become louder and more tormenting. Tom smokes cigarettes when he can afford them and drinks lots of caffeine.

Goals

(As determined in collaboration with Tom)

- Tom would like to go to McDonald's once a week on an outing.
- Tom would like to have control of his money.
- Tom would like to live independently.

Consumer information
Given name: Tom
Family name: Blake

Address: 35 Goosehound Drive, Kingslan, NSW

Parties involved

General practitioner	Joseph Yen	7 Singapore Rd, Ferntree	Ph: 95432198
Psychiatrist	Peter Fern	Evendale Clinic	Ph: 0435421101
Case manager	Lisa Brown	Evendale Clinic	Ph: 87213467
PHaMs worker	Jodie Fink	Waterdale	Ph: 0443675990

DESIRED OUTCOME	TIMELINE/ PERSONS RESPONSIBLE	CURRENT SITUATION	STRENGTHS	STRATEGIES/ INTERVENTIONS	DATE ACHIEVED
Tom to have social interaction with others in order to decrease social isolation	3 months Tom Jodie Fink (PHaMs)	Tom has no friends and minimal contact with others	Educated to Year 11 Has interest and knowledge in trains Is prepared to leave the SRS for the day with his worker	Initially take Tom to McDonald's once a week for 1:1 interaction Transition contact to assist him to meet with the local train enthusiasts society Encourage Tom to also attend the swimming activities provided by the council for residents of the SRS Tom to attend activities independently	1 week (DD/MM/20..) 4 weeks (DD/MM/20..) 8 weeks (DD/MM/20..) 12 weeks (DD/MM/20..)
Financial independence	Case manager Tom State Trustees financial administrator	State Trustees manages Tom's money	Has been able to be financially independent in the past Keen to gain this financial control Willing to work with administrator	Refer to budgeting program State Trustees Gradual financial control under the supervision of administrator Financial independence	Immediate (DD/MM/20..) Ongoing until independent 2 years (DD/MM/20..)
Independent living	Case manager	Lives in SRS	Has lived independently in the past Agrees to relearn skills that facilitate independence	Referral to community care unit for intensive assessment and skill development	Immediate referral Expected time of intake 3 months

REFLECTION ON LEARNING FROM PRACTICE

Jodie's experience with her first psychotic episode caused her significant losses and initially a high level of dysfunction in her relationships and community connections. Her mother's insistence and the eventual compulsory treatment and engagement of community services allowed her to receive early treatment and this resulted in a very good outcome. It is possible that Jodie may never experience another psychotic episode. Jodie was maintained on medication for 12 months as is the recommendation from evidence-based research and now is managing without medication and is symptom free.

CHAPTER RESOURCES

SUMMARY

- Deinstitutionalisation saw mental health care move from large institutions to the community and consumers could now receive support in their own homes. This led to the establishment of primary health care and federal government initiatives to increase the accessibility and equity to services for people with mental health issues, ensuring good-quality affordable care is delivered where it is needed most.

- The social determinants of health and mental health are the economic and social conditions that influence and impact the mental health of individuals and groups. These include factors such as discrimination, access to resources, personal and community safety, adverse early life experiences, poor education, lack of meaningful and appropriately remunerated employment, poor housing choice, inadequate nutrition and social exclusion.

- The Australian Government provides clinical and non-clinical delivery of mental services to consumers and both offer an assertive outreach approach that results in clinical staff being involved with consumers for extended periods of time or providing more episodic or crisis care.

- Mental health nurses employed in community mental health teams have several roles. They undertake clinical reviews, assessment and monitoring of a consumer's emotional and mental state, provide education and support with medication management as well as liaising with and referring to more generalist services, including GPs. Ongoing support and case management is also provided to consumers and teams may be involved in early transition from inpatient admissions to community-based mental health care. There are various types of community mental health teams, including acute community intervention services, mental health triage, crisis and assessment teams, community care teams and case management.

- Recognising and responding to specific mental health needs has seen the emergence of specialist mental health services to provide targeted care for specific populations: CALD refugees and asylum seekers, forensic, aged, child and adolescent, perinatal, homeless and Aboriginal and Torres Strait Islander peoples.

REVIEW QUESTIONS

1 What is deinstitutionalisation?
2 What is primary mental health care? Describe some of its advantages.
3 List 10 factors that would be considered to be social determinants of mental health.
4 John is a 75-year-old man experiencing an episode of depression and he is currently being treated on fluoxetine 40 mg by his local GP. John lost his spouse to cancer six months ago and is finding it difficult to cope with this loss. Suggest a primary care service and a clinical specialist service that may be helpful for John.

5 Crises and assessment teams provide:
  a Long-term clinical management for people with a mental health condition
  b Short-term crisis management and support for early hospital discharge for consumers with mental health issues
  c Inpatient care for consumers with a mental health condition
  d Case management services
6 Why is there a need for specialist CALD services?
7 Name some of the professionals who would comprise the multidisciplinary team involved in perinatal mental health services.

CRITICAL THINKING

1 What do you think are some of the advantages of deinstitutionalisation?
2 What do you think are some of the disadvantages of deinstitutionalisation?
3 Why is it important to consider the social determinants of health when planning strategies to address mental health needs?
4 Different areas of mental health services provide various services to consumers and different groups of consumers. Research the services that are available in your area.

5 Why would adult mental health and older (aged) care mental health teams require different skills?
6 What do you consider would be some of the barriers to immigrants, refugees and asylum seekers receiving needed mental health care?

USEFUL WEBSITES

- Asylum Seeker Resource Centre: https://www.asrc.org.au
- Australian Institute of Health and Welfare Mental Health Services in Australia: https://www.aihw.gov.au/reports/mental-health-services/mental-health-services-in-australia/report-contents/summary
- Embrace Multicultural Mental Health: https://mhaustralia.org/national-multicultural-mental-health-project
- National Aboriginal Community Controlled Health Organisation (NACCHO): http://www.naccho.org.au
- Orygen Youth Health: http://oyh.org.au
- World Health Organization: http://www.who.int/en

State and territory mental health services

- New South Wales: http://www.health.nsw.gov.au/mentalhealth/Pages/default.aspx
- Northern Territory: https://health.nt.gov.au/professionals/mental-health-information-for-health-professional
- Queensland: https://www.health.qld.gov.au/clinical-practice/guidelines-procedures/clinical-staff/mental-health/default.asp
- South Australia: https://www.sahealth.sa.gov.au/wps/wcm/connect/public+content/sa+health+internet/services/mental+health+and+drug+and+alcohol+services/mental+health+services/mental+health+services
- Tasmania: http://www.dhhs.tas.gov.au/mentalhealth
- Victoria: https://www2.health.vic.gov.au/mental-health
- Western Australia: https://www.wa.gov.au/information-about/health-wellbeing/mental-health

REFLECT ON THIS

Telehealth and mental healthcare

The COVID-19 pandemic has posed particular challenges for community mental health services due to social distancing precautions and the restrictions of home visits. One of the substitutes for in-person appointments is Telehealth. What was once seen as a necessary service for rural and remote health care became a common feature of inner-city health care during the pandemic. But how suitable is Telehealth in the mental health context?

1 Consider the barriers people may encounter to face-to-face appointments. Be sure to include sociodemographic considerations in your response, such as access to the internet and privacy. What do you think some of the benefits of Telehealth in a mental health context might be?

2 Traditionally, group-type meetings have had particular practical benefits in the mental health context. The reduced costs of running group sessions are one of the more obvious benefits, but there are other benefits to group therapy, such as sharing of experiences, making new support networks and exchanging ideas. Carers and people with a lived experience of mental illness have a unique and valuable experience to share that others in their situation may benefit from. Consider the positive and negative aspects of group therapy in the mental health context.

REFERENCES

Allen Consulting Group. (2012). *Police, Ambulance and Clinical Early Response (PACER) Evaluation: Final Report*. Retrieved from http://www.acilallen.com.au/cms_files/acgpacerevaluation2012.pdf.

American Psychiatric Association (APA). (2013). *Diagnostic and Statistical Manual of Mental Disorders (DSM-5)* (5th edn). Washington, DC: APA.

Australian Bureau of Statistics (ABS). (2007). *National Survey of Mental Health and Wellbeing: Highlights*. Canberra: ABS. Retrieved from https://www.health.gov.au/internet/main/publishing.nsf/Content/A24556C814804A99CA257BF0001CAC45/$File/mha2hig.pdf.

Australian Bureau of Statistics (ABS). (2013). *Australian Demographic Statistics. Aug 2013*. Cat. no. 33238.0.55.001. Canberra: ABS.

Australian Bureau of Statistics (ABS). (2014). *Mental Health and Experiences of Homelessness, Australia*. Canberra: ABS. Retrieved from http://www.abs.gov.au/ausstats%5Cabs@.nsf/0/51475D5561822F7FCA257FB1001DDBDA?Opendocument.

Australian Institute of Health and Welfare (AIHW). (2011). *The Health of Australia's Prisoners 2010*. Cat. no. PHE 149. Canberra: AIHW.

Australian Institute of Health and Welfare (AIHW). (2012). *Experience of Perinatal Depression: Data from the 2010 Australian National Infant Feeding Survey*. Information paper. Cat. no. PHE 161. Canberra: AIHW.

Australian Institute of Health and Welfare (AIHW). (2013). *Depression in Residential Aged Care 2008–2012. Aged Care Statistics Series No. 39*. Cat. no. AGE 73. Canberra: AIHW.

Australian Institute of Health and Welfare (AIHW). (2014). *Australia's Health*. Canberra: AIHW. Retrieved from http://www.aihw.gov.au/australias-health/2014/indigenous-health.

Australian Institute of Health and Welfare (AIHW). (2015a). *Mental Health Services – In Brief 2015*. Cat. no. HSE 169. Canberra: AIHW.

Australian Institute of Health and Welfare (AIHW). (2015b). *Specialist Homelessness Services 2014–15*. Canberra: AIHW. Retrieved from http://www.aihw.gov.au/homelessness/specialist-homelessness-services-2014-15.

Australian Institute of Health and Welfare (AIHW). (2015c). *The Health and Welfare of Australia's Aboriginal and Torres Strait Islander Peoples 2015*. Cat. no. IHW 147. Canberra: AIHW.

Australian Institute of Health and Welfare (AIHW). (2018). *Specialist Homelessness Services Annual Report 2017–18 (Web report)*. Retrieved from https://www.aihw.gov.au/reports/homelessness-services/specialist-homelessness-services-2017-18/contents/client-groups-of-interest/clients-with-a-current-mental-health-issue.

Bedell, J.R., Hunter, R.H. & Corrigan, P.W. (1997). Current approaches to assessment and treatment of persons with serious mental illness. *International Journal of Psychosocial Rehabilitation*. Retrieved from http://www.psychosocial.com/psr/assessment_treatment.html.

Commonwealth of Australia. (2015). *Aboriginal and Torres Strait Islander Health Performance Framework 2014 Report*. p. 18. Retrieved from https://www.dpmc.gov.au/sites/default/files/publications/Aboriginal_and_Torres_Strait_Islander_HPF_2014%20-%20edited%2016%20June2015.pdf. © Commonwealth of Australia (2015). Released under CC BY 4.0. Link to license: https://creativecommons.org/licenses/by/4.0/.

Compton, M.T. & Shim, R.S. (Eds.) (2015). *Social Determinants of Mental Health*. Arlington, VA: American Psychiatric Publishing, Inc. Retrieved from http://ACU.eblib.com/patron/FullRecord.aspx?p=2004575.

De Mendonça Lima, C.A. (2015). Abstracts of the 23rd European Congress of Psychiatry: Primary care mental health for older persons and the WHO Mental Health Plan 2013–2020. *European Psychiatry*, 30, 131. https://doi.org/10.1016/S0924-9338(15)30109-7

Department of Health. (2010). *Statewide Mental Health Triage Scale Guidelines*. Retrieved from https://www2.health.vic.gov.au/about/publications/policiesandguidelines/triage-scale-mental-health-services.

Department of Health. (2014a). *Acute Community Intervention Service Guidelines*. Retrieved from https://www2.health.vic.gov.au/about/publications/policiesandguidelines/Acute%20Community%20Intervention%20Service%20Guidelines%20-%20July%202014. © State of Victoria, Department of Health. Released under CC BY 3.0 AU. Link to license: https://creativecommons.org/licenses/by/3.0/au/.

Department of Health. (2014b). *ATAPS Suicide Prevention Service Initiative*. Retrieved from http://www.health.gov.au/internet/publications/publishing.nsf/Content/suicide-prevention-activities-evaluation~positioning-the-nspp~ataps.

Department of Health. (2014c). *Fact Sheet: Mental Health Services for People of Culturally and Linguistically Diverse (CALD) Backgrounds*. Retrieved from http://www.health.gov.au/internet/main/publishing.nsf/Content/mental-multi-fact.

Department of Health. (2014d). *Mental Health First Aid Training for Front Line Community Workers*. Retrieved from http://www.health.gov.au/internet/main/publishing.nsf/Content/mental-firstaid.

Department of Health. (2015a). *Better Access to Psychiatrists, Psychologists and General Practitioners through the MBS (Better Access) Initiative*. Retrieved from http://www.health.gov.au/mentalhealth-betteraccess.

Department of Health. (2015b). *Mental Health Services in Rural and Remote Areas (MHSRRA)*. Retrieved from http://www.health.gov.au/internet/main/publishing.nsf/Content/mental-rural.

Department of Health. (2015c). *Primary Mental Health Care Services Activities Grant Programme Guidelines*. Retrieved from http://www.health.gov.au/internet/main/publishing.nsf/Content/mental-pmhcsa-guidelines.

Department of Health. (2016). *Mental Health Nurse Incentive Program*. Retrieved from http://www.health.gov.au/internet/publications/publishing.nsf/Content/mental-pubs-m-mhnipro-toc.

Department of Health and Human Services (DHHS). (2015). *Koori Health Counts, Victoria*. Retrieved from https://www2.health.vic.gov.au/about/publications/data/Koori%20Health%20Counts%20201213.

Dezetter, A., Briffault, X., Bruffaerts, R., De Graaf, R., Alonso, J., König, H.H. & Kovess-Masféty, V. (2013). Use of general practitioners versus mental health professionals in six European countries: The decisive role of the organization of mental health-care systems. *Social Psychiatry and Psychiatric Epidemiology*, 48(1), 137–49. doi:http://dx.doi.org.ezproxy.lib.swin.edu.au/10.1007/s00127-012-0522-9.

Dudgeon, P., Milroy, H. & Walker, R. (2014). *Working Together: Aboriginal Health* (2nd edn). Department of the Prime Minister and Cabinet, Australia; Department of Health and Ageing; Telethon Institute for Child Health Research; Kulunga Research Network; University of Western Australia.

Elsayed, Y.A., Al-Zahrani, M. & Rashad, M.M. (2010). Characteristics of mentally ill offenders from 100 psychiatric court reports. *Annals of General Psychiatry*, 9, 4. Retrieved from http://ezproxy.lib.swin.edu.au/login?url=http://go.galegroup.com.ezproxy.lib.swin.edu.au/ps/i.do?id=GALE%7CA218620034&v=2.1&u=swinburne1&it=r&p=AONE&sw=w&asid=20e1ffb8d58438f25e5001ff45c381fe.

Evangelista, E., Lee, S., Gallagher, A., Peterson, V., James, J., Warren, N., ... Deveny, E. (2016). Crisis averted: How consumers experienced a police and clinical early response (PACER) unit responding to a mental health crisis. *International Journal of Mental Health Nursing*, 25(4), 367–76. doi:10.1111/inm.12218.

Haralambous, B., Lin, X., Dow, B., Jones, C., Tinney, J. & Bryant, C. (2009). *Depression in Older Age: A Scoping Study*. Melbourne: National Ageing Research Institute.

Harvey, C., Killackey, E., Groves, A. & Herrman, H. (2012). A place to live: Housing needs for people with psychotic disorders identified in the second Australian national survey of psychosis. *Australian and New Zealand Journal of Psychiatry*, 46(9), 840–50. doi:10.1177/0004867412449301.

Headspace National Youth Mental Health Foundation. (2016). *Understanding Substance Abuse – for Health Professionals*. Retrieved from http://headspace.org.au/health-professionals/understanding-substance-abuse-for-health-professionals.

Holmes, D. & Jacob, J.D. (2014). *Power and the Psychiatric Apparatus: Repression, Transformation, and Assistance*. Surrey: Routledge.

Hungerford, C., Hodgson, D., Clancy, R., Monisse-Redman, M., Bostwick, R. & Jones, T. (2015). *Mental Health Care: An Introduction for Health Professionals* (2nd edn). Sydney: John Wiley & Sons.

Johnson, G. & Chamberlain, C. (2011). Are the homeless mentally ill? *Australian Journal of Social Issues*, 46(1), 29–48. Retrieved from http://ezproxy.lib.swin.edu.au/login?url=http://go.galegroup.com.ezproxy.lib.swin.edu.au/ps/i.do?id=GALE%7CA260494127&v=

2.1&u=swinburne1&it=r&p=AONE&sw=w&asid=eaa00acba95969
ea95e8e4fa0f856975.

Kim, T.-W., Jeong, J.-H., Kim, Y.-H., Kim, Y., Seo, H.-J. & Hong, S.C. (2015). Fifteen-month follow up of an assertive community treatment program for chronic patients with mental illness. *BMC Health Services Research*, 15, 388.

Lee, S., Brunero, S., Fairbrother, G. & Cowan, D. (2008). Profiling police presentations of mental health consumers to an emergency department. *International Journal of Mental Health Nursing*, 17(5), 311–16. doi:10.1111/j.1447-0349.2008.00553.x.

Lee, S.J., Thomas, P., Doulis, C., Bowles, D., Henderson, K., Keppich-Arnold, S. & Stafrace, S. (2015). Outcomes achieved by and police and clinician perspectives on a joint police officer and mental health clinician mobile response unit. *International Journal of Mental Health Nursing*, 24(6), 538–46. doi:10.1111/inm.12153.

Martin, T., Ryan, J., Bawden, L., Maguire, T., Quinn, C. & Summers, M. (2012). *Forensic Mental Health Nursing Standards of Practice 2012*. Retrieved from http://www.forensicare.vic.gov.au/assets/pubs/Nursing%20Standards%202012.pdf.

McGorry, P.D., Purcell, R., Goldstone, R. & Amminge, G.P. (2011). Age of onset and timing of treatment for mental and substance use disorders: Implications for preventive intervention strategies and models of care. *Current Opinion in Psychiatry*, 24, 301–6.

Mental Health in Multicultural Australia (MHiMA). (2011). About us. Retrieved from http://www.mhima.org.au/about-us/the-project.

Minas, H., Kakuma, R., Too, L.S., Vayani, H., Orapeleng, S., Prasad-Ildes, R., Turner, G., Procter, N. & Oehm, D. (2013). *Mental Health Research and Evaluation in Multicultural Australia: Developing a Culture of Inclusion*. Brisbane: MIHMA. p. 14. Retrieved from http://www.mentalhealthcommission.gov.au/media/80646/2093%20mhima%20cald%20report_06.pdf.

Ministry of Health, NSW. (2012). *Mental Health Triage Policy*. Retrieved from http://www0.health.nsw.gov.au/policies/pd/2012/pdf/PD2012_053.pdf.

National Aboriginal Community Controlled Health Organization (NACCHO). (2016a). Definitions. Retrieved from http://www.naccho.org.au/about/aboriginal-health/definitions.

National Aboriginal Community Controlled Health Organization (NACCHO). (2016b). NACCHO Aboriginal Health News Alerts. Delivering better health is about more than healthcare. Retrieved from https://nacchocommunique.com/tag/social-determinants-of-health.

National Eating Disorders Collaboration (NEDC). (2010). *Eating Disorders Prevention, Treatment & Management: An Evidence Review*. Canberra: Commonwealth Department of Health and Ageing.

National Institute for Heath and Care Excellence (NICE). (2014). *Antenatal and Postnatal Mental Health: Clinical Management and Service Guidance. Clinical Guideline CG192*. Retrieved from https://www.nice.org.uk/guidance/cg192?unlid=2876033182016210223415.

National Mental Health Commission (NMHC). (2014). *The National Review of Mental Health Programmes and Services*. Sydney: NMHC. Retrieved from http://www.mentalhealthcommission.gov.au/media-centre/news/national-review-of-mental-health-programmes-and-services-report-released.aspx.

Northern Territory Primary Health Network (NTPHN). (2016). *Mental Health Services in Rural and Remote Areas (MHSRRA)*. Retrieved from http://www.ntphn.org.au/our-programs/mhsrra.

Orygen. (2015). *MythBuster Suicidal Ideation*. Retrieved from https://orygen.org.au/Campus/Expert-Network/Resources/Free/Mythbusters/Suicidal-Ideation/Orygen_Suicidal_Ideation_Mythbuster.aspx?ext=.

Palmer, C. (2013). Therapeutic interventions. In R. Elder, K. Evans & D. Nizette (eds), *Psychiatric and Mental Health Nursing* (3rd edn). Sydney: Mosby/Elsevier Australia.

Perinatal, Anxiety & Depression Australia (PANDA). (2012). *Fact Sheet 1: Anxiety & Depression in Pregnancy & Early Parenthood*. Retrieved from https://www.panda.org.au/images/resources/Resources-Factsheets/Anxiety-And-Depression-In-Early-Parenthood-And-Pregnancy.pdf.

Petrakis, M., Wilson, M. & Hamilton, B. (2013). Implementing the strengths model of case management: Group supervision fidelity outcomes. *Community Mental Health Journal*, 49(3), 331–7. doi:http://dx.doi.org.ezproxy.lib.swin.edu.au/10.1007/s10597-012-9546-.

Rapp, C.A. & Goscha, R.J. (2006). *The Strengths Model: Case Management with People with Psychiatric Disabilities* (2nd edn). New York: Oxford University Press.

Rosen, A. (2006). The Australian experience of deinstitutionalization: Interaction of Australian culture with the development and reform of its mental health services. *Acta Psychiatrica Scandinavica*, 113, 81–9. doi:10.1111/j.1600-0447.2005.00723.x.

Saugeres, L. (2011). (Un)accommodating disabilities: Housing, marginalization and dependency in Australia. *Journal of Housing and the Built Environment*, 26(1), 1–15. doi:http://dx.doi.org.ezproxy.lib.swin.edu.au/10.1007/s10901-010-9201-x.

Shim, R. & Rust, G. (2013). Primary care, behavioral health, and public health: Partners in reducing mental health stigma. *American Journal of Public Health*, 103(5), 774–6. doi:10.2105/AJPH.2013.301214.

Tilton, E. & Thomas, D. (2011). *Core Functions of Primary Health Care: A Framework for the Northern Territory*. Darwin: Northern Territory Aboriginal Health Forum.

Udechuku, A., Olver, J., Hallam, K., Blyth, F., Leslie, M., Nasso, M. & Burrows, G. (2005). Assertive community treatment of the mentally ill: Service model and effectiveness. *Australasian Psychiatry*, 13(2), 129–34. doi:10.1111/j.1440-1665.2005.02175.x.

Victorian Government Department of Human Services. (2008). *Refugee Health and Wellbeing Action Plan 2008–2010: Current and Future Initiatives*. Retrieved from http://library.bsl.org.au/jspui/bitstream/1/1043/1/Refugee_healthandwellbeing_plan.pdf.

Wheeler, C., Lloyd-Evans, B., Churchard, A., Fitzgerald, C., Fullarton, K., Mosse, L. & Johnson, S. (2015). Implementation of the crisis resolution team model in adult mental health settings: A systematic review. *BMC Psychiatry*, 15, 74.

Winkler, P., Barrett, B., McCrone, P., Csémy, L., Janoušková, M. & Höschl, C. (2016). Deinstitutionalised patients, homelessness and imprisonment: Systematic review. *British Journal of Psychiatry*, 208(5), 421–8.

World Health Organization (WHO). (1986). *Ottawa Charter for Health Promotion: First International Conference on Health Promotion. Ottawa, 21 November 1986*. Retrieved from https://www.healthpromotion.org.au/images/ottawa_charter_hp.pdf.

World Health Organization (WHO). (1993). *The ICD-10 Classification of Mental and Behavioural Disorders: Diagnostic Criteria for Research*. Geneva: WHO.

World Health Organization (WHO). (2010). *A Conceptual Framework for Action on the Social Determinants of Health*. Geneva: WHO.

Retrieved from http://www.who.int/sdhconference/resources/ConceptualframeworkforactiononSDH_eng.pdf.

World Health Organization (WHO). (2013). *Mental Health Action Plan 2013–2020*. Retrieved from https://apps.who.int/iris/bitstream/handle/10665/89966/9789241506021_eng.pdf;jsessionid=EC3536FDB3D5E49A5F56D81D46461DBA?sequence=1. © Copyright World Health Organization (WHO).

World Health Organization (WHO). (2016). *Social Determinants of Health*. Retrieved from http://www.who.int/social_determinants/sdh_definition/en.

World Health Organization and Calouste Gulbenkian Foundation (WHO). (2014). *Social Determinants of Mental Health*. Geneva: WHO.

CHAPTER 24

CHAPTER 25

CULTURAL CONTEXT IN PRACTICE IN AUSTRALIA

Doseena Fergie

LEARNING OUTCOMES

Upon completion of this chapter, you should be able to:

25.1 Examine the historical and cultural context of Aboriginal and Torres Strait Islander peoples

25.2 Identify the social determinants that impinge on the health and well-being of Aboriginal and Torres Strait Islander peoples

25.3 Understand the impact of colonisation on their social and emotional well-being

25.4 Understand the movement from being culturally aware to culturally safe practice when caring for Aboriginal and Torres Strait Islander peoples

LEARNING FROM PRACTICE

Michael, an Aboriginal liaison officer, was summoned urgently to the medical ward. As he approached the ward, he observed that all the staff were standing outside peering dubiously through the window in the door. Michael asked, 'What's going on here?' The nurse in charge replied, 'We've got a female patient and the husband is drunk. He just barged right into the ward. We're afraid he might do some damage and harm us!' Michael looked in and sure enough there was a dishevelled-looking Aboriginal man sitting on the edge of the bed of the female patient.

Michael walked in and noticed that the man was slightly drunk but not so intoxicated as had been relayed to him by the staff. He called out as he approached the couple, 'Hello brother, what's going on?' The female patient said, 'Bro, they (the staff) think my hubby was going to cause trouble and do something, so they want to kick him out! But he is lonely and needed to drink because he's afraid of coming up to the hospital.' Michael looked at the man who replied, 'I just want to come and see my wife, because I

haven't seen her for a week. I don't know how she's getting on. Yeah, I had a couple of drinks and that helped me to have the courage to walk straight in here.'

Michael told him that he would talk to the nurse in charge and suggested that next time he decided to visit his wife, the man should see him first and Michael would take him to the ward himself. The man was happy to do this in the future. He finished his visit with his wife and Michael and he walked to the exit of the hospital grounds. Meanwhile, the staff returned to the ward, with the nurse in charge declaring that what Michael did 'was nothing short of a miracle!' Michael, on the other hand, was annoyed that the staff had misjudged the real intent of the man and had chosen to 'make a mountain out of a molehill'.

This experience highlights a number of issues that Michael encountered in his role. What judgements and stereotypes do you think the charge nurse's response was based on?

INTRODUCTION

The First Nations people of Australia consist of two distinct ethnic groups: mainland Aboriginals and the Torres Strait Islanders. This chapter discusses the cultural context and historical background of Australian Aboriginal and Torres Strait Islander peoples in order to gain an understanding of the mental health issues that affect them in contemporary society. Compared with other Western countries, Australia is one of the wealthier nations, rich in resources and with a highly skilled health workforce. Yet the health disparity between non-Indigenous Australians and Aboriginal and Torres Strait Islanders remains significantly wide. The traumatic impact that **colonisation** had and continues to have on each generation is immense. In this chapter, the effects of historical, cultural and social determinants of health on Indigenous Australians will be discussed, as well as the risk factors and protective factors involved. British invasion is discussed, as well as the period of **colonialism** leading to the effect that government policies had on Aboriginal communities. Colonisation had a devastating effect on the social and emotional well-being of Indigenous Australians.

Indigenous Australians have a holistic view of mental health. Holistic health incorporates the physical, social, emotional, spiritual and cultural well-being of a person. Indigenous Australians demonstrate strength, perseverance and resilience in society and the environment.

CULTURAL CONSIDERATIONS

Terminology
The term 'Australian Aboriginal' is used to refer to Aboriginal people of Australia, noting the unique cultural differences of Aboriginal and/or Torres Strait Islander peoples. The term 'Indigenous' is used to refer to all Aboriginal and Torres Strait Islander peoples of Australia. There is also the occasional use of the terms 'Aboriginal', 'Indigenous', 'Aboriginal and Torres Strait Islander peoples' and 'First Nation'.

The term 'mental health' has negative connotations among Aboriginal people, and therefore it is usually referred to as their 'social and emotional well-being'.

HISTORICAL AND CULTURAL DETERMINANTS

Cultural values and practices along with the importance placed on kinship relationships are discussed within the historical context of Aboriginal histories. These include understanding the value of the Dreamtime, the centrality of land and sea in Aboriginal culture, and the development of rituals to express Indigenous Australian understanding.

Dreamtime

The Dreamtime is linked to the creation process and spiritual ancestors. Ceremonies, song and storytelling described the **lore** that was passed down through the ages, initiated by the creation of ancestor spirits. Through these spirits, the sacred land and waterways were formed and the ancestor spirits were believed to have been passed on through the generations in the form of animals, birds or sea creatures, such as kangaroo, eagle or stingray. These became known as their totems, from which Aboriginal people interpret their identity. These sacred Dreamings, from a term used by W.E. Stanner (1965) are timeless and came to represent the many names for the traditional belief systems; they were interpreted and implemented by designated Elders of the community as lore. This moral lore encouraged Aboriginals to respect and be responsible for the care of the land and waterways. It was an understanding that brought balance and harmony to the multiple layers of Aboriginal relationships in communities on the continent for over 60 000 years (Hampton & Toombs, 2013; Langton & Perkins, 2008).

CULTURAL CONSIDERATIONS

Connections with the Dreamtime
Zubrick and colleagues (2014, p. 76) wrote concerning the social and emotional well-being experience of Australian Aboriginals that 'it recognises the importance of connection to land, culture, spirituality, ancestry, family and community, and how these affect the individual'. The foundation of all these connections stems back to the Dreamtime.

Place and Country

Aboriginals have lived as hunter-harvesters on the Australian continent for approximately 60 000 years. This land, now known as Australia, but previously referred to in Latin as 'terra nullius' – that is, 'a land belonging to no-one' by the British colonists – is a sacred space and has special significance for Aboriginal and Torres Strait Islander peoples. For Indigenous Australians, their identity is strongly associated with their kinship, to whom they are related and their **Country** of origin – described by Rose (1996) as a 'nourishing terrain' or **place** (Dudgeon et al., 2010).

Kinship relationship

Traditionally, the intricate kinship structures that framed how family structure, the system of clans and then the formation of Nations were critical in the construction of what became the complex web of relationships in Aboriginal communities (Bourke, Bourke & Edwards, 2009). All of life was influenced by it, including relations to Dreaming stories, ancestral spirits, land and sacred sites, and fauna and flora. Each person depended on the other to live in the harsh Australian environment (Broome, 2010). Ceremonies and other cultural practices brought cohesion. There were separate roles for men and women. Kinships governed who individuals could marry and other daily behaviour like whom food was shared with (Bourke & Edwards, 1998; Broome, 2010). For instance, traditional foods like kangaroo and dugong were hunted by the men for ceremonial feasts, the food would be divided up and given according to the kinship hierarchy. Each person had a kin term that was not restricted to their genealogy; for example, a person could have many mothers, aunties and sisters. Kinship maintained respect and governed how people behaved and were polite towards, as well as to whom they had obligations. It was not uncommon within this communal context that children were cared for by a number of women. Their role as women and mothers provided a complex yet intimate relationship that bound the clan. This was different to the Western understanding of 'family' that tends to be confined to genealogical connections. This kinship relationship had enabled the Aboriginal population to be fully functional and stable for over 60 000 years until colonisation occurred (Bourke, Bourke & Edwards, 2009; Bourke & Edwards, 1998; Broome, 2010).

Rituals

Rituals were necessary to fulfil according to the stage of life (Dudgeon & Walker, 2011). Men and women, and each age group in traditional times, had particular roles and responsibilities that allowed a community and Indigenous society per se to maintain its economic viability and cultural stability (Broome, 2010). Traditional knowledge of cultural practices was passed on through ceremony and storytelling to stress the importance of men's and women's business.

A person went through rites of initiation carried out by Elders and recognised by the whole community as they went through the various life stages to reach adulthood. Women's business included all aspects of reproduction: menstruation, pregnancy, childbirth, contraception, abortion and female ceremonial business. Men's business involved hunting, conflicts, the land, male anatomy and male ceremonial business (Maher, 1999). Elders were held in high esteem and shown great respect as the holders of knowledge transferred down through the generations from the Ancestors.

Historical context

There was estimated to be approximately 300 000 to 500 000 Aboriginals, comprising approximately 260 distinct language groups and 500 dialects at the time of British colonisation. At no time did these First Nations people relinquish their sovereign rights to the British. They had maintained their independence and determined their own rules, regulations and way of life. Community members knew who they were, and where they belonged prior to the tall ships of colonisation arriving (Martin, 2003, 2008; Wilson 2008). Pre-British colonisation, Indigenous Australians had been in contact with external nations. For instance, they had traded for two centuries with South-East Asian fishermen (Macassans) who came to collect sea cucumber (trepang) from the northern shores. They had a considerable effect on Aboriginal people in those regions, influencing their language, culture and ceremonies.

The Spanish explorer Luis Vaez de Torres travelled through the Torres Strait in 1606. This area of sea, now named after him, lies between the Coral and Arafura Seas. Located at the beginning of the Great Barrier Reef, the Torres Strait consists of approximately 100 islands that were a part of the now submerged Sahul Shelf land bridge that connected mainland Australia with Papua New Guinea. However, it was after contact with the British that circumstances dramatically changed for Aboriginals and Torres Strait Islanders.

The different periods of colonisation

Aboriginal lands were invaded in 1788, beginning at Sydney Cove and expanding out to the rest of the sacred Land. As its peoples were displaced from their Country, despite violently resisting, diseases spread and the people's economic resources were deliberately removed from their possession. Aboriginal culture, languages and sovereign rights were destroyed. There was no official recognition of Aboriginal rights to occupy their Land. The British Crown allocated property through sale or grants to the settlers, and pastoralists and squatters often resented the presence of Aboriginal communities, and dispersed them using guns and poison (Hampton & Toombs, 2013). The Aboriginal population in the first generation was reduced by 85%, of which 75% was attributed to diseases (Broome, 2010). Aboriginals were relegated to 'the lowest levels of culture, intelligence and capability' under the 'Great Chain of Being' argument (Langton & Perkins, 2008), which claimed everything in the universe had a place within a hierarchy of relationships, of which it was regarded during the Renaissance and Enlightenment periods that Aboriginals were the lowest form of life.

After the initial occupation in 1788, the government dealt with Aboriginals through a number of policy eras that extended over the years to the present. However, down through the decades there were a number of communities and leaders such as Pemulwuy who resisted the invasion. They sought to uphold Aboriginal autonomy and self-determination.

Protection era

These political epochs included the Protection era from 1788 to 1890 in which, after the initial occupation, when Aboriginals were excluded from their land deliberately and forcefully, the Protection Act was introduced to 'protect' Aboriginals from the influence of Europeans. It attempted to allow the 'full blood' Aboriginals to naturally 'die out' or, as the anthropologist Daisy Bates described, 'to smooth the pillow' of a dying race (Hampton & Toombs, 2013). Western Arrernte scholar John Williams-Mozley argued that by doing so there would be no claim to land ownership or compensation (Williams-Mozley, 2012). The Act further isolated Aboriginals from accessing the emerging new society.

Segregation

From the late 1890s to 1950, segregation was introduced under state, territory and Commonwealth laws, in order to exclude and control Aboriginals with mixed descent through the establishment of reserves and missions. This began the plight of the stolen generation. The Australian Constitution was passed by the British Parliament as part of the *Commonwealth of Australia Constitution Act 1900*, and it took effect on 1 January 1901 (Commonwealth of Australia, 2014). It deliberately excluded Indigenous peoples in s. 127, which stated: 'In reckoning the numbers of the people of the Commonwealth, or of a State or other part of the Commonwealth, aboriginal natives should not be counted' (National Archives of Australia, 1999), and implemented the White Australia policy so that, according to writer David Day (2005, p. 205), an Anglo Australian's future 'in these 'settled' colonies' would be secured against the rising European and Asian races. Hampton and Toombs (2013, p. 41) highlighted that:

> Colonial attitudes and practices continued under state governments beyond the Racial Discrimination Act of 1975 as some authorities exercised total power over the lives of Indigenous Australians. They controlled where individuals lived, their access to education, employment, wages and dictated relationships and marriage.

If Aboriginals wanted to escape from these regulations, they had to apply for an Exemption Certificate with the requirement that all ties with their families were severed (Australian Archives Victorian Branch, 1993; Hampton & Toombs, 2013). Section 127 was not revoked until the 1967 Referendum, which changed the Constitution to allow Aboriginal and Torres Strait Islander peoples to be counted as full Australian citizens.

Assimilation

From 1950 to the 1960s, under assimilation policy, there began the movement to ensure all Australian residents assumed the Anglo-Celtic lifestyle, as many white Australians feared the rise of 'immigrants and "mixed" parentage of Aboriginal and Torres Strait Islanders' (Hampton & Toombs, 2013). The separation of Aboriginal children from their families for placement in white families continued, resulting in the continual erosion of Aboriginal cultures (Hampton & Toombs, 2013). This period of assimilation failed, leading in the 1960s to 1980s to the period of integration in which residents were expected to adopt 'Anglo-Australian characteristics while retaining their cultural and social experiences' (Hampton & Toombs, 2013, p. 43). This began to further transform into multiculturalism. However, in the 1970s Aboriginal Australians began to become politically active (Hampton & Toombs, 2013).

Given the insult of British invasion and resulting colonisation on First Australian sovereignty, Aboriginal and Torres Strait Islanders became determined to develop their own decisions (self-determination) and manage their own affairs (self-management).

Aboriginal representation

Aboriginal representative bodies have been formed in order to first, unify First Australians because of their diversity and, second, to enable Aboriginal Australians to manage their own affairs.

Despite the establishment of the Aboriginal and Torres Strait Islander Commission (ATSIC) in 1989, which was intended to ensure maximum participation of Indigenous Australians in government policy and promote self-management, the opportunities for self-determination remained limited. The Council for Aboriginal Reconciliation (CAR) was formed in 1992 and was 'designed to overcome Indigenous disadvantage and promote economic independence' (Hampton & Toombs, 2013, p. 43). Although this appeared to be a positive move towards Aboriginal self-determination, the recommendations of the final report have largely been ignored. ATSIC was dissolved in 2005 by the Liberal–National Government under John Howard. This was followed in 2007 with an act of contemporary colonialism on Aboriginal communities with the implementation of the government's response to child sexual abuse allegations and the Northern Territory Intervention (Hampton & Toombs, 2013).

The organisation 'Recognise' is a branch of Reconciliation Australia that has developed a social movement. It seeks to address the exemption of Indigenous Australians from the Australian Constitution and end the racial discrimination that exists within it. It has obtained a groundswell of support from the public arena. This aligns with discussions on the necessity of a Treaty. This would be an agreement negotiated by Aboriginal and Torres Strait Islanders with the Australian Government to determine certain binding obligations that must be adhered to. However, to amend the Constitution, a referendum needs to be held according to Westminster law. This would enable the Australian population to vote for or against a Bill of Motion at the time of a federal election. Aboriginal community consultation will be required beforehand for Aboriginal and Torres Strait Islanders to gain relevant information and voice their views.

The cultural, physical, emotional, social and spiritual isolation and trauma of Aboriginal Australians from British invasion to the present have had a significant impact on each generation. Sherwood (2013) has argued that the effect of colonisation is a determinant of health.

SOCIAL DETERMINANTS

According to the World Health Organization (2010), the social determinants of health – that is, the country's health system and the conditions into which individuals are born and live – are often shaped by how resources, power and finances are distributed. These, plus the influence of government policies, are responsible for inequities in health, both within and between countries. Given the historical trauma as a result of colonisation, Indigenous Australians have displayed characteristics of poor health inequalities.

Data collected in the National Aboriginal and Torres Strait Islander Health Survey 2004–05 indicated that Indigenous Australians in comparison with other Australians suffer greater emotional distress and therefore possibly increased mental health conditions, with females affected more than males (Trewin, 2006). Aboriginal men, although they are less than 2% of the general population, have the highest incarceration rate, constituting 25–30% of the overall Australian prison population (Steering Committee for the Review of Government Service Provision, 2011). According to the Australian Bureau of Statistics (2012) Aboriginal people are 15 times more likely to be imprisoned than their non-Aboriginal counterparts. Research indicates that offenders are more likely to have mental health problems with high risk alcohol and drug misuse being a common connection between crime and well-being (AIHW, 2008; Heffernan, Andersen, Dev & Kinner, 2012).

There are many factors that indicate Indigenous Australians are experiencing health disadvantages. For example, it has been established that there is a relationship between higher levels of income and socioeconomic status (SES) and health and well-being.

Conversely, people who experience lower income and more socioeconomic disadvantage have the highest rates of illness and death (Lynch, 2000). Indigenous Australians in comparison with other Australians are disadvantaged due to a range of social determinants such as education, employment, income and housing, and are therefore at an even greater risk of poor health (Lynch, 2000; Marmot, 2011; Marmot & Wilkinson, 2001).

Between 2010 and 2012, the large gap of 9.5 years less life expectancy remained between Indigenous females and non-Indigenous females, and the 10.6 years gap for males has only narrowed by 0.8% since 2007 (AIHW, 2015). Social determinants such as unemployment, rather than behavioural risk factors such as smoking, were the larger factors in prolonging this health gap (AIHW, 2014). According to the Australian Institute of Health and Welfare 2014 report, only one-fifth of Indigenous Australians were estimated to be in 'good health' compared with two-fifths of non-Indigenous Australians. However, conversely, four-fifths of Indigenous Australians and three-fifths of non-Indigenous Australians were estimated to be in 'not good health' (AIHW, 2014). In this context, the terms 'good health' and 'not good health' were in accordance with a composite self-assessment measurement undertaken between the physical and psychological dimensions of Indigenous Australians by the Australian Institute of Health and Welfare and the Australian Bureau of Statistics.

Increased stressors and emotional distress have led to higher risk behaviours such as smoking, consumption of alcohol at hazardous levels, greater exposure to family violence, lack of physical activity and obesity (AIHW, 2015; Bowen & Muhajarine, 2006; Manber, Blasey & Allen, 2008). Accessibility to health services and support is also limited due to factors such as proximity, availability, lack of transportation, cultural inappropriateness of the health service, lack of health insurance and health services affordability (Peachey, 2003). These factors have led to a greater risk of mortality, which finally spurred the development of the 'Close the Gap' in life expectancy initiative by the federal government (COAG, 2008).

Closing the Gap?

In March 2008, the federal government, representatives of Aboriginal health peak policy bodies and the Aboriginal and Torres Strait Islander Justice Commissioner signed a Statement of Intent on behalf of the government and Aboriginal peoples, with the aim of collaboratively working towards achieving equality in health status and life expectancy between the Aboriginal and non-Aboriginal Australian population by the year 2030 (Calma, 2009).

However, to date, in the forefront of Australian health and well-being statistics is the issue of persistent Aboriginal disadvantage despite the funding generated for and policies surrounding the Closing the Gap initiative. Communication barriers occur due to poor literacy and numeracy levels coupled with a marked history of discrimination within the health system (AIHW, 2009, 2011).

Racism and discrimination

Government and mission practice at the turn of the nineteenth century was steeped in racism and discrimination (Bourke, Bourke & Edwards, 2009).

Paradies, Harris and Anderson (2008) highlight the influence of systemic racism on Aboriginal Australians, recording that this underpins racial inequalities in health. It is racism's most pervasive form, extending from education, employment to housing by impacting negatively on Aboriginal health and well-being. There are correlations between racism and compromised social and emotional well-being such as 'psychological distress, depression and anxiety' (p. 3). There are also associations with risk behaviours such as smoking, alcohol and substance misuse (Paradies, 2006). Even so, racism is difficult to measure in any study and is particularly challenging in regard to Indigenous health.

The impact of colonisation has damaged the knowledge and identity of Aboriginals within the dominant society. Unfortunately, a negative view has been held by many dominating individuals in workplaces and within some institutions. A damaged identity is evident when Aboriginals are prevented from occupying roles or entering identity-building relationships. Their identity is further damaged when they internalise a negative view that other people have of them (Atkinson, 2002).

Identity

Identity is the understanding that we have of ourselves and others. This can be damaged when controlling people or institutions perceive that those they focus on are morally abnormal and there is an attempt to prevent roles and relationships from being established that would otherwise enhance a person's identity (Nelson, 2001).

Identity has been a contentious issue among Aboriginals given the genocidal history of colonisation and the attempt to 'smooth out the dying pillow'. An outcome of this oppression is the internalisation of dismissive views of others on that person (Atkinson, 2002; Nelson, 2001).

Aboriginal identity is declared on the premise of belonging to a people group, a community and a historical connection to a place or Country, and is not necessarily dependent on inherited genetic characteristics (Dudgeon et al., 2010; Morrissey, 2003). Dudgeon and colleagues (2010, p. 34) argue that:

[T]here has been considerable debate about how Indigenous identity has been constructed and imposed, manipulated and used in the creation of assimilationist policies and other destructive practices such as the removal of so-called 'half-caste' children. Part of the decolonising is for Indigenous peoples to challenge previously held assumptions about them and work towards creating new constructions of identity.

The Australian Government has defined who will and will not be regarded as Aboriginal in well-publicised fliers displayed within most health institutions in an attempt to quantify identity in order to receive more government funding to better support Aboriginals. Therefore, in order to access government services like housing, for example, a certificate of Aboriginality is required in which a person will need to identify themselves as of Aboriginal and/or Torres Strait Islander descent or prove that they have been accepted and are involved within the Aboriginal community (Aboriginal Housing Victoria, 2015). This process is reminiscent of times past when a certificate of exemption from the non-Indigenous Administrator was required in order for Aboriginals to be permitted to access their kin. This was yet another control measure imposed upon Aboriginals by the government of the day, another 'blow' to Aboriginal identity and freedom. The dominant order that had the resources controlled the minority who have little.

Intergenerational ramifications

Although a stressor event may be infrequent, events can be of such magnitude that they can cause change even within the family social system (Pariante & Lightman, 2008; Wagner 1997). Glass (2010) defined stressors as situations or events that create acute or chronic stress. Stress is a process, not only a situation, to which a person is exposed (Malia, 2006). There are 'environmental circumstances or conditions that threaten, challenge, exceed or harm the psychological or biological capacities of the individual' (Grant et al., 2003). These consist of an interrelated web of physical, social, spiritual or psychological stress. How an individual copes with stress will depend on their level of well-being and ability to cope at that moment (Blonna, 2005). The continual traumatic events of colonisation had an intergenerational impact, none more so than the removal of Aboriginal children from their families.

The Social Health Reference Group (2004, p. 9) highlighted that 'social and emotional well-being problems cover a broad range of problems that can result from unresolved grief and loss, trauma and abuse, domestic violence, removal from family, substance misuse, family breakdown, cultural dislocation, racism and discrimination and social disadvantage'. Social exclusion can constrict an individual's well-being.

Expressions of shaming

The expression of 'shame' to Indigenous Australians is a complex concept. It can mean fear, embarrassment, respect, tact or shyness. Horton (1994) suggests that 'shame' and the behaviour of shaming are social control mechanisms. Self-hate, doubt and a lack of purpose had developed as morale plunged among Aboriginals who lived in poverty under the colonial regime (Broome, 2010). Author Richard Broome (2010) emphasised that on a daily basis Aboriginals had to make choices about where their identity lay under the assimilation policy. An Aboriginal person commented: 'We got shame. We don't know whether we're black or whether we're white' (Broome, 2010). Generations of Aboriginals experienced poverty and denigration with many believing the prejudicial comments made by the dominant power that it was their fault. Some 'chose to imitate middle-class white Australians materially and culturally in order to escape poverty and the daily stigma of the caste barrier, thus creating division with the community' (Broome, 2010). Aboriginals were stigmatised as having no skills or independent thought (Hampton & Toombs, 2013). Legally, children of an Aboriginal mother were pronounced as 'neglected' from the time of birth (Hampton & Toombs, 2013). This led to the separation of families as children were removed, and these children became known as the stolen generation (Hampton & Toombs, 2013).

Stigma

The **stigma** of being diagnosed with a social and emotional illness can cause much anxiety for an Indigenous person, because of the fear of being judged and perhaps later held as a form of retribution by other community members.

Stigma can be defined as a negative attribute that links someone to characteristics that are perceived as undesirable in a society (Crocker et al., 1998). Furthermore, these negative attributes are understood as being of a discriminatory nature (Link & Phelan, 2001). There is no recognition of the individual and their needs. Moreover, it constricts the individual's sense of freedom to express themselves, and restricts their agency, while living within the expectations of others within society (Benson, 1994).

INDIGENOUS AUSTRALIANS' SOCIAL AND EMOTIONAL WELL-BEING

In Australia, wealthy and developed by world standards, the health status of Indigenous Australians since colonisation remains akin to that found in poor 'developing' countries. Despite successive government policies and initiatives purporting to address this gap, the gap remains.

The National Aboriginal and Torres Strait Islander Health Survey 2004–05 emphasised that if not addressed, serious psychological distress will lead to poor social and emotional well-being (SHRG, 2004). There will be increased rates of unhealthy behaviour and chronic illness and disability, and increased rates of suicide. The reason for this is that the determinants that impact Aboriginal and Torres Strait Islander lives, which include grief and loss, remain unresolved. Trauma and abusive situations such as family violence; the misuse of alcohol and other substances; physical health conditions and issues of identity; family breakdown; removal of children; incarceration; social disadvantage and cultural dislocation that are often due to racism and discrimination – all compromise the social and emotional well-being of Indigenous Australians (SHRG, 2004).

The stolen generation

Globally, child removal by government authorities affected many Indigenous women's perception of their identity and what was expected of them as mothers and as women (Fortin, 2005). Among community members it is possible, given the known statistics of higher numbers of Aboriginal child substantiations (i.e. the stage of reporting to an authority where a child is indicated to be at risk of neglect), that there remains a constant fear among women that their own family is at risk of being reported for negligence to the authorities (AIHW, 2015; DEECD, 2008). Therefore, families may remain committed to just their relatives and not towards others who are outside of their extended family.

In 1995, the federal Attorney-General established the national inquiry into the forcible removal of Aboriginal and Torres Strait Islander children from their families. Its report was published in 1997 and was known as the 'Bringing Them Home' report. This 680-page document consisted of stories that illustrated the gross violation of human rights of Indigenous communities and families, the traumatic intergenerational effect of which is still evident today. The 'Bringing Them Home' report in Australia illustrated that many Aboriginal women who had been 'stolen' were tenuous about motherhood (Dodson & Wilson, 1997). They did not understand what caring mothering practices were because as children they were often cited in records as having been taken from their Aboriginal mother who was deemed 'neglectful' (Dodson & Wilson, 1997). This description was a politically convenient excuse to remove children, who might well have ended up neglected because of the forced removal from their mothers. Child removal was a subtle way of 'smoothing the pillow [of the dying]'; that is, to rid the dominant society in the colonial era of Aboriginal peoples and their cultures

(Hampton & Toombs, 2013). See also the discussion of the protectionist era earlier in the chapter.

Contemporary child substantiation data

In the 2011 'Overcoming Indigenous Disadvantage' report, the rate of Aboriginal children from the ages of 0–16 years of age who had been notified to the authorities and substantiated as having been abused, neglected and harmed in their homes was seven times more than that of non-Aboriginal children in 2009–10 (Steering Committee for the Review of Government Service Provision, 2011). This was an outcome perpetuated through the generations of removing children from their families.

Long and Sephton (2011) argue that even today the ethnocentric view held among non-Aboriginal welfare workers on what they deem as in the 'best interests' of the child may be in stark contrast to the perception held by Aboriginal families. What is neglected is the context of Aboriginal self-determination, where Aboriginals are empowered to make their own decisions about their needs and the course of action that is required rather than being told what to do by non-Aboriginals (Long & Sephton, 2011; Victorian Aboriginal Child Care Agency, 2006).

CASE STUDY

FEAR OF CHILD PROTECTION SERVICES INTERVENTION

A mother recalled how when she recognised that she was depressed after having her baby, she decided to go to the local general practice to receive support and treatment. She said, 'I went to the doctor's and told her I had all these weird thoughts and she wanted to ring child protection straight away. That's when I got angry and walked out.' The doctor did not listen to the woman's entire story but assumed that because she was Aboriginal she was not coping and could not attend to her child's needs. The doctor instinctively decided to ring Child Protection Services.

Questions

1 What historical factors about Aboriginal people should have been considered before any adverse action was taken?
2 What culturally safe and appropriate actions should the doctor have taken?

Multiple stressors

Multiple stressors can also be attributed to transgenerational trauma. Indigenous Australians are deemed as being at a higher risk of acceleration in developing trauma given the detrimental effects of colonial history in Australia over 200 years (Atkinson, 2002; Swan & Raphael, 1995). This negatively affects individual Aboriginals and their family structure, and is exhibited in increased learning difficulties and negative behaviour patterns, decreased coping mechanisms and family dysfunction. Atkinson's traumagram – a measure that determines the amount of often 'compounded' trauma a person has endured in order to follow up on what is required for that person to recover – reported a six-generation account of the effects of violence on subsequent generations (Atkinson, 2002).

CASE STUDY

LIVING WITH MULTIPLE STRESSORS

This mother explained the stress she had to manoeuvre with her family. She recalled, 'The living situations we were in, was stressful, my partner was sleeping in the lounge room with our oldest child. I was in a room with the babies with no space or anything. He didn't have a job, I didn't have a job. Other people were living in the house.'

Questions

1 What historical and cultural issues needed to be considered here?
2 What support could you offer as a health practitioner?

Child removal and the disbanding of Indigenous families also took place among other nations such as Canada (Battiste, 2002). The dominant society in that country refused to acknowledge the devastating effects of colonialism.

Western notions of community are different from Aboriginal notions of community, in that to be a member of the community a person must be Aboriginal, identify accordingly and be known by that group so as to take on the various obligations and commitments of a member (Dudgeon et al., 2010). Aboriginal traditional culture can be claimed by some, while others such as Aboriginals residing in urban areas have either lost or had modified their traditional culture due to colonialism. Even so, they have not forgone their sense of who they are as Aboriginals; that is, their 'sense of Aboriginality' (Bourke, Bourke & Edwards, 2009). Instead, 'there are shared experiences, sharing the same relatives, stories, background, history, oppression, discrimination and a host of other factors' (Bourke, Bourke & Edwards, 2009, p. 118).

The transgenerational effect of trauma remains a source of psychological distress given the impact of colonialism on Indigenous Australians (Atkinson, Nelson & Atkinson, 2010).

The impact of colonisation upon First Australians' mental health

The government policies and practices that inflicted layer upon layer of grief and loss from first contact are not conducive to happiness, and neither are they overcome within a generation (Doyle, 2011). Aboriginal Australians, like other postcolonial peoples (i.e. Aboriginal Canadians, Indigenous North Americans and New Zealand Māori), share common experiences of colonisation that resulted in loss of cultural and community identity, marginalisation, prejudice and discrimination within their developed nation (National Aboriginal Health Strategy Working Party, 1989). However, Australian Aboriginals lag behind Canadian First Nations and Māori in most health statistics including life expectancy, mortality and burden of disease, chronic diseases and mental health indices (Stephens et al., 2005).

Depression

Over the past 30 years, depression has emerged as a major health concern. A survey conducted among Aboriginals in a community-controlled health organisation reported that just over half of the people who were tested with standard psychiatric rating scales were suffering from a psychiatric illness and that depression was the most common (McKendrick, Cutter, Mackenzie & Chiu, 1992). Depression was ranked as the fourth leading cause of disease burden globally and represents the single largest contributor to non-fatal burden (Üstün et al., 2004). Depressive disorders are a health priority, ranked as the leading cause of burden in the Global Burden of Disease 2010 study (Ferrari et al., 2013).

Death in custody

The Royal Commission into Aboriginal Deaths in Custody (Royal Commission & Muirhead, 1988) reported the growing problems of suicide among Aboriginals in custody. A large number of these deaths highlighted a history of having been forcibly separated from their families as children. Aboriginal Australians are also overrepresented in deaths in custody that are not related to suicide. Such deaths include those resulting from incidents occurring whilst in custody (e.g., becoming physically unwell but not receiving prompt treatment), or deaths related to the process of being detained (e.g., being shot, or dying whilst being physically restrained). As described by Silburn and colleagues (2010, p. 95), the 'interconnected issues of cultural dislocation, personal trauma and the ongoing stresses of disadvantage, racism, alienation and exclusion were all acknowledged by the Commission as contributing to the heightened risk of mental health problems, substance misuse and suicide'. There is a link between those Aboriginal men who have been incarcerated for violent offending and the experiences they had of childhood or adolescent trauma and violence (Zubrick et al., 2014).

Psychological distress in women

According to the Australian Bureau of Statistics (2012), Indigenous women are twice as likely to report high or very high levels of psychological distress in comparison to non-Indigenous women (Trewin, 2006). Community members still fear their children will be taken from their families, especially in medical settings, as this had been families' experiences since colonisation (Silburn et al., 2006). The stigma of 'cleanliness' may be an overflow from the distorted view of the colonisers, where the importance of cleanliness was stipulated to Indigenous Elders in their role of housekeepers in the 'white-fellas' homes in which they were employed.

However, statistics are a stark reminder of those stressors that continue to impact Aboriginal women. In a five-year period between 2006–10 Aboriginal babies died at twice the rate compared with non-Aboriginal babies from particular conditions that only arise in the perinatal period. These included birth trauma, foetal growth disorders, complications due to pregnancy, labour and delivery, and sudden infant death syndrome (SIDS) (HealthInfoNet, 2015).

The impact of trauma and stress on First Australian families

Reynolds (2000) emphasised that history and circumstances affect health and that over the past 220 years Indigenous Australians have suffered accumulating and persisting trauma. These effects are further exacerbated by exposure to continuing high levels of stress and trauma, including multiple bereavements and other losses (Milroy, 2008). The long-lasting effect of trauma to Aboriginal women, their families and community cannot be underestimated (Zubrick et al., 2014) as this is their lived experience. Moreton-Robinson (1998, p. 278) notes that for 'Aboriginal women, survival demands expertise in cultural translation and self-presentation within the dominant culture'.

In recent years, family resilience models have been pursued among Indigenous peoples in order to demonstrate the unique ways families respond positively by demonstrating characteristics of flexibility and the ability to 'bounce back' (McCubbin & McCubbin, 2005). These First Nations researchers previously identified family resilience as 'characteristics, dimensions, and properties of families which help them to be resistant to disruption in the face of change and adaptive in the face of crisis situations' (McCubbin & McCubbin, 1988, p. 247).

Recently, there has been significant research into predictors of resilience; that is, those circumstances that may give rise to resilience. This is believed to be determined by external factors like parenting styles and internal factors like biological and psychological factors, which determine the level of resilience (Zakeri, Jowkar & Razmjoee, 2010).

Protective factors

Protective factors that have been identified as easing the effectiveness of risks to the health and well-being of Aboriginal Australians have been the connection to Land, culture, ancestors and spirituality (Kelly, Dudgeon, Gee & Glaskin, 2009). For a community to function effectively, good leadership and community governance are important. The interdependent nature of family, kinship and community connectedness appears to offer some protection within many Aboriginal and Torres Strait Islander communities. Maintaining cultural beliefs and traditional practices encourages communities, especially among young people who need to maintain their sense of personal continuity and cultural identity in the face of development and cultural change within society (Zubrick et al., 2010). Interventions need to focus on reducing risk factors, including systematic discrimination, and increasing protective factors.

Given the historical trauma of the past, its intergenerational effect and the social determinants borne daily, health providers would do well to provide culturally appropriate service, and work with Aboriginal communities to ensure that Aboriginals feel safe, thus enabling trust to be developed.

CULTURALLY SAFE PRACTICE: RACIAL ISSUES

Often health workers in mental health services hold values and assumptions that reflect the norms of Western culture in the dominant majority of Australian society, such as cultural (colour) blindness, as well as racism. There is an inability to understand and appreciate the pervasive transgenerational impact of colonisation on Aboriginal and Torres Strait Islander communities, family and individuals.

CLINICAL OBSERVATIONS

Cultural inappropriateness
An Aboriginal mother remembered her treatment in hospital. She recalled, 'A nurse come in and she said, "Oh, you know if you get oil you can massage her nose straight". I said, "She's black!, so she's going to have a flat nose, plus all babies are born with flat noses".'

Racial issues are uncomfortable to discuss and full of challenges and controversy. Two issues, 'whiteness' and colour blindness, are discussed here.

'Whiteness' and colour blindness

In Australia, *whiteness* pertains to those characteristics that are attached to people with white skin and the white race. It marks those who are of Anglo and European descent. They may possess a variety of privileges and feel that they are 'normal' and 'belong'. They are often oblivious to this racially laden perspective. In comparison, they may regard those who are racially different to them as 'other', as people of 'colour' who are different, foreign, unusual and even exotic. The 'other', however, is usually dominated by the white race and is marginalised and oppressed. For example, British colonists (white and pure race) described Aboriginals (other) as 'savage, backward and stupid', while in contrast they saw themselves as civilised, intelligent and rational. 'Whiteness' is a loaded term that has political, social, economic and cultural connotations (Moreton-Robinson, 2004; Walter, Taylor, & Habibis 2011; Ziersch, Gallaher, Baum & Bentley, 2011). Contemporary research indicates that racism experienced by Aboriginals continues. Discrimination and racist attitudes that translate into behaviour, although seemingly less overt and more tolerable than they once were from the perpetrator's perspective, are still the experiences of everyday life for Aboriginals. Racism remains complex and painful for First Australians (Mellor, 2003).

Colour blindness is a sociological term, and is the racial ideology that treats each person as equal, disregarding their ethnic background, culture and race. However, this perspective of 'whiteness' refuses to celebrate the other's experiences, traditions and uniqueness. Colour blindness assumes that everyone has the same experience, but this ignores the historical causes of racial inequality as well as its existence today. There are those who dominate and subjugate others into becoming 'voiceless' and without **agency**. It then becomes uncomfortable to discuss the challenges of disadvantage, inequality and injustice (Walter, Taylor & Habibis, 2011).

Aboriginal workforce and Aboriginal community-controlled health services

The Aboriginal health workforce has become central to Aboriginal communities because of their ability to provide culturally appropriate health care to their people and therefore improve health (Adams & Spratling, 2001). They are vital components in 'Closing the Gap' of Indigenous disadvantage by providing user-friendly services that are accessible to Aboriginal community members (Fredericks,

CASE **STUDY**

THE IMPORTANCE OF THE MENTAL HEALTH ASSESSMENT

One Aboriginal mother recalled, 'If it wasn't for…the survey [the Edinburgh Postnatal Depression Scale Screening] that you have to do, I probably would not have even known I had it [postnatal depression]. It affects you more than you think it does. If I didn't have the support of family, friends and organisations, I was on my own doin' it. I was suicidal. It would've gone further if I didn't have the support of family. It's serious you know, it's not something you can just shrug away or forget about or try and deal with it yourself. You need to deal with it. You need help.'

Questions

1 What are the signs and symptoms of postnatal depression?

2 What is the Edinburgh Postnatal Depression Scale? When is this tool administered, and by whom?

3 What categories does the Edinburgh Postnatal Depression Scale cover?

4 How could it be adapted in order to be a culturally appropriate tool for First Australian families?

2008). Training this workforce in order to identify and implement culturally appropriate strategies is important (Adams & Spratling, 2001).

Culturally appropriate care and management

Health organisations that are under Indigenous control are perceived by the Indigenous community as places of identity where Aboriginal people are represented and defined among 'white' society. The capacity of Indigenous staff in these Aboriginal-specific organisations to spend adequate time with Aboriginal people so they can manage their issues themselves is a priority. This is carried out through 'yarning' and deep listening within a culturally appropriate and safe place.

Partnerships with communities through Aboriginal community-controlled organisations can lead to the development of health promotion resources by community that are culturally appropriate and specific to those communities. Existing services and approaches to improving the health and well-being of Aboriginal and Torres Strait Islander peoples have not been successful (AHMAC, 2004). It is important that health professionals consider the historical, cultural and environmental experiences and contemporary circumstances of Aboriginal and Torres Strait Islander peoples. The Australian Health Ministries' Advisory Council (2004) has developed the *National Cultural Respect Framework for Aboriginal and Torres Strait Islander Health 2004–09*, which sets out principles and examples of practices to guide health professionals when working with Aboriginal and Torres Strait Islanders.

Health professionals should recognise the limitations of access to care as a means of improving health. Warelow and Edward (2007) have suggested in their research that when a health professional, particularly in the mental health arena, develops their own sense of self and empowerment, then a caring ability involving empathy and support develops, which flows on to resilience. These workers are then better able to lead clients in a positive direction to develop their own sense of self and pursue their own personal goals. This is particularly important in the Indigenous health sector, where historically Aboriginal and Torres Strait Islander peoples have not been allowed control over the decisions that affect their health and lives.

REFLECTION ON LEARNING FROM PRACTICE

Aboriginal health workers, like Michael, are valued members of any health team because they bring a cultural perspective that enables the non-Aboriginal health staff to understand the 'other's' perspective. If the staff had acquired education on Aboriginal and Torres Strait Islander history and culture they would not have been fearful. They had made a number of false assumptions about the visitor, such as presuming the Aboriginal man was very intoxicated and had deliberately 'barged' his way into the ward. By understanding the negative impact colonisation has had on Aboriginal people's lives, they could have understood the fear Aboriginals have in approaching hospitals and the reason why the man drank alcohol before he had the courage to come in. They should have made a friendly approach to the man and inquired as to who he was visiting and escorted him to see his wife. By doing so in a friendly manner, they could have had an opportunity to explain the 'visiting hours' protocol for the ward, as the Aboriginal man would have listened carefully because he felt welcomed.

CHAPTER RESOURCES

SUMMARY

- In order to provide culturally safe care to Aboriginal and Torres Strait Islander peoples, it is essential to understand their historic and continuing context. This chapter introduced Indigenous Australians' historical issues and cultural perspectives.
- Colonisation has had a lasting impact on the social determinants that influence the health and well-being of Aboriginal and Torres Strait Islanders and their communities in contemporary times.

- The impact of colonisation on social determinants of health continue to impact upon the health and well-being of Aboriginal and Torres Strait Islander peoples. These include education, employment, income and housing, increased stressors and trauma resulting from colonisation.
- Reflective practice is essential in order for practitioners to provide culturally safe practice that is appropriate to the Aboriginal Australian consumer.

REVIEW QUESTIONS

1 The Dreamtime is a period when Aboriginals believe:
   a Spiritual ancestors roamed the Earth
   b British settlers introduced their stories
   c The creation process occurred and the land and waterways were formed
   d Was the time when native animals and the ancestors roamed the land in harmony.
2 What was the protection era of colonisation?
   a 1788, when the British tall ships landed at Sydney Cove
   b When Aboriginals were 'protected' under the Protection Acts from European influence
   c A period from 1850 to 1950 when Aboriginal and Torres Strait Islanders were allowed to control their lives
   d The time when Indigenous Australians were permitted to vote.
3 The social determinants of health are:
   a The conditions into which individuals are born and live accordingly
   b Not influenced by government policies

   c The Australian health system
   d The manner in which an Indigenous person interacts with other tribes.
4 Indigenous Australians' social and emotional well-being have been impacted by:
   a The colonisation period
   b Child removal policies
   c The Close the Gap strategy
   d All of the above.
5 Protective factors that influence First Australians' self-esteem are:
   a Having predominantly non-Indigenous staff to attend to Indigenous needs
   b Culturally safe practice
   c Culturally sensitive language when communicating
   d The government's development of Indigenous programs.

CRITICAL THINKING

1 Explain the relationship between racism and stereotyping in the context of Aboriginal Australia.
2 Why is it important to understand the significance of past history on Aboriginal and Torres Strait Islanders today?
3 What are some protective factors that enable Aboriginal Australians to survive and thrive in society today?

4 How does understanding the social determinants of health give the practitioner insight into the health and well-being of Aboriginal and Torres Strait Islanders?
5 What is meant by 'appropriating culturally safe practice' for an Aboriginal patient?

USEFUL WEBSITES

- ABC News: 'Ten Myer staff called on teenage boy who was shopping for school ball': https://apple.news/A8IpwkEsIRTKNbuVMcmVGXg
- 'First Australians: They Have Come to Stay. Sydney and NSW (1788–1824).' Episode 1 of 7: https://www.sbs.com.au/nitv/video/11721283804/First-Australians-S1-Ep1-They-Have-Come-To-Stay

- National Aboriginal Community Controlled Health Organisation: https://www.naccho.org.au

REFLECT ON THIS

Indigenous cultural awareness and competence

Ensuring the healthcare workforce has appropriate Indigenous cultural awareness and competence is an important responsibility of every service. As health professionals, it is our responsibility to ensure we practise in a culturally competent and sensitive manner, and this is also mandated by the regulatory bodies (e.g. AHPRA).

As a student in your health discipline:

1   What is your role in ensuring you practise in a culturally safe manner?
2   What steps will you take to ensure that you are informed and sensitive to the cultural needs of Aboriginal and Torres Strait Islander people when you begin working as a registered health professional?

REFERENCES

Aboriginal Housing Victoria. (2015). Application for housing form. Retrieved from http://www.ahvic.org.au/cms_uploads/docs/ahv-housing-application-form.pdf.

Adams, K. & Spratling, M. (2001). Keepin ya mob healthy: Aboriginal community participation and Aboriginal health worker training in Victoria. *Australian Journal of Primary Health*, 7(1), 116–19.

Atkinson, J. (2002). *Trauma Trails, Recreating Song Lines: The Transgenerational Effects of Trauma in Indigenous Australia.* Geelong: Spinifex Press.

Atkinson, J., Nelson, J. & Atkinson, C. (2010). Trauma, transgenerational transfer and effects on community wellbeing. In N. Purdie, P. Dudgeon & R. Walker (eds), *Working Together: Aboriginal and Torres Strait Islander and Mental Health and Wellbeing Principles and Practice* (pp. 135–44). Canberra: Australian Government, Department of Health and Ageing.

Australian Archives Victorian Branch. (1993). *My Heart Is Breaking: A Joint Guide to Records about Aboriginal people in the Public Record Office of Victoria and the Australian Archives, Victorian Regional Office.* Melbourne: Australian Archives Victorian Branch.

Australian Bureau of Statistics (ABS). (2012). *Prisoners in Australia 2012.* Canberra: ABS.

Australian Health Ministers' Advisory Council (AHMAC). Standing Committee for Aboriginal and Torres Strait Islander Health Working Party (2004). *Cultural Respect Framework for Aboriginal and Torres Strait Islander Health, 2004–2009.* Adelaide: Department of Health, South Australia. Retrieved from http://iaha.com.au/wp-content/uploads/2013/03/000211_culturalrespectframework.pdf.

Australian Institute of Health and Welfare (AIHW). (2008). *Australia's Health.* Canberra: AIHW. Retrieved from http://www.aihw.gov.au/WorkArea/DownloadAsset.aspx?id=6442453685.

Australian Institute of Health and Welfare (AIHW). (2009). *Aboriginal and Torres Strait Islander Health Performance Framework 2008.* Canberra: AIHW.

Australian Institute of Health and Welfare (AIHW). (2011). *The Health and Welfare of Australia's Aboriginal and Torres Strait Islander People 2011: An Overview.* Canberra: AIHW.

Australian Institute of Health and Welfare (AIHW). (2014). *Australia's Health 2014.* Canberra: AIHW.

Australian Institute of Health and Welfare (AIHW). (2015). *The Health and Welfare of Australia's Aboriginal and Torres Strait Islander Peoples: 2015.* Canberra: AIHW.

Battiste, M. (2002). *Indigenous Knowledge and Pedagogy in First Nations Education: A Literature Review with Recommendations.* Ottawa: Indian and Northern Affairs Canada.

Benson, P. (1994). Free agency and self-worth. *Journal of Philosophy*, (91)12, 650–68.

Blonna, R. (2005). *Coping with Stress in a Changing World.* New York: McGraw Hill.

Bourke, C., Bourke, E. & Edwards, B. (2009). *Aboriginal Australia: An Introductory Reader in Aboriginal Studies* (2nd edn). Adelaide: University of Queensland Press.

Bourke, C. & Edwards, B. (1998). Family and kinship. In C. Bourke, E. Bourke & B. Edwards (eds), *Aboriginal Australia: An Introductory Reader in Aboriginal Studies* (pp. 100–21). Brisbane: University of Queensland Press.

Bowen, A. & Muhajarine, N. (2006). Prevalence of antenatal depression in women enrolled in an outreach program in Canada. *Journal of Obstetric, Gynecologic, & Neonatal Nursing*, 35(4), 491–8.

Broome, R. (2010). *Aboriginal Australians. A History since 1788.* Melbourne: Allen & Unwin.

Calma, T. (2009). *Social Justice Report 2008: Aboriginal and Torres Strait Islander Social Justice Commissioner.* Sydney: Human Rights and Equal Opportunity Commission, pp. 62–76.

Commonwealth of Australia. (2014). *Fact Sheet: The Australian Constitution.* Canberra: Parliamentary Education Office.

Council of Australian Governments (COAG). (2008). *National Health Care Agreement: Intergovernmental Agreement on Federal Financial Relations.* Canberra: COAG.

Crocker, J. & Major, B.C. (1998). Social stigma. In D.T. Gilbert, S.T. Fiske & G. Lindzey (eds), *Handbook of Social Psychology* (vol. 2) (pp. 504–53). Boston, MA: McGraw-Hill.

Day, D. (2005). *Claiming a Continent.* Sydney: HarperCollins.

Department of Education and Early Childhood Development (DEECD). (2008). *Dardee Boorai: Victorian Charter of Safety and Wellbeing for Aboriginal Children and Young People.* Melbourne: DEECD, Statewide Outcomes for Children Division.

Dodson, M. & Wilson, R. (1997). *Bringing Them Home: Report of the National Inquiry into the Separation of Aboriginal and Torres Strait Islander Children from Their Families.* Human Rights and Equal Opportunity Commission. Canberra: Sterling Press.

Doyle, K. (2011). Modes of colonisation and patterns of contemporary mental health: Towards an understanding of Canadian Aboriginal, Australian Aboriginal and Maori peoples. *Aboriginal and Islander Health Worker Journal*, 31(1), 20–3.

Dudgeon, P. & Walker, R. (2011). The health, social and emotional wellbeing of Aboriginal women. In R. Thackrah, K. Scott & J. Winch (eds), *Indigenous Australian Health and Cultures: An Introduction for Health Professionals* (pp. 96–126). Sydney, Pearson Education.

Dudgeon, P., Wright, M., Paradies, Y., Garvey, D. & Walker, I. (2010). The social, cultural and historical context of Aboriginal and Torres Strait Islander Australians. In N. Purdie, P. Dudgeon & R. Walker (eds), *Working Together: Aboriginal and Torres Strait Islander and Mental*

Health and Wellbeing Principles and Practice (pp. 25–42). Canberra: Australian Government, Department of Health and Ageing.

Federal Register of Legislation. (2019). https://www.legislation.gov. au/Details/C2013Q00005/Html/Text. © Commonwealth of Australia. Commonwealth of Australia Constitution Act (The Constitution). For the latest information on Australian Government law please go to https://www.legislation.gov.au. Released under CC BY 4.0. Link to license: https://creativecommons.org/licenses/by/4.0/.

Ferrari, A.J., Charlson, F.J., Norman, R.E., Patten, S.B., Freedman, G., Murray, C.J.L., Vos, T. & Whiteford, H.A. (2013). Burden of depressive disorders by country, sex, age, and year: Findings from the Global Burden of Disease Study 2010. *PLoS Med*, 10(11), e1001547.

Fortin, N.M. (2005). Gender role attitudes and the labour-market outcomes of women across OECD countries. *Oxford Review of Economic Policy*, 21(3), 416–38.

Fredericks, B.L. (2008). Engaging with Aboriginal and Torres Strait Islander people. *Australian Institute of Health Policy Studies (AIHPS) National Citizen Engagement Forum*. Brisbane.

Glass, N. (2010). *Interpersonal Relating: Health Care Perspectives on Communication, Stress and Crisis*. Malaysia: Palgrave Macmillan.

Grant, K., Compas, B.E., Stuhlmacher, A.F., Thurm, A.E., McMahon, S.D. & Halpert, J.A. (2003). Stressors and child and adolescent psychopathology: Moving from markers to mechanisms of risk. *Psychological Bulletin*, 129(3), 447–66. © American Psychological Association.

Hampton, R. & Toombs, M. (2013). *Indigenous Australians and Health*. Melbourne: Oxford University Press.

HealthInfoNet (2015). Overview of Australian Indigenous health status, 2014. Retrieved from https://healthinfonet.ecu.edu.au/learn/health-facts/overview-aboriginal-torres-strait-islander-health-status.

Heffernan, E., Andersen, K., Dev, A. & Kinner, S. (2012). Prevalence of mental illness among Aboriginal and Torres Strait Islander people in Queensland prisons. *Medical Journal of Australia*, 197, 37–41. doi:10,5694/mja11.11352

Horton, D. (1994). *The Encyclopaedia of Aboriginal Australia*. Canberra: Aboriginal Press.

Kelly, K., Dudgeon, P., Gee, G. & Glaskin, B. (2009). *Living on the Edge: Social and Emotional Wellbeing and Risk and Protective Factors for Serious Psychological Distress among Aboriginal and Torres Strait Islander People. Discussion Paper Series: No. 10*. Darwin: Cooperative Research Centre for Aboriginal Health.

Langton, M. & Perkins, R. (2008). *The First Australians: An Illustrated History*. Melbourne: Melbourne University Press.

Link, B.G. & Phelan, J.C. (2001). Conceptualizing stigma. *Annual Review of Sociology*, 27(1), 363–85.

Long, M. & Sephton, R. (2011). Rethinking the 'best interests' of the child: Voices from Aboriginal child and family welfare practitioners [Abstract]. *Australian Social Work*, 64(1), 96–112.

Lynch, J.W. (2000). Income inequality and mortality: Importance to health of individual income, psychosocial environment, or material conditions. *British Medical Journal*, 320(7243), 1200–4.

Maher, P. (1999). A review of 'traditional' Aboriginal health beliefs. *Australian Journal of Rural Health*, 7(4), 229–36.

Malia, J.A. (2006). Basic concepts and models of family stress. *Stress, Trauma, and Crisis*, 9(3–4), 141–60.

Manber, R., Blasey, C. & Allen, J.J. (2008). Depression symptoms during pregnancy. *Archives of Women's Mental Health*, 11(1), 43–8.

Marmot, M. (2011). Social determinants and the health of Indigenous Australians. *Aboriginal and Islander Health Worker Journal*, 35(3), 21–2.

Marmot, M. & Wilkinson, R. (2001). Psychosocial and material pathways in the relation between income and health: A response to Lynch et al. *BMJ: British Medical Journal*, 322(7296), 1233.

Martin, K. (2003). Ways of knowing, being and doing: A theoretical framework and methods for Indigenous re-search and Indigenist research. *Journal of Australian Studies*, 27(76), 203–14.

Martin, K. (2008). *Please Knock Before You Enter: Aboriginal Regulation of Outsiders and the Implications for Researchers*. Brisbane: Post Pressed.

McCubbin, H.I. & McCubbin, M.A. (1988). Typologies of resilient families: Emerging roles of social class and ethnicity. *Family Relations*, 37(3), National Council on Family Relations. 247–54.

McCubbin, L.D. & McCubbin, H.I. (2005). Culture and ethnic identity in family resilience: Dynamic processes in trauma and transformation of indigenous people. In M. Ungar (ed.), *Handbook for Working with Children and Youth* (pp. 27–44). Sage Online.

McKendrick, J., Cutter, T., Mackenzie, A. & Chiu, E. (1992). The pattern of psychiatric morbidity in a Victorian urban Aboriginal general practice population. *Australian and New Zealand Journal of Psychiatry*, 26(1), 40–7. doi:10.3109/00048679209068308

Mellor, D. (2003). Contemporary racism in Australia: The experiences of Aborigines. *Personality and Social Psychology Bulletin*, 29(4), 474–86.

Milroy, H. (2008). *Children Are Our Future: Understanding the Needs of Aboriginal Children and Their Families*. Brisbane: Australian Academic Press.

Moreton-Robinson, A. (1998). When the object speaks: A postcolonial encounter: Anthropological representations and Aboriginal women's self-presentations. *Discourse: Studies in the Cultural Politics of Education*, 19(3), Taylor & Francis. 275–89.

Moreton-Robinson, A. (2004). *Whitening Race: Essays in Social and Cultural Criticism*. Canberra: Aboriginal Studies Press, AIATSI.

Morrissey, P. (2003). Aboriginality and corporatism. In M. Grossman (ed.), *Black lines: Contemporary Critical Writing by Indigenous Australians* (pp. 52–9). Melbourne: Melbourne University Press.

National Aboriginal Health Strategy Working Party. (1989). *A National Aboriginal Health Strategy*. Canberra: AGPS, pp. 207–17.

National Archives of Australia. (1999). Fact sheet 150 – the 1967 Referendum. Your story, our history. Retrieved from http://www.naa.gov.au/collection/fact-sheets/fs150.aspx.

Nelson, H.L. (2001). *Damaged Identities, Narrative Repair*. Ithaca, NY: Cornell University Press.

Paradies, Y. (2006). A systematic review of empirical research on self-reported racism and health. *International Journal of Epidemiology*, 35(4), 888–901.

Paradies, Y., Harris, R. & Anderson, I. (2008). *The Impact of Racism on Indigenous Health in Australia and Aotearoa: Towards a Research Agenda. Discussion Paper Series: No. 4*. Darwin: Cooperative Research Centre for Aboriginal Health.

Pariante, C.M. & Lightman, S.L. (2008). The HPA axis in major depression: Classical theories and new developments. *Trends in Neurosciences*, 31(9), 464–8.

Peachey, L.G. (2003). Indigenous health: It's time for a change. *Medical Journal of Australia*, 178(10), 503–4.

Purdie, N., Dudgeon, P. & Walker, R. (2010). *Working Together: Aboriginal and Torres Strait Islander and Mental Health and Wellbeing Principles and Practice*. Canberra: Australian Government, Department of Health and Ageing.

Reynolds, H. (2000). *Why Weren't We Told? A Personal Search for the Truth about Our History*. Melbourne: Penguin Books.

Rose, D.B. (1996). *Nourishing Terrains: Australian Aboriginal Views of Landscape and Wilderness.* Canberra: Australian Heritage Commission.

Royal Commission into Aboriginal Deaths in Custody & Muirhead, J.H. (1988). *Royal Commission into Aboriginal Deaths in Custody Interim Report.* Canberra: AGPS.

Sherwood, J. (2013). Colonisation – it's bad for your health: The context of Aboriginal health. *Contemporary Nurse*, 46(1), 28–40.

Silburn, S., Robinson, G., Leckning, B., Henry, D., Cox, A. & Kickett, D. (2010). Preventing suicide among indigenous Australians. In N. Purdie, P. Dudgeon & R. Walker (eds), *Working Together: Aboriginal and Torres Strait Islander and Mental Health and Wellbeing Principles and Practice* (pp. 91–104). Canberra: Australian Government, Department of Health and Ageing.

Silburn, S.R., Zubrick, S.R., De Maio, J.A., Shepherd, C., Griffin, J.A., Mitrou, F.G., … Pearson, G. (2006). *The Western Australian Aboriginal Child Health Survey: Strengthening the Capacity of Aboriginal Children, Families and Communities.* Perth: Curtin University of Technology and Telethon Institute for Child Health Research.

Social Health Reference Group (SHRG). (2004). *National Strategic Framework for Aboriginal and Torres Strait Islander Peoples' Mental Health and Social and Emotional Well Being 2004–2009.* Canberra: National Aboriginal and Torres Strait Islander Health Council and National Mental Health Working Group.

Stanner, W.E. (1965). Aboriginal territorial organisation: Estate, range, domain and regime. *Oceania*, 36(1), 1–26.

Steering Committee for the Review of Government Service Provision. (2011). *Overcoming Indigenous Disadvantage: Key indicators 2011.* Canberra: Productivity Commission.

Stephens, C., Nettleton, C., Porter, J., Willis, R. & Clark, S. (2005). Indigenous peoples' health: Why are they behind everyone, everywhere? *The Lancet*, 366, 10–13.

Swan, P. & Raphael, B. (1995). *Ways Forward: National Aboriginal and Torres Strait Islander Mental Health Policy. National Consultancy Report.* Canberra: AGPS.

Trewin, D. (2006). *2004–05 National Aboriginal and Torres Strait Islander Health Survey: Summary of Findings.* Canberra: ABS.

Üstün, T.B., Ayuso-Mateos, J.L., Chatterji, S., Mathers, C. & Murray, C.J. (2004). Global burden of depressive disorders in the year 2000. *British Journal of Psychiatry*, 184(5), 386–92.

Victorian Aboriginal Child Care Agency. (2006). *Working with Aboriginal Children and Families: A Guide for Child Protection and Child and Family Welfare Workers.* Melbourne: VACCA.

Wagner, B.M. (1997). Family risk factors for child and adolescent suicidal behavior. *Psychological Bulletin*, 121(2), 246–98.

Walter, M., Taylor, S. & Habibis, D. (2011). How white is social work in Australia? *Australian Social Work*, 64(1), 6–19.

Warelow, P. & Edward, K.I. (2007). Caring as a resilient practice in mental health nursing. *International Journal of Mental Health Nursing*, 16(2), 132–5.

Williams-Mozley, J. (2012). The stolen generations: What does this mean for Aboriginal and Torres Strait Islander children and young people today? In K. Price (ed.), *Aboriginal and Torres Strait Islander Education: An Introduction for the Teaching Professions* (pp. 21–34). New York: Cambridge University Press.

Wilson, S. (2008). *Research Is Ceremony: Indigenous Research Methods.* Nova Scotia: Fernwood Publishing.

World Health Organization (WHO). (2003). *Advocacy for Mental Health.* Geneva: WHO.

World Health Organization (WHO). (2010). *A Conceptual Framework for Action on the Social Determinants of Health.* Geneva: WHO. Retrieved from http://www.who.int/sdhconference/resources/ConceptualframeworkforactiononSDH_eng.pdf.

Zakeri, H., Jowker, B. & Razmjoee, M. (2010). Parenting styles and resilience. *Procedia – Social and Behavioral Sciences*, 5, 1067–70.

Ziersch, A.M., Gallaher, G., Baum, F. & Bentley, M. (2011). Responding to racism: Insights on how racism can damage health from an urban study of Australian Aboriginal people. *Social Science & Medicine*, 73(7), 1045–53.

Zubrick, S.R., Dudgeon, P., Gee, G., Glaskin, B., Kelly, K., Paradies, Y., Scrine, C. & Walker, R. (2010). Social determinants of Aboriginal and Torres Strait Islander social and emotional wellbeing. *Working together: Aboriginal and Torres Strait Islander Mental Health and Wellbeing Principles and Practice* (pp. 75–90). Canberra: Australian Government, Department of the Prime Minister and Cabinet.

Zubrick, S., Shepherd, C.J.C, Dudgeon, P., Gee, G., Paradies, Y., Scrine, C. & Walker, R. (2014). Social determinants of social and emotional wellbeing. In N. Purdie, P. Dudgeon & R. Walker (eds), *Working Together: Aboriginal and Torres Strait Islander and Mental Health and Wellbeing Principles and Practice* (pp. 93–112). Canberra: Australian Government, Department of Health and Ageing.

CHAPTER **26**

MENTAL HEALTH FIRST AID

Nygell Topp and Terry Froggatt

LEARNING OUTCOMES

Upon completion of this chapter, you should be able to:

26.1 Describe mental health first aid and how to apply it across the spectrum of mental health, including to specific mental health conditions such as anxiety, depression, psychosis, substance use and suicidality

26.2 Understand cultural considerations when providing mental health first aid to vulnerable groups

26.3 Discuss mental health first aid needs for carers and mental health first aid responders, and identify resources

INTRODUCTION

In order to identify the nature of **mental health first aid (MHFA)**, we first need to define the nature of mental health and well-being. The subject of mental health and well-being has been discussed in Chapter 2 – refer to that chapter for a comprehensive account. The following descriptor provides a synopsis of mental health and well-being as defined by the World Health Organization (WHO). Mental health is both an integral and essential component of good health. The WHO constitution states: 'Health is a state of complete physical, mental and social well-being and not merely the absence of disease or infirmity' (WHO, 1946). An important implication of this definition is that mental health is more than just the absence of mental health disorders or disabilities, either transient or permanent. It involves the promotion of and focus on recovery and hope. This is achieved by enlisting willingness and responsible action from both the individual, their carers and health workers using education, self-advocacy and various supports at both professional and personal levels.

Mental health is a state of well-being in which an individual realises their abilities, can cope with the normal stresses of life, can be resilient and adaptive to various life events, can work productively and is able to contribute to their community. Further, mental health is fundamental to both our collective and individual ability as humans to think, reason, emote and interact. This is in addition to earning a living and enjoying life in general. On this basis, the promotion, protection and restoration of mental health can be regarded as a vital concern to individuals, communities and the world (WHO, 2018).

A developing or worsening mental health problem necessitating MHFA can also be considered to be a broader term that seeks to encompass both a mental illness and symptoms of mental illness, but may not be acute enough to confer a diagnosis of a mental health condition. It can also include a mental health–related crisis; for example, an acute anxiety attack, psychosis

and post-traumatic stress disorder (PTSD). **Figure 26.1** illustrates the spectrum of interventions and where MHFA can best assist.

The importance of MHFA is made salient by the overall impact that mental health has throughout Australian society. This reality is illustrated by Australian Institute of Health and Welfare (AIHW) statistics indicating that one in five, or 20%, of Australians will experience a mental health crisis, issue or problem that would confer a diagnosis if they sought out a health care professional. This ranks mental illness as number three (after cancer and heart disease) on the disease burden scale (AIHW, 2011).

INTRODUCTION TO THE MHFA ACRONYM

In first aid courses, participants learn an action plan that prioritises steps to take and allows a series of interventions. Specifically, when applying physical first aid and prioritising interventions, there is an acronym: DRSABCD, which stands for danger, response, send for help, airway, breathing, circulation and defibrillation (Australian Resuscitation Council, 2016). This assists the first aid responder in prioritising the necessary sequence of steps in the correct order to assist in timely interventions. Similarly, MHFA also has an acronym. This action plan is used to assist a person experiencing a crisis or worsening of a mental health condition. However, the MHFA action plan differs slightly in that it outlines a series of actions that the mental health first aid responder utilises flexibly. This is in contrast to the compulsory sequence of steps initiated when providing physical first aid using the DRSABCD acronym. This action plan is called **ALGEE** (see **Figure 26.2**). The acronym ALGEE stands for:

- Approach the person
- Listen and communicate
- Give support and information
- Encourage the person to get help
- Encourage other supports.

Approach the person regarding your concerns

In understanding the MHFA action plan, the first action is to consider our approach. We need to identify any potential crisis, and where possible begin by assisting the consumer in managing it. The key identifiers for the MHFA responder are to determine a suitable time and space where both the mental health first aid responder and the person being assisted will feel comfortable.

If the person we approach is not initiating the conversation with us about their mood or thoughts, then the first aider should initiate this conversation. This conversation can be initiated by indicating what

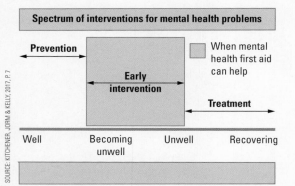

Spectrum of interventions for mental health problems

Prevention

Early intervention

When mental health first aid can help

Treatment

Well · Becoming unwell · Unwell · Recovering

FIGURE 26.1
Spectrum of interventions for mental health problems

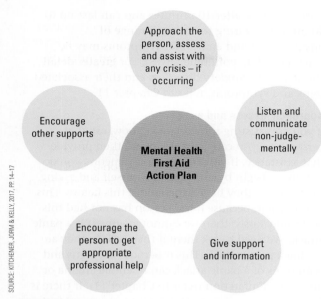

SOURCE: KITCHENER, JORM & KELLY 2017, PP. 14–17

FIGURE 26.2
ALGEE action plan

you have seen or heard that may be causing you concern. For example, 'Tegan, I can see you're really distressed right now and I'm worried about you.' It is paramount to respect the person's privacy and their confidentiality. This may need to be stated, and refers to the person's confidentiality being maintained and not disclosed to those not involved in the person's direct care or to non-health care providers.

However, in a situation where a crisis is unfolding and the person may hurt themselves by either attempting suicide and/or self-harm/non-suicidal self-injury, or is using substances and is possibly already intoxicated, then you will need to apply crisis first aid. A crisis can also include the person experiencing extreme distress such as an anxiety attack, a traumatic event or being in the midst of a severe psychotic episode. It can also include their behaviour, in that it may be disturbing others. This might also include aggression that is verbal and/or physical. A risk assessment should always be performed if you determine that a crisis is emerging or is already present. This includes assessing your own safety and whether you may need to withdraw from the environment and obtain immediate assistance.

For information pertaining to a specific condition, refer to the crisis information discussed for specific mental health first aid throughout this chapter. Moreover, if you have no concerns regarding the person being in crisis, then asking the person about their mood and thoughts and the length of time they have been experiencing these can also be used as an entry point into conversation to initiate MHFA (Kelly, Jorm & Wright, 2007).

Listen and communicate non-judgementally

When initiating communication and active listening with the person you are assisting, it is important to set aside any judgements you may have about the person or their situation. Most people you encounter who are experiencing a distressed mood or range of emotions and/or thoughts want to be listened to with empathy. This needs to occur before you offer resources and options that may assist them. The MHFA responder needs to adopt a certain attitude that uses both verbal and non-verbal skills for effective communication and listening. This can include active listening to allow you to really hear and understand what the person is saying. This also makes it easier for the person to talk freely without the sense of being judged while they are speaking.

Non-verbal cues such as open body language and maintaining eye contact (if culturally appropriate) can also assist in conveying active listening and non-judgemental communication. Remember, listening in this context is as an MHFA responder. Therefore, it is paramount to respect the person's privacy and confidentiality. This may need to be stated, and refers to the person's confidentiality being maintained, and therefore is a more specific form of listening and communicating, as opposed to a comprehensive mental state examination (MSE) that is undertaken by a mental health clinician. For more information on therapeutic communication skills and approaches, refer to Chapter 5.

Give support and information

It usually becomes easier for the MHFA responder to provide support and information once the person has felt they have been listened to. The support that is ideal at this time is that of empathy and also conveying hope of recovery. Additionally, offering practical assistance with tasks that may seem difficult or overwhelming can also provide a sense of support. Further, this can be an ideal time for the MHFA responder to provide information and resources about mental health issues, their personal impact and associated available resources (beyondblue, 2018).

Encourage the person to get professional help

Within this action, the MHFA responder can provide options for help and support, the nature of which will vary depending on the environment they are in. For example, in a community or primary health care setting this may mean contacting the crisis team, the person's general practitioner (GP), case manager or other health care provider in emergency situations. In a secondary health care setting, this may mean contacting their medical registrar or their consultant.

Ultimately, connection to a health professional is encouraged because the consumer may be unaware of the various options for support that are available to them due to the nature of their distress and possible impaired mood and/or thinking difficulties.

Encourage other supports
The MHFA responder can also encourage use of various self-help strategies. This can include initiating or increasing self-care activities. It can also be obtaining support from a partner, family member, friend, friendship group and other self-identified persons. This can assist by reinforcing awareness of the pre-existing help and support the person presently has, while aiding them in current and future recovery. Support groups also provide assistance that is useful for both those currently experiencing, and those recovering from a mental health challenge (Perry & Pescosolido, 2015).

HOW TO APPLY MHFA TO VARIOUS MENTAL HEALTH PROBLEMS
In this section, we look at how to apply MHFA to various mental health conditions. Additionally, we look at the MHFA response in both the context of a crisis and where there is no identified crisis. For each listed condition, we follow the ALGEE approach listed in **Figure 26.2**, which you should use as a reference point as you read through this section of the chapter.

Anxiety: crisis and no crisis
Anxiety as an umbrella term and its cohort of associated diagnoses include conditions such as: agoraphobia, generalised anxiety disorder (GAD), panic disorder, post-traumatic stress disorder (PTSD), obsessive-compulsive disorder (OCD) and social phobia. These conditions are described and discussed extensively in Section 2 of this book.

The MHFA plan is applied to the signs and symptoms you observe and not to the diagnosis. In many instances, a diagnosis may not have been established or may not be known. This is why the MHFA plan is a series of actions as opposed to steps. This allows for a greater flexibility when applying these skills in various settings and presentations to observed signs and symptoms.

Anxiety with crisis
A panic attack is characterised by a distinct episode of extreme anxiousness, discomfort and/or fear. The crisis situation being referred to here is that of a person experiencing an acute or extreme panic attack. These attacks are perceived as overwhelming and combine physical, emotional and/or psychological symptoms. These will normally peak after 10 minutes and can last up to 30 minutes. During this time, a range of physiological and emotional symptoms may be experienced (beyondblue, 2018). For greater detail about various anxiety disorders and their associated signs and symptoms, refer to Chapter 11.

Approach, assess and assist
If you are assisting someone you know, ask that person how you can assist them and then provide that assistance. If you are assisting someone you do not know, begin by introducing yourself and asking the person if they have experienced this before. This is important, because if the person has not had this occur previously, then we cannot assume it is a panic attack. We need to ask them if they believe they are having a panic attack. This is because the signs and symptoms of a panic attack can resemble angina or myocardial infarction (refer to Chapter 11). If there is any doubt, then you must default to a physical first aid response and observe for change in their level of consciousness, call for help, and monitor airway, breathing and circulation until professional help arrives (Australian Resuscitation Council, 2008).

Listen and communicate non-judgementally
It is paramount that you remain calm and do not panic. If you (or they) know they are experiencing a panic attack, then reassure them. Speak clearly, firmly and slowly by using simple and short sentences. You can also invite the person to sit somewhere – preferably a quiet place. Maintain neutral or open body language such as unfolded arms, and sitting next to the person as opposed to in front of them. Acknowledge that their panic and terror feel real to them. Remind the person that they are safe and that their feelings and their symptoms will pass. Also, be mindful not to diminish the person's feelings or experience by minimising or trivialising them.

Give support and information
Once the person's panic attack has fully subsided, you can then provide further support and information. Begin by asking whether they know where to obtain information and support about their panic attacks. If they are unaware of their options, offer a range of choices on where advice and support can be obtained. This is particularly important if the panic attacks continue to occur or are causing distress and functional impairment to the person.

Encourage appropriate professional help
As stated, if you or the person are unsure as to whether this is a panic attack then default to regular physical first aid and call emergency services and monitor airway, breathing and circulation until professional help arrives. If the person believes they are having a

panic attack, reassure them that there are effective treatments and interventions that are available for panic attacks and panic disorders. Perhaps they have practised deep-breathing exercises, or some other way of alleviating their anxiety, and reinstating these skills would be beneficial now.

Encourage the person to seek professional support and intervention. You may encounter resistance in this conversation and may find it beneficial to use probing questions that assist in identifying the nature of the resistance. This can then be met with factual statements to overcome the person's barriers to obtaining professional assistance. These may include: perceived financial barriers to accessing treatment, non-awareness that treatments such as cognitive behavioural therapy (CBT) exist, and medication resistance (e.g. believing medication will be necessary and conveying an unwillingness to take medication).

Encourage other supports

By assisting the person to identify other supports that exist, you can help them to begin or expand upon their pre-existing resources. These can include their close personal relationships, such as partners, siblings, parents, friends and friendship networks. Self-help books, internet resources, relaxation, meditation and mutual support groups can also assist, but may be more effective when used in conjunction with professional interventions and treatments.

Anxiety with no associated crisis

A person experiencing generalised anxiety without associated panic attacks may still experience distress and functional impairment. This is particularly so when their signs and symptoms have been occurring for some time, the length of which will vary between individuals, but is usually greater than 12 months before professional help is sought out (AIHW, 2018).

Approach, assess and assist

Assessment still needs to occur even when there is no apparent crisis. This is due to the need to identify a clear and specific approach for the person you are assisting. Identifying a time and a place where privacy and confidentiality can be maintained is also a necessary consideration. If you encounter resistance, it is suggested that you focus on your concerns, what you have seen and any distress you may have observed.

Listen and communicate non-judgementally

Active listening not only comprises verbal and non-verbal communication but also includes paraphrasing; that is checking for understanding what you have heard and confirming the person's statements. Allowing the person to tell their story without judgement or diminishing their experience is also paramount to active and engaged listening.

Give support and information

Once the person has finished speaking about their experience, providing support and information should occur. Remember to be realistic, treat the person with respect and accord them their dignity. What is not supportive, however, is enabling avoidance of anxiety-provoking situations as this can slow their journey to recovery and wellness. You may encounter resistance when providing support and information and this can be an opportunity to identify and address the potential barriers a person has to seeking professional help.

Encourage appropriate professional help

Only 38% of people with anxiety will seek treatment from a health care professional within the first 12 months of their symptom onset. Yet anxiety is the most common mental health issue for Australians (AIHW, 2018). This is why it is imperative to encourage connection to professional support and services. This will help to significantly reduce the development of secondary symptoms that can occur from prolonged avoidance. These can include substance use, and also developing signs and symptoms of depression. Again, it may be useful to identify the barriers that the person has to obtaining professional assistance and treatment. Identifying and countering these barriers can increase the likelihood of the person seeking professional intervention and treatment.

Encourage other supports

Prompt the person to identify existing support structures such as partners, parents, siblings, family, friends, friendship networks and support groups. You can encourage the person to make use of these pre-existing supportive structures. Further, there is some evidence that identifying supportive groups can be of benefit (Pistrang, Barker & Humphreys, 2008).

Depression: crisis and no crisis

A major depressive disorder often affects a person's ability to undertake activities of daily living, work and their enjoyment and satisfaction from both personal and intimate relationships. The spectrum of depressive disorders ranges from mild through to severe and their associated signs and symptoms have been discussed in depth in Chapter 10. The need for MHFA in the context of depression becomes important as depression is often recurrent. Also, outcomes can be poor for those waiting any length of time to receive therapeutic intervention, particularly with first onset depression (Ghio et al., 2014). This is why early intervention and a rapid MHFA response can lead to better outcomes.

Depression with associated crisis

As noted, depression exists on a spectrum from mild to moderate through to severe. It is normal for people experiencing depression to experience morbid thinking and to have occasional thoughts of death. From an MHFA perspective, what differentiates depression with crisis from depression with no associated crisis is whether the person's thoughts are preoccupied with death and have progressed to suicide and/or a plan of action and procurement of necessary resources to carry out that plan.

Approach, assess and assist

When approaching someone who has signs and symptoms of depression, it is salient to include an assessment of risk to self and others. Even if you are mildly unsure, it is important to still approach them. In some situations it is evident there is a crisis, while in others it may only become apparent after you have engaged the person in conversation. It is important to know that most people who are experiencing depression have morbid thoughts and behavioural changes.

Be aware that often the mental health worker can make a profound difference in a crisis situation, even in preventing someone taking their life. Knowing some of the warning signs and risk factors for suicide is the first step in being aware that someone might have thoughts of suicide. Once again, refer to Chapter 20 for comprehensive information regarding behaviours and risk of suicide in a person with moderate to severe depression. Finally, if it becomes apparent in conversation the person has thoughts of suicide with intent, then immediate intervention is required. For specific interventional information, refer to MHFA and suicide in this chapter.

Listen and communicate non-judgementally

Do your best to appear composed, tranquil, self-assured and empathic. By maintaining neutral body language and facial expressions, you can avoid negative or surprised reactions to the person's statements. It is important to listen with undivided attention and be supportive where you can. Asking open-ended questions can assist in encouraging the person to share their feelings and thoughts. You can also demonstrate listening by summarising what has been said and clarify key points to ensure clarity about what has been said.

Give support and information

Support in this instance centres around genuine empathy and realistic support. Accept the person as they are and be realistic about their current capacity to undertake activities of daily living. In many instances, cleaning the house, feeding pets and themselves may feel overwhelming. Acknowledging the impact and stating you think no less of them can be very supportive. Furthermore, the provision of support by assisting with practical tasks can be helpful.

Providing salient information is a key point. This needs to be both accurate and appropriate to the person's circumstances. Finally, consider what is unhelpful in this situation. This can include over-assistance, attempting to provide all the answers to their problems, nagging the person, minimising or belittling their feelings or becoming overprotective towards them.

Encourage appropriate professional help

It is vital to encourage the person to seek out professional assistance. This is to try to prevent secondary effects of depression becoming more entrenched and recovery prolonged as a result of delayed interventions. Introducing options in help seeking can assist in overcoming the person's resistance. For example, they may not know where to get help or their regular health care provider may not have recognised their symptoms as depression due to the person's non-disclosure. Furthermore, the person may not be aware of the multitude of treatment options that are currently available. Exploring the resistance the person has and countering it with factually accurate information can overcome their resistance.

If, however, all of their barriers have been explored and the person does not want to seek out professional assistance, we need to respect their right not to do so – if there is no risk of harm to self or others. Finally, let the person know the mental health service is available if they change their mind. This is important, because people are more likely to seek help if someone close to them suggests it (Kitchener, Jorm & Kelly, 2017). In a professional capacity (i.e., someone working in the role of a mental health clinician) legal responsibilities are as per indicated in the local jurisdiction's mental health act.

Encourage other supports

In recognising other supports, first and foremost is the need to ask the person to abstain from substance use, as concurrent usage can magnify feelings and simultaneously reduce personal insight. It can also enable acting out while disinhibited from the effects of the substance. If the person has previously made attempts at suicide, ask them what helped support them in those situations. Remember, in this instance other supports may be of value after the suicide intervention and when the person is on their path to recovery and wellness.

Depression with no associated crisis

The signs and symptoms of mild to moderate depression may not occur with a concurrent crisis. However, the symptoms affecting a person's behaviour, feelings, thinking and physical well-being can still interfere with and have a significant impact on their family, relationships and work.

Approach, assess and assist

It is important to consider the ideal time and place where you can speak with the person with minimal interruptions. This can allow for a more comfortable environment. However, if the person is not instigating conversation, then asking an open-ended question such as 'How are you feeling?' or 'How are you travelling?' can initiate this discussion. Be realistic – let the person know you wish to assist, but be careful not to 'take over' or encourage dependency. Offer consistent emotional support and understanding in your approach. Demonstrate genuine caring and do not be concerned about 'saying the wrong thing' when offering assistance. Do let the person know you are ready to talk when they are, if they are unwilling to open up at that time; let them choose the time. Finally, always respect the person's privacy and their confidentiality, unless you have assessed a risk of harm to self or to others.

Listen and communicate non-judgementally

It is important to listen to understand as opposed to listening to respond (Froggatt & Liersch-Sumskis, 2014). This can be paramount in being an effective, non-judgemental listener, as it requires paying attention to your personal attitudes and how you convey these in your interactions. It also means embracing a stance of acceptance by respecting the person's feelings, values and experiences. You can communicate this acceptance through avoiding the use of stigmatising language and attitudes and by choosing your words wisely. Realise also that the person may hold a stigmatising belief about mental illness. By being genuine in your communication, and displaying empathy in your verbal and non-verbal skills, you can role-model your acceptance and make it easier for the person to accept help.

Give support and information

Be realistic – let the person know you wish to assist by offering consistent emotional support, understanding and empathy.

Talking with someone who is depressed is helpful in itself. Although the person may be reluctant to speak with you, do not be put off by this. If they do choose to speak, listen carefully to what they are saying, listen to understand and try not to interrupt them. Moreover, you should seek clarification by asking the person to reiterate what they have said so that your understanding is accurate. Let the person know that you are concerned about them and you are willing to help. Let the person know that you have information for them to consider.

Finally, if thoughts of suicide have arisen in the MHFA conversation, work with the person to establish a **safety plan**. Essentially, this is an agreement you make with the person that, should these thoughts reoccur or if they are experiencing distress, they have a person or persons to call; this should include the contact details of who they can call (Stanley & Brown, 2012).

Encourage appropriate professional help

A person who is experiencing signs and symptoms of depression is more likely to seek out professional assistance if the health practitioner or someone close to them suggests this. Another possible way to encourage professional support is by encouraging (coaching) the person to talk about their thoughts and feelings with their GP as this can aid a speedier diagnosis. In most cases, people presenting to their GP discuss vague, non-specific physical symptoms as opposed to mood and thought content. Finally, identifying any resistance the person may have in seeking out professional services will assist you in overcoming their barriers to receiving professional care. This can be achieved by countering erroneous beliefs with factually accurate information.

Encourage other supports

Assist the person to identify supports they already have (both formal and informal). These may include family, friends, neighbours and community-based support groups. This can also include scheduling self-care activities and engagements with supportive persons. There is evidence that the perception and receipt of emotional support by the person experiencing depression can improve their recovery rate and personal outcome (Nasser & Overholser, 2005).

Psychosis: crisis and no crisis

There is a cluster of mental health conditions that fall broadly under the term psychosis. Learning about how to recognise some of the early signs may assist you to recognise whether a person is developing a psychotic illness. It is usually an amalgamation of these signs that suggests that something is 'not quite right'. Early intervention for a person developing psychosis is critical and you should act as soon as you are able, and not think that this is 'just a phase' or due to some other reason; for example, stress or substance use. The two predominant characteristics of psychosis are delusions and hallucinations. Other characteristics include disorganised thinking, speech impairment, blunted emotion and changes in behaviour. For a detailed account of delusions, hallucinations and other presenting signs and symptoms, refer to Chapter 8.

Psychosis: with associated crisis

Psychosis is usually episodic in nature. These episodes usually involve phases that vary in length in different individuals. They include premorbid, prodromal, acute, recovery and relapse phases and these concepts are discussed in greater detail in Chapter 8. What distinguishes a crisis event arising from psychosis is the impairment and distress the person is experiencing. The other crisis that may arise is the level of risk of harm a person may place themselves in from reduced or absent insight. This may include dangerous behaviour to self, and not just suicidal thoughts and/or behaviour. Refer to the section on suicide intervention in this chapter.

Approach, assess and assist

In a crisis situation, you should try to remain as calm as possible. Evaluate the situation by assessing the risks involved (e.g. whether there is any risk that the person will harm themselves or others). It is important to assess whether the person is at risk of suicide. Further, if the person has an advance directive or relapse prevention plan, you should locate this and follow those instructions. Alternatively, try to find out if the person has anyone they trust (e.g. close friends, family) and try to enlist their help. Also, assess whether it is safe for the person to be alone. If not, ensure that someone stays with the individual.

Be aware that the person might act upon a delusional belief or hallucination; this is called a command hallucination (refer to Chapter 8 for further information). Remember that your primary task is to de-escalate the situation and therefore you should not do anything to further agitate the person. This can be more easily achieved by focusing on the distress and the impairment the person is experiencing. If the person is at risk of harming themselves or others, then your immediate priority must be ensuring evaluation by a medical or mental health professional. If the crisis team is called, convey specific and concise observations about the severity of the person's distress, impairment and behaviour. However, if your concerns about the person are not addressed or are dismissed, persevere by seeking support for them through other sources.

Listen and communicate non-judgementally

It is important to communicate with the person in a clear and concise manner and to use short, simple sentences. Speak quietly in a non-threatening tone of voice at a moderate pace. If the person asks questions, answer them calmly. You should comply with requests, unless they are unsafe or unreasonable. This gives the person the opportunity to feel somewhat in control.

Give support and information

When a person is experiencing psychosis, providing information can be problematic and less than ideal. Instead, try to maintain safety and protect the person, yourself and others around you from harm. Make sure that you have access to an exit. Identify any unfamiliar people in the area and explain that they are there to help and how they are going to help.

Encourage appropriate professional help

Remain aware that you may not be able to de-escalate the situation and, if this is the case, you should be prepared to call for assistance. Where possible, involve the person in deciding whom to call. Ideally, this would be a health care provider who they know, such as their mental health clinician or GP. It could also be their case manager. If no consensus can be reached, the mental health crisis team can be the logical choice for both further guidance regarding management and potential intervention. Remember to focus on the person's distress and impairment as the reason why professional help is being sought.

Encourage other supports

In this instance, this action is best initiated when the person's acute episode has passed. When the person experiencing psychosis with crisis is recovering, then assisting them with practical assistance such as meals, cleaning and transportation can be of value. Also, encouraging the person to identify and reduce any stress in their life as much as is practicable can also be a supportive measure. It is also useful to suggest to the person to abstain from alcohol and other drugs that may heighten signs and symptoms and slow the progression to recovery.

Psychosis: with no associated crisis

A person experiencing the onset of early psychosis will often not identify thought or perceptual changes or seek out assistance. This is the very nature of psychotic illness and is due to their experience feeling unsettling or even frightening. Changes in thinking, perception, emotion and motivation can lead eventually to behavioural changes. There are a number of mental health conditions in which psychosis can occur; see Chapter 8 for further information.

Approach, assess and assist

Your approach needs to be well considered, in that a person experiencing psychosis can often withdraw as a result of fear, suspicion or mistrust. Therefore, where possible, approach the person privately about your concerns and their experiences, ideally in a place that is free from distractions. It is important to be specific about your concerns. Allow the person to set the tone and pace of the interaction. As the discussion unfolds, it is important to look for signs of crisis, suicidal thoughts and behaviour, and possible aggression. These are discussed in the crisis sections of this chapter. Finally, your approach and assessment will determine how you assist the person. They may be unwilling to talk with you because their thoughts and feelings may be frightening to them or they may feel very suspicious toward you. If this is the case, let them know you are available for when they would like to talk and that you will continue the discussion with them at a later date.

Listen and communicate non-judgementally

Listening in this context needs to be non-judgemental. It is likely that the person may be speaking and behaving differently due to their psychotic symptoms. It is important to avoid judgemental commentary about the person's experiences and beliefs. Rather, focus your concern on the distress and the impact this may be having on the person. Statements such as, 'I'm sure this is real for you but I cannot see or hear ...' can be helpful in listening and communicating. Also, the person's communication may be impaired and include disorganised speech, or you may need to repeat your sentences due to their impaired ability to concentrate.

Give support and information

It may be necessary to state to the person that you respect their privacy and confidentiality prior to listening and speaking with them; unless you have a concern about the person harming themself or another person. Moreover, consider the extent to which the person is able to decide autonomously or whether this function is impaired. Conveying a message of help, support and hope for recovery can assist. The information you provide needs to be accurate and relevant to the individual's situation. The ideal support is most likely to be practical support. Finally, identifying various ways to link the person to a health care provider is the optimal support in this instance.

Encourage appropriate professional help

There can be many reasons that a person may experience the signs and symptoms of psychosis. It is paramount that they are assessed by a health care professional as possible physical causes need to be ruled out. Further, it is well established that prolonged delays for those experiencing psychosis-type symptoms can often have poorer long-term outcomes for the person (NICE, 2014). For these reasons it is vital to assist the person in obtaining the necessary support. If the person does decide to obtain help, then provide practical and emotional support to assist them in actioning this decision. As discussed earlier, the person may be resistant to obtaining help and should this occur, encourage them to speak with someone they trust (if they are unwilling to speak with you). Your MHFA response will largely depend on the type and severity of the person's signs and symptoms. Finally, if they are not at risk of harming themself or others, then remain friendly and receptive to the likelihood that they may need your assistance another time.

Encourage other supports

When identifying supports, the most immediate support is asking the person to abstain from consuming alcohol and other drugs. Substance use can magnify unsettling thoughts, feelings, behaviours and further impair insight. Ask the person to identify pre-existing supports they have. These can be formal structures such as support groups and reducing

workloads. Informal support structures could include their partner, family, friends and other possible sources they have self-identified.

Substance use: crisis and no crisis

Substance use disorders are a serious and complex problem. They contribute annually to thousands of cases of illness, ongoing disease and death (AIHW, 2017). Substance use disorders have been substantially outlined and detailed in Chapter 14. The term 'substance use' is used in this chapter as opposed to alcohol and other drugs for a number of reasons. While various substances may have particular physical and/or psychological impacts on a person, the overall outcome can be similar. This is because repeated and sustained use can affect a person's family, friends, and social and work roles in similar ways. Second, it is important to note that the MHFA responder is not assessing a person's fit into certain diagnostic criteria for substance use disorder. Instead, MHFA responders are equipping themselves to have a conversation with a person they believe (or who states) is having a troublesome association with substance use.

Substance use: crisis

A crisis relating to substance use can occur across the spectrum of substance use; for example, a person may be unconscious and not rousable or highly agitated and potentially aggressive from the consumed substance. Both situations would necessitate intervention.

Approach, assess and assist

How you assess will be determined by the signs and symptoms that are evident as you approach the consumer. For example, alcohol intoxication or other central nervous depressants may cause a loss of coordination, slurred speech, altered gait, reduced consciousness or even episodic aggressive behaviour and loud speech. If the person is experiencing alcohol intoxication or poisoning, monitor for danger to themselves, ensuring you and others are also safe. The assistance you provide will be determined by your assessment of the person's condition. Remember that in this instance you may need to default to physical first aid by monitoring and providing support to the person's airway, breathing and circulation.

Listen and communicate non-judgementally

In the event the person is highly agitated, even with your best efforts it may be challenging to stay calm. Remember to communicate appropriately by using clear, concise and short statements. Use open and non-threatening body language. Speak with confidence in your tone of voice. Let the person talk and focus on the distress and the impairment the person may be experiencing. In the case of a semi-conscious or unconscious person, speak clearly and provide forewarning of touch by announcing your intention *prior* to doing it. For example, if you are going to place the person into the recovery position (see **Figure 26.3**), first state where you will touch them and why you are doing so. This will reduce a startled or combative response.

Give support and information

Remember to stay calm. Speak with the person in a relaxed tone, using simple and clear words. Avoid provoking the person through derision, sarcasm, shouting or frustration in your tone of voice. Furthermore, providing information at this time may generally be ineffective, not received or even retained. The focus in acute situations is on de-escalation of distress and impairment rather than overloading the person with un-retained information.

Encourage appropriate professional help

In a medical emergency, call an ambulance or take the person to a hospital. Do not be afraid to seek medical help for the person, even if there may be legal implications for them.

If an ambulance is called or medical help is sought, ensure that the person:

- is put in the recovery position if they are unconscious or semi-conscious (see **Figure 26.3**)
- is not left alone or given food or drink as they may choke even if partially conscious
- is kept warm to prevent hypothermia – although the person may feel warm, body temperature may actually be decreasing
- has their airway, breathing and circulation monitored.

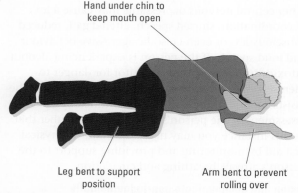

Hand under chin to keep mouth open

Leg bent to support position

Arm bent to prevent rolling over

FIGURE 26.3
Patient in a recovery position

It is beneficial if a friend or family member can accompany the person to hospital as they may be able to provide relevant information (Kingston et al., 2009).

Hostility in a mental health context is often associated with substance intoxication. If the person is combative or highly agitated, in the first instance the focus is on safety of yourself and of others (including the person where possible). If you are concerned the person is becoming increasingly hostile, the secondary focus will be on de-escalating the person's aggressive behaviour. Strategies for de-escalation can include:

- speaking, using the three Cs: clearly, calmly and confidently
- abstaining from physically restricting the person or their movement
- avoiding arguing with or threatening them
- avoiding responding in an aggressive, authoritarian or demanding manner.

Remember to take any threats or warnings seriously. If the person's hostility increases, you may need to withdraw and call the mental health crisis team or the police. If this occurs, describe the person's behaviour, their signs and symptoms, including any observed intoxication from substance use. This will assist in an optimised and tailored response.

Encourage other supports

In an acute situation this is best left until the person is not impaired or near recovery from their substance use. What is most helpful is to ask the person to abstain from any further use to reduce the effects of the current impact of their substance use. Remember, this is not asking them for complete abstinence, as this should never be attempted without the direct support and management of a health care provider due to the potential risk of withdrawal creating further harm.

Substance use: no crisis

A person can experience a substance use disorder, but not be presenting in a crisis situation such as that described above. However, their substance use may be contributing to other physical, social and/or emotional issues that the MHFA responder may have a conversation with the person about.

Approach assess and assist

Approaching a person who you believe may have a substance use problem requires thoughtfulness. If you are uncertain about how best to address this often very sensitive issue, you should consult a health professional who is competent in this field.

If you do feel a degree of confidence in being able to help, being non-judgemental, supportive and non-confrontational is critical. The amount of assistance you provide will depend on the circumstances in which you are providing the mental health first aid (Crisis Prevention Institute, 2019).

Listen and communicate non-judgementally

It is important to listen to the person without passing a moral judgement on their character, or assessing them as bad, weak or immoral. You may find that the person does not wish to acknowledge there is a problem or that anything is wrong. Lecturing, bribing, nagging, crying or even threatening will not bring about the change. Even in the most challenging circumstances, continue to treat the person with dignity and respect. Aim for a non-critical but concerned approach in your communication.

Give support and information
Some other effective communication strategies may include:

- staying calm and reasonable
- asking the person about their substance use rather than just making your own observations
- reiterating what they have said so that you have a clear understanding
- focusing on the problem instead of blaming the person
- expressing that you are concerned, worried for them and would like to assist them
- trying to keep to the point – do not argue or become defensive
- not criticising
- not using derogatory or stigmatising language.

There are effective interventions available to assist people with substance use issues. Providing a person with up-to-date and accurate information can be a great service. Be aware of what is available in your local community. Ultimately, it is an individual's decision whether they seek help; you can play an important role in assisting them, if they are prepared to do so. Also, your involvement may not be a 'one-off' encounter. Be prepared for the person to require your counsel at points along their journey of recovery.

Encourage appropriate professional help
It is necessary to be realistic in your expectations when giving support that encourages professional assistance. This is because changes in a person's thinking and behaviour will not occur immediately. When suggesting professional support, where possible try to identify local treatment options. Suggest that you will support the person in obtaining professional help by assisting them to make and keep appointments. Another possibility is to provide information regarding e-counselling or telephone counselling as a means of directing them towards professional help. Moreover, be prepared for the likelihood of a negative response. This can occur when a person's perspective of their substance use differs from others' perceptions of their use. If this transpires, remember to set boundaries on behaviour that you will not condone. Continue to remain supportive, however, and remind the person of the inherent risks. You may still be able to have a positive effect on their substance use.

Encourage other supports
Friends, family and support groups (both formal and informal) can provide other forms of support. Further, evidence suggests that stable relationships, an absence of criticism from within family support structures, and friends who are not substance users can encourage the person to abstain while they are initiating change (Kingston et al., 2009; Kingston et al., 2011).

Suicidality
It is important to differentiate between non-suicidal self-injury (NSSI; or self-harm) and suicide. A person who self-injures can be at risk of suicide. However, people can engage in NSSI over weeks, months and even years without becoming suicidal. The following MHFA response is for the provision of care and intervention for the person experiencing thoughts and/or behaviours of suicide.

Approach, assess and assist
The subject of suicide, including the signs and symptoms that a person may be suicidal, is covered in Chapter 20. The following is by no means exhaustive but serves as a brief recap from that chapter. Important signs and symptoms include:

- increase in substance use
- withdrawing from significant and supportive relationships
- sudden and/or dramatic changes to mood; for example, agitation, anxiety, anger and even mood improvement – particularly after a depressed mood
- hopelessness with no sense of life purpose
- finalising personal affairs
- threatening self-injury.

In considering your approach, be aware of your own attitudes about suicide and how they may be conveyed verbally and non-verbally in your conversation. Furthermore, consider if there are any cultural, religious or attitudinal beliefs that differ from your own – you may need to adjust your approach to optimise your MHFA response. If this is not possible, seek immediate assistance from someone else.

In shaping your approach, it is vital to act promptly, even if you suspect that someone has suicidal thoughts and not intent. This approach can be achieved through directly questioning the person. Unless the person has stated suicidal intent, the only way to be certain is by directly questioning them. This should always occur with neutral language. Do not use leading or judgemental language such as, 'Are you thinking of committing suicide?', 'Are you thinking of doing something stupid?' or 'You're not going to hurt yourself are you?' These types of questions are not helpful and may even cause the person to withdraw from your MHFA response. Instead, it is better to frame simple and direct questions, such as:

- 'Have you had thoughts of killing yourself?'
- 'How do you intend to suicide?'
- 'Have you previously attempted suicide or made plans?'

Assessment is vital in this instance. The urgency with which action is taken will be determined by the warning signs, the plan and its level of development – whether the resources have been procured, and whether a time and place have been determined. Those most at risk are people who have a plan and the resources to implement it. Remember, however, that the absence of a plan does not guarantee the person's safety.

Giving support is paramount. It is important to take all thoughts of suicide seriously and to take action. Identifying the nature of the support given is very much determined by the urgency of action that is needed. This is achieved by recognising all of the warning signs for suicide and further direct questioning.

The three key actions for helping a suicidal person are:

- If you think someone is suicidal, ask directly.
- Work together to keep the person safe, for now.
- Connect them to professional help (Kitchener, Jorm & Kelly, 2017, p. 126).

Listen and communicate non-judgementally

Genuine support and understanding are far more important than saying the correct thing at this time. Remain calm and patient while the person talks. It is not helpful to argue or debate about their thoughts and feelings concerning suicide. Moreover, minimising the person's problems, providing superficial reassurance such as saying, 'Cheer up', or providing your own stories is not helpful at this time. Do, however, clarify important points they have stated by paraphrasing to demonstrate both your empathy and understanding. Finally, thank the person for disclosing their thoughts and feelings, acknowledging the courage it takes to do this.

Give support and information

Acknowledging the distress and the personal impact the person is experiencing can illustrate reassurance. The fundamental support an MHFA responder can provide at this time is to 'work together to keep the person safe'. A safety plan can assist in this instance. This is an agreement between the MHFA responder and the person that involves undertakings to keep that person safe. This can include a plan of action such as who to call and their respective contact details. It also outlines what will be done and by whom. It is for a

specified length of time. Finally, find out who or what has supported the person previously and whether these supports are still current (Kitchener, Jorm & Kelly, 2017).

Encourage appropriate professional help

It is vital to take all thoughts of suicide seriously and to take action. If you think the person is not safe, contact their regular mental health professional. Ideally, the health care provider should be someone whom the consumer already knows and trusts. Where possible, involve the person experiencing suicidal thoughts and behaviour in the decision-making about who is contacted. However, if the person has a specific plan and/or the means to carry out the plan, call the mental health crisis team or mental health centre, or phone emergency services for advice and possible interventions (Kitchener, Jorm & Kelly, 2017).

If you think the suicidal person has a weapon, contact the police. Remember to inform the police of the suicidal intent to assist them in an optimal response to the situation. It is always important to act promptly even if you only have a slight impression that the person is having suicidal thoughts or intent. Finally, if the person has already harmed themselves, follow the DRSABCD of physical first aid.

Encourage other supports

In recognising other supports, first and foremost is the need for the individual to abstain from substance use as this can magnify feelings and enable acting out while disinhibited. If the person has previously made attempts at suicide, ask them what helped support them in those situations. Remember, in this instance other supports may be of value after the suicide intervention when the person is on the path to recovery and wellness.

Traumatic events

There is a substantial body of research with emerging evidence that trauma is a precursor to psychological distress (Bentall et al., 2012). Trauma is an event experienced by a person that *they have perceived* as being traumatic. There are many causes of trauma, some of which include a physical accident or assault or witnessing a terrible event. Psychological trauma may include sexual, physical or emotional abuse, torture, bullying or passive neglect (MHFA Australia, 2016).

Everyone is different in how they respond to trauma. The experience of trauma may result in some people experiencing its consequences for many years, while others may become more resilient as a result of their traumatic experiences. For more information on PTSD, see Chapter 18.

Approach, assess and assist

By their very nature, traumatic events involve risk to safety. In all circumstances, you must attend to your own safety before offering to assist someone else. You need to assess any risk or danger to yourself and to others. If anyone has injuries, these must be attended to as a priority. Always seek the assistance of professional first aid responders and do not try to take over their role.

Moreover, consider whether you are within a possible crime scene as this will require an increase in your situational awareness. Be mindful that evidence may need to be collected and certain actions and interactions could cause contamination.

Listen and communicate non-judgementally

When communicating with the person who has experienced trauma, you should be realistic and not make statements that you are unable to back up. Remember, when talking with someone who has experienced a traumatic event, it is important to demonstrate a caring attitude, respect the person's autonomy and treat them with dignity. Use their name as this can reorient them to their personhood and sense of self. The person may feel disconnected as a result of the preceding event, and hearing their name also helps connect them with you and the present moment. Ask the person how they would like to be helped.

Give support and information

In providing support, it is important to provide accurate information, but only if the person asks for it. This may include telling them about a fatality in a mindful, compassionate way. Further, it is vital that the person is protected from retelling their story if they are not able or ready to do so; that is, they should only retell their story if they are willing and able to. It is also important to normalise the situation by emphasising that there will be stress reactions and anxious responses, both immediately and shortly after, and the person has to be reassured that they are not 'losing their mind'. In most cases, the high anxiety state subsides within a few weeks.

Encourage appropriate professional help

After four weeks, some return to normal functioning should be expected. However, it is vital to seek appropriate professional help if the person is still:

- feeling very upset or fearful
- unable to escape intense, ongoing distressing feelings
- displaying unconventional withdrawal behaviours
- hypervigilant or having nightmares about the trauma
- unable to experience happiness or pleasure
- unable to carry out their usual activities.

Appropriate help can include making use of employee assistance programs at their workplace or seeing their GP for further support and intervention.

Encourage other supports

Encourage the person to self-identify other pre-existing supports they have. This includes increasing self-care activities, getting plenty of rest and participating in pleasurable activities. Remind the person to avoid unhelpful coping strategies such as working too hard or substance use during this time, as this can slow and impair their ability to personally integrate their experience of the traumatic event.

CULTURAL CONSIDERATIONS OF MHFA WITHIN VULNERABLE GROUPS

Cultural awareness allows the MHFA responder to understand how the concepts of health and illness are cognitively framed. This is important because it can guide the beliefs and views about health and well-being of the person being assisted. Simply stated, this involves significant considerations. The first is being aware that the person being assisted may have a different cultural background and hence an understanding that differs from our own. This consideration can be helpful when seeking to learn about underpinning beliefs a person's culture may contain surrounding mental health and mental illness. Second, it is also important to consider how our own cultural beliefs and the community we are from shapes and influences us. Questions we can ask ourselves include:

- Could there be conflict between our cultural beliefs and those of the consumer?
- Do we need to put our views to one side in order to be an effective MHFA responder? (For more information, refer to Chapter 5.)

Moreover, demonstrating cultural safety as an MHFA responder is equally important. This involves respect for the person's culture and using appropriate or neutral language in our communication. It also involves never shaming the person through our words or deeds. Supporting the individual's right to form decisions around obtaining culturally based care is vitally important.

Vulnerable population groups

A person's cultural identity and their connection to culture (both their own and the dominant culture at large) form an important function in their understanding and perception of health and the way they communicate about health. The following groups have been identified as requiring special consideration due to their overrepresentation of mental health conditions.

Aboriginal and Torres Strait Islander peoples

Aboriginal and Torres Strait Islander peoples are nearly three times more likely to be psychologically distressed than other Australians and twice as likely to die by suicide (ABS, 2015). Many Aboriginal and Torres Strait Islander peoples have different beliefs regarding health and well-being. A local Elder can provide cultural information specific to the region where you are practising MHFA. Generally, to practise cultural safety, ensure the person feels cared for, comfortable and respected.

Shame is a very important concept within many Aboriginal and Torres Strait Islander communities. This is because the experience of shame can be disempowering and overwhelming, and can act as a barrier to seeking professional help. Moreover, this experience of shame can be felt as a result of embarrassment or being singled out, or as a lack of respect from others or a breach of Aboriginal and Torres Strait Islander norms or taboos. Therefore, it is paramount that the MHFA responder avoids invoking feelings of shame in consumers.

Moreover, family and close friends are a cornerstone of Aboriginal and Torres Strait Islander culture. Therefore, you should expect involvement in caring for the person from family. However, always ask the person if they want family involvement, respecting that the person has the right to choose for themselves who they would like to be involved (Hart et al., 2009).

LGBTQ(IA+)

Sexual orientation, sexuality and gender identification are fluid and lie across a spectrum, as opposed to being fixed classifications. These factors can also change and evolve over a person's lifetime. The term LGBTQ(IA+) (lesbian, gay, bisexual, transgender, transexual, queer, intersex, asexual and more) is used to include all *non-identified* cisgender (individuals whose birth gender correlates to their personal identity) and/ or heterosexual people. This is an important point because it is a reminder not to make assumptions based on your own experience, understanding about or being LGBTQ(IA+). The LGBTQ(IA+) experience refers to people's experience of romantic, sexual attraction and/or behaviour in addition to their gender identity and in some cases intersex variation (MHFA Australia, 2016).

LGBTQ(IA+) experiences do not, in themselves, cause mental health conditions, but can be associated with specific stressors. These stressors include actual or potential abuse, discrimination, insensitive treatment, minority group status, prejudice and violence (MHFA Australia, 2016). When compared with heterosexual people, LGBTQ(IA+) are twice as likely to experience anxiety (31.5% compared with 14.1%) and three times as likely to experience depression and related conditions (19% compared with 6%) (ABS, 2008).

Moreover, not all people experience distress regarding their LGBTQ(IA+) experience. Therefore, never assume that LGBTQ(IA+) experiences are related to any mental health issues a person may have or distress that they are experiencing. What is important, however, is to consider how these factors may impact on your application of ALGEE and if it bears relevance to the distress that has been identified. This is of particular importance when giving support and information, encouraging support from a health professional (e.g. have you recommended an LGBTQ(IA+) sensitive health carer?) and even when identifying other supports (e.g. are their family aware and supportive versus rejecting and combative?).

Finally, if the person does not feel at ease disclosing to you or, conversely, you are not comfortable, then assist them to locate someone else – unless it is a crisis situation and you are the only person available. If this is the case, refer to specific MHFA crisis management previously discussed in this chapter.

Older adults

The WHO refers to an an older person as someone over the age of 60 (WHO, 2018b). It is a common misperception that depression is normal in the older adult; this is inaccurate. Depression however, is three-to-four times more common in people with dementia compared with older people without dementia (Dementia Australia, 2018). Physical and mental health, however, are intimately related; for example, depression can lead to poor physical health in older adults. Moreover, older adults with ischaemic heart disease have a higher incidence of depression (Gan et al., 2014; WHO, 2015). Consider the stressors in this cohort such as loss of independence due to ill health either chronic or acute, mobility challenges, bereavement, loss of financial status or independence, retirement and potential loss of meaning or purpose. All of these factors can result in psychological distress that can initiate a mental health issue. Further, it is equally important to consider that an older adult's mental health problem may not be related to their age or experiencing these challenges. Refer also to Chapter 16.

The use of MHFA in this instance needs to consider, and then incorporate the above factors into the application of MHFA for the older adult. This can be useful when identifying how to approach, assess and assist an older adult. Furthermore, it can illustrate the best way to give support and information in the provision of the MHFA response. Finally, it can also assist in fine-tuning the application of relevant resources for this cohort when applying ALGEE in these specific circumstances.

Youth

The adolescent phase of youth is the peak period of onset of mental health issues. Up to half of this cohort who experience a mental health condition will have had their first episode by 18 years of age. This age group also carries a low level of mental health literacy (understanding) and a high level of stigma towards individuals with mental health issues (Hart et al., 2016). Moreover, they are less willing to seek out health care providers and prefer to disclose their mental health status to peers rather than adults. The role of the MHFA responder in this instance is to assist the person in overcoming perceptions of stigma and to identify options for professional adult assistance and other supportive structures – usually peer based. The importance of this cannot be overstated due to this stage of life being pivotal in the development of foundation structures in a person's work, education, relationships and peer development.

MENTAL HEALTH FIRST AID FOR CARERS

Advocacy and care activities can be very rewarding to a carer. They can provide a sense of personal achievement and empowerment. However, they also carry with them some personal risk. These may include exposure to unfamiliar situations, expressing your views and having them challenged, a fear of failure creating inaction, and carer burnout. Different advocacy activities also require different personal characteristics, knowledge and resources. Moreover, recognising that not all advocacy activities will be successful is an important factor. All of these components can lead to harmful or prolonged levels of stress for the carer if not clearly identified.

Self-care practices

It is important to recognise the necessity of self-care practices. This is due to care-giving increasing the risk of the carer feeling depressed and developing physical health-related issues secondary to ongoing stress. You might find, after the provision of mental health first aid to a distressed person, that you feel worn out, frustrated, angry or even disrespected. What can assist at this time is identifying triggers and planning for times in the future when your care-giving will be needed in acute situations. This can assist you as the caregiver in having an enhanced sense of preparedness and serve to reduce stressful feelings that can arise in these crisis situations.

Additionally, you may need to respond to the feelings and reactions that you had set aside during your encounter as an MHFA responder. It can be helpful at these times to find a person or a trusted colleague with whom to debrief. Remember to respect the consumer's right to privacy and confidentiality if the colleague is not directly involved in the care of the person you are debriefing about.

Other useful practices that are known to improve personal mood and health include eating well, regular sleeping patterns, relaxation practices – including mindfulness, relaxed breathing and other relaxation techniques and meditation – and physical activity. Finally, scheduling enjoyable activities and undertaking activities that have previously assisted you are also helpful. These should be scheduled regularly and time allocated to ensure they are completed.

CHAPTER RESOURCES

SUMMARY

- Mental health first aid (MHFA) involves using a series of responses and actions to assist a person experiencing a crisis or worsening of a mental health condition. MHFA uses an acronym titled ALGEE to flexibly implement responses relevant to the individual's needs at the time. The ALGEE acronym is used to guide the health practitioner's thoughts, actions and interventions across the spectrum of common mental health conditions discussed in this chapter: anxiety, depression, psychosis, substance use and suicidality.
- MHFA involves respect for a person's culture and using appropriate or neutral language in communication. It also involves never shaming the person through words or deeds.

Supporting the individual's right to form decisions around obtaining culturally based care is essential.

- Advocacy and care activities can be very rewarding for a carer but can also be challenging. Exposure to unfamiliar situations, expressing views and having them challenged, a fear of failure creating inaction, and carer burnout can have emotional and/or physical impacts on carers. Seeking support/guidance from trusted people and maintaining your own health and well-being is essential.

REVIEW QUESTIONS

1 The three key interventions for assisting a suicidal person are:
   a Rationalise with them to change their mind, get them to focus on the positives in their life, tell them others have felt this way also
   b If you think they are suicidal, ask them directly, work together to keep them safe, connect them to professional help
   c Detain them in a room, call a family member from a separate room and give them space
   d None of the above
2 When applying mental health first aid to a person experiencing psychosis, it is best to:
   a Not rationalise with the person's delusions or hallucinations

   b Acknowledge the distress and impact they are experiencing
   c Avoid the use of humour and sarcasm to lighten the situation
   d All of the above
3 Cultural considerations to vulnerable groups are important because:
   a There is a statistical overrepresentation of mental health illness
   b Cultural safety is an important consideration when providing MHFA
   c Avoiding inducing shame can increase avoidance of professional help seeking
   d All of the above

CRITICAL THINKING

1 Can you correctly recall the acronym actions (in order) for the MHFA action plan?
2 Can you remember the names and prevalence (in order) of the most common mental health conditions?

3 What actions are undertaken in an MHFA crisis involving anxiety where a person has never experienced a panic attack before?

USEFUL WEBSITES

■ beyondblue: http://www.beyondblue.org.au
■ Head to Health: http://www.headtohealth.gov.au

■ Mental Health First Aid Australia: http://www.MHFA.com.au

REFLECT ON THIS

People's experience of anxiety during the COVID-19 pandemic

At the beginning of this chapter, Figure 26.1 presented a way of understanding the range of interventions for mental health issues and conditions. Many of the concepts explored in-depth through the book have been integrated and applied in this chapter.

1 If we consider anxiety with no associated crisis as one example presented in this chapter, how could you apply these ideas to people's experience of anxiety related to the COVID-19 pandemic?

2 Do the ideas in this chapter help you understand the factors and risks associated with the increase in substance use (such as alcohol) that has occurred during the pandemic? An interesting article to help you explore this issue further is the following: Colbert, S., Wilkinson, C., Thornton, L. & Richmond, R. (2020). COVID⊠19 and alcohol in Australia: Industry changes and public health impacts. *Drug and Alcohol Review*, 39, 435–40. https://doi-org.ezproxy1.acu.edu.au/10.1111/dar.13092

REFERENCES

Australian Bureau of Statistics (ABS). (2008). *National Survey of Mental Health and Wellbeing: Summary of Results, 2007*. Cat. no. 4326.0. Canberra: ABS. Retrieved from http://www.abs.gov.au/ausstats/abs@.nsf/mf/4326.0.

Australian Bureau of Statistics (ABS). (2015). *Australian Aboriginal and Torres Strait Islander Health Survey: First Results, 2012–13*.

Cat. no. 4727.0.55.001. Canberra: ABS. retrieved from http://www.abs.gov.au/ausstats/abs@.nsf/mf/4727.0.55.001.

Australian Institute of Health and Welfare (AIHW). (2011). *Australian Burden of Disease Study: Impact and Causes of Illness and Death in Australia*. Retrieved from https://www.aihw.gov.au/reports/

burden-of-disease/abds-impact-and-causes-of-illness-death-2011/contents/highlights.

Australian Institute of Health and Welfare (AIHW). (2017). *National Drug Strategy Household Survey 2016: Detailed Findings Drug Statistics Series No. 31*. Cat. no. PHE 214. Canberra: AIHW. Retrieved from https://www.aihw.gov.au/reports/illicit-use-of-drugs/ndshs-2016-detailed/contents/table-of-contents.

Australian Institute of Health and Welfare (AIHW). (2018). *Mental Health Services in Australia: In Brief 2018*. Canberra: AIHW. Retrieved from www.aihw.gov.au/reports/mental-health-services/mental-health-services-in-australia-in-brief-2018/contents/table-of-contents.

Australian Resuscitation Council. (2008). *ANZCOR Guideline 9.2.8: First Aid Management of Hyperventilation Syndrome*. Retrieved from https://resus.org.au/guidelines.

Australian Resuscitation Council. (2016). *ANZCOR Guideline 2: Managing an Emergency*. Retrieved from https://resus.org.au/guidelines.

Bentall, R.P., Wickham, S., Shevlin, M. & Varese, F. (2012). Do specific early-life adversities lead to specific symptoms of psychosis? A study from the 2007 The Adult Psychiatric Morbidity Survey. *Schizophrenia Bulletin*, 38(4), 734–40. doi:10.1093/schbul/sbs049

beyondblue. (2018). Homepage. Retrieved from https://www.beyondblue.org.au.

Colbert, S., Wilkinson, C., Thornton, L. & Richmond, R. (2020). COVID 19 and alcohol in Australia: Industry changes and public health impacts. *Drug and Alcohol Review*, 39, 435–40. https://doi-org.ezproxy1.acu.edu.au/10.1111/dar.13092

Crisis Prevention Institute. (2019). Homepage. Retrieved from https://www.crisisprevention.com.

Dementia Australia. (2018). Depression and dementia. Retrieved from https://www.dementia.org.au/national/support-and-services/carers/behaviour-changes/depression-and-dementia.

Froggatt, T. & Liersch-Sumskis, S. (2014). Assessment of mental health and mental illness. In N.G. Procter, H.P. Hamer, D. McGarry, R. Wilson & T. Froggatt (eds), *Mental Health: A Person-centred Approach*. Melbourne: Cambridge University Press.

Gan, Y., Gong, Y., Tong, X., Sun, H., Cong, Y., Dong, X., … Lu, Z. (2014). Depression and the risk of coronary heart disease: A meta-analysis of prospective cohort studies. *BMC Psychiatry*, 14, 371. doi:10.1186/s12888-014-0371-z

Ghio, L., Gotelli, S., Marcenaro, M., Amore, M. & Natta, W. (2014). Duration of untreated illness and outcomes in unipolar depression: A systematic review and meta-analysis. *Journal of Affective Disorders*, 152, 45–51.

Hart, L.M., Jorm, A.F., Kanowski, L.G., Kelly, C.M. & Langlands, R.L. (2009). Mental health first aid for Indigenous Australians: Using Delphi consensus studies to develop guidelines for culturally appropriate responses to mental health problems. *BMC Psychiatry*, 9(1), 47.

Hart, L.M., Mason, R.J., Kelly, C.M., Cvetkovski, S. & Jorm, A.F. (2016). 'Teen Mental Health First Aid': A description of the program and an

initial evaluation. *International Journal of Mental Health Systems*, 10(1), 3. doi:10.1186/s13033-016-0034-1

Kelly, C.M., Jorm, A.F. & Wright, A. (2007). Improving mental health literacy as a strategy to facilitate early intervention for mental disorders. *Medical Journal of Australia*, 187(7), S26.

Kingston, A.H., Jorm, A.F., Kitchener, B.A., Hides, L., Kelly, C.M., Morgan, A.J. & Lubman, D.I. (2009). Helping someone with problem drinking: Mental health first aid guidelines – a Delphi expert consensus study. *BMC Psychiatry*, 9(1), 79.

Kingston, A.H., Morgan, A.J., Jorm, A.F., Hall, K., Hart, L.M., Kelly, C.M. & Lubman, D.I. (2011). Helping someone with problem drug use: A Delphi consensus study of consumers, carers, and clinicians. *BMC Psychiatry*, 11(1), 3.

Kitchener, B.A., Jorm, A.F. & Kelly, C.M. (2017). *Mental Health First Aid Manual* (4th edn). Melbourne: Mental Health First Aid Australia.

Mental Health First Aid (MHFA) Australia. (2016). *Considerations When Providing Mental Health First Aid to an LGBTIQ+ Person*. Melbourne: Mental Health First Aid Australia. Retrieved from https://MHFA.com.au/mental-health-first-aid-guidelines.

Nasser, E.H. & Overholser, J.C. (2005). Recovery from major depression: The role of support from family, friends, and spiritual beliefs. *Acta Psychiatrica Scandinavica*, 111(2), 125–32.

National Collaborating Centre for Mental Health (NICE). (2014). *Psychosis and Schizophrenia in Adults: Treatment and Management. Updated Edition 2014. NICE Clinical Guidelines, No. 178*. Retrieved from https://www.ncbi.nlm.nih.gov/books/NBK248060.

Perry, B.L. & Pescosolido, B.A. (2015). Social network activation: The role of health discussion partners in recovery from mental illness. *Social Science & Medicine*, 125, 116–28.

Pistrang, N., Barker, C. & Humphreys, K. (2008). Mutual help groups for mental health problems: A review of effectiveness studies. *American Journal of Community Psychology*, 42(1–2), 110–21.

Stanley, B. & Brown, G.K. (2012). Safety planning intervention: A brief intervention to mitigate suicide risk. *Cognitive and Behavioural Practice*, 19(2), 256–64.

World Health Organization (WHO). (1946). Preamble to the Constitution of the World Health Organization as adopted by the International Health Conference, New York, 19–22 June, 1946; signed 22 July 1946 by the representatives of 61 States (Official Records of the World Health Organization, no. 2, p. 100) and entered into force on 7 April 1948.

World Health Organization (WHO). (2015). *World Report on Ageing and Health*. Geneva: WHO. Retrieved from http://apps.who.int/iris/bitstream/10665/186463/1/9789240694811_eng.pdf?ua=1.

World Health Organization (WHO). (2018). *Mental Health: Strengthening our Response*. Retrieved from http://www.who.int/news-room/fact-sheets/detail/mental-health-strengthening-our-response.

World Health Organization (2018b). Ageing and Health. Retrieved from https://www.who.int/news-room/fact-sheets/detail/ageing-and-health.

APPENDIX: MENTAL STATE EXAMINATION (MSE)

MSE DOMAIN	OBJECTIVE AND SUBJECTIVE DATA
General appearance and behaviour	
Speech	
Mood and affect (including sleep, appetite and libido)	
Thought Form/Processes: Content: Themes:	

Perception	
Cognition	
Judgement	
Orientation	
Memory	
Insight	
Risk assessment (includes risk to self, risk to others, risk from others (vulnerability)	

SUPPORTIVE NURSING INTERVENTIONS	RATIONAL INTERVENTIONS (HOW THE INTERVENTION(S) WILL SUPPORT THE CONSUMER)

Signature & designation: _____

Date: _____

GLOSSARY

A

active phase Follows the prodrome of schizophrenia and is characterised by a florid stage of symptoms where prominent features of the disorder (delusions, hallucinations, negative symptoms, thought disorder) are evident

acute dystonia A series of potentially fatal muscle spasms, which can occur early in treatment with antipsychotic medication

acute stress disorder Development of characteristic symptoms lasting from three days to one month following exposure to one or more traumatic events

affect The objective, observable expression of an individual's mood. Different terms used to describe affect include congruent, incongruent, restricted, blunted and flat

agency A person's ability to influence their lives and others within their sphere

aggressive communication To communicate in a way that one person's needs are belittled and disregarded. The outcome is that the aggressive communicator has their needs/goals met at the expense of another person

agnosia Complete or limited inability to recognise people or objects

agoraphobia An intense fear or anxiety state in response to being in open or enclosed spaces

agranulocytosis A bone marrow suppression disorder resulting in a lowered white blood cell count that is associated with antipsychotic treatment with clozapine. This serious condition renders the consumer unable to fight infection

akathisia An internal state of restlessness where the individual finds it difficult to sit still and feels the need to move. A common side effect from antipsychotic therapy

ALGEE Approach the person regarding your concerns; Listen and communicate non-judgementally; Give support and information; Encourage the person to get professional help; Encourage other supports

alleles Multiple forms of a gene developing from a genetic mutation and which are located in the same position on a chromosome

ambivalence A state of experiencing conflicting feelings towards a situation or person

anhedonia A lack of pleasure gained from previously pleasurable activities; for example, a man who used to love walking his dog no longer feels pleasure when doing this. Common to depression and is a negative symptom of schizophrenia

anorexia nervosa (AN) An eating disorder characterised by a failure to maintain normal weight (for age, gender, etc.) and impaired body image

anterograde Loss of ability to form new memories

anticholinergic side effects Usually occur in typical antipsychotic agents but do occur in atypical agents (namely clozapine) and include constipation, dry mouth, urinary incontinence, blurred vision, increased heart rate, decreased sweating, issues with memory and cognition and sedation

antidepressants Medications that elevate mood by enhancing the transmission of neurochemicals, particularly serotonin and noradrenaline. This occurs through blocking their reuptake at the synapse, inhibiting their metabolism and/or enhancing the activity of the receptors

antisocial personality disorder (APD) Disorder characterised by evidence of conduct disorder (CD) behaviours in the individual prior to the age of 15, and can only be diagnosed in individuals older than 18 years who have evident CD behaviours

anxiety A normal human response to a stressful situation which may involve worry and fear

anxiety disorder Overwhelming, prolonged worry or fear resulting in significant impact on an individual's life. Disordered anxiety impedes the individual from living their life, and can occur in the absence or presence of a stimulus

aphasia The loss of ability to communicate verbally due to damage to the area of the brain involved in understanding and expressing language

apraxia Loss of motor coordination and/or sensation in a particular group of muscles. This impacts on the person's capacity and independence to engage in purposeful activity or movements such as moving their arms, or speaking clearly because they cannot use their tongue or mouth

article synopses Structured summaries that provide an appraisal of an individual research study or review

assertive communication Communication between people that communicates needs and addresses issues in a respectful, direct and open way. It is communication that is not threatening, intimidating or bullying

assertive outreach A coordinated and flexible way of delivery care to hard-to-reach groups

asylum An institution where people with mental health conditions were housed

ataxia Lack of coordination

attendant An historical term for a male mental health nurse

attitudes A person's thoughts and feelings towards something that are then reflected in their communication and behaviour

autism spectrum disorder (ASD) Condition identified by persistent deficits in social interaction, social communication, and the presence of restricted, repetitive patterns of behaviour, interests or activities. A person diagnosed with ASD will experience these issues to varying degrees depending on their developmental level, age and the severity of the disorder

autonomy The right of an individual to be independent and to have the freedom to make their own choices (e.g. self-governing)

avoidant personality disorder (AVPD) Disorder characterised by a reluctance for social interactions and feelings of inadequacy

B

baby boomer A person born between 1946 and 1964

background question General clinical knowledge questions that help understanding of an issue in its broadest context and establish what is already known about a clinical issue

behavioural difficulties The observable responses of a person that are disruptive or difficult for others to tolerate

behavioural orientation A person's behaviour can be objectively observed and studied. Personality is determined by prior learning and shaped by the environment

belief A proposition that a person holds to be true

beneficence Our moral obligation to be charitable, and to show kindness and mercy towards others

best practice or clinical guidelines A critical appraisal of the best available evidence for a clinical practice issue intended to authoritatively inform clinical practice of the current state of knowledge

bilateral ECT Electrodes are placed on either both temporal or frontal areas of the scalp

binge-eating disorder (BED) The consumption of large quantities of food consumed in a short period of time (e.g. two hours)

biomedical orientation Physiological explanation of health and illness that categorises a condition based on a cluster of observable and measurable signs and symptoms

bipolar I disorder (BDI) A serious mental health condition characterised by episodes of mania, but is also commonly associated with episodes of depression and hypomania

bipolar II disorder (BDII) A milder form of BDI in which the individual experiences episodes of depression and hypomania, but never mania. There are no psychotic features to this disorder

bizarre delusion A delusion that could have no basis in reality (is impossible), such as a belief that a person can breathe in water and live under the sea or a male consumer who believes he is pregnant with God's baby

blood alcohol level (BAL) or concentration (BAC) The amount of alcohol in a person's bloodstream

blunted affect A lack of expression of emotional intensity that is more severe than a restricted affect

body mass index (BMI) A measurement of weight and height that is useful in the diagnosis of eating disorders

borderline personality disorder (BPD) A disorder characterised by unstable interpersonal relationships with others, impulsivity and poor self-image

bradycardia Low pulse rate measured at less than 60 beats per minute

bulimia nervosa (BN) An eating disorder characterised by behaviours such as eating excessive quantities of food, a feeling of lack of control over eating behaviours, actions that prevent weight gain (such as purging), and self-evaluation that hinges on idealised weight and body shape

bullying Behaviours from one or more person(s) that threaten or intimidate another individual or group

burden of disease The impact of a health condition as measured by the financial rates of disease and illness and death rates

burden of proof The obligation to offer evidence that a court or jury could reasonably believe in support of a contention

C

cardiovascular Pertaining to the heart and blood vessels

case-controlled studies Involve identifying patients (cases) with the outcome of interest and control patients without the same outcome, and then looking back over time to evaluate the exposure of interest

catatonia A rare condition seen in schizophrenia characterised by movement distortion

challenging behaviours Repeated behaviours that impact on a person's physical and emotional well-being, including their relationships with others

circumstantiality A form of thought disturbance where the consumer replies to questions in an indirect manner using overly inclusive or irrelevant or superfluous information

clanging Where words are chosen for their sound, not their meaning

classical conditioning Learning that results from the repeated combination of an unconditioned stimulus with a conditioned stimulus leading to a conditioned response

clinical decision A reasoned judgement involving complex problem-solving skills

clinical question Background or foreground question relevant to the situation, person, population or health care issue

clinical reasoning A decision-making process that applies critical thinking skills in a systematic and rigorous approach to clinical issues or questions

clinical review A multidisciplinary review of care given to consumers

cluster *A* personality disorders Characterised by behaviours that are odd, eccentric or paranoid and encompassing paranoid, schizotypal and schizoid personality disorders

cluster *B* personality disorders Characterised by behaviours that are emotional and dramatic, with strong manipulative tendencies encompassing antisocial, borderline, histrionic and narcissistic personality disorders

cluster *C* personality disorders Characterised by behaviours that are anxious or fearful, and usually associated with a high degree of stress

cognition Thought process experienced by a person shown through speech

cognitive behavioural therapy (CBT) A therapy based on the idea that a person experiences difficulty in life because of the way in which they perceive events in their lives and interactions with others, their thoughts and the thought patterns that result. CBT focuses on helping a person

to change their thinking patterns about themselves and/or events, to enable them to respond in a more positive way

cognitive functioning Higher level brain function incorporating the processing of information, acquisition and application of knowledge

cognitive symptoms Characterised by issues with executive functioning (EF), poor concentration and memory

cognitive theory (CT) Proposes links between thinking, attitudes, understanding and feelings with behaviour

cohort studies Involve identifying two groups (cohorts) where one group is the control group and the other is exposed to the experimental condition and outcomes evaluated over the time period

collateral history Obtaining pertinent assessment information for other key sources such as family

colonialism A practice of domination whereby one people or group assumes control over another

colonisation The process of settling among and establishing control over the Indigenous people of an area

command hallucinations Auditory hallucinations telling the individual to do something (e.g. 'Pick up the book and place it by the door')

communication The verbal, non-verbal or written exchange of information. When we communicate, we give and/or receive information

community treatment orders (CTOs) An order made by the responsible clinician to give a person supervised treatment in the community

compulsion A behaviour that is repetitive, and the act of undertaking it reduces anxiety; for example, handwashing continuously to rid the skin of germs or rechecking locks. Compulsions (or rituals) may include mental acts such as praying or counting

conditioned response A learnt response (see *conditioned stimulus*)

conditioned stimulus Condition when a neutral stimulus, after being repeatedly combined with an unconditioned stimulus, elicits a conditioned response

conduct disorder (CD) Disorder characterised by aggression towards people and animals, property destruction, theft, lying and the serious violation of the rights of others. Seen in childhood and adolescence

confabulation When a person makes up a story or part of a story to fill in the gaps in their memory. They recount the event in great detail and the details sound reasonable to the person listening

conscious mental processes Awareness of events, thoughts and feelings and ability to recall them

consumer Describes a person who identifies as having a lived experience of a mental health condition. This experience may be past or current

consumer consultant A person who has a lived experience of a mental health condition. They work within organisations and the community to provide consultation about issues and needs important to consumers. They also facilitate consumer involvement and connections with consumer organisations

conversion disorder Condition where the individual presents with various neurological symptoms suggestive of neurological impairment (e.g. Parkinson's disease). However, investigation yields negative results for a neurological basis for the symptoms

countertransference Where the therapist, or mental health nurse, has an emotional response to the person they are working with; for example, the nurse who is working with a consumer who reminds her of her brother, to whom she is very close

Country Can be described as both a geographic location and a 'nourishing terrain' with which Aboriginal and Torres Strait Islander peoples have physical, spiritual, cultural and social connections

critical appraisal A process of systematically evaluating and interpreting the validity and relevance of the research evidence

critical appraisal tools (CATs) Checklists that facilitate an objective, analytical and systematic evaluation of original research studies

culture shock A sense of unease, isolation and low mood when a person is confronted with a new culture and way of life

cyanosis Blueish discolouration of a person's extremities, especially the lips and skin, which is caused by a lack of oxygen.

cyclothymic disorder A mood disorder characterised by mild hypomania and mild depression that does not warrant official diagnosis of either presentation due to its chronicity, reduced severity and duration

D

de-escalation A communication style applied in interactions whereby the purpose is to prevent amplification of conflict (e.g. verbal aggression or physical violence). Clinicians working in mental health employ these techniques in communicating with consumers who are becoming increasingly distressed or agitated

defence mechanisms Unconscious responses by the ego used to reduce anxiety

and prevent the ego from being overwhelmed by the demands of the id and the superego

deinstitutionalisation The deliberate decision to move from institutional to community-based mental health care in the 1980s by closing large psychiatric hospitals and increasing the delivery of community-based treatment and co-location of mental health units into mainstream health care facilities.

deliberate self-harm (DSH) An intentional act of harm where the desire is to inflict pain or injury to the self, but not to die. See also *non-suicidal self-injury*

delusion A fixed, false belief that is held despite evidence to the contrary, and is not shared by a majority

dementia A group of disorders represented by progressive deterioration in cognition, behaviour and capacity to perform activities of daily living independently. Dementia is not a normal part of the ageing process

denial Refusal to accept the reality of a situation that the ego would find too threatening

dependent personality disorder (DPD) Disorder characterised by passiveness, deferring to others to make decisions, and separation anxiety

depersonalisation A feeling of unreality where a person may feel that parts of themselves, or entirely, do not exist

depressed mood Clinically assessed low mood that meets criteria for depression

derailment Thoughts progress in an illogical manner and are not logically connected. Also referred to as *loosening of associations*

derealisation Change in a person's sense of reality, where they may feel as if the world around them does not exist or that their surroundings have changed

descriptive design Typically uses observational or survey methods to provide an accurate summary or definition of a specified event, experience or participants

detention Describes the involuntary or compulsory apprehension of a person adhering to appropriate local legislation. Some mental health acts use the term 'custody' instead of detention. Consumers in detention are unable to leave a mental health facility

diagnostic overshadowing When symptoms of mental illness are mistakenly attributed to some cause/condition – commonly used in reference to physical symptoms, but originally used in relation to intellectual disability

dialectical behaviour therapy (DBT) Therapy that aims to enhance a person's capacity to deal with the difficulties they

experience in managing their emotional responses to interactions and events

diaphoresis Profuse, uncomfortable sweating

disinhibited reactive attachment disorder (RAD) Refers to a child who is not highly selective in their choice of attachment figures and is more likely to express attachment towards a stranger/new acquaintance than their own primary caregiver

disinhibited social engagement disorder (DSED) A condition related to severe neglect experienced by a child in the first two years of their life. DESD involves a pattern of inappropriate, overly familiar behaviour towards strangers by a child. This is seen in behaviours such as a lack of caution towards strangers and indiscriminate friendships

disorganised speech Characterised by speech that is almost incomprehensible and fragmented

displacement Transferring a strong emotion from the original object/person that would be unacceptable to express to another more socially acceptable (or 'safer') object or person

dissociation Distortion in imperative psychological states of functioning such as cognition, consciousness, memory, identity and situational awareness

dizygotic twins Twins that develop from the fertilisation of two eggs by two sperm

dopamine A neurotransmitter involved in motor coordination and control, cognition, attention and emotional behaviour; for example, overactivity of dopamine is understood to be associated with schizophrenia and mania

duty of care A responsibility held by all nurses whereby the nurse is accountable for reducing or limiting the potential harm or injury a patient may experience

dysphoria A feeling of unhappiness, anguish and distress

dysthymia Mild chronic symptoms of depression. Now referred to as persistent depressive disorder

E

echolalia A form of thought disturbance where the consumer mimics or echoes the words or actions of another (usually in a mocking manner)

ecomap A visual representation of the social and personal relations between family members and their environment

effect size (ES) Available research evidence to answer a specified question; a way of measuring the predicted strength that an intervention or treatment will have on a specific outcome

ego The component of Freud's personality structure that mediates between the demands of the id and superego and the external reality of a situation

electroconvulsive therapy (ECT) A medical procedure whereby an electrical current is passed through the brain to produce a modified seizure. Used to treat major depressive disorder

elevated mood Mood that is overtly cheerful or 'high'. On a self-rating scale, the consumer may rate their mood 10/10 or above. Seen in mania

emotional intelligence The extent to which a person is aware of, able to manage and express emotions in their interactions with others

emotional labour The effort required to suppress one's own emotions in order to effectively care for others and also care for oneself

empathy Understanding another person's experience of a situation through the use of active listening skills. The goal is to understand their situation, thoughts, feelings and behaviours

erotomanic delusions A delusional belief more common in women where the individual believes that someone else (who is usually of a higher 'status', such as a celebrity) is in love with them. Seen in mania and schizophrenia

evidence-based practice (EBP) The utilisation of critically appraised research-based information in nursing decisions

excoriation A compulsive skin-picking condition usually of the face, hands and arms resulting in skin damage and scarring

executive functioning (EF) Requires sustained and divided attention, and individuals experiencing difficulties with EF may exhibit issues with planning or implementing goals, problem solving and undertaking goal-directed behaviours. Seen in schizophrenia

expansive mood A mood state where individuals lack restraint in expressing their feelings or emotions and are often grandiose in their self-disclosure

extrapyramidal symptoms (EPS) A series of movement symptoms affecting the central nervous system, and a side effect of antipsychotic medication. EPS include akathisia, parkinsonism, tardive dyskinesia and acute dystonia

F

factitious disorder (formerly Munchausen by proxy) A condition where an individual will purposefully hurt or make another person (usually a child) ill (usually by poisoning them), seeking frequent medical attention or requesting a barrage of invasive, costly and painful tests

fatuous mood A mood state that is silly or foolish. Seen in mania

filtered (pre-appraised) information A systematic and defined appraisal of the research evidence for a specific topic, intervention or health care problem

flat affect An absence of emotional expression

flight of ideas A form of thought disorder where ideas rapidly change and are unable to be expressed completely, resulting in incomprehensible communication. Often seen in mania but can present in schizophrenia

foetal alcohol spectrum disorder (FASD) A range of physical and/or neuro-developmental issues that can lead to social, emotional, learning and behavioural issues. It is a result of exposure of the developing foetus during pregnancy

foetal alcohol syndrome (FAS) Sits under FASD as one of four conditions that are considered to be the consequence of exposure of the developing foetus to alcohol during pregnancy

foreground question Specific clinical question that drives the research strategy and directly informs clinical practice decisions

functional status The extent to which an older person can maintain their activities of daily living, which includes also *instrumental activities of daily living*

G

gender dysphoria A condition experienced by individuals who feel their gender identity differs from what they were assigned (or born) with; for example, a male who identifies more as a female. This incongruence results in dysphoria, or anguish and distress

genogram Visually records family members and their relations over a minimum of three generations, representing the nature of relationships between family members and the types of issues or patterns across generations

genuineness The congruence (or matching) of verbal and non-verbal behaviour seen in a person's interactions with others

grandiosity An inflated sense of self-esteem, self-worth, self-importance, knowledge or power. Often seen in mania and hypomania

H

half-life The amount of time needed for a quantity of a substance to decrease to half its original volume

hallucination A disorder of sensory perception characterised by experiences originating from internal origin. Hallucinations may be auditory, visual, olfactory, gustatory, tactile, somatic or kinaesthetic

health A dynamic process of holistic well-being across multiple domains, including emotional, interpersonal, physical, psychological, social, cultural, economic and spiritual

hidden agenda An ulterior or hidden goal or motive that a person does not share with the rest of a group, but takes action to meet

hierarchy of needs According to Maslow's theory of motivation, the order in which human needs emerge and need to be met

histrionic personality disorder (HPD) A disorder characterised by a need to be the centre of attention, in addition to sexually seductive behaviours and suggestibility

hoarding disorder (HD) A condition associated with the acquisition or collection of items (that others may consider rubbish) and storing these items, resulting in clutter, uninhabitable space and hygiene issues. The condition is also associated with difficulty parting with items

homeostasis A physiological process where the body seeks to achieve an internal state of balance or equilibrium

horizontal nystagmus Rapid and repetitive movement of the eye (nystagmus) from side to side (horizontal)

horizontal violence Hostile and/or aggressive behaviour from one or more members of a team to one or more other members of that group

hyperreflexia Overactive reflexes

hypersomnia Excessive sleepiness; inability to stay awake

hyperthermia Increased body temperature above normal parameters

hypomania A period of mania characterised by mood elevation and similar to mania, yet lacks the need for hospitalisation and presence of psychotic features

hypothesis testing Research designed to statistically test if the assumed relationship (hypothesis) is supported by the data

I

iatrogenic Adverse symptoms experienced by a person as a consequence of therapeutic treatment

id The component of Freud's personality structure that is focused on immediate gratification of needs

illusion A misinterpretation of a real stimulus

inappropriate affect Incongruence between emotional feeling, tone and the idea, thought or speech accompanying it

infarct Death of a localised area of tissue or an organ (such as the brain) as a result of interrupted blood flow that means the specific area is not oxygenated

informed consent A process for getting permission before conducting a health care intervention on a person; is a voluntary agreement with an action proposed by another

inhibited reactive attachment disorder (RAD) Refers to a child who is detached socially and emotionally

insight A person's ability to decipher the causes of their behaviour and is often assessed in the context of their understanding of their illness. A consumer demonstrating poor insight will attribute psychotic experiences as real, rather than as a symptom of their illness

insomnia Sleeplessness, or an inability to sleep

institutionalisation The commitment of individuals to a restricted care environment, such as an asylum

instrumental activities of daily living For example, shopping, using the telephone

interpersonal communication The exchange of information such as ideas, feelings, emotions and thoughts, which are expressed between people through both verbal and non-verbal (e.g. body language) interactions

intersex A person who is born with any of several variations in sex characteristics

intoxication A state where a person is affected physically and psychologically due to overconsumption of alcohol or other drug

involuntary patient Depending on the state or territory, an involuntary patient is also known as a compulsory patient, and there are subtle variations to the definition depending on location. Generally, a compulsory or involuntary patient is someone who has been subject to an order under a Mental Health Act. This means they meet appropriate criteria to be detained for treatment, and that if they refuse treatment, they may be subjected to it regardless, detained in a hospital, or subject to a community order living in their own premises

involuntary treatment Refers to medical treatment undertaken without consent; the commitment of individuals to a restricted care environment, such as an asylum

J

judgement The ability to learn from previous experiences and apply it to new learning; to understand the consequences of actions

justice Ethical principle that implies our moral obligation to be fair and equitable

L

labile affect An affect that moves rapidly between different states

labile mood Unstable mood characterised by rapid, often exaggerated, mood swings and intense reactions

libido (Chapter 2) A Freudian term used to describe an individual's emotional energy derived from the underlying instinct of eros

Libido (Chapter 6) A term used to describe an individual's sexual drive, or their desire for engaging in sexual activity

loosening of associations Distorted thinking where ideas are so poorly linked they lack logical connections

lore As understood by Aboriginal and Torres Strait Islander peoples, consists of the stories and customs to be lived by as passed on inter-generationally through ceremonies and song from the Dreamtime. On the other hand, the 'law' was introduced by the British during colonial times as the new English justice system that all people in Australian society were expected to abide by

M

magical thinking A concept best defined by the notion 'thinking equates to doing'; for example, 'If I wear a yellow top today, I will get a pay rise'

maintenance behaviours Are aimed at maintaining a climate for group activities, to reduce hostilities and to enlist everyone's contribution

malodorous Unpleasant smell often resulting from poor personal hygiene

mania A presentation representative of bipolar I disorder characterised by a persistent elevated, expansive or irritable mood coupled with a lack of need for sleep and engagement in goal-directed activity. May be accompanied by psychosis

manic switching Phenomenon where individuals with BD taking antidepressants revert to mania

marginalised housing Housing options that reinforce marginalisation of people with a lived experience of mental illness; for example, unstable living arrangements, high rental demands, shared accommodation that places vulnerable people at risk of increased stress and lack of appropriate support(s)

mental capacity A multidimensional construct that is central to an individual's ability to make autonomous decisions

mental health Represents how a person thinks, feels and behaves. It is about social and emotional well-being. Mental health is represented by such things as having meaningful social connections and relationships, contributing to one's community, feeling valued and being able to deal with normal stresses in life

mental health first aid (MHFA) A series of responses and actions used to assist a person experiencing a crisis or worsening of a mental health condition

Mental Health Tribunal An independent statutory tribunal established under a Mental Health Act

metabolic syndrome (or *MetSy*) A condition characterised by hypertension, increased waist circumference, elevated blood glucose and triglyceride levels. *MetSy* is often caused by the second-generation antipsychotics clozapine and olanzapine

methylphenidate Stimulant medication used to treat behavioural and attention disorders such as attention deficit/hyperactivity disorder, oppositional defiant disorder and conduct disorder

mini mental state examination (MMSE) A commonly used set of questions for screening cognitive function

monozygotic twins Twins that develop from the fertilisation of two eggs by two sperm

mood The subjective internal feelings experienced by a person expressed through their feelings and emotions. Mood is described to the nurse in the consumer's own words or phrases such as 'depressed' or 'low'

mood disorder Disorder characterised by an extreme fluctuation in a person's mood that impacts on their thinking, emotions and behaviour. This fluctuation can be either extremely heightened or lowered. Depression and bipolar disorder are two commonly known mood disorders

morality principle A function of the morality principle motivates a person to behave in a way that is answerable to the moral and social norms of society

motivational interviewing A person-focused directive counselling approach that aims to help a person engage in behaviour change

multidisciplinary team Members from a range of disciplines who work in parallel. There is coordination, collaboration and conferring

N

narcissistic personality disorder (NPD) Disorder characterised by grandiosity and a need to be idealised and admired by others

natal boy/girl Biologically assigned gender at birth

negative cognitive triad Thinking that reflects a negative view of oneself, the world and the future

negative reinforcement The removal of unpleasant/averse stimuli makes the desired response more likely to occur in the future

negative symptoms Occur in schizophrenia and are characterised by affective blunting, anhedonia, social withdrawal, apathy, poverty of speech and thought

neologisms A form of thought disorder displaying the development of new words (e.g. think-a-lator)

neurotransmitter A chemical substance that is used in the central nervous system to transmit messages across synapses between neurons. Serotonin, norepinephrine and dopamine are all neurotransmitters

non-adherence Describes behaviours associated with medication and or/treatment (e.g. counselling) refusal

non-assertive communication Communication that results in the person trying to avoid conflict by letting another person meet their needs first. Communication that is subservient

non-maleficence Ability to obtain a favourable outcome by adopting the least harmful approach; 'do no harm'

non-suicidal self-injury Act or behaviour that intentionally causes harm or injury to oneself, but does not result in a fatal outcome. Also referred to as self-injury

normal affect Reactive facial expressions that are harmonious to the situation

O

obsession An intrusive and unwanted repetitive thought that results in anxiety and distress. Seen in obsessive-compulsive disorder, examples of obsessions include fear of germs or worry that doors are not locked

obsessive-compulsive disorder (OCD) A condition characterised by both obsessions and compulsions that result in intrusive and unwanted thoughts that are repetitive and usually result in anxiety and distress

obsessive-compulsive personality disorder (OCPD) A condition associated with perfectionism, controlling behaviours and a need for uniformity, resulting in serious interpersonal and occupational dysfunction

Oedipus complex Psychodynamic concept whereby a child represses their desire for a parent of the opposite gender and identifies with the parent of the same gender. In Freudian terms this refers to the male child's attraction to his mother

operant behavioural therapy Focuses on the premise that behaviours are learnt responses and as such individuals can learn alternative behaviours that are more positive or productive

operant conditioning Learning that occurs in response to the consequences a certain behaviour elicits. The behaviour will be strengthened or weakened depending on the type of consequence elicited

oppositional defiant disorder (ODD) A condition seen in childhood which is characterised by behavioural disruption and impulsiveness, in addition to angry, irritable and argumentative behaviours and vindictiveness towards others

P

panic attack A distressing physiological and cognitive response often in the absence of a trigger or stimulus. Symptoms include palpitations, sweating, shaking, fear of dying and numbness

paranoia Mistrust, suspicion and wariness of others without logical reason

paranoid personality disorder (PPD) Disorder characterised by suspicion and mistrust of others' intentions, believing them to be malicious

parkinsonism Movement disorder characterised by fine tremor, shuffling gait, cogwheel rigidity, drooling, masklike facial features and rigidity. A side effect of antipsychotic therapy

peer worker Someone who has personal experience of mental distress/mental health issues. Their role is to support other people who experience mental health issues through sharing their own recovery journey

perinatal depression Depression that can be experienced at any point from conception through to 12 months post-delivery of an infant

perinatal period Antenatal through to postnatal period and includes breastfeeding considerations

perseveration A form of thought disturbance characterised by the repetition of words or ideas

personality The unique set of thoughts, emotions and feelings that a person brings to their interactions with the total environment

personality disorder An enduring, inflexible pattern of personal experiences and behaviours that lead to social, occupational and interpersonal impairment or distress

personality trait A person's consistent (or enduring) way of thinking, feeling and behaving

pharmaceuticals Mixture/compound developed for use in the treatment of medical conditions

PICO An acronym used to structure clinical foreground questions

place A particular locality with measured distances; a socially occupied space; or the feelings and shared emotions that are meaningful to an individual or community of people

pleasure principle Means by which the id seeks to avoid psychological tension, pain and achieve pleasure

polypharmacy The use of multiple medications (routinely four or more) at the same time. Polypharmacy includes the use of over-the-counter, prescribed and alternative medicines

positional asphyxia A medical emergency caused from being placed in a prone position (and restrained) for any period of time

positive reinforcement Where a pleasant or positive consequence to a behaviour makes the same response more likely to occur again

positive symptoms Occur in schizophrenia and are characterised by hallucinations, delusions, hostility, paranoia, suspicion, movement disorder and thought, speech and organisational difficulties

postnatal depression The experience of depression by a woman across the childbearing continuum from the antenatal period up to 12 months post-delivery

post-traumatic stress disorder A condition where a person experiences a particular range of symptoms as a reaction after a person or people around them have been through a traumatic event. This event leads to a range of stress responses

poverty of speech The consumer uses few words in their conversation

poverty of thought Reduction in the quantity of thoughts

poverty of thought content Where a person expresses minimal speech. It can be a reflection of slowed-down thought processes associated with depression and is also a negative symptom of schizophrenia. This is reflected in speech that lacks spontaneity and details

preceptorship Informal supervision by a registered nurse of a student while on clinical placement

pressured speech Speech that is intense, loud, rapid and highly emphatic. Seen in mania and schizophrenia

prodrome The early, pre-florid stage of schizophrenia where symptoms of the disorder are emerging, reduced in intensity, and do not warrant a clinical diagnosis

projection Attributing personal impulses or desires that are socially unacceptable onto another person

protective factors Those factors that are seen to safeguard an individual from a mental health condition and/or suicide risk

psychodynamic approach An approach to understanding how the 'human psyche' is in control of an individual's behaviour

psychoeducation An interactive and collaborative process whereby the mental health nurse, consumer and family members engage in information sharing and education on matters related to maintaining health and well-being. This includes education on medications, stress management, relapse signatures and prevention

psychomotor agitation Purposeless motor actions such as pacing, pulling at clothing, etc.

psychopathy A series or set of characteristics and behaviours affiliated with the exploitation of other people for personal gain

psychosis A condition characterised by delusions, hallucinations and thought disorder predominantly seen in schizophrenia and mania. Psychosis may also result after taking illicit drugs (such as crystal meth)

psychotropic Medications that are understood to influence an individual's mental state

puerperal psychosis (PP) (also referred to as postpartum psychosis) A rare and serious condition affecting women in the period after childbirth. May include delusional beliefs about the infant

punning Use of words that sound the same but have a different meaning. Seen in mania

purging behaviours A serious physiological response to starvation characterised by imbalances in serum levels of magnesium, potassium and sodium. Can be fatal

Q

qualitative studies Typically draw on interpretive methodologies to data analysis in order to obtain an in-depth understanding of the experience, meaning or phenomenon

quantitative research Uses objective measures and statistical analysis to test relationships between variables

R

randomised controlled trials (RCTs) Participants are randomly allocated into either a control group or experimental group and the outcomes evaluated over the trial period

rational emotive behaviour therapy (REBT) An action-oriented approach to emotional growth that emphasises an individual's capacity for creating their emotions by recognising irrational, disruptive thinking and replacing them with new ways of thinking

rationalisation Constructing plausible reasons/excuses to try and explain unreasonable behaviour

reaction formation an unconscious defense mechanism whereby a person expresses an impulse that is the opposite of what they are actually feeling/experiencing. This unacceptable impulse is threatening to the ego

reactive attachment disorder (RAD) A condition that is a potential consequence of insecure attachment due to severe neglect by the child's main caregiver(s). This neglect impacts on the child's ability to socially and emotionally engage with others

reality principle Operates when the individual's ego has matured and is able to develop an awareness of how the world functions. This then enables the ego to mediate between the demands of the id and superego

reciprocal determinism Environmental events, observable behaviour, and a person's thoughts and feelings influence each other, leading to behaviour

recovery Where a consumer experiences connectedness, hope and empowerment in their journey to reaching their own recovery goals. This process is non-linear and is not a medicalised notion of symptom amelioration; rather, it is a journey of individual discovery for the person with a lived experience

refeeding syndrome A serious physiological response to starvation characterised by imbalances in serum levels of magnesium, potassium and sodium. Can be fatal

reframing Looking at something from a new point of view and seeing it from different perspectives

regression Reverting to an earlier developmental level of responding to a situation or event

relapse Where a person who has commenced using substances after a period of abstinence. Relapse is impacted by a number of factors

repression Memories that are unacceptable/threatening to the ego are pushed into the unconscious

residual phase Follows the active phase of schizophrenia and is similar to the prodrome in intensity. The consumer is no longer classified as psychotic, but may continue to demonstrate strange or odd beliefs

resilience Used to describe an individual's ability to withstand challenges and to 'bounce back' from adversity. It is commonly believed that a lack of resilience is a risk factor associated with the development or worsening of a mental health condition

resistance A response from a person when they are not ready to take action towards making a change. Resistance is experienced in many ways and is an expected part of the change process

restraint A restrictive intervention where a consumer's free physical movement is confined through either physical (e.g. holding a person) or mechanical means (e.g. using hand restraints)

restricted affect A restricted expression of emotional intensity

retrograde Inability to recall existing memories

rumination Negative thoughts that are repetitive, increasingly intrusive and intense

S

safety plan A plan of action that a person develops to help them access support/resources at a time of emotional vulnerability and/or crisis

schizoaffective disorder A serious mental health condition where the individual has symptoms of schizophrenia in addition to affective symptoms (either mania, depression or a combination of both)

schizoid personality disorder (SZPD) Disorder characterised by disinterest in intimate relationships in addition to a limited emotional range

schizophrenia A severe mental health condition characterised by experiences of perceptual, behavioural, thought and speech disturbances

schizophreniform disorder Essentially 'pre-schizophrenia'; describes the period where symptoms of schizophrenia are present; however the time period (at least six months) has not been met for a diagnosis of schizophrenia

schizotypal personality disorder (STPD) Disorder characterised by unease with close, personal relationships, in addition to cognitive or perceptual oddities

self-concept The internal image a person has of themselves. It represents their beliefs regarding their nature, qualities and typical behaviour

self-efficacy The confidence and belief a person holds that their actions will help them achieve their desired goals/outcomes

serotonin Is implicated in sleep cycles, appetite and awareness, and dysfunction with this neurotransmitter is associated with depression and anxiety

sleep hygiene Describes practices and routines that promote well-balanced, effective sleep patterns

social determinants of health The social and economic conditions that populations experience that impact on individual and population health

social determinants of mental health Economic and social conditions that influence individual and group mental health status

somnolence Feeling drowsy or sleepy

Stevens-Johnson Syndrome (SJS) A rare and potentially life-threatening skin condition associated with use of the mood stabiliser lamotrigine. Indicators include flu-like symptoms and a prominent rash on the head, neck or trunk, genital/anal regions and mucous membranes

stigma Negative treatment of an individual, which is based on a set of characteristics that are believed to be distinguishable. For example, the incorrect belief that individuals with schizophrenia are dangerous and should be avoided

strengths-based Approach to working with people that focuses on their strengths and resources and how they can use these skills, resources and supports to promote well-being

structured problem solving Structured process in which consumers learn to implement practical strategies to solve issues related to their daily lives

sublimation A socially acceptable substitute replaces a socially unacceptable impulse

substance misuse Harmful use of substances (licit and illicit) that are not required for medical reasons

substance use disorders (SUDs) Recurrent use of substance(s) that lead to impaired control, risk taking behaviours, physical health problems, social, educational and/or occupational impairments

subsyndromal level Individuals who do not meet full diagnostic criteria of a mood episode such as mania, depression or hypomania

suicidal ideation The thoughts associated with how to end one's life. This can vary from fleeting thoughts to a detailed plan of suicide

suicide An intentional act of harm to self where the desire is to die

sundowning When a person with dementia becomes increasingly confused, agitated or restless later in the day. The person may become more disoriented and demanding. They may experience perceptual disturbances at night

superego The component of Freud's personality structure that is focused on society's values of what is right and wrong, good or bad. This element develops through the child's interaction with others such as parents

systematic review A rigorous, predetermined methodology to collate and critically appraise all the available research evidence to answer a specified question

T

talk therapy An umbrella term for CBT and interpersonal therapies, where a consumer is treated via conversations with a therapist

tangentiality Form of thought distortion whereby the consumer gives irrelevant or indirect answers to questions

tardive dyskinesia (TD) Distortion of facial features that responds poorly to treatment and is characterised by uncontrolled tongue withering, lip smacking and rapid blinking but can also involve involuntary movements of the limbs. A common side effect from antipsychotic therapy

task behaviours Behaviours that are helpful in getting the task completed

teratogenic effect The result of a teratogen; that is, anything that can negatively impact on normal foetal growth, including anatomic structures, physical functioning and postnatal development

therapeutic relationship A professional relationship between the nurse and the consumer where the focus is on helping. Therapeutic relationships foster a consumer's growth by working in partnership with them and respecting their ideas, experiences and feelings

thought blocking Abrupt gaps in the flow of thoughts

thought control or broadcasting The consumer believes others can control their thoughts, and their thoughts are broadcast for others to hear

topic syntheses A critical appraisal of the evidence aimed at addressing the clinical relevance of the research to the topic

tort A civil wrong that causes someone else to suffer loss or harm resulting in legal liability

transcranial magnetic stimulation (TMS) A treatment option for consumers who do not tolerate other forms of treatment, such as antidepressants, or to augment other treatment options such as antidepressants and psychotherapeutic interventions. TMS works by applying a magnetic field timed to be delivered rapidly and over the scalp. It is administered via a coil placed over the scalp that acts to stimulate brain activity

transference A process where a person (usually the consumer) transfers their feelings towards another person (often

someone from childhood) onto the therapist or mental health nurse; for example, the consumer whose nurse reminds her of her mother, whom she does not get along with, and these negative feelings are transferred to the nurse through their interactions

trauma-informed care/practice The recognition of the existence and impact of trauma on a person. This knowledge and understanding underpins practice through mental health clinicians practising in a way that does not re-traumatise the individual

trichotillomania A condition characterised by recurrent hair-pulling, and subsequent hair loss

U

unconditional positive regard The capacity to value and respect another person regardless of how they behave

unconditioned response Instinctive response to a stimulus

unconditioned stimulus A stimulus that produces an instinctive response. No learning is required

unconscious mental processes Thoughts and feelings are outside awareness and not remembered (but are argued to resurface through the experience of dreams)

unfiltered information Original research studies that have not been critically appraised

unilateral ECT Electrodes are placed on one hemisphere of the scalp (usually the right)

V

values What a person holds to be important in their life

vicarious trauma Trauma experienced from hearing about another person's story of trauma, or witnessing a traumatic event or situation

voluntary treatment Usually means that the consumer agrees to being treated at an inpatient facility

W

withdrawal Physical and mental symptoms experienced when a person ceases taking a substance (e.g. alcohol)

word salad A form of thought disorder where incomprehensible words and phrases are expressed in unintelligible speech

INDEX